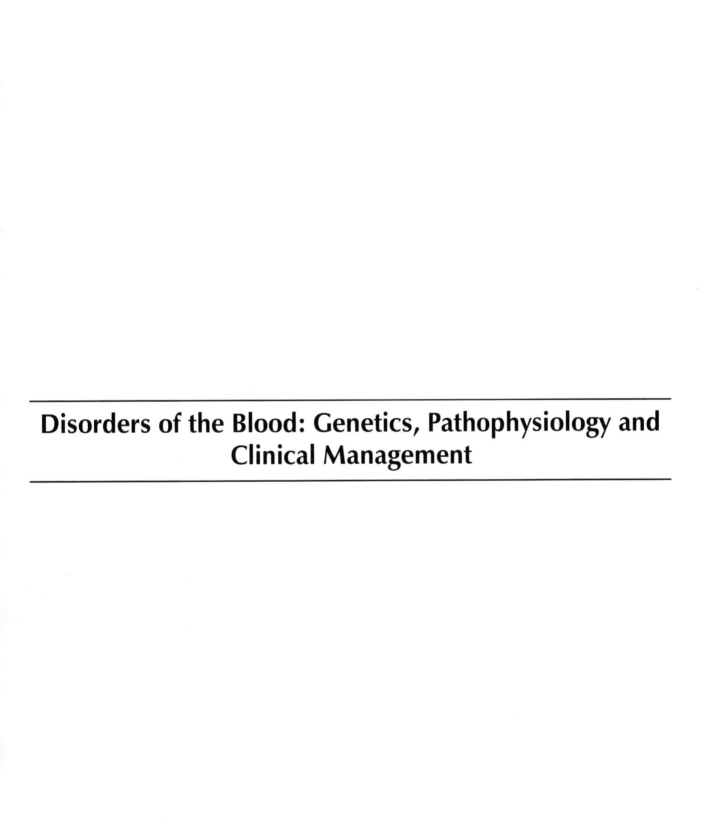

Disorders of the Blood: Genetics, Pathophysiology and Clinical Management

Disorders of the Blood: Genetics, Pathophysiology and Clinical Management

Editor: Martha Roper

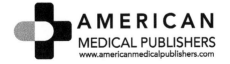

AMERICAN
MEDICAL PUBLISHERS
www.americanmedicalpublishers.com

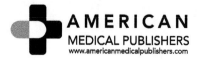

Cataloging-in-Publication Data

Disorders of the blood : genetics, pathophysiology and clinical management / edited by Martha Roper.
  p. cm.
Includes bibliographical references and index.
ISBN 979-8-88740-066-2
1. Blood--Diseases. 2. Blood--Diseases--Genetic aspects. 3. Blood--Diseases--Pathophysiology.
4. Blood--Diseases--Treatment. 5. Hematology. I. Roper, Martha.
RC636 .D57 2023
616.15--dc23

American Medical Publishers,
41 Flatbush Avenue,
1st Floor, New York,
NY 11217, USA

ISBN 979-8-88740-066-2 (Hardback)

Contents

Permissions

List of Contributors

Index

Preface

It is often said that books are a boon to mankind. They document every progress and pass on the knowledge from one generation to the other. They play a crucial role in our lives. Thus I was both excited and nervous while editing this book. I was pleased by the thought of being able to make a mark but I was also nervous to do it right because the future of students depends upon it. Hence, I took a few months to research further into the discipline, revise my knowledge and also explore some more aspects. Post this process, I begun with the editing of this book.

Blood disorders are a group of diseases that affect some part of the blood. Several organs and tissues play a major role in supporting blood and its function. These organs and tissues are bone marrow, lymphatic system, clotting proteins, spleen, liver and kidneys. The common types of blood disorders include different types of anemia, bleeding disorders, clotting disorders and blood cancers. The symptoms of blood disorders depend on which component of the blood is affected. Some major symptoms include fatigue, fever, infections and abnormal bleeding. There are several risk factors that affect the development of blood disorders. These factors incorporate aging, autoimmune diseases, exposure to certain drugs and chemicals, and liver, kidney or thyroid disease. Treatment and clinical management of blood disorders varies according to the type of disease. Some of the blood disorders are passed-down from one generation to another. Such disorders are called genetic blood disorders. Genetic defects result in red blood cells that do not perform their normal functions. Examples of genetic blood disorders include thalassemia and sickle cell anemia. The book is a valuable compilation of topics, ranging from the basic to the most complex advancements in the study of disorders of the blood. Its extensive content provides the readers with a detailed understanding of the genetics, pathophysiology and clinical management of these disorders.

I thank my publisher with all my heart for considering me worthy of this unparalleled opportunity and for showing unwavering faith in my skills. I would also like to thank the editorial team who worked closely with me at every step and contributed immensely towards the successful completion of this book. Last but not the least, I wish to thank my friends and colleagues for their support.

Editor

β-Hemoglobinopathies: The Test Bench for Genome Editing-Based Therapeutic Strategies

Gloria Barbarani, Agata Łabedz and Antonella Ellena Ronchi*

Dipartimento di Biotecnologie e Bioscienze, Università di Milano-Bicocca, Milan, Italy

*Correspondence:
Antonella Ellena Ronchi
antonella.ronchi@unimib.it

Hemoglobin is a tetrameric protein composed of two α and two β chains, each containing a heme group that reversibly binds oxygen. The composition of hemoglobin changes during development in order to fulfill the need of the growing organism, stably maintaining a balanced production of α-like and β-like chains in a 1:1 ratio. Adult hemoglobin (HbA) is composed of two α and two β subunits (α2β2 tetramer), whereas fetal hemoglobin (HbF) is composed of two γ and two α subunits (α2γ2 tetramer). Qualitative or quantitative defects in β-globin production cause two of the most common monogenic-inherited disorders: β-thalassemia and sickle cell disease. The high frequency of these diseases and the relative accessibility of hematopoietic stem cells make them an ideal candidate for therapeutic interventions based on genome editing. These strategies move in two directions: the correction of the disease-causing mutation and the reactivation of the expression of HbF in adult cells, in the attempt to recreate the effect of hereditary persistence of fetal hemoglobin (HPFH) natural mutations, which mitigate the severity of β-hemoglobinopathies. Both lines of research rely on the knowledge gained so far on the regulatory mechanisms controlling the differential expression of globin genes during development.

Keywords: β-hemoglobinopathies, genome editing, globin genes, hereditary persistence of fetal hemoglobin, programmable endonucleases

INTRODUCTION

Historically, because of the abundance and accessibility of red blood cells, globins served as a model for major discoveries later extended to other genes. In 1967, hemoglobin was the first human complex protein crystallized (Muirhead et al., 1967); in 1980, the β-locus was the first cloned gene cluster (Fritsch et al., 1980) and soon became the prototypical model of tissue-specific and developmentally regulated genes. In 1987, the β-locus control region (LCR) was the first long-distance position-independent enhancer characterized (Grosveld et al., 1987), and the current looping model for the interaction of far apart regulatory regions owes much to the study of globin gene sequential activation during development (Stamatoyannopoulos, 1991; Fraser and Grosveld, 1998). The wealth of data accumulated on globin genes put them now at the frontline of development of genome-editing approaches with therapeutic purposes.

THE GLOBIN GENES

In man, globin genes are organized in two clusters lying on chromosomes 16 (α cluster) and 11 (β cluster). A fine-tuned regulation maintains a 1:1 ratio of α-like and β-like chains during development to produce first HBZ ($\zeta 2\epsilon 2$, $\zeta 2\gamma 2$), then HbE ($\alpha 2\epsilon 2$), HbF ($\alpha 2\gamma 2$), and finally HbA ($\alpha 2\beta 2$) together with a small amount of HbA2 ($\alpha 2\delta 2$), in a process called hemoglobin switching.

At the molecular level, the hemoglobin switching involves the establishment of sequential long-range chromatin physical interactions between a common LCR and the different globin promoters active at a given developmental time (with inactive genes being looped out) in a structure called active chromatin hub (ACH) (Carter et al., 2002; Tolhuis et al., 2002; Palstra et al., 2003). The formation of ACH requires the presence of transcription factors/cofactors that, by binding with the correct affinity to their consensus on DNA, creates the favorable condition for the expression of the gene of interest (Wilber et al., 2011).

β-HEMOGLOBINOPATHIES

Qualitative or quantitative defects in the β-globin production cause the most common monogenic diseases: sickle cell disease (SCD) and β-thalassemia (Weatherall, 2008; Thein, 2013); both diseases, in particular β-thalassemias, are very severe in homozygous subjects, whereas symptoms are mild in carriers. In SCD, the amino acid β6Glu>Val substitution leads to the formation of long hydrophobic polymers of HbS that precipitate within the cell under hypoxic conditions, conferring the typical sickle shape. Sickle cells tend to stick, causing vessel obstruction and, because of their fragility, they frequently undergo hemolysis, finally leading to anemia.

In β-thalassemias, a wide spectrum of mutations causes the reduction of β-globin, which can range in severity from total absence (β^0) to partial reduction (β^+). Causative mutations vary from large deletions to small insertions or deletions (indels) and point mutations within the β gene. β-thalassemia mutations impact on all the different steps of the β gene expression regulation (Thein, 2013): transcription (mutations within regulatory regions), RNA processing (splicing mutations), and translation (ATG mutations, non-sense and missense mutations). In rare cases, β-thalassemia is caused by mutations outside the β-locus, in genes involved in the basal transcription machinery XPD (Viprakasit et al., 2001) or in the erythroid-specific transcription factor GATA1 (Yu et al., 2002). The common output of β-thalassemia mutations is a reduced production of functional β chains with the consequent precipitation of the excess α chains causing hemolysis and anemia. The presence of dysfunctional erythroid progenitors causes ineffective erythropoiesis (Rivella, 2012) and impacts on hematopoietic stem cells (HSCs) self-renewal (Aprile et al., 2020).

The definitive cure for β-hemoglobinopathies is HSC transplantation, a treatment available only for the few patients who have an HLA-matched donor. Despite intense efforts, the only drug of some efficacy remains hydroxyurea (Yu et al., 2020), used to treat SCD (Platt, 2008) and, less successfully, β-thalassemia (Koren et al., 2008; Pourfarzad et al., 2013). Although the condition of β-diseased patients have greatly improved in the last years (Taher et al., 2009), there is a clear need

of new approaches, the most innovative of them being based on genome modifications.

THE LESSON FROM NATURE: HEREDITARY PERSISTENCE OF FETAL HEMOGLOBIN

The term hereditary persistence of fetal hemoglobin (HPFH) indicates a heterogeneous spectrum of spontaneous mutations, collectively named by their effect, i.e., the maintenance of the expression of fetal γ-globin in adult stages (Forget, 1998). HPFH alleles, when coinherited with β-hemoglobinopathies, greatly improve the condition of patients, 30% of HbF expression being considered a significant curative threshold able to prevent α free chains polymerization in β-thalassemias and HbS precipitation in SCD (Steinberg et al., 2014). Moreover, δβ-thalassemias, in which δ and β genes are deleted and γ-globin is reactivated, in general to a lesser extent than in HPFH, show that even a relatively low level of γ-globin has beneficial effects on β-thalassemias (Ottolenghi et al., 1982).

HPFH mutations can be broadly divided in three categories: large deletions affecting the structure of the β-locus; point mutations within the γ promoter that identify "hot-spot" HPFH sequences (−200, −175, −158, -distal CCAAT box); and mutations non-linked with the β-locus (Forget, 1998). Two of these non-linked loci, identified by genome-wide association analysis (GWAS), correspond to BCL11A gene, the most important repressor of γ-globin (Menzel et al., 2007; Sankaran et al., 2008; Uda et al., 2008) and to its key activator KLF1 (Borg et al., 2010; Zhou et al., 2010). More recently, knock-out studies in HUDEP cells led to the identification of LRF gene (also known as ZBTB7A), which represses γ-globin independently from BCL11A (Masuda et al., 2016). HPFH mutations within the β-locus greatly increase the expression of one or both γ genes in cis, whereas non-linked HPFH are associated with lower γ-globin levels (Forget, 1998).

The integration of the genetic data on HPFH with molecular studies led to the identification of the target sequences amenable for therapeutic genome editing (see below). In 1992, a pioneer study in mice transgenic for the human β-locus first demonstrated that it is indeed possible to reproduce HPFH (Berry et al., 1992).

THERAPEUTIC GENOME MODIFICATIONS: THE CHOICE OF THE MODIFICATION

In principle, different therapeutic genomic modifications can be envisaged to cure β-hemoglobinopathies (**Figure 1A**):

(1) The addition to the defective cell of an intact β gene, that, once delivered and integrated in the genome of the target hematopoietic stem cell, will produce the missing β chain under the control of an exogenous regulatory cassette, designed to ensure stable, erythroid-specific, and high-level expression. This approach (not discussed in this review), thanks to intensive efforts in developing safe and efficient vectors and in the improvement of their delivery, reached very significant results

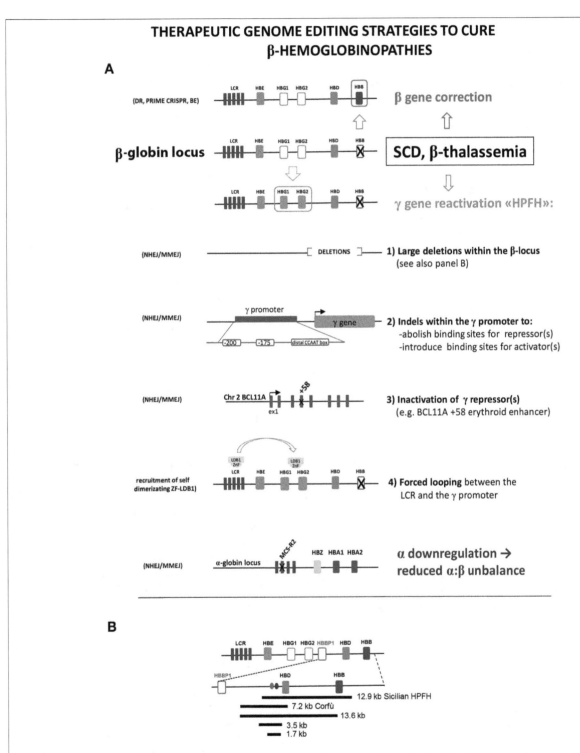

FIGURE 1 | **(A)** Schematic representation of the different editing strategies developed to cure β-hemoglobinopathies. These approaches are oriented to correct the mutated β-globin gene, to reactivate the expression of the fetal γ gene in adult cells or to lower α-globin expression. The reactivation of γ can be obtained via the introduction of different modifications mimicking HPFH caused by large deletions within the β locus or by mutations within the γ promoter that disrupt the binding site of a repressor or create the binding site of an activator. As an alternative, the disruption of the erythroid-specific enhancer of the γ repressor BCL11A abolishes its expression in erythroid cells, thus resulting in γ overexpression. A different approach relies on the forced interaction of the LCR with the γ promoter obtained by exploiting the self-dimerization property of a fusion ZnF-LDB1 protein recruited on these regions. The detrimental effect of the α:β chain imbalance can be mitigated by mutating the MCS-R2 α-globin enhancer, in order to reduce α expression. These different strategies exploit different enzymes/cellular pathway described in the text: HDR, homology-directed repair; BE, base editing; NHEJ, non-homologous end joining; MMEJ, microhomology end joining. **(B)** Schematic representation of the deletions within the β-locus discussed in the text. Ovals represent the BCL11A (red) and the polypyrimidine (gray) sites thought to be responsible for γ repression.

(Ikawa et al., 2019; Magrin et al., 2019). Importantly, the optimization of protocols developed by gene addition approaches represents a knowledge asset fundamental for bringing genome editing approaches to clinical application.

(2) The exact correction of the mutation causing the disease (gene editing), with the advantage of having the β gene expressed under the endogenous regulatory sequences, thus ensuring a perfectly regulated and stable expression with no risk of insertional mutagenesis. This procedure is particularly attractive for point mutations such as the β6Glu>Val SCD-causing mutation or for some β-thalassemia mutations, with the caveat that their extreme heterogeneity would require the design of patient-specific editing strategies. Under this aspect, this approach is worth only for mutations with high frequencies in given populations, as for the *HBB* −28A>G β-thal mutation in Southeast Asia or for the β⁰39C>T and β⁺thal IVS-I-110G>A mutations in the Mediterranean area (https://www.ithanet.eu/) (Kountouris et al., 2014).

In an extended perspective, the substitution of the mutated β gene with a wild-type β gene by homologous recombination could combine gene addition and gene editing to create a "universal" substitution cassette, which would minimize the risk of insertional mutagenesis (Cai et al., 2018).

(3) The introduction within the genome of modifications mimicking HPFH, in order to reactivate the expression of the fetal γ-globin gene and to compensate for the missing/defective β-globin expression.

(4) The reduction of the expression of α-globin, an important β-thalassemia modifier, as demonstrated by the milder clinical outcome of patients coinheriting α- and β-thalassemia (Thein, 2008; Mettananda et al., 2015). Reduced α levels indeed reduce the α:β chain imbalance, which represent a major problem in β-hemoglobinopathies. This effect has been achieved experimentally by deleting the MCS-R2 α enhancer (Mettananda et al., 2017).

THE ADVENT OF PROGRAMMABLE ENDONUCLEASES IN THE EDITING OF GLOBIN GENES: THE SEARCH FOR THE BEST COMPROMISE BETWEEN PRECISION AND EFFICIENCY

In 1985, Oliver Smithies first exploited homologous recombination (HR) to introduce an exogenous DNA sequence within the β-locus (Smithies et al., 1985), demonstrating the feasibility of this approach. Since then, HR was used to generate gene knock-out models (including the KO of GATA1 (Pevny et al., 1991) and KLF1 (Nuez et al., 1995; Perkins et al., 1995)), by inserting exogenous DNA in the desired target. However, the very low efficiency of gene targeting, the consequent need of selecting the modified cells, and the technical difficulties of the method discouraged clinical applications (Vega, 1991).

The scenario radically changed with the advent of programmable endonucleases: zinc finger (ZnF) and TALENs first and now, CRISPR/Cas9 and its derivatives (Cornu et al.,

2017; Komor et al., 2017). These nucleases introduce double-strand breaks (DSBs) with extreme specificity at the target genomic position. CRISPR/Cas9 is the most flexible system: its cutting specificity relies on a short guide RNA (sgRNA) and only requires the additional presence of an adjacent genomic proto-spacer adjacent motif (PAM) for its cut [this limit is actually being solved by the "near-PAM-less"-engineered CRISPR-Cas9 variants (Walton et al., 2020)]. In order to minimize possible off targets, different solutions are under study: better algorithms for the prediction of optimal DNA targets, optimized sgRNAs, engineered proto-spacers and Cas enzymes improved on the basis of thermodynamical models (Chen, 2019).

Once generated, DSBs are resolved by different DNA repair cellular pathways:

(i) The homology-directed repair (HDR) high-fidelity system that uses a donor template (the sister identical chromatid in physiological conditions) to repair DSBs when cells are in S and G2 phases. The implication is that HDR is poorly efficient in non-dividing HSC (Dever and Porteus, 2017), the target cell for therapeutic correction of β-hemoglobinopathies.

(ii) The non-homologous end joining (NHEJ) error-prone system acting in all cell cycle phases that inserts small indels at the site of the lesion, resulting in the disruption of the target sequence.

(iii) The microhomology end-joining (MMEJ) (Wang and Xu, 2017) error-prone system, which exploits small homology domains to align the broken filaments and close the gap. This molecular mechanism introduces deletions encompassing the microhomology regions flanking the break sites.

On these premises, the design of HDR recombination-based therapeutic strategies is difficult because of the requirement for a codelivered donor DNA template, of the low efficiency of HDR in HSCs and of the competition of the unwanted NHEJ and MMEJ error-prone repair systems. Despite these problems, the correction of the SCD mutation in HSCs was obtained by using both ZnF (Hoban et al., 2015) and CRISPR nucleases (Dever et al., 2016). However, the efficiency of the correction, assessed in HSCs *in vitro*, dramatically decreased after transplantation *in vivo*, confirming that HSCs are more resistant to HDR-based editing than more mature progenitors (Hoban et al., 2015) and that a selection step could be required to enrich for HSC-edited cells, capable of long-term correction *in vivo* (Dever et al., 2016). Instead, NHEJ is more flexible and allow to reach an efficiency up to ≈90% of edited HSCs that is maintained *in vivo* (Genovese et al., 2014; Chang et al., 2017; Charlesworth et al., 2018; Psatha et al., 2018; Wu et al., 2019).

The "perfect" editing should leave no trace, to avoid unintended off-target mutations and should at the same time guarantee high editing efficiency with reduced toxicity for HSCs. To reach this goal, an intense optimization work has been focused on the different steps of the genome editing procedure: the development of new editing reagents [single-strand DNA donor templates (Park et al., 2019), modified sgRNA (De Ravin et al., 2017; Park et al., 2019), pre-complexed ribonucleoproteins (RNPs) (Gundry et al., 2016)] and their integration in improved platforms for their delivery (Lino et al., 2018; Lattanzi et al., 2019; Schiroli et al., 2019). This massive effort finally led to the generation of selection-free HSCs of therapeutic potential (Genovese et al., 2014; DeWitt et al., 2016; Porteus, 2016; Yu et al., 2016; Wu et al., 2019).

THE EDITING OF GLOBIN GENES INSPIRED BY HPFH

NHEJ has been used to generate two classes of HPFH-inspired mutation: large deletions within the β-locus, to remove putative γ-globin repressive regions, and small indels within the γ-globin promoter or within the regulatory regions driving the erythroid expression of the γ-globin repressor BCL11A (Bauer et al., 2013; Canver et al., 2015). Large deletions focus around the critical "HPFH γδ-region" 5′ to the δ gene, deleted with different breakpoints in several HPFH [https://www.omim.org/entry/141749; https://www.ithanet.eu/; (Kountouris et al., 2014)]. This region is generally lost in deletions involving δ and β genes and causing HPFH, whereas it is retained in δβ-thalassemia deletions, which similarly remove δ and β genes but with little increase of γ-globin expression. This observation led to hypothesize that this region contains an element capable to repress the γ genes in *cis*. The CRISPR-mediated deletion corresponding to the 12.9-kb Sicilian HPFH, spanning from 3.2 kb upstream of the δ gene to the 3′ flanking region of the β gene, gave indeed a HPFH phenotype (increase in γ-globin with concomitant drop of β-globin expression) in HUDEP cells and in human *ex vivo* HSC-derived erythroblasts (Ye et al., 2016). The same result (γ-globin increased and β-globin decreased) was obtained by the CRISPR-mediated deletion (or inversion) of a large 13.6-kb region starting downstream to the pseudo-β1 (HBBP1) gene and extending into the β gene (Antoniani et al., 2018). The 5′ border of this deletion corresponds to the 5′ breakpoint of the Corfù δβ-thal 7.2-kb deletion (Wainscoat et al., 1985) that ends in the δ gene and is not associated with HPFH *in vivo* in humans (except in some rare cases, in homozygotes, in which an additional independent mutation in the downstream β gene is present (Kulozik et al., 1988). The CRISPR-mediated deletion of the 7.2-kb Corfù region and of two smaller internal regions of 3.5 and 1.7 kb, centered around a BCL11A binding site and a polypyrimidine stretch (**Figure 1B**), thought to mediate γ-globin repression (Sankaran et al., 2011), resulted in a very little γ-globin increase (Antoniani et al., 2018; Chung et al., 2019). These results indicate that the 1.7-kb element and its surrounding sequences *per se* are not an autonomous γ-globin silencer, as also suggested by previous studies (Galanello et al., 1990; Calzolari et al., 1999; Gaensler et al., 2003; Chakalova et al., 2005). Instead, they suggest a more complex scenario, where the competition with β-globin expression, the perfect distance/order between intergenic enhancer/repressor, and the enhancers delimiting the locus (the LCR and the 3′ DNAseI hypersensitive site), all together concur to the correct γ/β gene expression (and to γ-globin increase, when perturbed in HPFH).

The effects of distorting the architecture of the β-locus can be turned in an advantage: Dr. Blobel and colleagues obtained a great increase in γ-globin (with β-globin reduction) by tethering

LDB1 to the LCR and to the γ-globin promoter, thus forcing their looping (Deng et al., 2014). This result again highlights the importance of the competition between γ and β genes for the LCR.

HPFH mutation mapping within the γ-globin promoter alters the binding of transcription factors/cofactors. Theoretically, the γ-globin upregulation can be obtained either by increasing the binding of an activator or by decreasing the binding of a repressor. Both cases are observed in HPFH. Mutations at positions −198, −175, and −113 create new binding sites for erythroid transcriptional activators [KLF1 (Wienert et al., 2017), TAL1 (Wienert et al., 2015), GATA1 (Martyn et al., 2019), respectively]. Other mutations clustered around position −200 and around the distal CCAAT box (−115) reduce the binding of the γ-globin repressors LRF and BCL11A, respectively (Liu et al., 2018; Martyn et al., 2018).

Consistently, the CRISPR-mediated disruption of these two binding sites resulted in a relevant increase in γ-globin expression (Traxler et al., 2016; Weber et al., 2020). Of note, the editing of the −158 ("XmnI-Gγ-site"), known to be influenced by a QTL on chromosome 8 (Garner et al., 2002), only marginally increased γ-globin expression (Weber et al., 2020), suggesting that possible background effects might be taken into account when considering editing for therapeutic purposes.

The existence of two highly homologous γ-globin genes poses specific editing issues: the double-stranded DNA cut at the gRNA recognition sites in the HBG2 and HBG1 promoters could result in NHEJ-mediated joining of the two ends with loss of the intergenic (≈5 kb) genomic sequence in variable proportion (Traxler et al., 2016; Antoniani et al., 2018). Thus, the editing of these γ-globin regions can result either in the mutation of a single or both HBG genes or in the deletion of the intergenic region, with different resulting percentages of γ-globin induction. Moreover, given the presence of short repeats within the promoter, MMEJ can also occur (Traxler et al., 2016; Weber et al., 2020).

NHEJ can also be used to destroy the specific erythroid expression of repressors, such as BCL11A or, in principle, of LRF (both proteins have important roles in other hematopoietic cell types that must be preserved). On this front, four clinical trials based on targeting a GATA1-binding site within the intronic +58 (Canver et al., 2015) erythroid-specific BCL11A enhancer are ongoing (Hirakawa et al., 2020).

Theoretically, all the different genes involved in the γ-globin repression identified so far, including BCL11A, LRF, SOX6, and DRED are possible targets for genome editing, with the general caveat that their ablation should not perturb stem cell viability, their engraftment and differentiation potential. For example, the ubiquitous knockdown of BCL11A impairs normal HSC function and lymphopoiesis (Luc et al., 2016); LRF (Maeda et al., 2009), SOX6 (Cantu et al., 2011), and KLF1 (Nuez et al., 1995; Perkins et al., 1995) are instead required for proper erythroid differentiation. In this latter case, the need of fine-tuning the downregulation of the γ-globin repressor in order to lead to an appreciable γ-globin increase while maintaining a correct erythroid differentiation could represent an insurmountable obstacle.

Overall, the success obtained in reactivating γ-globin expression at therapeutic levels demonstrates that this strategy can work. Theoretically, the possibility to generate multiple HPFH mutations could further increase γ-globin expression.

Importantly, beside the final goal of its clinical application, the relative ease-of-use of the CRISPR-based editing techniques represents a formidable tool to answer the unsolved questions on the molecular mechanisms regulating the hemoglobin switching.

BEYOND CRISPR/CAS9: PRIME-CAS AND BE-CAS

The use of HDR to correct β-disease mutations is limited by its low efficiency and by the downstream activation of p53, which can induce toxicity and, even worse, the possible selection of potentially harmful p53low cells (Haapaniemi et al., 2018; Ihry et al., 2018). To overcome this problem, a new generation of engineered Cas9 that do not introduce DBSs (also avoiding unwanted NHEJ/MMEJ events triggered by the DBSs) and do not require donor DNA are under development. They rely on catalytically inactive Cas9 fused to a modified reverse transcriptase (prime editing) or to base-specific DNA deaminase enzymes [base editors (BEs)]. As for many innovations, these newcomers in the CRISPR toolbox

have been tested on β-disease mutations. Prime editing has been used to correct the β6Glu>Val SCD mutation artificially introduced in HEK-293T cells (Anzalone et al., 2019). Dr. Bauer and colleagues recently demonstrated the versatility of BE by disrupting the GATA1-binding site within the +58 BCL11A erythroid-specific enhancer. The obtained HSC-edited cells express HbF at levels similar to those obtained by the NHEJ-mediated disruption of the same site and are capable of multi-lineage repopulation in serial transplantation experiments (Zeng et al., 2020). In addition, the simultaneous multiplex edit of the β-thal −28 A>G mutation in the TATA box of the β promoter increased β-globin production in the same cells.

Instead, Beam Therapeutics recently presented data relative to two therapeutic approaches based on BE, the first recreating an HPFH mutation and the second converting HbS into HbG-Makassar, a naturally occurring human variant that does not cause sickling[1].

Although at present the issues of unwanted bystander/off target mutations remain to be explored, it is clear that Prime editing and BE represent important new instruments for genome

---

[1]https://investors.beamtx.com/news-releases/news-release-details/beam-therapeutics-reports-additional-data-asgct-annual-meeting

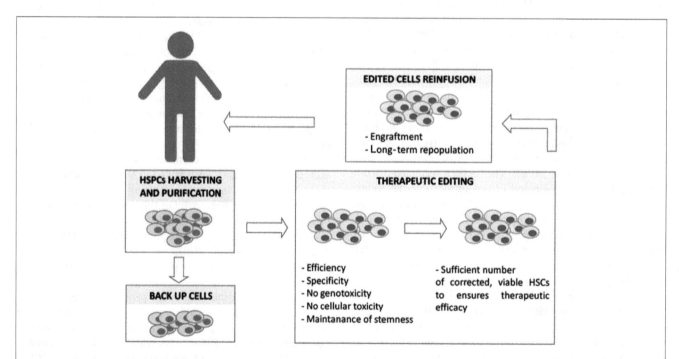

FIGURE 2 | Overview of the different steps of HSC autologous transplantation and of its major critical issues. In the case of β-hemoglobinopathies, ineffective erythropoiesis and a compromised bone marrow microenvironment sensibly reduce the yield of CD34+HSCs amenable for the editing process, posing a serious problem in a clinical-scale setting. Different mobilization protocols are currently used to maximize the yield of harvested hematopoietic stem progenitor cells (HSPCs) that must also include backup cells to be reinfused into the patient in case of engraftment failure. Editing should ensure efficiency (in terms of complete allelic correction and percentage of edited cells) and, at the same time, minimize the exposure to editing reagents, to reduce the risk of unwanted mutations. Editing manipulations must preserve the population of CD34+ long-term repopulating cells. Before the reinfusion of the edited cells, the patient is treated with myeloablative agents to maximize the engraftment of the edited cells within the bone marrow niche. The conditioning regimen should be designed to guarantee the optimal risk-benefit balance between toxicity and efficacy of the engraftment, in order to achieve a stable, long-term therapeutic bone marrow repopulation.

editing, with the perspective to become even more attractive with the ongoing development of BE enabling more transition substitutions (Komor et al., 2018).

CONCLUDING REMARKS

The number of genome-editing tools is rapidly increasing (Papasavva et al., 2019; Doudna, 2020), holding the promise to reach in the near future a safe, precise, and efficient editing of β-disease mutations, via different strategies. The availability of different molecular options (HDR, NHEJ, and BE based, **Figure 1**) poses the problem of the evaluation of the pros and cons of each strategy (Ikawa et al., 2019; Papasavva et al., 2019): HDR-based approaches could ensure a higher precision at the expenses of HSC correction efficiency, whereas NHEJ is more efficient but less precise. Base editing, which does not require double-strand breaks, could be a safer option when a nucleotide substitution is required. Beside the choice of the optimal genetic modification, other issues remain open, first of all those related to unforeseeable genotoxicity (with the serious concern of inducing hyperproliferative/leukemic mutations in HSCs), the efficiency of the correction and the optimization of the delivery of genome editing reagents to target cells in conditions that preserve their stemness. Moreover, the clinical translation of these approaches requires the definition of scalable protocols to obtain under non-invasive conditions, a sufficient number of autologous HSCs amenable for the editing procedures and capable of optimal engraftment (in addition to backup cells to be reinfused in the patient in the case of engraftment failure) (**Figure 2**). This last point involves the identification of the best preparative conditioning regimen of the patient to allow efficient engraft of the corrected HSCs within the recipient niche (Psatha et al., 2016). Despite these difficulties, the recent announcement of the curative response of the first three patients (carrying a transfusion-dependent

β-thalassemia and the SCD mutation) with CRISPR-Cas9-edited cells targeting BCL11A (CRISPR Therapeutics and Vertex CTX001 clinical trial[2&3]), clearly highlights the clinical potential of gene therapy. The advent of this new era urges the need to make these approaches affordable and available in low-resource settings/countries, where a large number of patients is waiting for a cure.

AUTHOR CONTRIBUTIONS

AR conceived and wrote the manuscript. GB contributed with ideas and discussion. GB and AŁ contributed in the organization of the manuscript. All authors contributed to the article and approved the submitted version.

ACKNOWLEDGMENTS

We are indebted with Dr. Sergio Ottolenghi for the generous sharing of his deep knowledge of the β-locus and of its mutations and with Christina Pitsillidou and Sarah Stucchi for their suggestions in preparing figures.

---

[2]https://www.globenewswire.com/news-release/2020/06/12/2047260/0/en/CRISPR-Therapeutics-and-Vertex-Announce-New-Clinical-Data-for-Investigational-Gene-Editing-Therapy-CTX001-in-Severe-Hemoglobinopathies-at-the-25th-Annual-European-Hematology-Associ.html (accessed October 5, 2020).

---

[3]http://ir.crisprtx.com/news-releases/news-release-details/crispr-therapeutics-and-vertex-pharmaceuticals-announce-priority (accessed October 5, 2020).

REFERENCES

Antoniani, C., Meneghini, V., Lattanzi, A., Felix, T., Romano, O., Magrin, E., et al. (2018). Induction of fetal hemoglobin synthesis by CRISPR/Cas9-mediated editing of the human beta-globin locus. *Blood* 131, 1960–1973. doi: 10.1182/blood-2017-10-811505

Anzalone, A. V., Randolph, P. B., Davis, J. R., Sousa, A. A., Koblan, L. W., Levy, J. M., et al. (2019). Search-and-replace genome editing without double-strand breaks or donor DN. A. *Nature* 576, 149–157. doi: 10.1038/s41586-019-1711-4

Aprile, A., Gulino, A., Storto, M., Villa, I., Beretta, S., Merelli, I., et al. (2020). Hematopoietic stem cell function in beta-thalassemia is impaired and is rescued by targeting the bone marrow niche. *Blood* 136–610–22. doi: 10.1182/blood.2019002721

Bauer, D. E., Kamran, S. C., Lessard, S., Xu, J., Fujiwara, Y., Lin, C., et al. (2013).An erythroid enhancer of BCL11A subject to genetic variation determines fetal hemoglobin level. *Science* 342, 253–257. doi: 10.1126/science.1242088

Berry, M., Grosveld, F., and Dillon, N. (1992). A single point mutation is the cause of the Greek form of hereditary persistence of fetal haemoglobin. *Nature* 358, 499–502. doi: 10.1038/358499a0

Borg, J., Papadopoulos, P., Georgitsi, M., Gutierrez, L., Grech, G., Fanis, P., et al. (2010). Haploinsufficiency for the erythroid transcription factor KLF1

causes hereditary persistence of fetal hemoglobin. *Nat. Genet.* 42, 801–805. doi: 10.1038/ng.630

Cai, L., Bai, H., Mahairaki, V., Gao, Y., He, C., Wen, Y., et al. (2018). A universal approach to correct various HBB gene mutations in human stem cells for gene therapy of beta-thalassemia and sickle cell disease. *Stem Cells Transl. Med.* 7, 87–97. doi: 10.1002/sctm.17-0066

Calzolari, R., McMorrow, T., Yannoutsos, N., Langeveld, A., and Grosveld, F. (1999). Deletion of a region that is a candidate for the difference between the deletion forms of hereditary persistence of fetal hemoglobin and deltabeta-thalassemia affects beta- but not gamma-globin gene expression. *EMBO J.* 18, 949–958. doi: 10.1093/emboj/18.4.949

Cantu, C., Ierardi, R., Alborelli, I., Fugazza, C., Cassinelli, L., Piconese, S., et al. (2011). Sox6 enhances erythroid differentiation in human erythroid progenitors. *Blood* 117, 3669–3679. doi: 10.1182/blood-2010-04-282350

Canver, M. C., Smith, E. C., Sher, F., Pinello, L., Sanjana, N. E., Shalem, O., et al. (2015). BCL11A enhancer dissection by Cas9-mediated *in situ* saturating mutagenesis. *Nature* 527, 192–197. doi: 10.1038/nature15521

Carter, D., Chakalova, L., Osborne, C. S., Dai, Y. F., and Fraser, P. (2002). Long-range chromatin regulatory interactions *in vivo*. *Nat. Genet.* 32, 623–626. doi: 10.1038/ng1051

Chakalova, L., Osborne, C. S., Dai, Y. F., Goyenechea, B., Metaxotou-Mavromati, A., Kattamis, A., et al. (2005). The Corfu deltabeta thalassemia deletion disrupts gamma-globin gene silencing and reveals post-transcriptional regulation of HbF expression. *Blood* 105, 2154–2160. doi: 10.1182/blood-2003-11-4069

Chang, K. H., Smith, S. E., Sullivan, T., Chen, K., Zhou, Q., West, J. A., et al. (2017). Long-term engraftment and fetal globin induction upon BCL11A gene editing in bone-marrow-derived CD34(+) hematopoietic stem and progenitor cells. *Mol Ther Methods Clin Dev.* 4, 137–148. doi: 10.1016/j.omtm.2016.12.009

Charlesworth, C. T., Camarena, J., Cromer, M. K., Vaidyanathan, S., Bak, R. O., Carte, J. M., et al. (2018). Priming human repopulating hematopoietic stem and progenitor cells for Cas9/sgRNA gene targeting. *Mol. Ther. Nucleic Acids* 12, 89–104. doi: 10.1016/j.omtn.2018.04.017

Chen, S. J. (2019). Minimizing off-target effects in CRISPR-Cas9 genome editing. *Cell Biol. Toxicol.* 35, 399–401. doi: 10.1007/s10565-019-09486-4

Chung, J. E., Magis, W., Vu, J., Heo, S. J., Wartiovaara, K., Walters, M. C., et al. (2019). CRISPR-Cas9 interrogation of a putative fetal globin repressor in human erythroid cells. *PLoS ONE* 14:e0208237. doi: 10.1371/journal.pone.0208237

Cornu, T. I., Mussolino, C., and Cathomen, T. (2017). Refining strategies to translate genome editing to the clinic. *Nat. Med.* 23, 415–423. doi: 10.1038/nm.4313

De Ravin, S. S., Li, L., Wu, X., Choi, U., Allen, C., Koontz, S., et al. (2017). CRISPR-Cas9 gene repair of hematopoietic stem cells from patients with X-linked chronic granulomatous disease. *Sci Transl Med.* 9, 1–10. doi: 10.1126/scitranslmed.aah3480

Deng, W., Rupon, J. W., Krivega, I., Breda, L., Motta, I., Jahn, K. S., et al. (2014). Reactivation of developmentally silenced globin genes by forced chromatin looping. *Cell* 158, 849–860. doi: 10.1016/j.cell.2014.05.050

Dever, D. P., Bak, R. O., Reinisch, A., Camarena, J., Washington, G., Nicolas, C. E., et al. (2016). CRISPR/Cas9 beta-globin gene targeting in human haematopoietic stem cells. *Nature* 539, 384–389. doi: 10.1038/nature20134

Dever, D. P., and Porteus, M. H. (2017). The changing landscape of gene editing in hematopoietic stem cells: a step towards Cas9 clinical translation. *Curr. Opin. Hematol.* 24, 481–488. doi: 10.1097/MOH.0000000000000385

DeWitt, M. A., Magis, W., Bray, N. L., Wang, T., Berman, J. R., Urbinati, F., et al. (2016). Selection-free genome editing of the sickle mutation in human adult hematopoietic stem/progenitor cells. *Sci. Transl. Med.* 8:360ra134. doi: 10.1126/scitranslmed.aaf9336

Doudna, J. A. (2020). The promise and challenge of therapeutic genome editing. *Nature* 578, 229–236. doi: 10.1038/s41586-020-1978-5

Forget, B. G. (1998). Molecular basis of hereditary persistence of fetal hemoglobin. *Ann. N. Y. Acad. Sci.* 850, 38–44. doi: 10.1111/j.1749-6632.1998.tb10460.x

Fraser, P., and Grosveld, F. (1998). Locus control regions, chromatin activation and transcription. *Curr. Opin. Cell Biol.* 10, 361–365. doi: 10.1016/S0955-0674(98)80012-4

Fritsch, E. F., Lawn, R. M., and Maniatis, T. (1980). Molecular cloning and characterization of the human beta-like globin gene cluster. *Cell* 19, 959–972. doi: 10.1016/0092-8674(80)90087-2

Gaensler, K. M., Zhang, Z., Lin, C., Yang, S., Hardt, K., and Flebbe-Rehwaldt, L. (2003). Sequences in the (A)gamma-delta intergenic region are not required for stage-specific regulation of the human beta-globin gene locus. *Proc. Natl. Acad. Sci. U.S.A.* 100, 3374–3379. doi: 10.1073/pnas.0634132100

Galanello, R., Melis, M. A., Podda, A., Monne, M., Perseu, L., Loudianos, G., et al. (1990). Deletion delta-thalassemia: the 7.2 kb deletion of Corfu delta beta-thalassemia in a non-beta-thalassemia chromosome. *Blood* 75, 1747–1749. doi: 10.1182/blood.V75.8.1747.1747

Garner, C. P., Tatu, T., Best, S., Creary, L., and Thein, S. L. (2002). Evidence of genetic interaction between the beta-globin complex and chromosome 8q in the expression of fetal hemoglobin. *Am. J. Hum. Genet.* 70, 793–799. doi: 10.1086/339248

Genovese, P., Schiroli, G., Escobar, G., Tomaso, T. D., Firrito, C., Calabria, A., et al. (2014). Targeted genome editing in human repopulating haematopoietic stem cells. *Nature* 510, 235–240. doi: 10.1038/nature13420

Grosveld, F., van Assendelft, G. B., Greaves, D. R., and Kollias, G. (1987). Position-independent, high-level expression of the human beta-globin gene in transgenic mice. *Cell* 51, 975–985. doi: 10.1016/0092-8674(87)90584-8

Gundry, M. C., Brunetti, L., Lin, A., Mayle, A. E., Kitano, A., Wagner, D., et al. (2016). Highly efficient genome editing of murine and human hematopoietic progenitor cells by CRISPR/Cas9. *Cell Rep.* 17, 1453–1461. doi: 10.1016/j.celrep.2016.09.092

Haapaniemi, E., Botla, S., Persson, J., Schmierer, B., and Taipale, J. (2018). CRISPR-Cas9 genome editing induces a p53-mediated DNA damage response. *Nat. Med.* 24, 927–930. doi: 10.1038/s41591-018-0049-z

Hirakawa, M. P., Krishnakumar, R., Timlin, J. A., Carney, J. P., and Butler, K. S. (2020). Gene editing and CRISPR in the clinic: current and future perspectives. *Biosci. Rep.* 40, 1–37. doi: 10.1042/BSR20200127

Hoban, M. D., Cost, G. J., Mendel, M. C., Romero, Z., Kaufman, M. L., Joglekar, A. V., et al. Correction of the sickle cell disease mutation in human hematopoietic stem/progenitor cells. *Blood* (2015). 125, 2597–604. doi: 10.1182/blood-2014-12-615948

Ihry, R. J., Worringer, K. A., Salick, M. R., Frias, E., Ho, D., Theriault, K., et al. (2018). p53 inhibits CRISPR-Cas9 engineering in human pluripotent stem cells. *Nat. Med.* 24, 939–946. doi: 10.1038/s41591-018-0050-6

Ikawa, Y., Miccio, A., Magrin, E., Kwiatkowski, J. L., Rivella, S., and Cavazzana, M. (2019). Gene therapy of hemoglobinopathies: progress and future challenges. *Hum. Mol. Genet.* 28:R24–30. doi: 10.1093/hmg/ddz172

Komor, A. C., Badran, A. H., and Liu, D. R. (2017). CRISPR-based technologies for the manipulation of eukaryotic genomes. *Cell* 168, 20–36. doi: 10.1016/j.cell.2016.10.044

Komor, A. C., Badran, A. H., and Liu, D. R. (2018). Editing the genome without double-stranded DNA breaks. *ACS Chem. Biol.* 13, 383–388. doi: 10.1021/acschembio.7b00710

Koren, A., Levin, C., Dgany, O., Kransnov, T., Elhasid, R., Zalman, L., et al. (2008). Response to hydroxyurea therapy in beta-thalassemia. *Am. J. Hematol.* 83, 366–370. doi: 10.1002/ajh.21120

Kountouris, P., Lederer, C. W., Fanis, P., Feleki, X., Old, J., and Kleanthous, M. (2014). IthaGenes: an interactive database for haemoglobin variations and epidemiology. *PLoS ONE* 9:e103020. doi: 10.1371/journal.pone.0103020

Kulozik, A. E., Yarwood, N., and Jones, R. W. (1988). The Corfu delta beta zero thalassemia: a small deletion acts at a distance to selectively abolish beta globin gene expression. *Blood* 71, 457–462. doi: 10.1182/blood.V71.2.457.457

Lattanzi, A., Meneghini, V., Pavani, G., Amor, F., Ramadier, S., Felix, T., et al. (2019). Optimization of CRISPR/Cas9 delivery to human hematopoietic stem and progenitor cells for therapeutic genomic rearrangements. *Mol. Ther.* 27, 137–150. doi: 10.1016/j.ymthe.2018.10.008

Lino, C. A., Harper, J. C., Carney, J. P., and Timlin, J. A. (2018). Delivering CRISPR: a review of the challenges and approaches. *Drug Deliv.* 25, 1234–1257. doi: 10.1080/10717544.2018.1474964

Liu, N., Hargreaves, V. V., Zhu, Q., Kurland, J. V., Hong, J., Kim, W., et al. (2018). Direct promoter repression by BCL11A controls the fetal to adult hemoglobin switch. *Cell* 173, 430–42 e17. doi: 10.1016/j.cell.2018.03.016

Luc, S., Huang, J., McEldoon, J. L., Somuncular, E., Li, D., Rhodes, C., et al. (2016). Bcl11a Deficiency leads to hematopoietic stem cell defects with an aging-like phenotype. *Cell Rep.* 16, 3181–3194. doi: 10.1016/j.celrep.2016.08.064

Maeda, T., Ito, K., Merghoub, T., Poliseno, L., Hobbs, R. M., Wang, G., et al. (2009). LRF is an essential downstream target of GATA1 in erythroid development and regulates BIM-dependent apoptosis. *Dev. Cell.* 17, 527–540. doi: 10.1016/j.devcel.2009.09.005

Magrin, E., Miccio, A., and Cavazzana, M. (2019). Lentiviral and genome-editing strategies for the treatment of beta-hemoglobinopathies. *Blood* 134, 1203–1213. doi: 10.1182/blood.2019000949

Martyn, G. E., Wienert, B., Kurita, R., Nakamura, Y., Quinlan, K. G. R., and Crossley, M. (2019). A natural regulatory mutation in the proximal promoter elevates fetal globin expression by creating a de novo GATA1 site. *Blood* 133, 852–856. doi: 10.1182/blood-2018-07-863951

Martyn, G. E., Wienert, B., Yang, L., Shah, M., Norton, L. J., Burdach, J., et al. (2018). Natural regulatory mutations elevate the fetal globin gene via disruption of BCL11A or ZBTB7A binding. *Nat. Genet.* 50, 498–503. doi: 10.1038/s41588-018-0085-0

Masuda, T., Wang, X., Maeda, M., Canver, M. C., Sher, F., Funnell, A. P., et al. (2016). Transcription factors LRF and BCL11A independently repress expression of fetal hemoglobin. *Science* 351, 285–289. doi: 10.1126/science.aad3312

Menzel, S., Garner, C., Gut, I., Matsuda, F., Yamaguchi, M., Heath, S., et al. (2007). A QTL influencing F cell production maps to a gene encoding a zinc-finger protein on chromosome 2p15. *Nat. Genet.* 39, 1197–1199. doi: 10.1038/ng2108

Mettananda, S., Fisher, C. A., Hay, D., Badat, M., Quek, L., Clark, K., et al. (2017). Editing an alpha-globin enhancer in primary human hematopoietic stem cells as a treatment for beta-thalassemia. *Nat. Commun.* 8:424. doi: 10.1038/s41467-017-00479-7

Mettananda, S., Gibbons, R. J., and Higgs, D. R. (2015). alpha-Globin as a molecular target in the treatment of beta-thalassemia. *Blood* 125, 3694–3701. doi: 10.1182/blood-2015-03-633594

Muirhead, H., Cox, J. M., Mazzarella, L., and Perutz, M. F. (1967). Structure and function of haemoglobin. 3. A three-dimensional fourier synthesis of human deoxyhaemoglobin at 5.5 Angstrom resolution. *J. Mol. Biol.* 28, 117–56. doi: 10.1016/S0022-2836(67)80082-2

Nuez, B., Michalovich, D., Bygrave, A., Ploemacher, R., and Grosveld, F. (1995). Defective haematopoiesis in fetal liver resulting from inactivation of the EKLF gene. *Nature* 375, 316–318. doi: 10.1038/375316a0

Ottolenghi, S., Giglioni, B., Taramelli, R., Comi, P., and Gianni, A. M. (1982). Delta beta-Thalassemia and HPF. H. *Birth Defects Orig. Artic. Ser.* 18, 65–67.

Palstra, R. J., Tolhuis, B., Splinter, E., Nijmeijer, R., Grosveld, F., and de Laat, W. (2003). The beta-globin nuclear compartment in development and erythroid differentiation. *Nat. Genet.* 35, 190–194. doi: 10.1038/ng1244

Papasavva, P., Kleanthous, M., and Lederer, C. W. (2019). Rare opportunities: CRISPR/Cas-based therapy development for rare genetic diseases. *Mol. Diagn. Ther.* 23, 201–222. doi: 10.1007/s40291-019-00392-3

Park, S. H., Lee, C. M., Dever, D. P., Davis, T. H., Camarena, J., Srifa, W., et al. (2019). Highly efficient editing of the beta-globin gene in patient-derived hematopoietic stem and progenitor cells to treat sickle cell disease. *Nucleic Acids Res.* 47, 7955–7972. doi: 10.1093/nar/gkz475

Perkins, A. C., Sharpe, A. H., and Orkin, S. H. (1995). Lethal beta-thalassaemia in mice lacking the erythroid CACCC-transcription factor EKL. F. *Nature* 375, 318–322. doi: 10.1038/375318a0

Pevny, L., Simon, M. C., Robertson, E., Klein, W. H., Tsai, S. F., D'Agati, V., et al. (1991). Erythroid differentiation in chimaeric mice blocked by a targeted mutation in the gene for transcription factor GATA-1. *Nature* 349, 257–260. doi: 10.1038/349257a0

Platt, O. S. (2008). Hydroxyurea for the treatment of sickle cell anemia. *N. Engl. J. Med.* 358, 1362–1369. doi: 10.1056/NEJMct0708272

Porteus, M. (2016). Genome editing: a new approach to human therapeutics. *Annu. Rev. Pharmacol. Toxicol.* 56, 163–190. doi: 10.1146/annurev-pharmtox-010814-124454

Pourfarzad, F., von Lindern, M., Azarkeivan, A., Hou, J., Kia, S. K., Esteghamat, F., et al. (2013). Hydroxyurea responsiveness in beta-thalassemic patients is determined by the stress response adaptation of erythroid progenitors and their differentiation propensity. *Haematologica* 98, 696–704. doi: 10.3324/haematol.2012.074492

Psatha, N., Karponi, G., and Yannaki, E. (2016). Optimizing autologous cell grafts to improve stem cell gene therapy. *Exp. Hematol.* 44, 528–539. doi: 10.1016/j.exphem.2016.04.007

Psatha, N., Reik, A., Phelps, S., Zhou, Y., Dalas, D., Yannaki, E., et al. (2018). Disruption of the BCL11A erythroid enhancer reactivates fetal hemoglobin in erythroid cells of patients with beta-thalassemia major. *Mol Ther Methods Clin Dev* 10, 313–326. doi: 10.1016/j.omtm.2018.08.003

Rivella, S. (2012). The role of ineffective erythropoiesis in non-transfusion-dependent thalassemia. *Blood Rev.* 26(Suppl. 1):S12–S15. doi: 10.1016/S0268-960X(12)70005-X

Sankaran, V. G., Menne, T. F., Xu, J., Akie, T. E., Lettre, G., Van Handel, B., et al. (2008). Human fetal hemoglobin expression is regulated by the developmental stage-specific repressor BCL11A. *Science* 322, 1839–1842. doi: 10.1126/science.1165409

Sankaran, V. G., Xu, J., Byron, R., Greisman, H. A., Fisher, C., Weatherall, D. J., et al. (2011). A functional element necessary for fetal hemoglobin silencing. *N. Engl. J. Med.* 365, 807–814. doi: 10.1056/NEJMoa1103070

Schiroli, G., Conti, A., Ferrari, S., Della Volpe, L., Jacob, A., Albano, L., et al. (2019). Precise gene editing preserves hematopoietic stem cell function following transient p53-mediated DNA damage response. *Cell Stem Cell* 24, 551–65 e8. doi: 10.1016/j.stem.2019.02.019

Smithies, O., Gregg, R. G., Boggs, S. S., Koralewski, M. A., and Kucherlapati, R. S. (1985). Insertion of DNA sequences into the human chromosomal beta-globin locus by homologous recombination. *Nature* 317, 230–234. doi: 10.1038/317230a0

Stamatoyannopoulos, G. (1991). Human hemoglobin switching. *Science* 252:383. doi: 10.1126/science.2017679

Steinberg, M. H., Chui, D. H., Dover, G. J., Sebastiani, P., and Alsultan, A. (2014). Fetal hemoglobin in sickle cell anemia: a glass half full? *Blood* 123, 481–485. doi: 10.1182/blood-2013-09-528067

Taher, A. T., Musallam, K. M., and Cappellini, M. D. (2009). Thalassaemia intermedia: an update. *Mediterr. J. Hematol. Infect. Dis.* 1:e2009004. doi: 10.4084/MJHID.2009.004

Thein, S. L. (2008). Genetic modifiers of the beta-haemoglobinopathies. *Br. J. Haematol.* 141, 357–366. doi: 10.1111/j.1365-2141.2008.07084.x

Thein, S. L. (2013). The molecular basis of beta-thalassemia. *Cold Spring Harb. Perspect. Med.* 3:a011700. doi: 10.1101/cshperspect.a011700

Tolhuis, B., Palstra, R. J., Splinter, E., Grosveld, F., and de Laat, W. (2002). Looping and interaction between hypersensitive sites in the active beta-globin locus. *Mol. Cell* 10, 1453–1465. doi: 10.1016/S1097-2765(02)00781-5

Traxler, E. A., Yao, Y., Wang, Y. D., Woodard, K. J., Kurita, R., Nakamura, Y., et al. (2016). A genome-editing strategy to treat beta-hemoglobinopathies that recapitulates a mutation associated with a benign genetic condition. *Nat. Med.* 22, 987–990. doi: 10.1038/nm.4170

Uda, M., Galanello, R., Sanna, S., Lettre, G., Sankaran, V. G., Chen, W., et al. (2008). Genome-wide association study shows BCL11A associated with persistent fetal hemoglobin and amelioration of the phenotype of beta-thalassemia. *Proc. Natl. Acad. Sci. U.S.A.* 105, 1620–1625. doi: 10.1073/pnas.0711566105

Vega, M. A. (1991). Prospects for homologous recombination in human gene therapy. *Hum. Genet.* 87, 245–253. doi: 10.1007/BF00200899

Viprakasit, V., Gibbons, R. J., Broughton, B. C., Tolmie, J. L., Brown, D., Lunt, P., et al. (2001). Mutations in the general transcription factor TFIIH result in beta-thalassaemia in individuals with trichothiodystrophy. *Hum. Mol. Genet.* 10, 2797–2802. doi: 10.1093/hmg/10.24.2797

Wainscoat, J. S., Thein, S. L., Wood, W. G., Weatherall, D. J., Metaxotou-Mavromati, A., Tzotos, S., et al. (1985). A novel deletion in the beta-globin gene complex. *Ann. N. Y. Acad. Sci.* 445, 20–27. doi: 10.1111/j.1749-6632.1985.tb17171.x

Walton, R. T., Christie, K. A., Whittaker, M. N., and Kleinstiver, B. P. (2020). Unconstrained genome targeting with near-PAMless engineered CRISPR-Cas9 variants. *Science* 368, 290–296. doi: 10.1126/science.aba8853

Wang, H., and Xu, X. (2017). Microhomology-mediated end joining: new players join the team. *Cell Biosci.* 7:6. doi: 10.1186/s13578-017-0136-8

Weatherall, D. J. (2008). Hemoglobinopathies worldwide: present and future. *Curr. Mol. Med.* 8, 592–599. doi: 10.2174/156652408786241375

Weber, L., Frati, G., Felix, T., Hardouin, G., Casini, A., Wollenschlaeger, C., et al. (2020). Editing a gamma-globin repressor binding site restores fetal hemoglobin synthesis and corrects the sickle cell disease phenotype. *Sci Adv.* 6:eaay9392. doi: 10.1126/sciadv.aay9392

Wienert, B., Funnell, A. P., Norton, L. J., Pearson, R. C., Wilkinson-White, L. E., Lester, K., et al. (2015). Editing the genome to introduce a beneficial naturally occurring mutation associated with increased fetal globin. *Nat. Commun.* 6:7085. doi: 10.1038/ncomms8085

Wienert, B., Martyn, G. E., Kurita, R., Nakamura, Y., Quinlan, K. G. R., and Crossley, M. (2017). KLF1 drives the expression of fetal hemoglobin in British HPF. H. *Blood* 130, 803–807. doi: 10.1182/blood-2017-02-767400

Wilber, A., Nienhuis, A. W., and Persons, D. A. (2011). Transcriptional regulation of fetal to adult hemoglobin switching: new therapeutic opportunities. *Blood* 117, 3945–3953. doi: 10.1182/blood-2010-11-316893

Wu, Y., Zeng, J., Roscoe, B. P., Liu, P., Yao, Q., Lazzarotto, C. R., et al. (2019). Highly efficient therapeutic gene editing of human hematopoietic stem cells. *Nat. Med.* 25, 776–783. doi: 10.1038/s41591-019-0401-y

Ye, L., Wang, J., Tan, Y., Beyer, A. I., Xie, F., Muench, M. O., et al. (2016). Genome editing using CRISPR-Cas9 to create the HPFH genotype in HSPCs:

an approach for treating sickle cell disease and beta-thalassemia. *Proc. Natl. Acad. Sci. U.S.A.* 113, 10661–10665. doi: 10.1073/pnas.1612075113

Yu, C., Niakan, K. K., Matsushita, M., Stamatoyannopoulos, G., Orkin, S. H., and Raskind, W. H. (2002). X-linked thrombocytopenia with thalassemia from a mutation in the amino finger of GATA-1 affecting DNA binding rather than FOG-1 interaction. *Blood* 100, 2040–2045. doi: 10.1182/blood-2002-02-0387

Yu, K. R., Natanson, H., and Dunbar, C. E. (2016). Gene editing of human hematopoietic stem and progenitor cells: promise and potential hurdles. *Hum. Gene Ther.* 27, 729–740. doi: 10.1089/hum.2016.107

Yu, L., Myers, G., and Engel, J. D. (2020). Small molecule therapeutics to treat the beta-globinopathies. *Curr. Opin. Hematol.* 27, 129–140. doi: 10.1097/MOH.0000000000000579

Zeng, J., Wu, Y., Ren, C., Bonanno, J., Shen, A. H., Shea, D., et al. (2020). Therapeutic base editing of human hematopoietic stem cells. *Nat. Med.* 26, 535–541. doi: 10.1038/s41591-020-0790-y

Zhou, D., Liu, K., Sun, C. W., Pawlik, K. M., and Townes, T. M. (2010). KLF1 regulates BCL11A expression and gamma- to beta-globin gene switching. *Nat. Genet.* 42, 742–744. doi: 10.1038/ng.637

2

Mesenchymal Stromal Cells as a Cellular Target in Myeloid Malignancy: Chances and Challenges in the Genome Editing of Stromal Alterations

Bella Banjanin [1,2] and Rebekka K. Schneider [1,2,3]*

[1] Department of Hematology, Erasmus Medical Center Cancer Institute, Rotterdam, Netherlands, [2] Oncode Institute, Erasmus Medical Center Cancer Institute, Rotterdam, Netherlands, [3] Department of Cell Biology, Faculty of Medicine, Institute for Biomedical Engineering, Rheinisch-Westfälische Technische Hochschule (RWTH) Aachen University, Aachen, Germany

Correspondence:
Rebekka K. Schneider
reschneider@ukaachen.de

The contribution of bone marrow stromal cells to the pathogenesis and therapy response of myeloid malignancies has gained significant attention over the last decade. Evidence suggests that the bone marrow stroma should not be neglected in the design of novel, targeted-therapies. In terms of gene-editing, the focus of gene therapies has mainly been on correcting mutations in hematopoietic cells. Here, we outline why alterations in the stroma should also be taken into consideration in the design of novel therapeutic strategies but also outline the challenges in specifically targeting mesenchymal stromal cells in myeloid malignancies caused by somatic and germline mutations.

Keywords: genome-editing, BM MSCS, myeloid malignancies, stromal alterations, BM niche

INTRODUCTION

Under physiological conditions, hematopoietic stem cells (HSCs) are regulated by their bone marrow microenvironment (BMM) through cellular interactions and secreted factors to maintain a continuous pool of hematopoietic cells (Morrison and Scadden, 2014; Pinho and Frenette, 2019). This crosstalk between the hematopoietic system with its surroundings is essential for the proper functioning of HSCs throughout life and becomes deregulated in hematological malignancies. The main constituents of the BMM are bone marrow mesenchymal stromal cells (MSCs), osteolineage cells (OLCs), endothelial cells, amongst various other cells including adipocytes, neural, and hematopoietic cells (Pinho and Frenette, 2019; Méndez-Ferrer et al., 2020). MSCs are a heterogenous group of non-hematopoietic cells that express key hematopoiesis-supporting factors such as stem cell factor (SCF) and CXC motif ligand (CXCL)-12. In humans the surface markers CD271 and CD146 have been shown to enrich for cells that can form fibroblast colonies (CFU-F) (Kfoury and Scadden, 2015). MSCs have been described in mouse models using numerous Cre-drivers and surface markers outlined in **Figure 1**.

Historically, the development of myeloid malignancies was considered to be HSC-intrinsic, be it driven by germline or somatic mutation. The BMM can either facilitate oncogenesis by supporting the expansion of malignant cells, and suppressing normal hematopoiesis, or induce oncogenesis by acquiring mutations or functional alterations that pre-dispose for oncogenesis. These two theories are not mutually exclusive, as is amply exemplified in the pathogenesis of myeloid malignancies including myeloproliferative neoplasms (MPN), myelodysplastic syndromes (MDS) and acute myeloid leukemia (AML) (Medyouf, 2017; Fathi et al., 2019; Behrmann et al., 2020). Thus, the mutual interaction between mutated HSCs and the BMM has further evolved as an attractive novel therapeutic target.

In this article, we will outline the role of stromal cells (specifically BM MSCs) in myeloid malignancies in somatic disease, as well as germline conditions, and describe recent progress in dissecting the HSC-stroma crosstalk. Finally, we discuss possible application of the established murine disease models and future challenges in developing genetically targeted therapies for the BM stroma.

THE ROLE OF THE STROMA IN LEUKEMIA PRE-DISPOSITION SYNDROMES

The World Health Organization (WHO) introduced a new category of "myeloid malignancies with germline predisposition" to the 2016 Classification of hematopoietic tumors. Given that these "rare" mutations are only coming to light with increased use of parallel sequencing platforms in population and family studies (Porter, 2016; Miller et al., 2018; Kim et al., 2020), it can be speculated that germline stromal mutations exist which have yet to be discovered. An exemplary disease is Shwachman-Diamond syndrome (SDS); a rare autosomal recessive bone marrow failure disorder caused by mutation in the *SBDS* gene with a cumulative probability of leukemic progression of >30% at the age of 30 years (Dale et al., 2006; Nelson and Myers, 2018). Hematopoietic cell specific deletion of *Sbds* did not result in MDS or AML in two murine disease models (Rawls et al., 2007; Zambetti et al., 2015), whereas exposure of wildtype HSCs to *Sbds*-deficient osteolineage MSCs led to an MDS phenotype and genotoxic stress in HSCs (Zambetti et al., 2016). The prominent clinical feature of skeletal abnormalities in SDS patients was recapitulated through the niche-specific deletion of *Sbds* (Zambetti et al., 2016). Importantly, the alarmin heterocomplex S100A8/9 secreted by the niche was identified as a candidate driver of inflammatory stress in HSCs, highlighting that the crosstalk between stroma and HSCs is of particular interest as a possible therapy target. Targeted deletion of *Dicer1* in osteolineage MSCs resulted in reduced expression of *Sbds* in transplanted WT HSCs (Raaijmakers et al., 2010). The resulting phenotype displayed key features of human MDS and a tendency to develop AML; clearly showing that alterations in BM stromal cells can induce malignancy and stress in HSCs (Raaijmakers et al., 2010). Intriguing case studies of donor cell-derived leukemia (DCL) development upon allogeneic HSC transplantation in humans have brought about the possibility of oncogenesis driven by the diseased recipient BMM (Berger et al., 2016; Engel et al., 2018).

In line, numerous genetic modifications (deletions) in non-hematopoietic, stromal cells were reported to give rise to a myeloproliferative phenotype *in vitro* and *in vivo* (Rupec et al., 2005; Walkley et al., 2007; Xiao et al., 2018), but also activation of e.g., Notch signaling (Kim et al., 2008; Dong et al., 2016). Inflammation seems to play an important role in the pathogenesis of these myeloid malignancies. As an example, IL-1B propagates

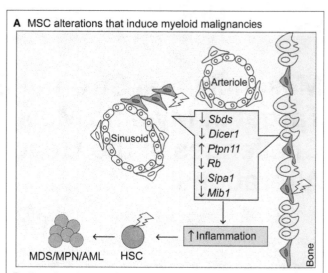

FIGURE 1 | MSC niche in myeloid malignancies. **(A)** Schematic representation of MSC niche alterations that promote the leukemic transformation. Lightning bolt indicates genetic lesion in MSC-like cells that have been shown to promote oncogenesis through increased inflammation and increased (genotoxic) stress of HSCs. Deletion of *Dicer1* and *Sbds* in Osterix+ osteoprogenitor MSCs leads to a MDS phenotype with sporadic AML upon *Dicer1* deletion (Raaijmakers et al., 2010; Zambetti et al., 2016). Activating mutations in tyrosine-protein phosphatase non-receptor type 11 (*Ptpn11*) in Nestin-Cre+ cells induces a MPN phenotype. A MDS/MPN phenotype was also seen in activating *Ptpn11* in *Mx1*-Cre+, *Prx1*-Cre+, *Lepr*-Cre+, *Osx1*-Cre+ cell-type specific knock-in mice, highlighting that MSCs and osteoprogenitors can induce MPN and that there is probably overlap in cells populations targeted by the Cre-drivers, whereas differentiated osteoblasts (Oc-Cre+) and endothelial cells (VE-Cadherin-Cre+-ERT2) could not induce MPN (Dong et al., 2016). *Rb* (encodes RB protein) (Walkley et al., 2007) and *Mib1* (encodes mind bomb 1 protein) (Kim et al., 2008) promote an MPN-like phenotype in a Mx1-Cre+ driver. The Mx1-Cre+ driver traces MSC-like cells that are located within the bone marrow but also at the periosteum (Ortinau et al., 2019), and have limited *in vivo* adipogenic differentiation potential, making them more osteoprogenitor-like (Park et al., 2012). *Sipa1* expression is most abundant in CD31+ BM endothelial cells, but also found in MSCs (CD45−Lin−CD31−CD51+Sca1+) (Xiao et al., 2018). Deletion of *Sipa1* results in the development of MDS/MPN and *Sipa1*−/− MSCs cultured *in vitro* show increased adipogenic and chrondrogenic differentiation potential, but impaired osteogenic differentiation (Xiao et al., 2018). **(B)** Upon exposure of a mutated hematopoietic cell within the niche, MSCs are functionally altered

(Continued)

FIGURE 1 | through cytokine stimulation, direct cell-cell contact and activation of inflammatory pathways, promoting the survival of the mutant HSC in favor of WT HSCs and increase in inflammatory signatures. Specifically, Lepr-Cre[+] (Decker et al., 2017) and Gli1-Cre[+] (Schneider et al., 2017) cells expand and proliferate in an MPN setting and produce extracellular matrix. Nestin-Cre[+] cells proliferate in AML and provide chemotherapy resistance (Forte et al., 2020), whereas they become apoptotic in MPN disease due to neural damage and Schwann cell death triggered by interleukin-1β production by the mutated HSC. AML cells seem to induce osteogenic differentiation and block adipogenesis of MSCs, as well as blocking maturation of osteolineage-MSCs into mature osteoblasts (Battula et al., 2017; Pievani et al., 2020b). MSCs, mesenchymal stem cells; HSC, hematopoietic stem cells; AML, acute myeloid leukemia; MPN, myeloproliferative neoplasm; MDS, myelodysplastic syndrome; ECM, extracellular matrix; Lepr, Leptin receptor; Prx1, Paired related homeobox 1; Mx-1, Myxovirus Resistance-1.

an inflammatory BMM as it activates HSCs to differentiate toward myeloid cells and monocytes (Rupec et al., 2005). Early stages of MPN disease are also characterized by increased IL-1β expression, which triggers pro-inflammatory damage to the BMM and advances disease progression (Arranz et al., 2014). This showcases that stromal drivers influence the hematopoietic system and can result in secondary neoplasms (schematically depicted in **Figure 1A**).

CROSSTALK BETWEEN NON-MUTATED STROMA AND HEMATOPOIETIC CELLS WITH SOMATIC MUTATIONS

It is becoming evident that the BMM is functionally altered by exposure to hematopoietic cells harboring somatic mutations, creating a proinflammatory environment that seems to propagate leukemic disease development and supresses normal hematopoiesis (**Figure 1B**). Overall differences in MSC compartments have been noted in myeloid malignancies compared to normal bone marrow. In AML, there is generally a reduction of bulk MSCs. However, Nestin[+] cells, as well-documented MSCs in the BM (Mendez-Ferrer et al., 2010), have been shown to be 4–5-fold more abundant in human AML patients, in line with expansion of Nestin[+] cells in the murine iMLL-AF9 AML model (Hanoun et al., 2014; Forte et al., 2020). This is in striking contrast to the decrease in Nestin[+] cells in murine models and human MPN (Arranz et al., 2014; Drexler et al., 2019), suggesting that the same group of niche cells can behave differently in various myeloid malignancies and/or stages of leukemic disease. Conditional depletion of Nestin[+] cells upon AML development in iMLL-AF9 mice lead to a significantly extended mouse survival, suggesting that Nestin[+] cells promote leukemogenesis *in vivo* (Forte et al., 2020). Importantly, in a competitive transplant setting, depletion of Nestin[+] cells during AML development selectively diminished the number of leukemic cells, while leaving normal hematopoiesis unaffected (Forte et al., 2020), which is one of the major challenges in the treatment of AML.

The direct effect of a mutated hematopoietic clone on the bone microenvironment is evidently illustrated in murine models but also patient samples with bone marrow fibrosis. In a murine model of CML, endosteal OLCs expanded upon expression of BCR/ABL in the hematopoietic compartment leading to deposition of extracellular matrix (Schepers et al., 2013). In response to MPN clones, Gli1[+] stromal cells are activated from their normal endosteal and perivascular niches and significantly expand in murine models and patient samples (Schneider et al., 2017). Importantly, their genetic ablation ameliorates fibrosis, proving functional proof that they play a central role in the fibrotic transformation. Another stromal subset of Lepr[+] MSCs has been shown to expand in fibrosis (Decker et al., 2017). Conditional deletion of platelet-derived growth factor receptor a (Pdgfra) from Lepr[+] cells or the administration of the tyrosine kinase inhibitor imatinib suppressed Lepr[+] cell expansion and mitigated fibrosis. There seems to be a common initial pro-inflammatory stromal response to the malignant MPN clone that poises the stroma to become pro-fibrotic (Gleitz et al., 2020; Leimkuhler et al., 2020). This is in line with the observation of a diseased niche characterized by cellular stress and an increased inflammatory signature in bulk RNA-sequencing of prospectively sorted mesenchymal cells from human low-risk MDS patients (Chen et al., 2016). Additionally, human MDS MSCs produce inflammatory cytokines (IL-1β, IL-6, and TNFα) compared to control *in vitro* cultured MSCs (Flores-Figueroa et al., 2002, 2008). Notably, IL-6 knockout in the BM reduces fibrosis in a MPN setting (Gleitz et al., 2020). Likewise, our group demonstrated increased expression of the inflammatory S100A8 alarmin in the stromal niche in murine models and patient samples of del(5q) MDS (Ribezzo et al., 2018). This increased expression of S100A8 in MSCs resulted in decreased hematopoiesis-support *in vitro*, indicating that mutated hematopoietic cells can initiate a vicious cycle of inflammation in the niche, leading to decreased support of normal hematopoiesis and fuelling the progression of haematopoietic malignancy. The common denominator in hematological malignancies driven by somatic or germline mutations thus seems to be an inflammatory "mutagenic" microenvironment that precedes malignant transformation and disease progression (Craver et al., 2018; Gleitz et al., 2018; Leimkühler and Schneider, 2019; Pronk and Raaijmakers, 2019).

CHALLENGES OF GENETIC EDITING IN THE BONE MARROW STROMA

As outlined, the bone marrow stroma seems to play a significant role in the initiation, maintenance and progression of myeloid malignancies and murine models indicate that MSCs are a highly attractive therapeutic target. The importance of targeting the stroma is highlighted by the fact that despite improvements in the treatment of AML, long-term survival is <30% in adults (Ferrara and Schiff, 2013). In murine models, specific subsets of stromal cells can be modified by using stromal Cre-drivers. The correlate to this procedure in the human setting would optimally be genome editing of stromal cells. Nuclease-based site-specific genome editing has provided an unprecedented opportunity to artificially modify genetic information within mammalian cells (Romito et al., 2019). The clustered regularly interspersed short palindromic repeats (CRISPR)/Cas9 system has been used to create germline and somatic mouse models, and has the benefits of relatively easy design and high mutational efficiency (Mou et al., 2015; González-Romero et al., 2019; Broeders et al., 2020; Lee et al., 2020). The HSC has been the most relevant cell type to edit, with major advances in Cas9 clinical translation made, particularly in the monogenetic disorders sickle cell disease and β-thalassemia (Dever and Porteus, 2017).

In this section we highlight some of the key challenges hampering the development of targeted genetic therapy of BM stromal populations: (1) identification of specific MSC population to edit, (2) targeting MSCs in their *in situ* location vs. *ex vivo*, (3) indirect targeting of MSC function *in vivo* through genome editing of hematopoietic cells and cell-to-cell interactions, and (4) *in vitro* functional characterization of MSCs and potential therapeutic targets through CRISPR screens and 3D models.

IDENTIFICATION AND TARGETING MSCs *IN SITU* – DIRECT VS. INDIRECT STRATEGIES

Much of our understanding of the BM MSCs has originated from genetic-fate tracing mouse models in which MSC populations have been labeled via a stromal Cre-driver (Kfoury and Scadden, 2015). Functionality of these Cre-drivers has been shown by conditional deletion using diphteria-toxin receptor based mechanisms (Schneider et al., 2017; Pinho and Frenette, 2019). Additionally, Cre-drivers of MSC populations provide spatial information when combined with a fluorescent-reporter. Nevertheless, the current widely-used Cre-drivers likely label heterogeneous groups of MSCs, outlined in a recent review (Al-Sabah et al., 2020). The recombination efficacy in Cre-drivers has resulted in variable results (Chen et al., 2017), while conditional Cre-lines result in higher specificity compared to constitutive Cre-lines and allow fate-tracing experiments in health and disease setting (Méndez-Ferrer et al., 2020). Recent advancements in single-cell RNA sequencing (scRNAseq) have for the first time allowed us to zoom in on heterogeneous populations within the murine BMM (Schroeder et al., 2016; Baryawno et al., 2019; Tikhonova et al., 2019; Wolock et al., 2019; Baccin et al., 2020; Leimkuhler et al., 2020). Tikhonova et al. have shown that the Lepr[+] Cre-driver previously studied as one MSC population, contains four subclusters of MSCs, with functional differences between them as current evidence suggests. As we gain knowledge of functionally distinct MSCs and their possibly common progenitors, it will become possible to target them. Importantly, the location of MSCs in relation to (mutant) HSPCs seems to predict biological functionality and these sinusoidal and CXCL12 niches will need to be further investigated (Gomariz et al., 2018; Baccin et al., 2020; Kokkaliaris et al., 2020). Perhaps the use of multiplexed imaging (Kokkaliaris et al., 2020) in combination with laser-capture techniques to isolate specific BM populations (Baccin et al., 2020) can aid in inferring spatial and signaling relationships between cells from single cell transcriptomic data.

Specifically, these new techniques can help identify new druggable pathways through, for example, ligand-receptor analysis between mutated hematopoietic cells and the stromal counterpart in myeloid malignancies (Efremova et al., 2020). This method was very recently employed in the unbiased scRNAseq paper showing populations of murine and human MSCs interacting with hematopoietic populations in MPN (Leimkuhler et al., 2020). A druggable alarmin axis was identified in the fibrotic transformation both in murine models and patients and treatment with Tasquinimod, inhibiting the binding of the alarmins S100A8/S100A9 to TLR4, ameliorated the MPN phenotype in mice.

Due to the lack of evident genetic modifications and a prominent cell of origin, a clear-cut molecular target for BM MSCs is not apparent. It is possible, however, to target HSPCs as they are relatively easily accessible for genome editing. The use of gene therapy for neurometabolic disorders using HSPC transplantation has shown that overexpression of therapeutic proteins has cross-correction capacity as also non-hematopoietic cells are being exposed to the therapeutic effect (Ferrari et al., 2020). This could be useful if loss-of-function mutations are found in MSCs.

One could imagine that mutated hematopoietic cells can be examined for specific receptors that are not vital for their physiological function but are unique for their malignant interaction with stroma (Kokkaliaris and Scadden, 2020; Pievani et al., 2020a). The α4β1 integrin–VCAM1 axis between stroma and the AML mutant cell aids in chemoresistance (Jacamo et al., 2014; Carter et al., 2016). AML chemo-resistant cells also have high expression of very late antigen 4 (VLA4) which facilitates adherence to the stroma through VCAM1 activated NF-kB signaling (Jacamo et al., 2014). Indeed, patients with VLA-4-negative AML have a more favorable prognosis, highlighting the role of stroma-HSCPs cross-talk (Matsunaga et al., 2003). Within the CXCL12-CXCR4 axis, CXCL12 is expressed by MSCs and interacts with HSCs via the binding to CXCR4, regulating their mobilization (Greenbaum et al., 2013). Blockade of this axis can release leukemic cells from their chemoprotective niches (Nervi et al., 2009). Recently, an elegant *in vivo* pooled CRISPR screen targeting selected cell surface genes was performed in murine *MLL-AF9* AML cells and identified CXCR4 as a positive regulator of leukemic cells, indispensable for their growth and survival *in vivo* (Ramakrishnan et al., 2020). CXCR4 is essential for the development of AML independently of its interaction with CXCL12 on MSCs or endothelial cells. In contrast, $Cxcr4^{-/-}$ normal HSCs are capable of long-term hematopoiesis (Nie et al., 2008), highlighting the different biology in homeostasis and malignant disease and possible targeting avenues.

As an example, inflammation within the BM niche, specifically the erythroblastic niche, can be targeted by genetically editing the hematopoietic cell. In our previous work, we applied CRISPR-Cas9 technology in a murine MDS model to genetically inactivate *S100a8* and improve the defective erythropoiesis characteristic for the disease. Compared to control non-targeting sgRNA, CRISPR-mediated inactivation of *S100a8* in MDS cells restored erythropoiesis and restored a normal erythroid niche by interrupting the cycle of inflammation (Schneider et al., 2016).

Ideally, the complex interplay between the hematopoietic system and the stroma could be modeled more efficiently with CRISPR-Cas9 based techniques in mice (Heckl et al., 2014; Tothova et al., 2017). With advancements in deep-sequencing, novel germline/somatic mutations in stroma of patients might be identified. More complex models could then be made to mimic the different mutations identified in the hematopoietic and the stromal compartment in mice, to search for druggable targets. The genome-editing efficiency is also consistently being improved, with DNA-free systems being developed that are more suitable for human trials as there is no risk for random insertional mutagenesis (Shapiro et al., 2020).

GENETIC EDITING OF STROMAL CELLS *EX VIVO*: FEASIBILITY OF DELIVERY

A commonly used CRISPR/Cas9- based technique for gene editing *ex vivo* is the isolation of the target cell and delivery of the gene-editing machinery via electroporation, microinjection, or virus-based vehicles before injecting the corrected cells back into patients or mice (Broeders et al., 2020). MSCs in general have been widely investigated for use in multiple diseases due to the ease of their isolation (plastic adherence and self-renewal properties), their low immunity potential, and their ability to secrete factors (Kean et al., 2013). The production of inflammatory cytokines such as PDGF, TNFa, CCR8, and CCR2 within the solid organ tumor microenvironment, has been shown to enhance homing of MSCs to the tumor location (Marofi et al., 2017). Primary MSCs can express CRISPR/Cas9 proteins through nucleofection, lentivirus, and non-integrating adeno-associated virus (Golchin et al., 2020). However, the homing of edited MSCs to the bone marrow niche has not been formally tested yet.

A possible technique by which CRISPR-based strategies on the BM stroma could be performed, is by injecting complete CRISPR-proteins through intrafemoral injections. Intrafemoral injection has been used to model osteosarcoma in orthotopic mouse models (Sasaki et al., 2016). The only downside is that off-target effects on surrounding (hematopoietic) cells can occur. To circumvent this, a possibility could be to expand MSCs *ex vivo* and genetically alter them using CRISPR *in vitro*, and then inject them back through an intrafemoral injection. It has been shown that donor MSCs injected via intramarrow injection also contribute to the reconstitution of the stromal niche in the ablated bone marrow of recipient mice (Muguruma et al., 2006; Ahn et al., 2010; Zhou et al., 2014). Intraosseal therapy could pose clinical challenges, with an invasive procedure that has an increased chance of complications (in particular infections), compared to intravenous or intraarterial administration. However, the intravenously administered MSCs easily get trapped in the lung circulation and have limited engraftment of about a week, whereas arterially administered MSCs seem to engraftment better at the site of injury, e.g., hind leg bone irradiation in mice (Kean et al., 2013). First, proof of

principle studies using intrafemoral/intraosseal injections need to be performed where candidate genes can be knocked out or mutations introduced within the mouse or even specifically in the stroma by using floxed Cas9 mice crossed to specific stromal Cre-drivers. The beauty of this method in mice is additionally that one leg can be edited while one leg serves as a non-targeted control. A major point to consider, however, is the determination of recombination efficiency within the bone marrow stroma as MSCs are difficult to obtain as single-cell suspension cells. A possible read-out here could be *in situ* hybridization of mRNA of the targeted genes in a multiplex imaging set-up.

Cas proteins need specially designed delivery vehicles for tissue-specific delivery as they cannot cross biological barriers themselves and have a high positive charge and molecular mass. Extracellular vesicles (EVs) are used as possible packing devices for sgRNA:Cas9 ribonucleoprotein complexes. It has been shown however that EVs are mainly taken up by the liver (~84%), whereas roughly 1.6% are found back in the bone marrow 4 h upon systemic administration, making delivery to the bone marrow quite challenging (Kostyushev et al., 2020). Progress is made on engineering functionalized exosomes (M-CRISPR-Cas9 exosome) which encapsulate CRISPR-Cas9 components more efficiently (Ye et al., 2020). Recently, the interest for vesicle nanoparticles containing the Cas9 machinery has been growing. While traditionally nanoparticles can mainly be found in the liver and lung after injection, a recent breakthrough study (Krohn-Grimberghe et al., 2020), reported the design and *in vivo* performance of systemically injected lipid–polymer nanoparticles encapsulating small interfering RNA (siRNA), for the silencing of genes specifically in bone-marrow endothelial cells. Using nanoparticle enabled RNAi, the group targeted stromal-derived factor 1 (*Sdf1*) resulting in stem cell liberation into the blood, and monocyte chemotactic protein 1 (*Mcp1*) whose silencing retained monocytes in the BM. These modified nanoparticles lay the ground for editing non-hematopoietic cells in the bone marrow with a high efficacy and show that HSPCs biology can be altered through stroma alterations.

FUNCTIONAL TESTING OF GENETIC MODIFICATION OF MSCs *IN VITRO* AND *IN VIVO*

Isolation of MSCs directly from the BM remains a challenge as stromal cells are closely associated with extracellular matrix within the marrow and single-cell suspensions are difficult to obtain even after digestion of bone (Gomariz et al., 2018). Most often, MSCs are left to grow out from bone chips or human aspirates and selected for on the basis of their plastic adherence. Cultured human MSCs are minimally characterized by their trilineage differentiation potential, expression of surface markers that enhance CFU-F potential, and plastic adherence *in vitro* (Dominici et al., 2006; Kfoury and Scadden, 2015; Agha et al., 2017). Murine MSCs are often identified by a panel of typical surface markers and have a less stringent definition (Agha et al., 2017). Nevertheless, functional characterization of *in vitro* isolated cells still needs to be optimized, as even a short-term (passage 0) *ex vivo* culturing environment greatly reprograms MSCs compared to direct sorting of primary cells for microarray analysis (Ghazanfari et al., 2017). Despite retaining their *in vitro* clonogenicity and tri-lineage differentiation potential (Pevsner-Fischer et al., 2011), culture-induced gene expression changes are present and raise the question of comparability of primary and cultured cells, as well as the possibility that only specific subsets of MSCs are selected for in adherent culture (Tormin et al., 2009). BM MSCs cultured as non-adherent 3D sphere colonies termed mesenspheres, have been reported to retain MSC surface markers, tri-lineage potential, and to have an increased self-renewal potential in serial transplantations into immunodeficient NOD scid gamma mice compared to adherent cultured cells (Ghazanfari et al., 2016). Gene expression in cultured MSC mesenspheres was still altered compared to primary sorted MSCs, but 3D cultured cells had more osteogenic and adipogenic transcription factor expression compared to 2D adherent cells (Ghazanfari et al., 2017). This difference in culturing conditions might be confounding as Forte et al. have shown that in MSCs derived from the same AML donors, only mesenspheres provided enhanced chemoprotection of human AML blasts, whereas plastic-adherent MSCs did not (Forte et al., 2020). The improved fitness of 3D cultured MSCs advocates for its use. Ideally, there will be a standardized protocol for the isolation of murine and human BM MSCs so that results from different groups can be compared easily (Stroncek et al., 2020).

Patient derived cultured MSCs however, in 2D but also 3D cultures, can serve as a platform for personalized screening approaches to detect alterations which hamper therapy or find potential targets. As an example, a genome-scale CRISPR knock-out screen was used to uncover imatinib-sensitizing genes *in vitro* on K562 cells (Lewis et al., 2020). Although this was performed on cell lines, one can imagine broadening the application and do similar tests in smaller format (due to the high cell number needed) on patient derived cells.

These methods could be used as proof-of-principle platforms to identify candidate proteins for genome editing. Recently, human mesenchymal stromal cells were shown to endure nucleofection with Cas9-adeno-associated virus serotype 6 (AAV-6) and genome-editing including gene disruption and targeted integration of up to 3.2 kb of DNA with stable transgene expression, while retaining their *in vitro* tri-lineage differentiation potential and phenotypical signature (Srifa et al., 2020). Through integration of PDGF-BB, VEGFA, and IL-10 transgenes at the *HBB* locus they successfully created hypersecreting hMSC which actively improved wound healing in diabetic wounds of mice. Specifically the combination of scaffolds coated with human MSCs could be modified with the Cas9-AAV-6 system to model normal and malignant human hematopoiesis by subcutaneous implantation in immunodeficient mice (Vaiselbuh et al., 2010; Abarrategi et al., 2017; Passaro et al., 2017). The benefit of such a system is that patient-derived leukemic cells can grow in the hMSC scaffolds as they form ectopic humanized BMM and can be followed up for long periods of time in an *in vivo* setting. Similarly, human femur-derived bone fragments from AML patients were transplanted into NSG mice using Matrigel as a carrier and were vascularized 4 weeks post implantation (Battula et al., 2017). These systems could allow for easily-accessible and controllable *in vivo* gene-editing of multiple relevant human BMM populations in the presence of clonal xenografted AML cells.

FUTURE OUTLOOK

As we gain knowledge of the different functional subcomponents of the bone marrow niche, the disease model of myeloid malignancies will become more complex. It is evident that oncogenesis can arise from two non-mutually exclusive theories: niche-induced and niche-facilitated. In patients, we envision a future of personalized medicine in which the stroma can be pharmacologically targeted in combination with a hematopoietic cell-based therapy. We can use the accumulating knowledge with genome editing by (1) generation of murine disease models *in vivo* on the basis of new possible germline/somatic mutations within the niche found with targeted sequencing in human disease to study disease pathogenesis, (2) targeting MSCs *in vivo* directly through MSC/EV-based approaches, (3) indirectly through modulation of hematopoietic cells, (4) modeling of the human hematopoietic niche using ossified scaffolds in xenotransplantations, and (5) *in vitro* Cas9-based screening methods. Targeted genome-editing will most likely become more feasible as we characterize the true MSCs as the target cell and improve engineering of carriers which will deliver the sgRNA:Cas9 cargo with high efficacy to the bone marrow.

AUTHOR CONTRIBUTIONS

All authors listed have made a substantial, direct and intellectual contribution to the work, and approved it for publication.

REFERENCES

Abarrategi, A., Foster, K., Hamilton, A., Mian, S. A., Passaro, D., Gribben, J., et al. (2017). Versatile humanized niche model enables study of normal and malignant human hematopoiesis. *J. Clin. Invest.* 127, 543–548. doi: 10.1172/JCI89364

Agha, E., El, Kramann, R., Schneider, R. K., Li, X., Seeger, W., and Humphreys, B. D. (2017). Mesenchymal stem cells in fibrotic disease. *Stem Cell* 21, 166–177. doi: 10.1016/j.stem.2017.07.011

Ahn, J., Park, G., and Shim, J. (2010). Intramarrow injection of β-catenin-activated, but not naïve mesenchymal stromal cells stimulates self-renewal of hematopoietic stem cells in bone marrow. *Exp. Mol. Med.* 42, 122–131. doi: 10.3858/emm.2010.42.2.014

Al-Sabah, J., Baccin, C., and Haas, S. (2020). Single-cell and spatial transcriptomics approaches of the bone marrow microenvironment. *Curr. Opin. Oncol.* 32, 146–153. doi: 10.1097/CCO.0000000000000602

Arranz, L., Sanchez-Aguilera, A., Martin-Perez, D., Isern, J., Langa, X., Tzankov, A., et al. (2014). Neuropathy of haematopoietic stem cell niche is essential for myeloproliferative neoplasms. *Nature* 512, 78–81. doi: 10.1038/nature1 3383

Baccin, C., Al-sabah, J., Velten, L., Helbling, P. M., Grünschläger, F., Hernández-Malmierca, P., et al. (2020). Combined single-cell and spatial transcriptomics reveal the molecular, cellular and spatial bone marrow niche organization. *Nat. Cell Biol.* 22, 38–48. doi: 10.1038/s41556-019-0439-6

Baryawno, N., Przybylski, D., Kowalczyk, M. S., Kfoury, Y., Severe, N., Gustafsson, K., et al. (2019). A cellular taxonomy of the bone marrow stroma in homeostasis and leukemia. *Cell* 177, 1915–1932.e16. doi: 10.1016/j.cell.2019.04.040

Battula, V. L., Le, P. M., Sun, J. C., Nguyen, K., Yuan, B., Zhou, X., et al. (2017). AML-induced osteogenic differentiation in mesenchymal stromal cells supports leukemia growth. *JCI Insight* 2:e90036. doi: 10.1172/jci.insight.90036

Behrmann, L., Wellbrock, J., and Fiedler, W. (2020). The bone marrow stromal niche: a therapeutic target of hematological myeloid malignancies. *Expert Opin. Ther. Targets* 24, 451–462. doi: 10.1080/14728222.2020.1744850

Berger, G., Berg, E., Van Den Abbott, K. M., Sinke, R. J., Bungener, L. B., Mulder, A. B., et al. (2016). Re-emergence of acute myeloid leukemia in donor cells following allogeneic transplantation in a family with a germline DDX41 mutation. *Leukemia* 31, 520–522. doi: 10.1038/leu.2016.310

Broeders, M., Herrero-hernandez, P., Ernst, M. P. T., and Van Der Ploeg, A. T. (2020). Sharpening the molecular scissors : advances in gene-editing technology. *iScience* 23:100789. doi: 10.1016/j.isci.2019.100789

Carter, B. Z., Mak, P. Y., Chen, Y., Mak, D. H., Mu, H., Ruvolo, V., et al. (2016). Anti-apoptotic ARC protein confers chemoresistance by controlling leukemia-microenvironment interactions through a NFκB/IL1β signaling network. *Oncotarget* 7:7911. doi: 10.18632/oncotarget.7911

Chen, K. G., Johnson, K. R., and Robey, P. G. (2017). Mouse genetic analysis of bone marrow stem cell niches: technological pitfalls, challenges, and translational considerations. *Stem Cell Rep.* 9, 1343–1358. doi: 10.1016/j.stemcr.2017.09.014

Chen, S., Zambetti, N. A., Bindels, E. M. J., Kenswil, K. J. G., Mylona, M. A., Adisty, N., et al. (2016). Massive parallel RNA sequencing of highly purified mesenchymal elements in low-risk MDS reveals tissue- context-dependent activation of inflammatory programs. *Leukemia* 30, 1938–1942. doi: 10.1038/leu.2016.91

Craver, B. M., Alaoui, K., El Scherber, R. M., and Fleischman, A. G. (2018). The critical role of inflammation in the pathogenesis and progression of myeloid malignancies. *Cancers* 10:104. doi: 10.3390/cancers10040104

Dale, D. C., Bolyard, A. A., Schwinzer, B. G., Pracht, G., Bonilla, M. A., Boxer, L., et al. (2006). The severe chronic neutropenia international registry : 10-year follow-up report. *Support. Cancer Ther.* 3, 220–231. doi: 10.3816/SCT.2006.n.020

Decker, M., Martinez-morentin, L., Wang, G., Lee, Y., Liu, Q., Leslie, J., et al. (2017). Leptin receptor-expressing bone marrow stromal cells are myofibroblasts in primary myelofibrosis. *Nat. Cell. Biol.* 19, 677–688. doi: 10.1038/ncb3530

Dever, D. P., and Porteus, M. H. (2017). The changing landscape of gene editing in hematopoietic stem cells: a step towards cas9 clinical translation daniel. *Curr. Opin. Hematol.* 24, 481–488. doi: 10.1097/MOH.0000000000000385

Dominici, M., Blanc, K., Le Mueller, I., Marini, F. C., Krause, D. S., Deans, R. J., et al. (2006). Minimal criteria for defining multipotent mesenchymal stromal cells. International society for cellular therapy position statement. *Cytotherapy* 8, 315–317. doi: 10.1080/14653240600855905

Dong, L., Yu, W., Zheng, H., Loh, M. L., Bunting, S. T., Pauly, M., et al. (2016). Leukaemogenic effects of Ptpn11 activating mutations in the stem cell microenvironment. *Nat. Publ. Gr.* 539, 304–308. doi: 10.1038/nature20131

Drexler, B., Passweg, J. R., Tzankov, A., Bigler, M., Theocharides, A. P. A., Cantoni, N., et al. (2019). The sympathomimetic agonist mirabegron did not lower JAK2-V617F allele burden, but restored nestin-positive cells and reduced reticulin fibrosis in patients with myeloproliferative neoplasms: results of phase II study SAKK 33/14. *Haematologica* 104, 710–716. doi: 10.3324/haematol.2018.200014

Efremova, M., Vento-tormo, M., and Teichmann, S. A. (2020). CellPhoneDB : inferring cell – cell communication from combined expression of multi-subunit ligand – receptor complexes. *Nat. Protoc.* 15, 1484–1506. doi: 10.1038/s41596-020-0292-x

Engel, N., Rovo, A., Badoglio, M., Labopin, M., Basak, G. W., Beguin, Y., et al. (2018). European experience and risk factor analysis of donor cell-derived leukaemias / MDS following haematopoietic cell transplantation. *Leukemia* 33, 508–517. doi: 10.1038/s41375-018-0218-6

Fathi, E., Sanaat, Z., and Farahzadi, R. (2019). Mesenchymal stem cells in acute myeloid leukemia: a focus on mechanisms involved and therapeutic concepts. *Blood Res.* 54, 165–174. doi: 10.5045/br.2019.54.3.165

Ferrara, F., and Schiff, C. A. (2013). Acute myeloid leukaemia in adults. *Lancet* 381, 484–495. doi: 10.1016/S0140-6736(12)61727-9

Ferrari, G., Thrasher, A. J., and Aiuti, A. (2020). Gene therapy using haematopoietic stem and progenitor cells. *Nat. Rev. Genet.* doi: 10.1038/s41576-020-00298-5. [Epub ahead of print].

Flores-Figueroa, E., Gutiérrez-Espindola, G., José Montesinos, J., Maria Arana-Trejo, R., and Mayani, H. (2002). *In vitro* characterization of hematopoietic microenvironment cells from patients with myelodysplastic syndrome. *Leuk. Res.* 26, 677–686. doi: 10.1016/S0145-2126(01)00193-X

Flores-Figueroa, E., Montesinos, J. J., Flores-guzm, P., Espindola, G. G., Arana-Trejo, R. M., Hernandez-Estevez, E., et al. (2008). Functional analysis of myelodysplastic syndromes-derived mesenchymal stem cells. *Leuk. Res.* 32, 1407–1416. doi: 10.1016/j.leukres.2008.02.013

Forte, D., Fernandez, M. G., Sanchez-Aguilera, A., Stavropoulou, V., Fielding, C., Martin-Perez, D., et al. (2020). Bone marrow mesenchymal stem cells support acute myeloid leukemia bioenergetics and enhance antioxidant defense and escape from chemotherapy. *Cell Metab.* 32, 829–843.e9. doi: 10.1016/j.cmet.2020.09.001

Ghazanfari, R., Li, H., Zacharaki, D., Lim, H. C., and Scheding, S. (2016). Human non-hematopoietic CD271pos/CD140alow/neg bone marrow stroma cells fulfill stringent stem cell criteria in serial transplantations. *Stem Cells Dev.* 25, 1652–1658. doi: 10.1089/scd.2016.0169

Ghazanfari, R., Zacharaki, D., Li, H., Lim, H. C., Soneji, S., and Scheding, S. (2017). Human primary bone marrow mesenchymal stromal cells and their *in vitro* progenies display distinct transcriptional profile signatures. *Sci. Rep.* 7:10338. doi: 10.1038/s41598-017-09449-x

Gleitz, H., Dugourd, A. J. F., Leimkühler, N. B., Snoeren, I. A. M., Fuchs, S. N. R., Menzel, S., et al. (2020). Increased CXCL4 expression in hematopoietic cells links inflammation and progression of bone marrow fibrosis in MPN. *Blood* 136, 2051–2064. doi: 10.1182/blood.2019004095

Gleitz, H. F. E., Kramann, R., and Schneider, R. K. (2018). Understanding deregulated cellular and molecular dynamics in the haematopoietic stem cell niche to develop novel therapeutics for bone marrow fibrosis. *J. Pathol.* 245, 138–146. doi: 10.1002/path.5078

Golchin, A., Shams, F., and Karami, F. (2020). Advancing mesenchymal stem cell therapy with CRISPR/Cas9 for clinical trial studies. *Adv. Exp. Med. Biol.* 1247, 89–100. doi: 10.1007/5584_2019_459

Gomariz, A., Helbling, P. M., Isringhausen, S., Suessbier, U., Becker, A., Boss, A., et al. (2018). Quantitative spatial analysis of haematopoiesis-regulating stromal cells in the bone marrow microenvironment by 3D microscopy. *Nat. Commun.* 9:2532. doi: 10.1038/s41467-018-04770-z

González-Romero, E., Martínez-Valiente, C., García-Ruiz, C., Vázquez-Manrique, R. P., Cervera, J., and Sanjuan-Pla, A. (2019). CRISPR to fix bad blood : a new tool in basic and clinical hematology. *Haematologica* 104, 881–893. doi: 10.3324/haematol.2018.211359

Greenbaum, A., Hsu, Y.-M. S., Day, R. B., Schuettpelz, L. G., Christopher, M. J., Borgerding, J. N., et al. (2013). CXCL12 production by early mesenchymal progenitors is required. *Nature* 495, 227–230. doi: 10.1038/nature11926

Hanoun, M., Zhang, D., Mizoguchi, T., Pinho, S., Pierce, H., Kunisaki, Y., et al. (2014). Acute myelogenous leukemia-inducedsympathetic neuropathy promotes malignancyin an altered hematopoietic stem cell niche. *Cell Stem Cell* 15, 365–375. doi: 10.1016/j.stem.2014. 06.020

Heckl, D., Kowalczyk, M. S., Yudovich, D., Belizaire, R., Puram, R. V., Mcconkey, M. E., et al. (2014). Generation of mouse models of myeloid malignancy with combinatorial genetic lesions using CRISPR-Cas9 genome editing. *Nat. Biotechnol.* 32, 941–946. doi: 10.1038/nbt.2951

Jacamo, R., Chen, Y., Wang, Z., Wencai, M., Zhang, M., Spaeth, E. L., et al. (2014). Reciprocal leukemia-stroma VCAM-1/VLA-4-dependent activation of NF-κB mediates chemoresistance. *Blood* 123, 2691–2702. doi: 10.1182/blood-2013-06-511527

Kean, T. J., Lin, P., Caplan, A. I., and Dennis, J. E. (2013). MSCs : delivery routes and engraftment, cell-targeting strategies, and immune modulation. *Stem Cells Int.* 2013:732742. doi: 10.1155/2013/732742

Kfoury, Y., and Scadden, D. T. (2015). Mesenchymal cell contributions to the stem cell niche. *Stem Cell* 16, 239–253. doi: 10.1016/j.stem.2015.02.019

Kim, B., Yun, W., Lee, S. T., Choi, J. R., Yoo, K. H., Koo, H. H., et al. (2020). Prevalence and clinical implications of germline predisposition gene mutations in patients with acute myeloid leukemia. *Sci. Rep.* 10:14297. doi: 10.1038/s41598-020-71386-z

Kim, Y. W., Koo, B. K., Jeong, H. W., Yoon, M. J., Song, R., Shin, J., et al. (2008). Defective notch activation in microenvironment leads to myeloproliferative disease. *Blood* 112, 4628–4638. doi: 10.1182/blood-2008-03-148999

Kokkaliaris, K. D., Kunz, L., Cabezas-Wallscheid, N., Christodoulou, C., Renders, S., Camargo, F., et al. (2020). Adult blood stem cell localization reflects the abundance of reported bone marrow niche cell types and their combinations. *Blood* 136, 2296–2307. doi: 10.1182/blood.2020006574

Kokkaliaris, K. D., and Scadden, D. T. (2020). Cell interactions in the bone marrow microenvironment affecting myeloid malignancies. *Blood Adv.* 4, 3795–3803. doi: 10.1182/bloodadvances.2020002127

Kostyushev, D., Kostyusheva, A., Brezgin, S., Smirnov, V., Volchkova, E., Lukashev, A., et al. (2020). Gene editing by extracellular vesicles. *Int. J. Mol. Sci.* 21, 1–34. doi: 10.3390/ijms21197362

Krohn-Grimberghe, M., Mitchell, M. J., Schloss, M. J., Khan, O. F., Courties, G., Guimaraes, P. P. G., et al. (2020). Nanoparticle-encapsulated siRNAs for gene silencing in the haematopoietic stem-cell niche. *Nat. Biomed. Eng.* 4, 1076–1089. doi: 10.1038/s41551-020-00623-7

Lee, J., Bayarsaikhan, D., Bayarsaikhan, G., Kim, J., Schwarzbach, E., and Lee, B. (2020). Pharmacology & therapeutics recent advances in genome editing of stem cells for drug discovery and therapeutic application. *Pharmacol. Ther.* 209:107501. doi: 10.1016/j.pharmthera.2020.107501

Leimkuhler, N. B., Gleitz, H., Ronghui, L., Snoeren, I. A. M., Fuchs, S. N. R., Nagai, J. S., et al. (2020). Heterogeneous bone-marrow stromal progenitors drive myelofibrosis via a druggable alarmin axis. *Cell Stem Cell* 28, 1–16. doi: 10.1016/j.stem.2020.11.004

Leimkühler, N. B., and Schneider, R. K. (2019). Inflammatory bone marrow microenvironment. *Hematol. Am. Soc. Hematol. Educ. Program* 2019, 294–302. doi: 10.1182/hematology.2019000045

Lewis, M., Florence, V. P., Iggo, R., Turcq, B., Richard, E., Iggo, R., et al. (2020). A genome-scale CRISPR knock-out screen in chronic myeloid leukemia identifies novel drug resistance mechanisms along with intrinsic apoptosis and MAPK signaling. *Cancer Med.* 9, 6739–6751. doi: 10.1002/cam4.3231

Marofi, F., Vahedi, G., Biglari, A., Esmaeilzadeh, A., and Athari, S. S. (2017). Mesenchymal stromal / stem cells : a new era in the cell-based targeted gene therapy of cancer. *Front. Immunol.* 8:1770. doi: 10.3389/fimmu.2017.01770

Matsunaga, T., Takemoto, N., Sato, T., Takimoto, R., Tanaka, I., Fujimi, A., et al. (2003). Interaction between leukemic-cell VLA-4 and stromal fibronectin is a decisive factor for minimal residual disease of acute myelogenous leukemia. *Nat. Med.* 9, 1158–1165. doi: 10.1038/nm909

Medyouf, H. (2017). The microenvironment in human myeloid malignancies: emerging concepts and therapeutic implications. *Blood* 129, 1617–1626. doi: 10.1182/blood-2016-11-696070

Méndez-Ferrer, S., Bonnet, D., Steensma, D. P., Hasserjian, R. P., Ghobrial, I. M., Gribben, J. G., et al. (2020). Bone marrow niches in haematological malignancies. *Nat. Rev. Cancer* 20, 285–298. doi: 10.1038/s41568-020-0245-2

Mendez-Ferrer, S., Michurina, T. V., Ferraro, F., Mazloom, A. R., Macarthur, B. D., Lira, S. A., et al. (2010). Mesenchymal and haematopoietic stem cells form a unique bone marrow niche. *Nature* 466, 829–834. doi: 10.1038/nature09262

Miller, L. H., Qu, C. K., and Pauly, M. (2018). Germline mutations in the bone marrow microenvironment and dysregulated hematopoiesis. *Exp. Hematol.* 66, 17–26. doi: 10.1016/j.exphem.2018.07.001

Morrison, S. J., and Scadden, D. T. (2014). The bone marrow niche for haematopoietic stem cells. *Nature* 505, 327–334. doi: 10.1038/nature12984

Mou, H., Kennedy, Z., Anderson, D. G., Yin, H., and Xue, W. (2015). Precision cancer mouse models through genome editing with CRISPR-Cas9. *Genome Med.* 7:53. doi: 10.1186/s13073-015-0178-7

Muguruma, Y., Yahata, T., Miyatake, H., Sato, T., Uno, T., Itoh, J., et al. (2006). Reconstitution of the functional human hematopoietic microenvironment derived from human mesenchymal stem cells in the murine bone marrow compartment. *Blood* 107, 1878–1887. doi: 10.1182/blood-2005-06-2211

Nelson, A. S., and Myers, K. C. (2018). Diagnosis, treatment, and molecular pathology of shwachman-diamond syndrome. *Hematol. Oncol. Clin. North Am.* 32, 687–700. doi: 10.1016/j.hoc.2018.04.006

Nervi, B., Ramirez, P., Rettig, M. P., Uy, G. L., Holt, M. S., Ritchey, J. K., et al. (2009). Chemosensitization of acute myeloid leukemia (AML) following mobilization by the CXCR4 antagonist AMD3100. *Blood* 113, 6206–6214. doi: 10.1182/blood-2008-06-162123

Nie, Y., Han, Y. C., and Zou, Y. R. (2008). CXCR4 is required for the quiescence of primitive hematopoietic cells. *J. Exp. Med.* 205, 777–783. doi: 10.1084/jem.20072513

Ortinau, L. C., Wang, H., Lei, K., Deveza, L., Jeong, Y., Hara, Y., et al. (2019). Identification of functionally distinct Mx1+αSMA+ periosteal skeletal stem cells. *Cell Stem Cell* 25, 784–796.e5. doi: 10.1016/j.stem.2019.11.003

Park, D., Spencer, J. A., Koh, B. I., Kobayashi, T., Fujisaki, J., Clemens, T. L., et al. (2012). Endogenous bone marrow MSCs are dynamic, fate-restricted participants in bone maintenance and regeneration. *Cell Stem Cell* 10, 259–272. doi: 10.1016/j.stem.2012.02.003

Passaro, D., Abarrategi, A., Foster, K., Ariza-McNaughton, L., and Bonnet, D. (2017). Bioengineering of humanized bone marrow microenvironments in mouse and their visualization by live imaging. *J. Vis. Exp.* 2017:55914. doi: 10.3791/55914

Pevsner-Fischer, M., Levin, S., and Zipori, D. (2011). The origins of mesenchymal stromal cell heterogeneity. *Stem Cell Rev. Rep.* 7, 560–568. doi: 10.1007/s12015-011-9229-7

Pievani, A., Biondi, M., Tomasoni, C., Biondi, A., and Serafini, M. (2020a). Location first: targeting acute myeloid leukemia within its niche. *J. Clin. Med.* 9:1513. doi: 10.3390/jcm9051513

Pievani, A., Donsante, S., Tomasoni, C., Corsi, A., Dazzi, F., Biondi, A., et al. (2020b). Acute myeloid leukemia shapes the bone marrow stromal niche *in vivo*. *Haematologica* 2020:247205. doi: 10.3324/haematol.2020.247205

Pinho, S., and Frenette, P. S. (2019). Haematopoietic stem cell activity and interactions with the niche. *Nat. Rev. Mol. Cell Biol.* 20, 303–320. doi: 10.1038/s41580-019-0103-9

Porter, C. C. (2016). Germ line mutations associated with leukemias. *Hematol. Am. Soc. Hematol. Educ. Program* 2016, 302–308. doi: 10.1182/asheducation-2016.1.302

Pronk, E., and Raaijmakers, M. H. G. P. (2019). The mesenchymal niche in MDS. *Blood* 133, 1031–1038. doi: 10.1182/blood-2018-10-844639

Raaijmakers, M. H. G. P., Mukherjee, S., Guo, S., Zhang, S., Kobayashi, T., Schoonmaker, J. A., et al. (2010). Bone progenitor dysfunction induces myelodysplasia and secondary leukaemia. *Nature* 464, 852–857. doi: 10.1038/nature08851

Ramakrishnan, R., Peña-Martínez, P., Agarwal, P., Rodriguez-Zabala, M., Chapellier, M., Högberg, C., et al. (2020). CXCR4 signaling has a CXCL12-independent essential role in murine MLL-AF9-driven acute myeloid leukemia. *Cell Rep.* 31:107684. doi: 10.1016/j.celrep.2020.107684

Rawls, A. S., Gregory, A. D., Woloszynek, J. R., Liu, F., and Link, D. C. (2007). Lentiviral-mediated RNAi inhibition of Sbds in murine hematopoietic progenitors impairs their hematopoietic potential. *Blood* 110, 2414–2422. doi: 10.1182/blood-2006-03-007112

Ribezzo, F., Snoeren, I. A. M., Ziegler, S., Stoelben, J., Olofsen, P. A., Henic, A., et al. (2018). Rps14, Csnk1a1 and miRNA145/miRNA146a deficiency cooperate in the clinical phenotype and activation of the innate immune system in the 5q-syndrome. *Leukemia* 33, 1759–1772. doi: 10.1038/s41375-018-0350-3

Romito, M., Rai, R., Thrasher, A. J., and Cavazza, A. (2019). Genome editing for blood disorders : state of the art and recent advances. *Emerg. Top. Life Sci.* 3, 289–299. doi: 10.1042/ETLS20180147

Rupec, R. A., Jundt, F., Rebholz, B., Eckelt, B., Weindl, G., Herzinger, T., et al. (2005). Stroma-mediated dysregulation of myelopoiesis in mice lacking IκBα. *Immunity* 22, 479–491. doi: 10.1016/j.immuni.2005.02.009

Sasaki, H., Iyer, S. V., Sasaki, K., Tawfik, O. W., Iwakuma, T., City, K., et al. (2016). An improved intrafemoral injection with minimized leakage as an orthotopic mouse model of osteosarcoma. *Anal. Biochem.* 486, 70–74. doi: 10.1016/j.ab.2015.06.030

Schepers, K., Pietras, E. M., Reynaud, D., Flach, J., Binnewies, M., Garg, T., et al. (2013). Myeloproliferative neoplasia remodels the endosteal bone marrow niche into a self-reinforcing leukemic niche. *Cell Stem Cell* 13, 285–299. doi: 10.1016/j.stem.2013.06.009

Schneider, R. K., Mullally, A., Dugourd, A., Peisker, F., Hoogenboezem, R., Van Strien, P. M. H., et al. (2017). Gli1+ mesenchymal stromal cells are a key driver of bone marrow fibrosis and an important cellular therapeutic target. *Cell Stem Cell* 20, 785–800.e8. doi: 10.1016/j.stem.2017.03.008

Schneider, R. K., Schenone, M., Ferreira, M. V., Kramann, R., Joyce, C. E., Hartigan, C., et al. (2016). Rps14 haploinsufficiency causes a block in erythroid differentiation mediated by S100A8 and S100A9. *Nat. Med.* 22, 288–297. doi: 10.1038/nm.4047

Schroeder, T., Geyh, S., Germing, U., and Haas, R. (2016). Mesenchymal stromal cells in myeloid malignancies. *Blood Res.* 51, 225–232. doi: 10.5045/br.2016.51.4.225

Shapiro, J., Iancu, O., Jacobi, A. M., McNeill, M. S., Turk, R., Rettig, G. R., et al. (2020). Increasing CRISPR efficiency and measuring its specificity in HSPCs using a clinically relevant system. *Mol. Ther. Methods Clin. Dev.* 17, 1097–1107. doi: 10.1016/j.omtm.2020.04.027

Srifa, W., Kosaric, N., Amorin, A., Jadi, O., Camarena, J., Gurtner, G. C., et al. (2020). Cas9-AAV6-engineered human mesenchymal stromal cells improved cutaneous wound healing in diabetic mice. *Nat. Commun.* 11:2470. doi: 10.1038/s41467-020-16065-3

Stroncek, D. F., Jin, P., McKenna, D. H., Takanashi, M., Fontaine, M. J., Pati, S., et al. (2020). Human mesenchymal stromal cell (MSC) characteristics vary among laboratories when manufactured from the same source material : a report by the cellular therapy team of the biomedical excellence for safer transfusion (BEST) collaborative. *Front. Cell Dev. Biol.* 8:458. doi: 10.3389/fcell.2020.00458

Tikhonova, A. N., Dolgalev, I., Hu, H., Sivaraj, K. K., Hoxha, E., Cuesta-domínguez, Á., et al. (2019). The bone marrow microenvironment at single-cell resolution. *Nature* 569, 222–228. doi: 10.1038/s41586-019-1104-8

Tormin, A., Brune, J. C., Olsson, E., Valcich, J., Neuman, U., Olofsson, T., et al. (2009). Characterization of bone marrow-derived mesenchymal stromal cells (MSC) based on gene expression profiling of functionally defined MSC subsets. *Cytotherapy* 11, 114–128. doi: 10.1080/14653240802716590

Tothova, Z., Krill-burger, J. M., Popova, K. D., Landers, C. C., Sievers, Q. L., Yudovich, D., et al. (2017). Multiplex CRISPR-Cas9 based genome editing in human hematopoietic stem cells models clonal hematopoiesis and myeloid neoplasia. *Cell Stem Cell* 21, 547–555. doi: 10.1016/j.stem.2017.07.015

Vaiselbuh, S. R., Edelman, M., Lipton, J. M., and Liu, J. M. (2010). Ectopic human mesenchymal stem cell-coated scaffolds in NOD/SCID mice: an *in vivo* model of the leukemia niche. *Tissue Eng. C Methods* 16, 1523–1531. doi: 10.1089/ten.tec.2010.0179

Walkley, C. R., Shea, J. M., Sims, N. A., Purton, L. E., and Orkin, S. H. (2007). Rb regulates interactions between hematopoietic stem cells and their bone marrow microenvironment. *Cell* 129, 1081–1095. doi: 10.1016/j.cell.2007.03.055

Wolock, S. L., Krishnan, I., Tenen, D. E., Tenen, D. G., Klein, A. M., Welner, R. S., et al. (2019). Mapping distinct bone marrow niche populations and their differentiation paths. *Cell Reports* 28, 302–311.e5. doi: 10.1016/j.celrep.2019.06.031

Xiao, P., Dolinska, M., Sandhow, L., Kondo, M., Johansson, A. S., Bouderlique, T., et al. (2018). Sipa1 deficiency-induced bone marrow niche alterations lead to the initiation of myeloproliferative neoplasm. *Blood Adv.* 2, 534–548. doi: 10.1182/bloodadvances.2017013599

Ye, Y., Zhang, X., Xie, F., Xu, B., Xie, P., Yang, T., et al. (2020). An engineered exosome for delivering sgRNA:Cas9 ribonucleoprotein complex and genome editing in recipient cells. *Biomater. Sci.* 8, 2966–2976. doi: 10.1039/D0BM00427H

Zambetti, N. A., Bindels, E. M. J., Strien, P. M. H., Van Valkhof, M. G., Adisty, M. N., Remco, M., et al. (2015). Deficiency of the ribosome biogenesis gene Sbds in hematopoietic stem and progenitor cells causes neutropenia in mice by attenuating lineage progression in myelocytes. *Haematologica* 100, 1285–1293. doi: 10.3324/haematol.2015.131573

Zambetti, N. A., Ping, Z., Chen, S., Loosdrecht, A. A., Van De Vogl, T., Raaijmakers, M. H. G. P., et al. (2016). Mesenchymal inflammation drives genotoxic stress in hematopoietic stem cells and predicts disease evolution in human pre-leukemia. *Stem Cell* 19, 613–627. doi: 10.1016/j.stem.2016.08.021

Zhou, B. O., Yue, R., Murphy, M. M., Peyer, J. G., and Morrison, S. J. (2014). Leptin-receptor-expressing mesenchymal stromal cells represent the main source of bone formed by adult bone marrow. *Cell Stem Cell* 15, 154–168. doi: 10.1016/j.stem.2014.06.008

3

Gene Editing and Genotoxicity: Targeting the Off-Targets

Georges Blattner, Alessia Cavazza, Adrian J. Thrasher and Giandomenico Turchiano *

Infection, Immunity and Inflammation Research and Teaching Department, Zayed Centre for Research into Rare Disease in Children, Great Ormond Street Institute of Child Health, University College London, London, United Kingdom

Correspondence:
Giandomenico Turchiano
g.turchiano@ucl.ac.uk

Gene editing technologies show great promise for application to human disease as a result of rapid developments in targeting tools notably based on ZFN, TALEN, and CRISPR-Cas systems. Precise modification of a DNA sequence is now possible in mature human somatic cells including stem and progenitor cells with increasing degrees of efficiency. At the same time new technologies are required to evaluate their safety and genotoxicity before widespread clinical application can be confidently implemented. A number of methodologies have now been developed in an attempt to predict expected and unexpected modifications occurring during gene editing. This review surveys the techniques currently available as state of the art, highlighting benefits and limitations, and discusses approaches that may achieve sufficient accuracy and predictability for application in clinical settings.

Keywords: gene editing, CRISPR, genotoxicity, off-target, DSB = double-strand break, DNA damage, translocation, chromosomal aberration

INTRODUCTION

Therapeutic approaches relying on the genetic engineering of cells for the treatment of hereditary diseases has long been a promising strategy to overcome the shortcomings of conventional drug therapies. The principle of these gene therapies is to counteract, correct, or replace a malfunctioning gene within cells that are most severely affected by the caused condition. However, any process affecting DNA integrity or causing DNA or chromosomal damage bears the risk of genotoxicity (Bohne and Cathomen, 2008).

While viral vectors utilized for gene addition-based strategies showed encouraging initial results (Anderson, 1990; Rosenberg et al., 1990; Gaspar et al., 2004), subsequent trials targeting hematopoietic stem and progenitor cells (HSPCs) exposed the risk of therapy-related toxicities, particularly insertional activation of proto-oncogenes leading to malignant cell transformation. Indeed, the activation of MDS1-EVI1 and LMO2 oncogenes caused by the integration of the gamma retroviral vector led to clonal skewing and development of malignancies in patients enrolled in several gene therapy clinical trials. (Hacein-Bey-Abina et al., 2003; Raper et al., 2003; Ott et al., 2006; Cattoglio et al., 2007; Schwarzwaelder et al., 2007; Howe et al., 2008; Metais and Dunbar, 2008; Stein et al., 2010; Zhou et al., 2016). These issues have been partly addressed through development of next generation vectors including in particular lentiviruses (Naldini et al., 1996; Aiuti et al., 2013; Hacein-Bey-Abina et al., 2014; Kohn et al., 2020) and adeno-associated virus (AAV) (Nathwani et al., 2011) lowering, but not eliminating, the risk of insertional mutagenesis and immunogenicity.

Besides the risk of insertional mutagenesis and immunogenicity (Cavazzana-Calvo et al., 2010), viral vectors have additional drawbacks, including their inability to address dominant mutations and their potential influence on the host cell's gene expression (Maeder and Gersbach, 2016).

Further attempts to address these issues have been made, for example by using chimeric proteins to retarget lentiviral integration to sites with reduced transcriptional activity (Gijsbers et al., 2010; Vranckx et al., 2016).

Many of these limitations can however be overcome by gene therapy approaches that rely on genome editing techniques which enable more precise, targeted genomic modifications to restore wild-type sequences, while preserving the temporal and tissue-specific control of the afflicted gene, or to specifically knock out genes.

Initially the four main families of nucleases–meganucleases (Chevalier et al., 2001; Epinat et al., 2003), zinc finger nucleases (ZFNs) (Urnov et al., 2005), transcription activator-like effector nucleases (TALENs) (Bogdanove and Voytas, 2011), and Clustered Regularly Interspaced Short Palindromic Repeats (CRISPR)-associated nucleases (Cas) (Jinek et al., 2012) were used to induce targeted DNA double-strand breaks (DSBs). Meganucleases, ZFNs, and TALENS are tethered toward specific DNA sequences by means of DNA-binding protein domains while the CRISPR-Cas system is based on a nuclease protein guided by an RNA molecule complementary to the targeted DNA sequence (gRNA) via Watson-Crick base pairing. The introduction of DSBs activates one of the two main endogenous cellular repair pathways, including the error prone non-homologous end joining (NHEJ) and the homology directed repair (HDR) pathways. Some repurposed derivatives of the engineered nucleases, in particular of Cas, have been developed to fulfill different tasks. Nickases, which are Cas9 proteins with only one functional nuclease domain (Sapranauskas et al., 2011; Jinek et al., 2012), are used to induce DNA single-stranded breaks (SSBs), combined with base editors (BEs) fused to a cytidine or an adenine deaminase to induce precise transition mutations (Komor et al., 2016, 2017; Gaudelli et al., 2017; Kurt et al., 2020). In addition, the prime editing strategy uses a nickase fused with a reverse transcriptase complexed with a prime editing guide RNA (pegRNA) to mediate targeted insertions of few bases, deletions, and base conversions (Anzalone et al., 2019).

Similar to viral vectors, genome editing techniques have been rapidly adopted and they have proven suitable for clinical application in various fields. So far, seven patients have been infused with CRISPR-Cas9 modified autologous CD34+ HSPCs for the treatment of beta-hemoglobinopaties, showing encouraging results; among those, two patients affected by beta thalassemia are transfusion independent after 5 and 15 months after infusion while one patient affected by sickle cell disease is free of vaso-occlusive crises at 9 months after treatment (NCT03655678; NCT03745287). CRISPR-Cas9 or TALENs have also been applied to engineer patient or Universal Chimeric Antigen Receptor (CAR)T lymphocytes for improved antitumor immunity (Qasim et al., 2017; Stadtmauer et al., 2020) (NCT02735083; NCT02808442; NCT02746952; NCT03081715; NCT02793856; NCT04244656; NCT04035434). Moreover, TALENs have been used to create allogenic CS1, CD123, or CD22-specific CAR-T cells (NCT04142619; NCT03190278; NCT04150497) and ZFNs helped to engineer T cells with a C-C motif chemokine receptor 5 knockout to induce resistance to HIV infection (Tebas et al., 2014) (NCT03617198). In addition,

AAV vectors together with ZFN-mediated genome editing were applied for the insertion of a correct copy of the α-L-iduronidase gene for subjects with attenuated Mucopolysaccharidosis type I (MPS I) (NCT02702115).

While genome editing techniques address certain limitations and reduce particular risks of genotoxicity in viral vector-based gene therapy, they entail new complications. Off-target activity, the induction of DNA modifications at unintended sites, is a concern with all designer nucleases (Fu et al., 2013; Koo et al., 2015). Such off-target activity can potentially lead to point mutations, deletions, insertions or inversions. Besides off-targeting due to a sequence similarity to the targeted site, there can also be collateral cleavage activity. This has been observed for CRISPR-Cas12a, which, upon RNA-guided on-target DNA binding, non-specifically cleaves single-stranded DNA molecules (Chen et al., 2018). While high fidelity variants of the Cas9 protein have successfully been developed to reduce off-target activity (Kleinstiver et al., 2016; Vakulskas et al., 2018) they still bear the risk of inducing on-target damage after cleavage in the form of large deletions spanning several kilobases or translocations (Kosicki et al., 2018; Connelly and Pruett-Miller, 2019; Turchiano et al., 2020). As those large deletions can bring relatively distant elements close together, they could have a genotoxic potential similar to the insertional mutagenesis caused by viral vectors. A key prerequisite for the clinical application of genome editing tools is the monitoring of their safety before, during and after the administration of the treatment. However, while gene therapy and genome editing are advancing at a rapid pace, the application of appropriate assays to evaluate unintended genomic effects suffers from a lack of standardized methods and guidelines (Corrigan-Curay et al., 2015). A multitude of techniques have been developed in the recent years to detect small insertions and deletions (Indels), potential off-target DNA breaks, translocations, or viral integration sites but the lack of standardized analyses that allow an absolute quantification of those modifications makes a direct comparison among these tools cumbersome. The aim of this review is to give an overview of the drawbacks and benefits of the currently available tools to assess the safety of gene editing applications and of the parameters that need to be taken into account for a correct safety assessment of a gene therapy approach.

BIASED DETECTION METHODS

A major step for the successful use of designer nucleases is the choice of the target site and the according nuclease or gRNA design following criteria of editing efficiency and specificity. Potential off-targets can be predicted in-silico (Grau et al., 2013; Bae et al., 2014; Cradick et al., 2014; Montague et al., 2014; Concordet and Haeussler, 2018) or identified on cultured cells (in cellula) or in vitro assays for DSB detection. The list of potential off-target sites identified must be subsequently verified in the target cell type/tissue alongside the detection of on-target cleavage. There are three common types of approach to quantify indels formation at the selected sites, all of which rely on polymerase chain reactions (PCR) performed on genomic DNA treated with the designer nuclease of choice. After denaturation and rehybridization of the PCR products, hetero-duplex DNA containing a mutated and a wild-type strand can form, which can then be cleaved by mismatch-detection nucleases such as Surveyor nuclease or T7 endonuclease I (Mashal et al., 1995; Qiu et al., 2004), enabling the quantification of the cleavage products by electrophoresis. While cost-effective and simple, a drawback of those techniques is that single nucleotide polymorphisms are poorly recognized. Quantification of Indels in the PCR products can also be determined by methods such as Tracking of Indels by Decomposition (TIDE) or Inference of CRISPR Edits (ICE) analyses, which compare the Sanger sequence chromatograms of an untreated control against a treated sample at the intended editing site (Brinkman et al., 2014; Hsiau et al., 2019). Moreover, Indels can also be directly quantified using deep sequencing of the PCR products (Pinello et al., 2016). As all of these approaches are based on PCR amplicons of around 200–700 base pairs (bp) from the potential target loci, they all suffer from the same shortcoming, that is the missed detection of larger deletions or other aberrations that could encompass at least one of the PCR primer binding sites. While it is commonly accepted that most of the indels fall in a size spectrum of under 50 bp (Koike-Yusa et al., 2014; van Overbeek et al., 2016), it has been shown that genome editing can also lead to large deletions of several kilobases (kb) (Kosicki et al., 2018; Chakrabarti et al., 2019; Turchiano et al., 2020). Moreover, even in the case of deletions being amplified/detected by PCR, a minimal sequence length of sufficient quality, required for the alignment with either a control sequence or a reference genome, might not be reached.

Indel assessment by deep sequencing requires additional consideration. Artifactual sequencing errors produce a background signal that is usually filtered out by setting an arbitrary threshold to define the relevant modified loci. This kind of analysis can produce either false-positives or false-negatives since every amplicon can present higher or lower background levels, respectively. Statistically more robust approaches are needed, but they can be laborious particularly when a multitude of targets are investigated. Performing the analysis on a large set of replicates and untreated controls in order to compare the mean editing frequencies using a t-test would be the preferable procedure (Zeng et al., 2020). Alternatively a two-sample test for equality of proportions or a Fisher's exact test can be performed to detect differences between the mutation rates of edited and untreated samples. In order for this approach to be robust, a high number of reads is desirable. Moreover, when different assays are employed, these statistical tests can account for the variability of the NGS measurements to better define the null hypothesis or introduce a false discovery rate correction (e.g., Benjamini–Hochberg; Kuscu et al., 2014; Turchiano et al., 2020). This would be a more traceable practice compared to indel values subtractions between the treated and the relative untreated samples (Cameron et al., 2017) or to simply assuming a background noise level (Yang et al., 2014; Kim et al., 2016; Kim and Kim, 2018). This approach allows compensation for sequencing errors, especially for challenging regions with repetitive elements, which might produce a considerable amount of indel-like reads and that might even require a visual inspection

to evaluate potential sequencing or alignment artifacts (Zeng et al., 2020).

Alternatively, oligo integration analysis rather than indel detection allows dramatic reduction in background noise in the untreated control of about 100 fold, enabling off-target detection at <0.001% rates (Tsai et al., 2017). It is worth noting that the reliability of this method is dependent on the oligo integration efficiency in the cell type of interest, generally higher in cell lines as compared to primary cells; moreover this technique cannot be applied to samples that are meant to be infused into patients, since this would imply integrations of non-therapeutically relevant exogenous sequences into the genome.

UNBIASED DETECTION METHODS

DSB Detection

While *in silico* off-target prediction is a fast and cheap option, it suffers from high false-positive rates as it is mostly based on the similarity of a sequence to the target site and does not consider differences due to genetic variants; moreover, it has a limited sensitivity in the detection of bona fide off-targets (Tsai et al., 2015; Kim et al., 2019b). This bias can be overcome with the use of *in vitro* methods that are based upon the incubation of purified genomic DNA with the designer nuclease of choice. The DSBs induced by the nuclease are then detected in various ways, either by the circularization of the created DNA fragments in CIRCLE-seq (circularization for *in vitro* reporting of cleavage effects by sequencing) or CHANGE-seq (circularization for high-throughput analysis of nuclease genome-wide effects by sequencing) (Tsai et al., 2017; Lazzarotto et al., 2020), the ligation of adapters in SITE-seq (selective enrichment and identification of adapter-tagged DNA ends by sequencing) (Cameron et al., 2017) or End-seq (DNA end sequencing) (Canela et al., 2016), or deep sequencing and identification of identical 5' DNA fragments in Digenome-seq (*in vitro* Cas9-digested whole-genome sequencing) (Kim et al., 2015). While being sensitive, a common drawback of these approaches is a tendency to overestimate the number of sites that are actually modified in cells (Cho et al., 2014), as the influence of the chromatin structure in determining the DNA accessibility is widely disregarded (Kim and Kim, 2018). Moreover, the impact of the nuclease concentration inside the cell (Wu et al., 2014) and of the delivery method on the cleavage footprint are not considered by *in vitro* assays (Kim et al., 2014; Cameron et al., 2017). Those *in vitro* techniques are usually returning the highest number of sites, but their relative validation rates disregard at least half of them in the best case scenario. The *in cellula* derived deep sequencing validation deserves some additional considerations: (1) it is usually performed only on the top performing sites disregarding the ones close to the cutoff thresholds; (2) it cannot be sensitive enough to detect rare indel events; (3) some DSBs can be perfectly repaired without creating any mutation and therefore could be missed during the validation process.

A more representative assessment can hence be expected from methods where designer nucleases are applied directly in cellula. In GUIDE-seq (genome-wide, unbiased identification of DSBs

Enabled by sequencing; Tsai et al., 2015), IDLV (integrative-deficient lentiviral vectors) capture (Gabriel et al., 2011) and ITR-seq (Inverted Terminal Repeat sequencing; Breton et al., 2020) the DSBs are marked by insertion of exogenous sequences, which are subsequently exploited as specific primer binding sites and then amplified via linker mediated PCR. Instead techniques like BLESS (direct *in situ* breaks labeling, enrichment on streptavidin and next-generation sequencing; Crosetto et al., 2013; Ran et al., 2015), its variant DSB Capture (Lensing et al., 2016) or BLISS (Breaks Labeling *in situ* and Sequencing; Yan et al., 2017, 2019) are based on *in situ* processing of the DNA at the open DSB ends and ligation of biotinylated adapters or adaptors for *in vitro* transcription. For DSB-seq high molecular weight genomic DNA is isolated from treated cells and the DNA ends are 3'-end tailed with biotinylated nucleotides by terminal deoxynucleotidyl transferase (TdT) before sonication, capturing, and sequencing (Baranello et al., 2014). An alternative approach based on Chromatin immunoprecipitation sequencing (ChIP-seq) targets the phosphorylated histone variant H2A.X or other repair factors that are recruited to cleaved sites (Iacovoni et al., 2010). However, as those factors can spread several kb around DSBs, an identification of the cleavage sites at nucleotide resolution is difficult. In DISCOVER-seq (discovery of *in situ* Cas off-targets and verification by sequencing), detection of the MRE11 subunit of the MRN complex binding by ChIP-seq returns a more specific and sensitive information filtered by a custom algorithm that retains cleaved sites followed by the protospacer-adjacent motif (PAM) and the putative protospacer binding site (Wienert et al., 2019, 2020). It is worth mentioning here that unbiased DSB discovery is also performed by some of the techniques described in section "Translocation and Other Chromosomal Aberration Detection."

SSB/BE Detection

Compared to the variety of assays for DSB detection, methods to monitor SSBs induced by designer nickases and/or base editors are less abundant. This type of gene editors is generally thought to be less harmful than designer nucleases generating DSBs (Hu et al., 2016; Bothmer et al., 2017) but thorough and more specific analyses could report a higher genome and RNA mutational rate with some BEs (Rees et al., 2019; Xin et al., 2019).

Detection techniques designed for and tested on samples treated with designer nickases linked to BEs are EndoV-seq (Endonuclease V-based sequencing; Liang et al., 2019) and Digenome-seq (Kim et al., 2017, 2019a, 2020) (**Supplementary Table 2**). Both techniques rely on an *in vitro* nicking, base modification and subsequent DNA end repairing in order to obtain a particular pattern after whole genome sequencing (WGS). This approach and its respective bioinformatic analysis help to filter out the majority of the natural occurring DNA nicks, but requires a good WGS coverage (>30×), which makes these techniques expensive and only applicable to studies in a pre-clinical phase.

The validation rate for these techniques can vary greatly compared to DSB detection methods. Since SSBs cannot be directly revealed by indel quantification, base editing frequencies at potential off-target sites can be measured by NGS or, in alternative, DSBs induced by an active designer nuclease can be employed as surrogates.

Other techniques are showing great potential but they have not been tested on designer editors/nickases. Among those, SSB-seq (Baranello et al., 2014), SSiNGLe (single-strand break mapping at nucleotide genome level) (Cao et al., 2019), GLOE-seq (genome-wide ligation of 30-OH ends followed by sequencing) (Sriramachandran et al., 2020), and Nick-seq (Cao et al., 2020) are able to return data from an in cellula approach.

The "Prime editors" strategy instead presents a new challenge for this kind of techniques since its nickase activity is coupled with a reverse transcriptase that could potentially introduce indels at off-target sites or cause retrotransposon activations and integrations of random reverse transcribed RNA sequences into the genomic DNA (Anzalone et al., 2019). A recent work using Digenome-seq (Kim et al., 2020) exploited the aspecific capacity of the dCas9-H840A protein, utilized in the PE, to cleave also the non-targeted strand, resulting in a characteristic signature after WGS and enabling the use of an analysis compatible with the Digenome-seq bioinformatic pipeline. The authors showed that not all the off-target sites detected by Digenome-seq and validated for the presence of indels are prime-edited, confirming the importance of the pegRNA specific priming activity. In support of this, a different work recently showed the presence of unexpected large deletions after prime editing in mice embryos, mainly ascribed to the dCas9-H840A activity (Aida et al., 2020). However, this proposed strategy do not allow the detection of all the possible mutations that this system may induce *in cellula* and therefore it is not completely exhaustive.

Translocation and Other Chromosomal Aberration Detection

Off-target mutations and insertional mutagenesis are considered to be harmful because they can perturb the expression of nearby genetic elements by means of different mechanisms (McCormack and Rabbitts, 2004). While this dysregulation is usually localized, rare or innocuous, major concerns derive from general genomic instability and the several chromosomal aberrations that we may or may not detect after editing. Increasing evidences are showing how those gross chromosomal aberrations generate after designer nucleases activity (Weinstock et al., 2008; Kosicki et al., 2018; Turchiano et al., 2020). Oncongenic translocations have been reproduced *in vivo* in lung tissues of mouse models by the simultaneous introduction of two DSBs, confirming this major concern (Blasco et al., 2014). Large deletions, loss of heterozygosity, large inversions, or translocations may also impact the 3D genomic organization and cause dysregulations of entire topological associated domains (median size ~880 kb) usually organized to be transcriptionally active or repressed (Dixon et al., 2012; Bonev and Cavalli, 2016).

Recent studies also observed on-target related chromosomal aberrations with formation of micronuclei and chromosome bridges leading to copy number variation, telomeric portion loss, and chromotripsis (Cullot et al., 2019; Leibowitz et al., 2020) rising further concerns for the safety of designer nucleases in clinic.

The portfolio of translocation detection techniques developed to recognize those mutations with increasing sensitivity comprises TC-seq (translocation capture sequencing; Klein et al., 2011), UDiTaS (UniDirectional Targeted Sequencing; Giannoukos et al., 2018), AMP-seq (anchored multiplexed PCR sequencing; Zheng et al., 2014), LAM-HTGTS (linear amplification-mediated high-throughput genome-wide sequencing; Frock et al., 2015), and CAST-seq (chromosomal aberration analysis by single targeted LM-PCR sequencing; Turchiano et al., 2020).

All of these methods are based on nested PCRs with primers binding between a known target site and fused unknown sites marked by an adapter. NGS sequencing is then used to identify the fusion partners. Differences among these techniques include in particular the adapter attachment via tagmentation (UDiTas), bridge adaptor ligation (LAM-HTGTS), or dsDNA ligation (CAST-seq and AMP-seq). Besides, the amount of input DNA and the bioinformatic pipeline can differ substantially for these techniques as shown in **Supplementary Table 3**. For designer nucleases, the validation of translocation sites can be performed by looking for off-target cleavage at the fused sites by deep sequencing. On the other hand, translocations can also be directly validated through PCR or ddPCR with specific primers recognizing the two fusion partners (Bak et al., 2017). As translocations themselves exhibit a distinguishable element in the form of the specific point of fusion, the quantification of individual events becomes easier even without the addition of unique molecular identifiers (UMIs) barcodes.

TECHNICAL CHALLENGES

All of these techniques have potential drawbacks in their methodology or bioinformatic analysis as summarized in **Supplementary Tables 1–3** (excluding techniques not optimized to describe designer nucleases activity). Besides the above mentioned biological biases, the distinction between *in vitro* and *in cellula* assays is essential due to their expected difference in sensitivity and hence in the number of returned off-target sites; for *in vitro* techniques, the introduction of an arbitrary threshold (e.g., the amount of reads per element) to select a smaller subset of sites could be an option, even though it may introduce a significant bias in the off-target detection. In a clinical setting, this bias could be reduced by further validating some of the sites that have been discarded by the arbitrary threshold, as for example those that are found close to oncogenic elements within a window of 50–100 kb of distance.

Another aspect that is crucial from the perspective of clinical application is the required amount of DNA or cell input, since attainable patient samples are limited. Some techniques might not be suitable for the analysis of the most clinically relevant samples. The introduction of additional elements (IDLV, DNA oligonucleotides) into the cell makes approaches like GUIDE-seq and IDLV capture unsuitable for performing the off-target screening directly on the cells intended for the treatment. When using these techniques, off-target detection must be performed in surrogate cell lines hence the cleavage footprint might not be accurate for a particular patient or the particular treatment due to diverging sequences, chromatin state, or DNA accessibility.

While the qualitative description of the off-target sites is an important information, their cleavage frequencies, and their reliable ranking can be equally of value, especially when monitoring the clonal expansion of modified cells in patients. Barcode sequences can be introduced at the cleavage site or upon adapter ligation prior to amplification steps in order to quantify individual events in an unambiguous manner. On the other hand, a semiquantitative/quantitative information might still be retrieved, without barcoding, by calculating the relative reads amount of a certain mutation over the total amount of reads (Crosetto et al., 2013; Wienert et al., 2019) or by utilizing other unique molecular signatures such as the linker ligation point and the translocation fusion point (Zheng et al., 2014; Frock et al., 2015; Turchiano et al., 2020).

Not least the bioinformatic pipelines are of major importance due to the potential biases they can introduce or remove. Sequences filtering process is mainly borne by the reads/alignments quality and the reads amount counted in a defined genomic region. In order to avoid false positive results, the comparison with an untreated control can be beneficial, as it limits the biases coming from sequence misalignment or indexing hopping phenomena (Kircher et al., 2012) in multiplex NGS. A problematic practice is filtering out sites that do not reach a defined degree of homology to the on-target site. This kind of filtering, sometimes arbitrarily defined, can have a particular impact in case of differences between the patient's and the reference genome. Additionally, unspecific cleavage phenomena such as collateral activity of Cas12a (Li et al., 2018) would never be observed with this kind of filtering. This approach can be difficult to be applied when using other heterodimeric designer nucleases such as TALENs or ZFNs, especially if homodimers or other unintended dimers orientations and distances that can lead to cleavage are considered.

The parameters that may be used to define the potency of an assay could be the sensitivity and the accuracy. For a well-founded sensitivity assessment a known amount of potentially detectable events is ideally present within a sample or where a specific detected event can be quantified by other means and tested in a dilution series. Estimating the sensitivity based on measurements of indels for example suffers from the aforementioned uncertainty of the NGS analysis itself. It is also worth noting that the sensitivity of a technique depends also on the experimental conditions, and could be directly proportional to the numbers of cells treated, the amount of input material and the sequencing depth. The accuracy of this kind of technique relies on the ability to detect off-targeted sites with a minimal error rate or bias and is dependent by the amount of validated false positive and false negative sites. The validation process usually relies on deep sequencing of the inquired genomic regions to discern the false positive sites with all the drawbacks beforehand described. **Supplementary Tables 1–3** reports the validation rates for the described techniques; however we do not have an objective and complete overview of all the mutations induced by the genome editing tools therefore calculating the false negative rate parameter is impossible with the current state of the art.

In this scenario, we also have to include the possibility of a designer nuclease having off-target activity in some genome widespread repetitive elements. Genomic instability events in these regions would be worrisome as they can be abundant, difficult to align and might be filtered out by the relative bioinformatic pipelines. In this case, use of unmasked reference genomes and a tolerant alignment algorithm together with the comparison with the untreated control would help mitigating the bias and finding a balance with the accuracy rate.

CONCLUSIONS AND OUTLOOKS

Gene therapy based on integrating viral vector evolved in the last decades together with techniques and analyses that can at least in part evaluate safety (Modlich et al., 2006; Montini et al., 2006; Zhou et al., 2016; Biasco, 2017). In the same way, the different gene editing strategies are shaping novel reagents, techniques and strategies to improve their safety and efficiency for clinical application (Miller et al., 2007; Kleinstiver et al., 2016; Casini et al., 2018; Gao et al., 2018; Vakulskas et al., 2018; Rai et al., 2020). Further studies are required to understand and analyse the genotoxicity of new therapeutic strategies, and compare it with existing technologies. So far, the genotoxic effects of retroviral vectors employed in gene therapy approaches have been linked to insertional mutagenesis events mediated by viral enhancers (Bohne and Cathomen, 2008; Hacein-Bey-Abina et al., 2014), while designer nucleases act differently and may be more detrimental in regards to cell viability and genome integrity (Schiroli et al., 2019; Leibowitz et al., 2020). Delivery methods were also shown to impact differently on the mutational capacity of designer nucleases and the scientific community is moving toward a hit-and-run approach, utilizing ribonucleoproteins, or mRNA, that ensures a quick clearance of the exogenous nuclease and a more specific activity (Hendel et al., 2015). A balanced discussion should also consider the different impact of mutations in stem or in differentiated cells, with the latter likely to bear a lower risk of genotoxicity due to their shorter lifespan.

In light of these observations we can derive a new definition for genotoxicity which can be described as the property of an agent able to alter the genetic function within a cell causing unwanted mutations/effects, which may lead to functional impairment (e.g., cancer, therapy impairment, differentiation impairment).

CRISPR-Cas technology has largely democratized and accelerated the gene editing field but there are not yet standard techniques that can evaluate all the possible mutations induced directly or indirectly by the editing procedure. Recent publications revealed that off-targeting is responsible only for a minor portion of mutations characterized in edited cells, while there are on-target related mutations that justify careful

evaluation (Kosicki et al., 2018; Connelly and Pruett-Miller, 2019; Cullot et al., 2019; Turchiano et al., 2020).

Hence, a combination of an *in cellula* technique for the discovery of off-targets sites (DISCOVER-seq, BLISS) and one for all other chromosomal aberrations (CAST-seq, HTGTS) would likely detect most of the unexpected mutations without the need to modify the current ex-vivo clinical procedures. *In vitro* techniques can describe a worst-case-scenario of off-target editing in a pre-clinical setting but require in addition a thorough validation via deep sequencing to exclude the abundant false positive sites that can be returned by the analysis, even when using base editors (see **Supplementary Tables 2, 3**). In clinical settings, where hundreds of millions of cells need to be edited, the deep sequencing indel detection threshold of 0.01–0.1% may not be sufficient to detect the actual off-target activity. CAST-seq shows an increased sensitivity reaching 0.006% (1 mutation out of 15,000 genome haplotypes) when compared with the absolute ddPCR quantification capacity, and hopefully also DSB detection techniques may be improved in the near future to achieve or lower that threshold in therapeutic settings.

In this review, we have highlighted the currently available techniques to detect DSBs, SSBs, translocations, and other chromosomal aberrations and the methods to quantify cleavage of designer nucleases. Overall, the amount of input DNA, the reliable quantification of events, an unbiased bioinformatic pipeline, the traceable sensitivity and the validation rate assessment are critical to evaluate the suitability of a technique.

The gene therapy field is moving fast; new molecular strategies are being proposed or are now under investigation in order to expand the applications and improve the editing efficiency. Prime editing (Anzalone et al., 2019), for example, could entail new potential. Alternatively, a new site specific and scareless integrative strategy could be developed soon by harnessing the transposase activity (Voigt et al., 2012; Klompe et al., 2019; Kovac et al., 2020), making another giant leap forward in the field. Advanced methods to assess genotoxicity of such technologies must be devised and will hopefully incorporate additional sensitivity and capacity to quantify all genetic modifications introduced by current and next-generation gene editing platforms.

AUTHOR CONTRIBUTIONS

GB, AC, AT, and GT contributed to the final version of the manuscript. All authors contributed to the article and approved the submitted version.

REFERENCES

Aida, T., Wilde, J. J., Yang, L., Hou, Y., Li, M., Xu, D., et al. (2020). Prime editing primarily induces undesired outcomes in mice. *bioRxiv* 2020.2008.2006.239723. doi: 10.1101/2020.08.06.239723

Aiuti, A., Biasco, L., Scaramuzza, S., Ferrua, F., Cicalese, M. P., Baricordi, C., et al. (2013). Lentiviral hematopoietic stem cell gene therapy in patients with Wiskott-Aldrich syndrome. *Science* 341:1233151. doi: 10.1126/science.1233151

Anderson, W. F. (1990). September 14, 1990: the beginning. *Hum. Gene Ther.* 1, 371–372. doi: 10.1089/hum.1990.1.4-371

Anzalone, A. V., Randolph, P. B., Davis, J. R., Sousa, A. A., Koblan, L. W., Levy, J. M., et al. (2019). Search-and-replace genome editing without double-strand breaks or donor DNA. *Nature* 576, 149–157. doi: 10.1038/s41586-019-1711-4

Bae, S., Park, J., and Kim, J. S. (2014). Cas-OFFinder: a fast and versatile algorithm that searches for potential off-target sites of Cas9 RNA-guided endonucleases. *Bioinformatics* 30, 1473–1475. doi: 10.1093/bioinformatics/btu048

Bak, R. O., Dever, D. P., Reinisch, A., Cruz Hernandez, D., Majeti, R., and Porteus, M. H. (2017). Multiplexed genetic engineering of human hematopoietic stem and progenitor cells using CRISPR/Cas9 and AAV6. *Elife* 6. doi: 10.7554/eLife.27873.025AQ

Baranello, L., Kouzine, F., Wojtowicz, D., Cui, K., Przytycka, T. M., Zhao, K., et al. (2014). DNA break mapping reveals topoisomerase II activity genome-wide. *Int. J. Mol. Sci.* 15, 13111–13122. doi: 10.3390/ijms150713111

Biasco, L. (2017). Integration site analysis in gene therapy patients: expectations and reality. *Hum. Gene. Ther.* 28, 1122–1129. doi: 10.1089/hum.2017.183

Blasco, R. B., Karaca, E., Ambrogio, C., Cheong, T. C., Karayol, E., Minero, V. G., et al. (2014). Simple and rapid *in vivo* generation of chromosomal rearrangements using CRISPR/Cas9 technology. *Cell Rep.* 9, 1219–1227. doi: 10.1016/j.celrep.2014.10.051

Bogdanove, A. J., and Voytas, D. F. (2011). TAL effectors: customizable proteins for DNA targeting. *Science* 333, 1843–1846. doi: 10.1126/science.1204094

Bohne, J., and Cathomen, T. (2008). Genotoxicity in gene therapy: an account of vector integration and designer nucleases. *Curr. Opin. Mol. Ther.* 10, 214–223.

Bonev, B., and Cavalli, G. (2016). Organization and function of the 3D genome. *Nat. Rev. Genet.* 17, 661–678. doi: 10.1038/nrg.2016.112

Bothmer, A., Phadke, T., Barrera, L. A., Margulies, C. M., Lee, C. S., Buquicchio, F., et al. (2017). Characterization of the interplay between DNA repair and CRISPR/Cas9-induced DNA lesions at an endogenous locus. *Nat. Commun.* 8:13905. doi: 10.1038/ncomms13905

Breton, C., Clark, P. M., Wang, L., Greig, J. A., and Wilson, J. M. (2020). ITR-seq, a next-generation sequencing assay, identifies genome-wide DNA editing sites *in vivo* following adeno-associated viral vector-mediated genome editing. *BMC Genomics* 21:239. doi: 10.1186/s12864-020-6655-4

Brinkman, E. K., Chen, T., Amendola, M., and van Steensel, B. (2014). Easy quantitative assessment of genome editing by sequence trace decomposition. *Nucleic. Acids Res.* 42:e168. doi: 10.1093/nar/gku936

Cameron, P., Fuller, C. K., Donohoue, P. D., Jones, B. N., Thompson, M. S., Carter, M. M., et al. (2017). Mapping the genomic landscape of CRISPR-Cas9 cleavage. *Nat. Methods* 14, 600–606. doi: 10.1038/nmeth.4284

Canela, A., Sridharan, S., Sciascia, N., Tubbs, A., Meltzer, P., Sleckman, B. P., et al. (2016). DNA breaks and end resection measured genome-wide by end sequencing. *Mol. Cell* 63, 898–911. doi: 10.1016/j.molcel.2016.06.034

Cao, B., Wu, X., Zhou, J., Wu, H., Liu, L., Zhang, Q., et al. (2020). Nick-seq for single-nucleotide resolution genomic maps of DNA modifications and damage. *Nucleic Acids Res.* 48, 6715–6725. doi: 10.1093/nar/gkaa473

Cao, H., Salazar-Garcia, L., Gao, F., Wahlestedt, T., Wu, C. L., Han, X., et al. (2019). Novel approach reveals genomic landscapes of single-strand DNA breaks with nucleotide resolution in human cells. *Nat. Commun.* 10:5799. doi: 10.1038/s41467-019-13602-7

Casini, A., Olivieri, M., Petris, G., Montagna, C., Reginato, G., Maule, G., et al. (2018). A highly specific SpCas9 variant is identified by *in vivo* screening in yeast. *Nat. Biotechnol.* 36, 265–271. doi: 10.1038/nbt.4066

Cattoglio, C., Facchini, G., Sartori, D., Antonelli, A., Miccio, A., Cassani, B., et al. (2007). Hot spots of retroviral integration in human CD34+ hematopoietic cells. *Blood* 110, 1770–1778. doi: 10.1182/blood-2007-01-068759

Cavazzana-Calvo, M., Payen, E., Negre, O., Wang, G., Hehir, K., Fusil, F., et al. (2010). Transfusion independence and HMGA2 activation after gene therapy of human beta-thalassaemia. *Nature* 467, 318–322. doi: 10.1038/nature09328

Chakrabarti, A. M., Henser-Brownhill, T., Monserrat, J., Poetsch, A. R., Luscombe, N. M., and Scaffidi, P. (2019). Target-specific precision of CRISPR-mediated genome editing. *Mol. Cell* 73, 699–713.e696. doi: 10.1016/j.molcel.2018.11.031

Chen, J. S., Ma, E., Harrington, L. B., Da Costa, M., Tian, X., Palefsky, J. M., et al. (2018). CRISPR-Cas12a target binding unleashes indiscriminate single-stranded DNase activity. *Science* 360, 436–439. doi: 10.1126/science.aar6245

Chevalier, B. S., Monnat, R. J. Jr., and Stoddard, B. L. (2001). The homing endonuclease I-CreI uses three metals, one of which is shared between the two active sites. *Nat. Struct. Biol.* 8, 312–316. doi: 10.1038/86181

Cho, S. W., Kim, S., Kim, Y., Kweon, J., Kim, H. S., Bae, S., et al. (2014). Analysis of off-target effects of CRISPR/Cas-derived RNA-guided endonucleases and nickases. *Genome Res.* 24, 132–141. doi: 10.1101/gr.162339.113

Concordet, J. P., and Haeussler, M. (2018). CRISPOR: intuitive guide selection for CRISPR/Cas9 genome editing experiments and screens. *Nucleic. Acids Res.* 46, W242–W245. doi: 10.1093/nar/gky354

Connelly, J. P., and Pruett-Miller, S. M. (2019). CRIS.py: a versatile and high-throughput analysis program for CRISPR-based genome editing. *Sci. Rep.* 9:4194. doi: 10.1038/s41598-019-40896-w

Corrigan-Curay, J., O'Reilly, M., Kohn, D. B., Cannon, P. M., Bao, G., Bushman, F. D., et al. (2015). Genome editing technologies: defining a path to clinic. *Mol. Ther.* 23, 796–806. doi: 10.1038/mt.2015.54

Cradick, T. J., Qiu, P., Lee, C. M., Fine, E. J., and Bao, G. (2014). COSMID: a web-based tool for identifying and validating CRISPR/Cas off-target sites. *Mol. Ther. Nucleic Acids* 3:e214. doi: 10.1038/mtna.2014.64

Crosetto, N., Mitra, A., Silva, M. J., Bienko, M., Dojer, N., Wang, Q., et al. (2013). Nucleotide-resolution DNA double-strand break mapping by next-generation sequencing. *Nat. Methods* 10, 361–365. doi: 10.1038/nmeth.2408

Cullot, G., Boutin, J., Toutain, J., Prat, F., Pennamen, P., Rooryck, C., et al. (2019). CRISPR-Cas9 genome editing induces megabase-scale chromosomal truncations. *Nat. Commun.* 10:1136. doi: 10.1038/s41467-019-09006-2

Dixon, J. R., Selvaraj, S., Yue, F., Kim, A., Li, Y., Shen, Y., et al. (2012). Topological domains in mammalian genomes identified by analysis of chromatin interactions. *Nature* 485, 376–380. doi: 10.1038/nature11082

Epinat, J. C., Arnould, S., Chames, P., Rochaix, P., Desfontaines, D., Puzin, C., et al. (2003). A novel engineered meganuclease induces homologous recombination in yeast and mammalian cells. *Nucleic Acids Res.* 31, 2952–2962. doi: 10.1093/nar/gkg375

Frock, R. L., Hu, J., Meyers, R. M., Ho, Y. J., Kii, E., and Alt, F. W. (2015). Genome-wide detection of DNA double-stranded breaks induced by engineered nucleases. *Nat. Biotechnol.* 33, 179–186. doi: 10.1038/nbt.3101

Fu, Y., Foden, J. A., Khayter, C., Maeder, M. L., Reyon, D., Joung, J. K., et al. (2013). High-frequency off-target mutagenesis induced by CRISPR-Cas nucleases in human cells. *Nat. Biotechnol.* 31, 822–826. doi: 10.1038/nbt.2623

Gabriel, R., Lombardo, A., Arens, A., Miller, J. C., Genovese, P., Kaeppel, C., et al. (2011). An unbiased genome-wide analysis of zinc-finger nuclease specificity. *Nat. Biotechnol.* 29, 816–823. doi: 10.1038/nbt.1948

Gao, X., Tao, Y., Lamas, V., Huang, M., Yeh, W. H., Pan, B., et al. (2018). Treatment of autosomal dominant hearing loss by *in vivo* delivery of genome editing agents. *Nature* 553, 217–221. doi: 10.1038/nature25164

Gaspar, H. B., Parsley, K. L., Howe, S., King, D., Gilmour, K. C., Sinclair, J., et al. (2004). Gene therapy of X-linked severe combined immunodeficiency by use of a pseudotyped gammaretroviral vector. *Lancet* 364, 2181–2187. doi: 10.1016/S0140-6736(04)17590-9

Gaudelli, N. M., Komor, A. C., Rees, H. A., Packer, M. S., Badran, A. H., Bryson, D. I., et al. (2017). Programmable base editing of A*T to G*C in genomic DNA without DNA cleavage. *Nature* 551, 464–471. doi: 10.1038/nature24644

Giannoukos, G., Ciulla, D. M., Marco, E., Abdulkerim, H. S., Barrera, L. A., Bothmer, A., et al. (2018). UDiTaS, a genome editing detection method for indels and genome rearrangements. *BMC Genomics* 19:212. doi: 10.1186/s12864-018-4561-9

Gijsbers, R., Ronen, K., Vets, S., Malani, N., De Rijck, J., McNeely, M., et al. (2010). LEDGF hybrids efficiently retarget lentiviral integration into heterochromatin. *Mol. Ther.* 18, 552–560. doi: 10.1038/mt.2010.36

Grau, J., Boch, J., and Posch, S. (2013). TALENoffer: genome-wide TALEN off-target prediction. *Bioinformatics* 29, 2931–2932. doi: 10.1093/bioinformatics/btt501

Hacein-Bey-Abina, S., Pai, S. Y., Gaspar, H. B., Armant, M., Berry, C. C., Blanche, S., et al. (2014). A modified gamma-retrovirus vector for X-linked severe combined immunodeficiency. *N. Engl. J. Med.* 371, 1407–1417. doi: 10.1056/NEJMoa1404588

Hacein-Bey-Abina, S., Von Kalle, C., Schmidt, M., McCormack, M. P., Wulffraat, N., Leboulch, P., et al. (2003). LMO2-associated clonal T cell proliferation in two patients after gene therapy for SCID-X1. *Science* 302, 415–419. doi: 10.1126/science.1088547

Hendel, A., Bak, R. O., Clark, J. T., Kennedy, A. B., Ryan, D. E., Roy, S., et al. (2015). Chemically modified guide RNAs enhance CRISPR-Cas genome editing in human primary cells. *Nat. Biotechnol.* 33, 985–989. doi: 10.1038/nbt.3290

Howe, S. J., Mansour, M. R., Schwarzwaelder, K., Bartholomae, C., Hubank, M., Kempski, H., et al. (2008). Insertional mutagenesis combined with acquired somatic mutations causes leukemogenesis following gene therapy of SCID-X1 patients. *J. Clin. Invest.* 118, 3143–3150. doi: 10.1172/JCI35798

Hsiau, T., Conant, D., Rossi, N., Maures, T., Waite, K., Yang, J., et al. (2019). Inference of CRISPR edits from Sanger Trace Data. *bioRxiv* 251082. doi: 10.1101/251082

Hu, J., Meyers, R. M., Dong, J., Panchakshari, R. A., Alt, F. W., and Frock, R. L. (2016). Detecting DNA double-stranded breaks in mammalian genomes by linear amplification-mediated high-throughput genome-wide translocation sequencing. *Nat. Protoc.* 11, 853–871. doi: 10.1038/nprot.2016.043

Iacovoni, J. S., Caron, P., Lassadi, I., Nicolas, E., Massip, L., Trouche, D., et al. (2010). High-resolution profiling of gammaH2AX around DNA double strand breaks in the mammalian genome. *EMBO J.* 29, 1446–1457. doi: 10.1038/emboj.2010.38

Jinek, M., Chylinski, K., Fonfara, I., Hauer, M., Doudna, J. A., and Charpentier, E. (2012). A programmable dual-RNA-guided DNA endonuclease in adaptive bacterial immunity. *Science* 337, 816–821. doi: 10.1126/science.1225829

Kim, D., Bae, S., Park, J., Kim, E., Kim, S., Yu, H. R., et al. (2015). Digenome-seq: genome-wide profiling of CRISPR-Cas9 off-target effects in human cells. *Nat. Methods* 12, 237–243, 231 p following 243. doi: 10.1038/nmeth.3284

Kim, D., Kim, D. E., Lee, G., Cho, S. I., and Kim, J. S. (2019a). Genome-wide target specificity of CRISPR RNA-guided adenine base editors. *Nat. Biotechnol.* 37, 430–435. doi: 10.1038/s41587-019-0050-1

Kim, D., and Kim, J. S. (2018). DIG-seq: a genome-wide CRISPR off-target profiling method using chromatin DNA. *Genome Res.* 28, 1894–1900. doi: 10.1101/gr.236620.118

Kim, D., Kim, S., Kim, S., Park, J., and Kim, J. S. (2016). Genome-wide target specificities of CRISPR-Cas9 nucleases revealed by multiplex Digenome-seq. *Genome Res.* 26, 406–415. doi: 10.1101/gr.199588.115

Kim, D., Lim, K., Kim, S. T., Yoon, S. H., Kim, K., Ryu, S. M., et al. (2017). Genome-wide target specificities of CRISPR RNA-guided programmable deaminases. *Nat. Biotechnol.* 35, 475–480. doi: 10.1038/nbt.3852

Kim, D., Luk, K., Wolfe, S. A., and Kim, J.-S. (2019b). Evaluating and enhancing target specificity of gene-editing nucleases and deaminases. *Ann. Rev. Biochem.* 88, 191–220. doi: 10.1146/annurev-biochem-013118-111730

Kim, D. Y., Moon, S. B., Ko, J. H., Kim, Y. S., and Kim, D. (2020). Unbiased investigation of specificities of prime editing systems in human cells. *Nucleic Acids Res.* 48, 10576–10589. doi: 10.1093/nar/gkaa764

Kim, S., Kim, D., Cho, S. W., Kim, J., and Kim, J. S. (2014). Highly efficient RNA-guided genome editing in human cells via delivery of purified Cas9 ribonucleoproteins. *Genome Res.* 24, 1012–1019. doi: 10.1101/gr.171322.113

Kircher, M., Sawyer, S., and Meyer, M. (2012). Double indexing overcomes inaccuracies in multiplex sequencing on the Illumina platform. *Nucleic Acids Res.* 40:e3. doi: 10.1093/nar/gkr771

Klein, I. A., Resch, W., Jankovic, M., Oliveira, T., Yamane, A., Nakahashi, H., et al. (2011). Translocation-capture sequencing reveals the extent and nature of chromosomal rearrangements in B lymphocytes. *Cell* 147, 95–106. doi: 10.1016/j.cell.2011.07.048

Kleinstiver, B. P., Pattanayak, V., Prew, M. S., Tsai, S. Q., Nguyen, N. T., Zheng, Z., et al. (2016). High-fidelity CRISPR-Cas9 nucleases with no detectable genome-wide off-target effects. *Nature* 529, 490–495. doi: 10.1038/nature 16526

Klompe, S. E., Vo, P. L. H., Halpin-Healy, T. S., and Sternberg, S. H. (2019). Transposon-encoded CRISPR-Cas systems direct RNA-guided DNA integration. *Nature* 571, 219–225. doi: 10.1038/s41586-019-1323-z

Kohn, D. B., Booth, C., Kang, E. M., Pai, S. Y., Shaw, K. L., Santilli, G., et al. (2020). Lentiviral gene therapy for X-linked chronic granulomatous disease. *Nat. Med.* 26, 200–206. doi: 10.1038/s41591-019-0735-5

Koike-Yusa, H., Li, Y., Tan, E. P., Velasco-Herrera Mdel, C., and Yusa, K. (2014). Genome-wide recessive genetic screening in mammalian cells with a lentiviral CRISPR-guide RNA library. *Nat. Biotechnol.* 32, 267–273. doi: 10.1038/nbt.2800

Komor, A. C., Kim, Y. B., Packer, M. S., Zuris, J. A., and Liu, D. R. (2016). Programmable editing of a target base in genomic DNA without double-stranded DNA cleavage. *Nature* 533, 420–424. doi: 10.1038/nature17946

Komor, A. C., Zhao, K. T., Packer, M. S., Gaudelli, N. M., Waterbury, A. L., Koblan, L. W., et al. (2017). Improved base excision repair inhibition and bacteriophage Mu Gam protein yields C:G-to-T:A base editors with higher efficiency and product purity. *Sci. Adv.* 3:eaao4774. doi: 10.1126/sciadv.aao4774

Koo, T., Lee, J., and Kim, J. S. (2015). Measuring and reducing off-target activities of programmable nucleases including CRISPR-Cas9. *Mol. Cells* 38, 475–481. doi: 10.14348/molcells.2015.0103

Kosicki, M., Tomberg, K., and Bradley, A. (2018). Repair of double-strand breaks induced by CRISPR-Cas9 leads to large deletions and complex rearrangements. *Nat. Biotechnol.* 36, 765–771. doi: 10.1038/nbt.4192

Kovac, A., Miskey, C., Menzel, M., Grueso, E., Gogol-Doring, A., and Ivics, Z. (2020). RNA-guided retargeting of sleeping beauty transposition in human cells. *Elife* 9:53868. doi: 10.7554/eLife.53868

Kurt, I. C., Zhou, R., Iyer, S., Garcia, S. P., Miller, B. R., Langner, L. M., et al. (2020). CRISPR C-to-G base editors for inducing targeted DNA transversions in human cells. *Nat. Biotechnol.* doi: 10.1038/s41587-020-0609-x

Kuscu, C., Arslan, S., Singh, R., Thorpe, J., and Adli, M. (2014). Genome-wide analysis reveals characteristics of off-target sites bound by the Cas9 endonuclease. *Nat. Biotechnol.* 32, 677–683. doi: 10.1038/nbt.2916

Lazzarotto, C. R., Malinin, N. L., Li, Y., Zhang, R., Yang, Y., Lee, G., et al. (2020). CHANGE-seq reveals genetic and epigenetic effects on CRISPR-Cas9 genome-wide activity. *Nat. Biotechnol.* doi: 10.1038/s41587-020-0555-7

Leibowitz, M. L., Papathanasiou, S., Doerfler, P. A., Blaine, L. J., Yao, Y., Zhang, C.-Z., et al. (2020). Chromothripsis as an on-target consequence of CRISPR-Cas9 genome editing. *bioRxiv.* 2020.2007.2013.200998. doi: 10.1101/2020.07.13.200998

Lensing, S. V., Marsico, G., Hansel-Hertsch, R., Lam, E. Y., Tannahill, D., and Balasubramanian, S. (2016). DSBCapture: in situ capture and sequencing of DNA breaks. *Nat. Methods* 13, 855–857. doi: 10.1038/nmeth.3960

Li, S. Y., Cheng, Q. X., Liu, J. K., Nie, X. Q., Zhao, G. P., and Wang, J. (2018). CRISPR-Cas12a has both cis- and trans-cleavage activities on single-stranded DNA. *Cell Res.* 28, 491–493. doi: 10.1038/s41422-018-0022-x

Liang, P., Xie, X., Zhi, S., Sun, H., Zhang, X., Chen, Y., et al. (2019). Genome-wide profiling of adenine base editor specificity by EndoV-seq. *Nat. Commun.* 10:67. doi: 10.1038/s41467-018-07988-z

Maeder, M. L., and Gersbach, C. A. (2016). Genome-editing technologies for gene and cell therapy. *Mol. Ther.* 24, 430–446. doi: 10.1038/mt.2016.10

Mashal, R. D., Koontz, J., and Sklar, J. (1995). Detection of mutations by cleavage of DNA heteroduplexes with bacteriophage resolvases. *Nat. Genet.* 9, 177–183. doi: 10.1038/ng0295-177

McCormack, M. P., and Rabbitts, T. H. (2004). Activation of the T-cell oncogene LMO2 after gene therapy for X-linked severe combined immunodeficiency. *N. Engl. J. Med.* 350, 913–922. doi: 10.1056/NEJMra032207

Metais, J. Y., and Dunbar, C. E. (2008). The MDS1-EVI1 gene complex as a retrovirus integration site: impact on behavior of hematopoietic cells and implications for gene therapy. *Mol. Ther.* 16, 439–449. doi: 10.1038/sj.mt.6300372

Miller, J. C., Holmes, M. C., Wang, J., Guschin, D. Y., Lee, Y. L., Rupniewski, I., et al. (2007). An improved zinc-finger nuclease architecture for highly specific genome editing. *Nat. Biotechnol.* 25, 778–785. doi: 10.1038/nbt1319

Modlich, U., Bohne, J., Schmidt, M., von Kalle, C., Knoss, S., Schambach, A., et al. (2006). Cell-culture assays reveal the importance of retroviral vector design for insertional genotoxicity. *Blood* 108, 2545–2553. doi: 10.1182/blood-2005-08-024976

Montague, T. G., Cruz, J. M., Gagnon, J. A., Church, G. M., and Valen, E. (2014). CHOPCHOP: a CRISPR/Cas9 and TALEN web tool for genome editing. *Nucleic Acids Res.* 42, W401–407. doi: 10.1093/nar/gku410

Montini, E., Cesana, D., Schmidt, M., Sanvito, F., Ponzoni, M., Bartholomae, C., et al. (2006). Hematopoietic stem cell gene transfer in a tumor-prone mouse model uncovers low genotoxicity of lentiviral vector integration. *Nat. Biotechnol.* 24, 687–696. doi: 10.1038/nbt1216

Naldini, L., Blomer, U., Gage, F. H., Trono, D., and Verma, I. M. (1996). Efficient transfer, integration, and sustained long-term expression of the transgene in adult rat brains injected with a lentiviral vector. *Proc. Natl. Acad. Sci. U. S. A.* 93, 11382–11388. doi: 10.1073/pnas.93.21.11382

Nathwani, A. C., Tuddenham, E. G., Rangarajan, S., Rosales, C., McIntosh, J., Linch, D. C., et al. (2011). Adenovirus-associated virus vector-mediated gene transfer in hemophilia B. *N. Engl. J. Med.* 365, 2357–2365. doi: 10.1056/NEJMoa1108046

Ott, M. G., Schmidt, M., Schwarzwaelder, K., Stein, S., Siler, U., Koehl, U., et al. (2006). Correction of X-linked chronic granulomatous disease by gene therapy, augmented by insertional activation of MDS1-EVI1, PRDM16 or SETBP1. *Nat. Med.* 12, 401–409. doi: 10.1038/nm1393

Pinello, L., Canver, M. C., Hoban, M. D., Orkin, S. H., Kohn, D. B., Bauer, D. E., et al. (2016). Analyzing CRISPR genome-editing experiments with CRISPResso. *Nat. Biotechnol.* 34, 695–697. doi: 10.1038/nbt.3583

Qasim, W., Zhan, H., Samarasinghe, S., Adams, S., Amrolia, P., Stafford, S., et al. (2017). Molecular remission of infant B-ALL after infusion of universal TALEN gene-edited CAR T cells. *Sci. Transl. Med.* 9. doi: 10.1126/scitranslmed.aaj2013

Qiu, P., Shandilya, H., D'Alessio, J. M., O'Connor, K., Durocher, J., and Gerard, G. F. (2004). Mutation detection using surveyor nuclease. *Biotechniques* 36, 702–707. doi: 10.2144/04364PF01

Rai, R., Romito, M., Rivers, E., Turchiano, G., Blattner, G., Vetharoy, W., et al. (2020). Targeted gene correction of human hematopoietic stem cells for the treatment of Wiskott–Aldrich syndrome. *Nat. Commun.* 11:4034. doi: 10.1038/s41467-020-17626-2

Ran, F. A., Cong, L., Yan, W. X., Scott, D. A., Gootenberg, J. S., Kriz, A. J., et al. (2015). *In vivo* genome editing using *Staphylococcus aureus* Cas9. *Nature* 520, 186–191. doi: 10.1038/nature14299

Raper, S. E., Chirmule, N., Lee, F. S., Wivel, N. A., Bagg, A., Gao, G. P., et al. (2003). Fatal systemic inflammatory response syndrome in a ornithine transcarbamylase deficient patient following adenoviral gene transfer. *Mol. Genet. Metab.* 80, 148–158. doi: 10.1016/j.ymgme.2003.08.016

Rees, H. A., Wilson, C., Doman, J. L., and Liu, D. R. (2019). Analysis and minimization of cellular RNA editing by DNA adenine base editors. *Sci. Adv.* 5:eaax5717. doi: 10.1126/sciadv.aax5717

Rosenberg, S. A., Aebersold, P., Cornetta, K., Kasid, A., Morgan, R. A., Moen, R., et al. (1990). Gene transfer into humans–immunotherapy of patients with advanced melanoma, using tumor-infiltrating lymphocytes modified by retroviral gene transduction. *N. Engl. J. Med.* 323, 570–578. doi: 10.1056/NEJM199008303230904

Sapranauskas, R., Gasiunas, G., Fremaux, C., Barrangou, R., Horvath, P., and Siksnys, V. (2011). The *Streptococcus thermophilus* CRISPR/Cas system provides immunity in *Escherichia coli*. *Nucleic Acids Res.* 39, 9275–9282. doi: 10.1093/nar/gkr606

Schiroli, G., Conti, A., Ferrari, S., Della Volpe, L., Jacob, A., Albano, L., et al. (2019). Precise gene editing preserves hematopoietic stem cell function following transient p53-mediated DNA damage response. *Cell Stem Cell* 24, 551–565.e558. doi: 10.1016/j.stem.2019.02.019

Schwarzwaelder, K., Howe, S. J., Schmidt, M., Brugman, M. H., Deichmann, A., Glimm, H., et al. (2007). Gammaretrovirus-mediated correction of SCID-X1

is associated with skewed vector integration site distribution *in vivo*. *J. Clin. Invest.* 117, 2241–2249. doi: 10.1172/JCI31661

Sriramachandran, A. M., Petrosino, G., Mendez-Lago, M., Schafer, A. J., Batista-Nascimento, L. S., Zilio, N., et al. (2020). Genome-wide nucleotide-resolution mapping of DNA replication patterns, single-strand breaks, and lesions by GLOE-seq. *Mol. Cell* 78, 975–985.e977. doi: 10.1016/j.molcel.2020.03.027

Stadtmauer, E. A., Fraietta, J. A., Davis, M. M., Cohen, A. D., Weber, K. L., Lancaster, E., et al. (2020). CRISPR-engineered T cells in patients with refractory cancer. *Science* 367. doi: 10.1126/science.aba7365

Stein, S., Ott, M. G., Schultze-Strasser, S., Jauch, A., Burwinkel, B., Kinner, A., et al. (2010). Genomic instability and myelodysplasia with monosomy 7 consequent to EVI1 activation after gene therapy for chronic granulomatous disease. *Nat. Med.* 16, 198–204. doi: 10.1038/nm.2088

Tebas, P., Stein, D., Tang, W. W., Frank, I., Wang, S. Q., Lee, G., et al. (2014). Gene editing of CCR5 in autologous CD4 T cells of persons infected with HIV. *N. Engl. J. Med.* 370, 901–910. doi: 10.1056/NEJMoa1300662

Tsai, S. Q., Nguyen, N. T., Malagon-Lopez, J., Topkar, V. V., Aryee, M. J., and Joung, J. K. (2017). CIRCLE-seq: a highly sensitive *in vitro* screen for genome-wide CRISPR-Cas9 nuclease off-targets. *Nat. Methods* 14, 607–614. doi: 10.1038/nmeth.4278

Tsai, S. Q., Zheng, Z., Nguyen, N. T., Liebers, M., Topkar, V. V., Thapar, V., et al. (2015). GUIDE-seq enables genome-wide profiling of off-target cleavage by CRISPR-Cas nucleases. *Nat. Biotechnol.* 33, 187–197. doi: 10.1038/nbt.3117

Turchiano, G., Andrieux, G., Blattner, G., Pennucci, V., Klermund, J., Monaco, G., et al. (2020). Quantitative evaluation of chromosomal rearrangements in primary gene-edited human stem cells by preclinical CAST-seq. *Cell Stem Cell*. doi: 10.2139/ssrn.3565007

Urnov, F. D., Miller, J. C., Lee, Y. L., Beausejour, C. M., Rock, J. M., Augustus, S., et al. (2005). Highly efficient endogenous human gene correction using designed zinc-finger nucleases. *Nature* 435, 646–651. doi: 10.1038/nature03556

Vakulskas, C. A., Dever, D. P., Rettig, G. R., Turk, R., Jacobi, A. M., Collingwood, M. A., et al. (2018). A high-fidelity Cas9 mutant delivered as a ribonucleoprotein complex enables efficient gene editing in human hematopoietic stem and progenitor cells. *Nat. Med.* 24, 1216–1224. doi: 10.1038/s41591-018-0137-0

van Overbeek, M., Capurso, D., Carter, M. M., Thompson, M. S., Frias, E., Russ, C., et al. (2016). DNA Repair profiling reveals nonrandom outcomes at Cas9-mediated breaks. *Mol. Cell* 63, 633–646. doi: 10.1016/j.molcel.2016.06.037

Voigt, K., Gogol-Doring, A., Miskey, C., Chen, W., Cathomen, T., Izsvak, Z., et al. (2012). Retargeting sleeping beauty transposon insertions by engineered zinc finger DNA-binding domains. *Mol. Ther.* 20, 1852–1862. doi: 10.1038/mt.2012.126

Vranckx, L. S., Demeulemeester, J., Debyser, Z., and Gijsbers, R. (2016). Towards a safer, more randomized lentiviral vector integration profile exploring artificial LEDGF chimeras. *PLoS One* 11:e0164167. doi: 10.1371/journal.pone.0164167

Weinstock, D. M., Brunet, E., and Jasin, M. (2008). Induction of chromosomal translocations in mouse and human cells using site-specific endonucleases. *J. Natl. Cancer Inst. Monogr.* 39, 20–24. doi: 10.1093/jncimonographs/lgn009

Wienert, B., Wyman, S. K., Richardson, C. D., Yeh, C. D., Akcakaya, P., Porritt, M. J., et al. (2019). Unbiased detection of CRISPR off-targets in vivo using DISCOVER-seq. *Science* 364, 286–289. doi: 10.1101/469635

Wienert, B., Wyman, S. K., Yeh, C. D., Conklin, B. R., and Corn, J. E. (2020). CRISPR off-target detection with DISCOVER-seq. *Nat. Protoc.* 15, 1775–1799. doi: 10.1038/s41596-020-0309-5

Wu, X., Scott, D. A., Kriz, A. J., Chiu, A. C., Hsu, P. D., Dadon, D. B., et al. (2014). Genome-wide binding of the CRISPR endonuclease Cas9 in mammalian cells. *Nat. Biotechnol.* 32, 670–676. doi: 10.1038/nbt.2889

Xin, H., Wan, T., and Ping, Y. (2019). Off-targeting of base editors: BE3 but not ABE induces substantial off-target single nucleotide variants. *Signal. Transduct. Target Ther.* 4:9. doi: 10.1038/s41392-019-0044-y

Yan, W., Mirzazadeh, R., Garnerone, S., Scott, D., Schneider, M., Kallas, T., et al. (2019). Breaks labeling *in situ* and sequencing (BLISS). *Res. Square*. doi: 10.21203/rs.2.1448/v2

Yan, W. X., Mirzazadeh, R., Garnerone, S., Scott, D., Schneider, M. W., Kallas, T., et al. (2017). BLISS is a versatile and quantitative method for genome-wide profiling of DNA double-strand breaks. *Nat. Commun.* 8:15058. doi: 10.1038/ncomms15058

Yang, L., Grishin, D., Wang, G., Aach, J., Zhang, C. Z., Chari, R., et al. (2014). Targeted and genome-wide sequencing reveal single nucleotide variations impacting specificity of Cas9 in human stem cells. *Nat. Commun.* 5:5507. doi: 10.1038/ncomms6507

Zeng, J., Wu, Y., Ren, C., Bonanno, J., Shen, A. H., Shea, D., et al. (2020). Therapeutic base editing of human hematopoietic stem cells. *Nat. Med.* 26, 535–541. doi: 10.1038/s41591-020-0790-y

Zheng, Z., Liebers, M., Zhelyazkova, B., Cao, Y., Panditi, D., Lynch, K. D., et al. (2014). Anchored multiplex PCR for targeted next-generation sequencing. *Nat. Med.* 20, 1479–1484. doi: 10.1038/nm.3729

Zhou, S., Fatima, S., Ma, Z., Wang, Y. D., Lu, T., Janke, L. J., et al. (2016). Evaluating the safety of retroviral vectors based on insertional oncogene activation and blocked differentiation in cultured thymocytes. *Mol. Ther.* 24, 1090–1099. doi: 10.1038/mt.2016.55

4

Baboon Envelope Pseudotyped "Nanoblades" Carrying Cas9/gRNA Complexes Allow Efficient Genome Editing in Human T, B and CD34+ Cells and Knock-in of AAV6-Encoded Donor DNA in CD34+ Cells

Alejandra Gutierrez-Guerrero [1†], Maria Jimena Abrey Recalde [1,2†], Philippe E. Mangeot [1], Caroline Costa [1], Ornellie Bernadin [1], Séverine Périan [1], Floriane Fusil [1], Gisèle Froment [1], Adriana Martinez-Turtos [3], Adrien Krug [3], Francisco Martin [4], Karim Benabdellah [4], Emiliano P. Ricci [1,5], Simone Giovannozzi [6,7], Rik Gijsbers [6], Eduard Ayuso [8], François-Loïc Cosset [1] and Els Verhoeyen [1,3*]

[1] CIRI–International Center for Infectiology Research, Inserm, U1111, Université Claude Bernard Lyon 1, CNRS, UMR5308, Ecole Normale Supérieure de Lyon, Université Lyon, Lyon, France, [2] Laboratory of Lentiviral Vectors and Gene Therapy, University Institute of Italian Hospital, National Scientific and Technical Research Council (CONICET), Buenos Aires, Argentina, [3] Université Côte d'Azur, INSERM, Nice, France, [4] Centre for Genomics and Oncological Research (GENYO), Genomic Medicine Department, Pfizer/University of Granada/Andalusian Regional Government, Granada, Spain, [5] Laboratory of Biology and Modeling of the Cell (LBMC), Université de Lyon, Ecole Normale Supérieure de Lyon (ENS de Lyon), Université Claude Bernard, Inserm, U1210, CNRS, UMR5239, Lyon, France, [6] Laboratory for Viral Vector Technology & Gene Therapy, Department of Pharmaceutical and Pharmacological Sciences, Faculty of Medicine, Katholieke Universiteit Leuven, Leuven, Belgium, [7] KU Leuven, Department of Microbiology, Immunology and Transplantation, Allergy and Clinical Immunology Research Group, Leuven, Belgium, [8] INSERM UMR1089, University of Nantes, Centre Hospitalier Universitaire, Nantes, France

*Correspondence:
Els Verhoeyen
els.verhoeyen@ens-lyon.fr;
els.verhoeyen@unice.fr

[†] These authors have contributed equally to this work

Programmable nucleases have enabled rapid and accessible genome engineering in eukaryotic cells and living organisms. However, their delivery into human blood cells can be challenging. Here, we have utilized "nanoblades," a new technology that delivers a genomic cleaving agent into cells. These are modified murine leukemia virus (MLV) or HIV-derived virus-like particle (VLP), in which the viral structural protein Gag has been fused to Cas9. These VLPs are thus loaded with Cas9 protein complexed with the guide RNAs. Highly efficient gene editing was obtained in cell lines, IPS and primary mouse and human cells. Here, we showed that nanoblades were remarkably efficient for entry into human T, B, and hematopoietic stem and progenitor cells (HSPCs) thanks to their surface co-pseudotyping with baboon retroviral and VSV-G envelope glycoproteins. A brief incubation of human T and B cells with nanoblades incorporating two gRNAs resulted in 40 and 15% edited deletion in the Wiskott-Aldrich syndrome (WAS) gene locus, respectively. CD34+ cells (HSPCs) treated with the same nanoblades allowed 30–40% exon 1 drop-out in the WAS gene locus. Importantly, no toxicity was detected upon nanoblade-mediated gene editing of these blood cells. Finally, we also treated HSPCs with nanoblades in combination with a donor-encoding rAAV6 vector resulting in up to 40% of stable expression cassette knock-in into the WAS gene locus. Summarizing, this new technology is simple to implement, shows high flexibility for different targets including primary immune cells of human and murine origin, is relatively inexpensive and therefore gives important prospects for basic and clinical translation in the area of gene therapy.

Keywords: hematopoietic stem cells, T cell, B cell, gene editing, CRISPR/Cas9, nanoblade, immunotherapy, gene therapy

INTRODUCTION

Gene-editing approaches aim at directly manipulating the genome allowing gene disruption, gene correction, or transgene integration at a precise endogenous genomic locus. In contrast to ectopic gene expression, gene editing has the advantage of allowing a spacio-temporal and thus physiological regulation of transgene expression (Gilbert et al., 2014; Antony et al., 2018; Kuo et al., 2018). An additional advantage over gene addition using integrating viral vectors is that gene editing avoids insertional mutagenesis and gene silencing. Thus, precise genetic manipulation of cells provides unpreceded opportunities for research (Tothova et al., 2017; Chen et al., 2018; Ting et al., 2018) and therapeutic applications (Lombardo and Naldini, 2014; De Ravin et al., 2017; Diez et al., 2017; Kuo et al., 2018; Gentner and Naldini, 2019). Gene editing is based on the induction of DNA double-strand breaks (DSBs) at a specific site in the genome by endonucleases. There are various specific engineered nucleases used as gene editing tools such as zinc finger nucleases (ZFN), transcription activator-like effector nucleases (TALENs), and more recently clustered regularly interspaced short palindromic repeats (CRISPR)/associated protein 9 (Cas9) (Jinek et al., 2012; Gaj et al., 2013; Osborn et al., 2020). The most frequent DNA repair pathway that takes place after DSB is non-homologous end-joining (NHEJ). In this case DNA ends are fused without a repair template and this leads to insertion or deletion of nucleotides, often introducing frame shift mutations, totally or partially blocking gene transcription and translation (Doudna and Charpentier, 2014; Sander and Joung, 2014; Shalem et al., 2014). In contrast, homology-directed repair (HDR) results in complete gene correction by homologous recombination with the sister chromatid or delivery of a donor DNA repair template. The DSB induced by endonucleases at a specific locus can be sealed by HDR when an exogenous DNA template is provided carrying homology arms to the site of the DSB. This template is provided either by integration-deficient lentiviral vectors (IDLVs), recombinant adeno-associated viruses serotype 6 (rAAV6) or by electroporation of single-stranded DNA, or oligonucleotides (ODN) (Hendel et al., 2015a; Wang et al., 2015; Antony et al., 2018). However, since HDR is restricted to the S/G2 phase of the cell cycle, gene modification in primary cells remains a challenge for the scientific community.

In particular, the bacteria-originated CRISPR/Cas9 system has revolutionized the methodology to produce knock-out and knock-in genome editing due to its high specificity, activity and easy design to perform efficient gene editing in cell lines but also in primary cells (Chen et al., 2018; Daniel-Moreno

et al., 2019; Hartweger et al., 2019; Moffett et al., 2019). The CRISPR/Cas9 component can be introduced in the cell of interest using different methods, e.g., by using CRISPR/Cas9 encoding retroviral vectors (Heckl et al., 2014) or plasmids (Mandal et al., 2014) and RNAs (Hendel et al., 2015a) encoding for these components introduced by electroporation. Currently though, the method of choice is electroporation of ribonucleoproteins (RNPs), incorporating guide RNA(s) (gRNA), and Cas9 proteins to obtain efficient gene editing in primary human T and B cells and HSPCs (Bak et al., 2018; Wu et al., 2018; Hultquist et al., 2019). This offers a major advantage since the Cas9/gRNAs are only transiently present in the cell, thereby avoiding insertional mutagenesis as reported for integrative vectors (Howe et al., 2008; Patiroglu et al., 2016), implying a safety benefit essential for clinical applications. CRISPR/Cas9 applications cover various fields in biotechnology, biological investigation and human medicine (Gaj et al., 2013; Gupta and Musunuru, 2014). Here we focus on the value of this tool for genome editing in primary gene therapy targets such as T, B and hematopoietic stem and progenitor cells (HSPCs).

Anti-cancer strategies have been revolutionized since the invention of TCR engineered T-cell and chimeric antigen receptor T-cell (CAR-T) therapy. CAR-T cell therapy involves changing a patient's own immune cells to augment the immune reponse to cancer cells (June et al., 2015). Along with CD19 CAR-T cells for B cell malignancies (Porter et al., 2011; Kochenderfer et al., 2012), other CAR-T cells are under evaluation for hematological malignancies (HM) directed against CD5, CD33, CD70, CD123, CD38, and B cell maturation antigen (BCMA) (Townsend et al., 2018). However, CAR T cell immunotherapy is associated with toxicities, exhaustion, immune suppression, lack of long-term persistence, and low CAR T-cell tumor infiltration. Major efforts to overcome these hurdles are currently on the way (Mhaidly and Verhoeyen, 2020). This involves gene editing-mediated knockouts of immune checkpoint regulators such as PD-1, the endogenous TCR and histocompatibility leukocyte antigen (HLA) complex to avoid the graft-versus-host-disease (GvHD) and to generate universal allogeneic CAR-T cells (Ren et al., 2017). Thus, gene editing to generate therapeutic T cells permits the immunotherapy field to move forward quickly.

B cells are also interesting targets for gene editing given their involvement in B-cell dysfunctions, autoimmune diseases and infectious diseases. Indeed, B cells have the potential to induce specific immune activation. Their downstream effectors plasmablasts and plasma cells are specialized antibody-secreting cells and central to humoral immune response (Radbruch et al., 2006; Forthal, 2014). Long-lived plasma cells (LLPCs) can persist a lifetime and assure a continuous supply of serum antibodies (Amanna and Slifka, 2010). Primary B cells and plasma cells were engineered to produce therapeutic antibodies and proteins, such as antibodies against hepatitis C, anti-HIV broadly neutralizing antibodies, and the human clotting factor IX (FIX) (Luo et al., 2009; Fusil et al., 2015; Vasileva et al., 2015; Levy et al., 2016; Hung et al., 2018; Voss et al., 2019). To reprogram B cells for ectopic antibody expression, it would be advantageous to include the transition from the B-cell receptor (BCR) form to secreted immunoglobulins (Ig). To achieve this goal, genome editing in B cells can place the ectopic anti-body expression under the control of endogenous regulatory elements. More recently, CRISPR/Cas9 was used for precision editing in primary human B cells by using Cas9 mRNA or protein combined with chemically modified gRNAs (Hendel et al., 2015a; Johnson et al., 2018). This method was combined with an rAAV6 vector providing the HDR donor template to obtain efficient knock-in in primary B cells (Hung et al., 2018; Johnson et al., 2018; Feng et al., 2019). In contrast to T cells, B cells have received little attention for therapeutic gene editing purposes. Recently though, reprogramming of B cell antigen specificity to specific pathogens has been successful to protect against infections or to secrete anti-PD1 for immune check point inhibition using CRISPR/Cas9 technology (Moffett et al., 2019; Voss et al., 2019; Luo et al., 2020).

Hematopoietic stem cells are "the gene therapy target cells of choice" for cure of many genetic diseases since they will pass on the gene correction in the stem cell to all derived blood lineages. Using lentiviral gene transfer in HSCs, X-linked Severe Combined Immunodeficiency (SCID-X1) gene therapy led to 100% survival rates and over 80% efficiency (Gaspar et al., 2011). However, gene therapy using integrative vectors in HSCs is associated with safety concerns since the integration profiles of these vectors can give rise to genotoxicity or dysregulated transgene expression as detected in the SCID-X1 trials (Demeulemeester et al., 2015), Wiskott-Aldrich syndrome (WAS; Boztug et al., 2006) and X-linked chronic granulomatous disease (X-CGD, (Grez et al., 2011). For this reason, the emerging gene therapy approach of choice for HSCs is gene editing. The correction of genes at their endogenous locus in HSCs can potentially define a safer curative strategy for hematological diseases without the risk of insertional mutagenesis and assure tightly regulated expression of the transgenes by endogenous regulatory elements in all the hematopoietic cell lineages. Schiroli et al. achieved functional gene correction for the interleukin-2 receptor gamma (IL2RG) in HSCs from SCID-X1 using ZFN nucleases and an AAV6 vector encoding for a donor DNA repair template (Schiroli et al., 2017). Pavel-Dinu et al. used a CRISPR/Cas9/AAV6-based strategy to introduce the correcting cDNA into the genome under the control of the IL2RG promoter in HSCs (Pavel-Dinu et al., 2019). This approach has the benefit of maintaining the cell intrinsic expression pattern, thereby reducing the likelihood of side effects and may represent therefore a new therapeutic opportunity for SCID-X1 patients. Kuo et al. also used the CRISPR/Cas9 platform to correct another primary immunodeficiency, the X-linked hyper IgM syndrome, by introducing a normal copy of the CD40L cDNA downstream of the endogenous promoter (Kuo et al., 2018). Further, De Ravin et al. used CRISPR/Cas9-based gene editing to obtain successful gene repair of HSCs from GCD patients, by confining transgene expression to the myeloid lineage (De Ravin et al., 2017). Gene-editing strategies for β-hemoglobinopathies (β-thalassemia and sickle cell disease) have rather focused on disruption of silencing factors and regulators such as BCL11A to induce *de novo* expression of fetal hemoglobin (Canver et al., 2015; Antoniani et al., 2018; Martyn et al., 2018). Additionally, HIV infection is one of the most studied diseases using gene editing therapy approaches (Mandal et al., 2014). Strategies based on NHEJ as evoked here for β-hemoglobinopathies and HIV are attractive since NHEJ events occur more frequently in HSCs than HDR, which requires HSCs to cycle (Antony et al., 2018).

For the previously mentioned studies, different methods to deliver the gene editing tools such as electroporation, adenoviruses, AAVs, and lentiviral vectors (LVs) have been used, conferring different degrees of efficiency, toxicity, and off-target effects. Ideally, perfect gene editing tool delivery be fast, precise, non-toxic, and associated with low off-target effects. Recently, we described a vehicle for Cas9/gRNA by which the ribonucleoprotein (RNPs) are packed into a virus-like particle (VLP) from a murine leukemia virus (MLV), called "nanoblade" (Mangeot, 2019; Mangeot et al., 2019). These nanoblades contain Cas9 protein associated with gRNAs and are devoid of a viral genome, which allows thus a transient and rapid RNP delivery into the target cells. We previously have shown that these nanoblades were able to induce DSB more rapidly and efficiently than other delivery methods and they were able to deliver their cargo not only to immortalized cells but also to primary fibroblast and induced pluripotent stem cells (Mangeot et al., 2019). More interestingly, since these are viral-vector-derived particles, they carry an enveloped vector capsid and can be pseudotyped as their counterpart viral vectors with different envelope glycoproteins (gps). We have previously shown that the baboon endogenous virus (BaEV) envelope gp incorporated into a LV, allowed efficient cell entry into human T, B and HSPCs (Girard-Gagnepain et al., 2014; Levy et al., 2016; Bernadin et al., 2019). Here we evaluated if the BaEV envelope gps was as able to confer efficient nanoblade attachment to and fusion with the target cell to release the Cas9-sgRNA complexes they incorporated into relevant human T, B cells and HSPCs and permit efficient gene editing in these primary target cells.

MATERIALS AND METHODS

Plasmids

To construct the GagMLV-CAS9 fusion, sequential insertions of PCR-amplified fragments in an expression plasmid harboring the human cytomegalovirus early promoter (CMV), the rabbit beta-globin intron and polyadenylation signals were performed. For the construction of the MA-CA-NC sequence from Friend Murine Leukemia virus (Accession Number: M93134) the MA/p12 protease-cleavage site (9 aa) and the Flag-nls-spCas9 (*Streptococcus pyogenes* Cas9) amplified from pLenti CRISPR were fused (Mangeot et al., 2019). HIV-CAG-CAS9 (KLAP 229) was constructed by replacing the MA/CA/NC sequence from MLV in BIC-GAG-CAS9 (Addgene #119942) by MA/CA/NC PCR amplified from the HIV sequence

(NL4-3) using XhoI and AgeI sites. A protease cleavage site (KARVLAEAMS corresponding to MA/CA HIV-protease site) was inserted upstream the flag-CAS9sp sequence. BaEVRless envelope glycoproteins were previously described (Girard-Gagnepain et al., 2014). All envelope glycoproteins were expressed in the phCMV-G expression plasmid (Maurice et al., 2002).

The cassette containing SFFV-GFP DNA flanked by the WASP gene 3′ and 5′ homologous arms was excised from pDonor-SFFV-GFP plasmid by Sbf1/Pac1 digestion, blunted and cloned into plasmid vector pAAV-MCS-spA (Stratagene), that was previously digested by Pst1/Mfe1 and restriction sites were blunted. The resulting plasmid pAAV-SFFV-GFP contained the ITR2 sequences from AAV serotype 6 flanking the donor DNA cassette.

Cell Lines
The HEK293T cells (CRL11268; American Type Culture Collection; Rockville, MD) were maintained in Dulbecco's Modified Eagle's Medium (DMEM, Invitrogen, Edinburgh, Scotland) supplemented with 10 % Fetal Bovine Serum (FBS) (PAA Laboratories GmbH, Austria) and penicillin/streptomycin (Gibco, Invitrogen, Auckland, New Zeeland). The human erythroleukaemic cell line K562 (ATCC, Manassas, VA; CCL-243) and the Raji cell line (ATCC; Manassas, VA; CCL-86) were maintained in RPMI 1640 media (Gibco-BRL, Middlesex, UK), supplemented with 10% FBS and penicillin/streptomycin.

Nanoblade Production
Nanoblades particles were generated by transient transfection of HEK293T cells using $CaPO_4$ method. For MLV-derived nanoblade production, 3 μg of Cas9-MLV-gag encoding plasmid (BicCas9) was added. For HIV-derived nanoblades, 3 μg of Cas9-HIV-gag encoding plasmid (KLAP229) was added. Five micro gram of either BaEVRLess (BRL) or VSVG envelope gp-encoding plasmids were transfected for BRL or VSVG gp pseudotyping of nanoblades. For co-pseudotyping of nanoblades with BRL and VSVG, 2 μg of each envelope encoding plasmid was used. Three micro gram of each plasmid coding for a gRNA (301-agcctcgccagagaagacaa and 305-gatgcttggacgaaaatgct) was added as well as 3 μg of the HIV or MLV gag-pol encoding plasmid either for HIV- or MLV-based nanoblade production, respectively. Medium was replaced by Optimen supplemented with Hepes (Gibco, Invitrogen, Auckland, New Zealand) and penicillin/streptomycin 18 h post-transfection. Nanoblades were harvested 48 h post-transfection, centrifuged and filtered through 0.45 μm. Low speed concentration of the nanoblades was performed overnight at 3,000 g and 4°C. The concentrated nanoblades were collected the following morning and stored at 4°C.

Cas9 Quantification in the Nanoblades by ELISA
Recombinant Cas9 (New England Biolabs, USA) was used to generate a standard curve (20μM, 6 serial dilutions of 1/2), while the nanoblade supernatants were diluted 1/200 and 1/400. The dilutions were performed in coating buffer (1%

Triton) and were then coated onto 96-well-plates by incubation overnight at 4°C. The following day, the wells were incubated with washing buffer (PBS/0.05% Tween) and blocked with PBS/0.05%Tween/3%BSA (Sigma). Subsequently the wells were washed and the primary anti-Cas9 antibody (Cas9-7A9-3A3, 14697P; Cell signaling Technology, Inc., USA) was added at 1/1,000 dilution in PBS/3% BSA, and incubated at RT for 1 h, while shaking. Before and after 1 h incubation with a secondary anti-mouse HRP (F6009-X639F South biotech, USA) diluted 1/10,000 in PBS/3%BSA, a wash-step was performed. Finally, the mixed TMB substrate solution, containing HRP substrate was added for 20 min (Bethyl, Inc., Texas, USA). Stop reaction was added in each well and protein was measured at 450 nm in a Multiskan FC (Thermo Scientific).

Production of AAV6 Vectors
The pAAV-SFFV-GFP contained the ITR2 sequences from AAV serotype 6 flanking the donor DNA cassette and was used to produce recombinant AAV2/6 vectors as described previously (Ayuso et al., 2010). Briefly, HEK293 cells in CellStack-5 chambers (CS5) were transfected with two plasmids (pDG6 containing rep2cap6 sequences and adenovirus genes, and the vector plasmid pAAV-SFFV-GFP) by the calcium phosphate precipitation method, cells were harvested 72 h post-transfection by centrifugation. The cell pellet was resuspended in TBS buffer and AAV particles were extracted by freeze-thaw cycles. Upon centrifugation, the supernatant was PEG-precipitated, then purified by double CsCl density gradient ultracentrifugation, and finally formulated in 1 × DPBS containing Ca^{2+} and Mg^{2+} through dialysis in Slide-A-Lyzer 10 K cassettes (Thermo Scientific, Illkirch, France). Vector genomes were titrated by quantitative PCR as followed: 3 μl of purified AAV vectors were treated with 4U of DNase I (Sigma-Aldrich) in DNase buffer (13 mM Tris pH7.5, 0.12 mM $CaCl_2$, and 5 mM $MgCl_2$) for 45 min at 37°C. Then, DNase I-resistant nucleic acids were purified by the NucleoSpin RNA Virus kit (Macherey-Nagel, Hoerdt, France), and vector genomes were quantified by TaqMan qPCR in Premix Ex Taq probe qPCR master mix (TaKaRa Bio, Saint-Germain-en-Laye, France). Primers were targeted to ITR2 sequence and the standard curve was prepared as described previously (D'Costa et al., 2016).

Primary Lymphocyte Isolation
Peripheral blood samples were obtained from healthy donors after informed consent and approval was obtained by the ethical committee of the hospital according to the Helsinki declaration. PBMCs were isolated using Ficoll gradient (Sigma-Aldrich, St Louis, MO). $CD19^+$ B cells and $CD3^+$ T cells were purified by negative selection using the B cell isolation Kit II (Miltenyi Biotec) for $CD19^+$ B cells and the human Pan T cells isolation kit (Miltenyi Biotec) for the $CD3^+$ T cells following manufacturer's instructions followed by separation through the Automacs pro-separator (Miltenyi Biotec). Purity of isolated B and T cells was monitored using anti-hCD19APC and anti-hCD3PE antibodies (Miltenyi Biotec), respectively, and was analyzed by flow cytometry (MACSQuant VYB, Milteny Biotech).

CD34$^+$ Cells Isolation

Umbilical cord blood (CB) samples from full-term pregnancies (provided by Lyon Sud Hospital, Lyon) were collected in bags containing anti-coagulant after informed consent of donors and approval was obtained by the ethics committees of the hospitals according to the Helsinki Declaration. Low-density cells were separated by Ficoll gradient (Sigma-Aldrich, St Louis, MO). CD34$^+$ purification was performed by positive magnetic cell separation using the Automacs pro-separator (Miltenyi Biotech) after staining of the cells with the human CD34$^+$ MicroBead Kit (Miltenyi Biotec). Purity of the selected CD34$^+$ cell fraction was evaluated by FACS analysis (FACSCanto, BD) with APC-conjugated anti-CD34 antibody (Miltenyi Biotech). Cells were frozen in FCS 10% DMSO for later use.

Transduction of Cells With Nanoblades

For nanoblade transduction into cell lines: 2E5 293T, K562, or Raji cells were plated in 6- (293T) or 24-well plates (K562, Raji) and nanoblades, equivalent to 4 μm of Cas9 protein, were added. Cells were pelleted 48 h post-transduction for subsequent DNA extraction and PCR. For nanoblade transduction of lymphocytes: freshly isolated unstimulated lymphocytes were seeded in RPMI 1640 medium (Gibco Invitrogen, Auckland, New Zeland) supplemented with 10% FSC (Lonza, Verviers, Belgium) and penicillin/streptomycin (Gibco, Invitrogen, Auckland, New Zealand). B cells were stimulated for 24 h with 200 ng/ml Pansorbin A [Staph. Protein A (SpA; Sigma)] and 100 ng/ml IL-2. T cells were activated for 3 days with IL-7 (20 ng/ml; Miltenyi Biotech) or stimulated through the TCR using TransAct CD3/CD28 beads (Miltenyi Biotech) supplemented with IL-2 (100 ng/ml) in RPMI medium as previously described (Bernadin et al., 2019). CD34$^+$ cells were thawed and seeded in Cellgro medium (Cell genix, Germany) and stimulated with cytokines (human thrombopoietin (hTPO), 20 ng/ml; human stem cell factor (hSCF), 100 ng/ml; human FMS-like tyrosine kinase 3 ligand (hFlt3-L),100ng/ml) for 24 h before incubation with nanoblades. Viability was determined before and after nanoblade incubation (see below).

For nanoblade transduction of primary cells, 1.5 × 10^5 CD34$^+$, T and B cells were seeded in 48-well-plates coated with RetroNectin® (Clontech/Takara; 12 μg/ml PBS according to manufacturer's recommendations) to which nanoblades (4 μm of Cas9 protein), were added. After 8–16 h of incubation with nanoblades, fresh media was added. 8 h later cells were pelleted for DNA extraction. T cells preactivated for 3 days with IL-7 (20 ng/ml; Miltenyi Biotech) and incubated with nanoblades or not as described above, were continued in culture supplemented with rIL-7 or in the presence of TransAct CD3/CD28 beads (Miltenyi Biotech) supplemented with IL-2 (100 ng/ml) in RPMI. Cells were replenished with IL-7 or IL-2, respectively every 3 days. Cell viability (DAPI staining), proliferation rates, gene editing, and phenotyping was performed by FACS for detecting surface expression of CD4, CD8, CD45RA, CD45RO day 3, day 6, and day 10 of culture.

For pro T cell differentiation, CB CD34$^+$ cells were cultured in 48-well plates coated with a Dll4 Fc fusion protein (Dll4-Fc, 5 mg/mL; PX9Therapeutics, Grenoble, France). Cultures were initiated at 3 × 10^4 CD34$^+$ cells per well in X-VIVO-20 medium (Lonza, Basel, Switzerland) and supplemented with 20% defined fetal calf serum (Hyclone; Thermo Fisher Scientific, Illkirch, France) and cytokines: hIL-7, hFlt3-L, hSCF, and hTPO (each at 100 ng/mL; Miltenyi Biotech). Nanoblades preincubated with vectofusin (12 μg/mL; Miltenyi Biotech) were added to the pro T cell cultures at day 5 of differentiation for 24 h, then pelleted for DNA extraction and PCR. At day 3, 7, and 14 of culture, the cells were analyzed by flow cytometry for surface expression of CD34, CD7, and CD5 to distinguish the T cell subpopulations.

Viability

Viability of T, B, and CD34$^+$ cells upon nanoblade incubation was determined using Annexin V/ propidium iodide staining and was then analyzed by flow cytometry.

Quantification of DNA Editing Efficacy

Genomic DNA extraction for cell lines and primary cells was performed using the NucleoSpin tissue kit (Macherey-Nagel, GmBH & Co.) The genomic region flanking the cleavage site targeted by the nanoblades with two gRNAs (301 and 305) was amplified by PCR with the WASFw/WASRv primers (AGGGTTCCAATCTGATGGCG/TTGAGAACTGGCTTGCAAGTCC) or the WAS2Fw/WAS2Rv(ATTGCGGAAGTTCCTCTTCTTACCCTG/TTCCTGGGAAGGGTGGATTATGACGGG). The PCR product was run on a 1% agarose gel. With the WASFw/WASRv primer pair one observed one fragment of 811 bp when no cleavage or only 1 DSB occurred and an additional fragment of 647 bp when the two gRNA (301 and 305) target sites were cut simultaneously in the WAS gene. With the WAS2Fw/WAS2Rv primer pair we observed a 351 bp band when no cleavage or only 1 DSB occurred and an additional fragment of 227 bp was observed when the two gRNA (301 and 305) target sites were cut simultaneously in the WAS gene. The percentage of cleavage was determined by densitometry with FluorChem Sp (Alfpha Inmotech) of the two bands. Note that the gel blots for the PCR products shown in the figures were in some cases overexposed and contrast was increased to better see the two PCR bands but the original unsaturated images were used for quantification.

Detection of Single gRNA On-target Efficiency

In addition, upon nanoblade incubation, genomic DNA of the cells was isolated and the genomic region flanking the cleavage site targeted by the nanoblades with two gRNAs (301 and 305) was amplified by PCR with the hWASFw/hWASRv primers. The fragment of 811 bp generated using the hWASFw/hWASRv primer pair englobing the two gRNA target sites was separated from the 647 bp band present when both gRNA target sites were cut (**Figure 6**). The residual single cuts at target sequences for gRNA301 or gRNA305 were evaluated in the 811 pb PCR band by Sanger sequencing using following primers: Fw-target 1 (GCCCAAGCTCAGCCTAACG) for gRNA301 target site and RV-Target 2 (GAAATGCCGGAAGTCCACTGG) for gRNA305 target site. The chromatograms were analyzed by the online tool ICE (https://ice.synthego.com) and TIDE (https://tides.deskgen.

com) (Brinkman et al., 2014). ICE analysis allows for +40bp/-40pb INDEL detections while by default the TIDE algorithm allows +10 bp/−10 bp INDEL detection.

Off-target Detection

Genomic loci that were similar to the gRNA 301 and gRNA 305 target sequence were identified through CRISPR Seek (http://www.bioconductor.org). We selected the two most probable off-target genomic sites for gRNA301 target sequence and the two most probable off target for gRNA 305 target sequence. PCR primers were designed to amplify a 400 bp fragment around the genomic region of these off-target site (See **Supplementary Tables 1, 2**). Firstly, genomic DNA was extracted from nanoblade-treated cells using the Nucleospin gDNA extraction kit (Macherey-Nagel). Then, 50 ng of genomic DNA was used for PCR amplification. The PCR products were verified for off-target cuts by performing the surveyor assay: PCR products were diluted by a factor 2 and complemented with Buffer 2 (New England Biolabs) to a final concentration of 1X. Diluted PCR amplicons were then heat denatured at 95°C and cooled down to 20°C with a 0.1°C/second ramp. Heteroduplexes were incubated for 30 min at 37°C in presence of 10 units of T7 Endonuclease I (NEB). Samples were finally run on a 2.5% agarose gel or on a BioAnalyzer chip (Agilent) to assess editing efficiency. In parallel, the obtained PCR-products for off-target sites, were purified for Sanger sequencing using a kit (Nucleospin Gel and PCR Clean up kit, Macherey Nagel, ref 740609). Sanger sequencing used the same primers as for the Surveyor assay (**Supplementary Tables 1, 2**). The obtained sequences were then analyzed for INDELs at the off-target sites using ICE (https://ice.synthego.com) and TIDE analysis (Brinkman et al., 2014).

Combined Nanoblades and AAV6 Treatment of K562 Cells and Human CD34+ Cells

K562 cells and CD34+ cells were treated with nanoblades as described above. Together with the nanoblades, the rAAV6 vectors encoding for the donor cassette were added to the cells at indicated MOIs. CD34+ cells were pre-stimulated 72 h in Cellgro medium supplemented with cytokines (hTPO, 20 ng/ml; hSCF, 100 ng/ml; hFlt3-L; 100 ng/ml) and seeded on plates coated with RetroNectin® (Clontech/Takara; 12 µg/ml PBS) according to manufacturer's recommendations, prior to nanoblade (4 µmoles of Cas9 protein) and rAAV6 addition. Eight hours later the medium was changed for Cellgro medium supplemented with cytokines and cultured for 48 h. The cells were washed, counted, and used for flow cytometry analysis, pelleted for genomic DNA isolation to confirm stable integration of the donor cassette or seeded in methyl cellulose medium (STEMCELL Technologies) to perform a colony forming cell (CFC) assay according manufacturer's recommendation (Levy et al., 2017). CFCs were analyzed at day 14 of culture for GFP expression and DNA was isolated from these CFCs to confirm stable integration of the donor cassette by PCR.

Analysis of Stable Integration of Donor Cassette in K562 and CD34+ Cells

Genomic DNA isolated from K562 or CD34+ cells or CFCs was subjected to PCR with 1 forward primer situated in the endogenous WAS locus, WAS-FW (AGGGGCTCGCTCTGTAATTA) and a reverse primer in the reporter GFP, REV-GFP (AACTTGTGGCCGTTTACGTC).

Statistical Analysis

We have applied the unpaired t-test to compare two sample groups of the experiment which are performed at least three times using for each experiment a different primary cell donor and a different nanoblade preparation.

RESULTS

BaEV and VSV-G gp Co-pseudotyped Nanoblades Confer High Level Gene Editing in Cell Lines

Earlier, we developed the nanotechnology called nanoblades, which are virus-like particles (VLPs) derived from the murine leukemia virus (MLV) (Mangeot et al., 2019). These MLV-based nanoblades are composed of a gag polyprotein fused to a flag-tagged version of *Streptococcus pyogenes* Cas9 (Gag-Cas9) and separated by a proteolytic cleavage site borrowed from the MA/p12 MLV junction (**Figures 1A–C**). These particles can incorporate one or more guide RNAs through association with Cas9. Here, we developed the corresponding HIV-derived nanoblades by fusing Cas9 to the HIV gag protein. To allow release of the Cas9 into the cells, a proteolytic site situated between HIV MA and CA was inserted between Gag and Cas9, which can be cleaved by the HIV protease in the HIV-based nanoblades (**Figure 1C**). Nanoblade cell entry is conferred by surface display of envelope gps equivalent to pseudotyping of γ-retroviral and LV particles (VSVG, BaEVRless, **Figure 1D**) (Girard-Gagnepain et al., 2014). To produce the nanoblades, we utilized a protocol similar as used for MLV retroviral or LV production. HEK-293T cells were transfected by the CaPO4 method with plasmids coding for MLV or HIV Gag-Cas9, Gag-pol and plasmids coding for one or more single-guide RNA (gRNA) and viral envelope glycoproteins (**Figure 1A**), which then released the pseudotyped nanoblades in the culture medium (**Figure 1B**).

Previously, it became clear that MLV-based nanoblades co-pseudotyped with VSV-G and BaEV gps were more efficacious for gene editing in cell lines than single gp pseudotyped nanoblades Interestingly, we quantified the amount of Cas9 protein in the nanoblades by ELISA and detected that when both envelopes were present on the MLV-based nanoblades, more than two-fold higher Cas9 protein levels had incorporated than when either of the two envelopes (BaEV or VSVG) was present alone (**Figure 2A**). Equivalent results were obtained in the context of HIV-based nanoblades (**Figure 2A**). This observation suggested that the combination of both envelope glycoproteins

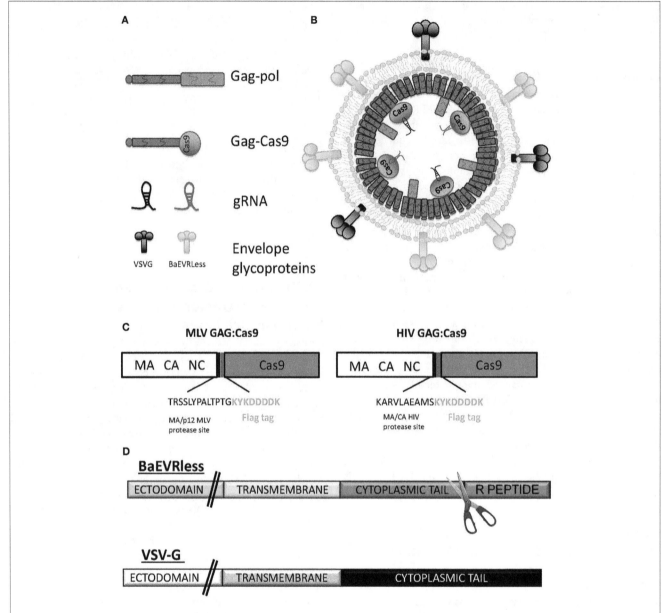

FIGURE 1 | Schematic presentation of nanoblades. **(A)** Representation of the different components of the nanoblades: gag-pol, the gag-Cas9 fusion protein, the different gRNA and the envelope glycoproteins (gps), **(B)** Schematic representation of the assembly of a nanoblade particle, **(C)** Scheme of the MLV GAG:Cas9 fusion (left) and HIV GAG:Cas9 fusion (right) indicating the inserted MLV or HIV protease site followed by a Flag tag. **(D)** Schematic representation of the mutant BaEV envelope gp (BaEVRless) and the VSV-G envelope gp. The R-peptide of the cytoplasmic tail of BaEVwt was deleted resulting in the BaEVRLess mutant gp.

helped recruiting Cas9 protein and the associated gRNAs into the nanoblades.

To evaluate the efficiency of the MLV- and HIV-based nanoblades, we first targeted the 293T cell line for induction of genomic DSB. We designed two gRNA targeting the exon 1 of the WASP gene, which will result in a 170 bp deletion in the WAS locus. This NHEJ-mediated dropout of exon 1, can readily be detected by PCR using the primer pair, WASFw and WASRv, indicated in **Figure 2B**. To assess if the higher incorporation of Cas9 also induced more gene editing, we incubated 293T cells with the different MLV- and

HIV-based nanoblades displaying either of the two envelope gps (BaEV or VSVG) or each one alone. We isolated genomic DNA and performed a PCR using WASFw and WASRv primers to amplify the WAS gene locus, 48 h post-treatment. Coinciding with higher Cas9 incorporation in MLV nanoblades, we observed that the percentage of gene editing was higher when both envelopes were present (up to a 60% of exon 1 deletion for V+B, **Figures 2C,D**) as compared to BaEV alone (up to 31% exon1 deletion) and VSV-G alone (up to 25% exon 1 deletion) (**Figures 2C,D**). HIV-derived nanoblades showed a similar result (**Figures 2C,D**). Moreover, no toxicity

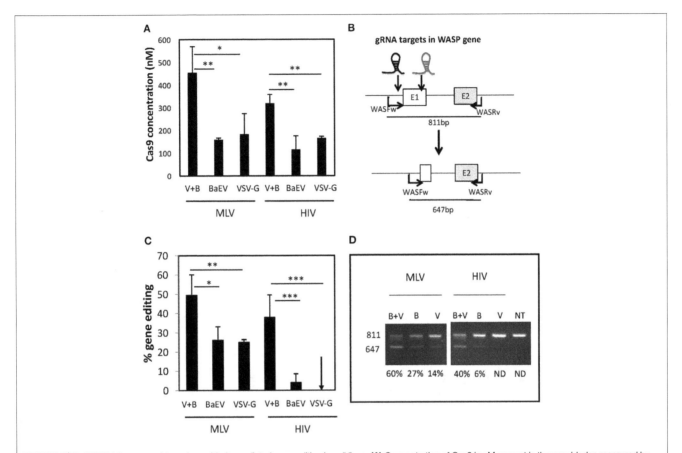

FIGURE 2 | BaEV/VSV-G gp pseudotyped nanoblade-mediated gene editing in cell lines. **(A)** Concentration of Cas9 in nM present in the nanoblades measured by ELISA in MLV and HIV-derived nanoblades co-pseudotyped with BaEV- and VSVG-gps (B + V) or pseudotyped only with BAEV-gp or VSVG-gp (V) (means ± SD, $n = 3$; student t-test, *$p < 0.05$ and **$p < 0.01$) **(B)** Schematic representation of expected band sizes of WAS PCR product with WASFw/WASRv primers before the cleavage (811 bp), which represent the intact WAS gene and the edited WAS gene after the deletion upon DSB at both gRNA targets (647 bp); the gRNA-301 and−305 target sites are indicated as a black and red gRNA, respectively; **(C)** Graph summarizing percentage of cleavage (right) (means ± SD; MLV B + V $n = 17$, MVL B $n = 4$, MLV V $n = 5$, HIV B + V $n = 16$, HIV B $n = 7$, HIV V $n = 6$; student t-test, *$p < 0.05$, **$p < 0.01$, and ***$p < 0.001$). **(D)** Representative electrophoresis gel of the PCR products on genomic DNA from 293T cells transduced with MLV or HIV nanoblades co-pseudotyped with B + V, B, or V gps; quantification of gene editing is indicated for each lane (left).

of nanoblades was detected on 293T cells and gene editing was stable (**Supplementary Figure 1**).

BaEV and VSV-G gp Co-pseudotyped Nanoblades Permit Efficient Gene Editing in Human T and B Cells

Since the BaEV and VSV-G gp co-pseudotyped nanoblades, outperformed the single pseudotypes for gene editing in 293T cells, we set out to evaluate them on valuable primary gene therapy targets such as human T and B cells. These cells are not easy to transfect and electroporation of Cas9/gRNA RNPs is toxic to some extent. Importantly, the BaEV envelopes have been shown in the context of lentiviral vectors to allow efficient entry in T cells as well as B cells without affecting their survival (Levy et al., 2016; Bernadin et al., 2019). As depicted in **Figure 3A**, T cells were pre-stimulated through the T cell receptor (TCR) using anti-CD3/anti-CD28-coated beads or alternatively with the T cell survival cytokine, IL-7, and then transduced with the MLV- and HIV-derived nanoblades loaded with Cas9 associated

with the 2 gRNAs directed again exon 1 of WAS (**Figure 3B**). Following 24 h nanoblade incubation genomic DNA was isolated and gene editing was evaluated by PCR using the WAS2Fw and WAS2Rv primer pair resulting in a 351 bp band when none or only one of the gRNAs target site was cut or a 227 bp band when both target sites were cut simultaneously (**Figure 3B**). For T cells stimulated through the TCR, we detected up to 40% of genomic deletion with the MLV nanoblades while HIV nanoblades resulted maximum in 25% deletion (**Figure 3C**). Upon a much milder stimulation with survival cytokine IL7, no difference between the two nanoblade systems (MLV or HIV), was detected resulting in up to 35% of WAS gene deletion (**Figure 3D**). Of note, we are revealing here by PCR only the cells that were cut at both gRNA target sites simultaneously. We verified stability of gene editing in two different culture conditions for T cells: (1) IL-7 (survival cytokine) culture and (2) CD3/CD28 stimulation inducing proliferation for 10 days. We evaluated for these cultures, gene editing, cell survival and proliferation, as also the % CD4 and % CD8 memory (CD45RO+) and naïve (CD45RA+

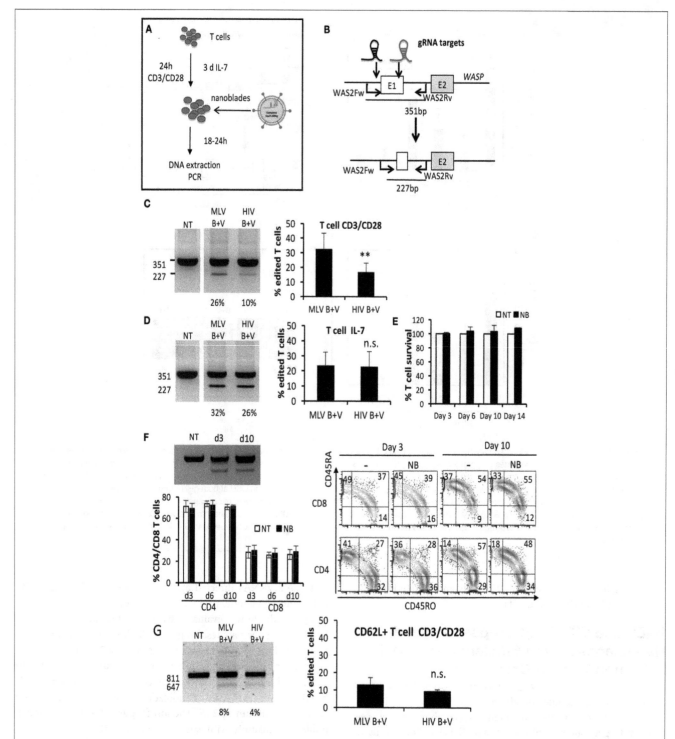

FIGURE 3 | BaEV/VSV-G gp displaying nanoblades allow efficient gene-editing in human T cells. **(A)** Outline of T cell activation and incubation with nanoblades for evaluation of CRISPR/CAS9 gene editing. **(B)** Schematic representation of expected band sizes of the PCR products using the WAS2Fw/WAS2Rv primer pair without cleavage (351 bp) and after gene-edited deletion into the WAS gene (227 bp); gRNA-301 and−305 target sites are indicated as black and red gRNA, respectively. CD3/CD28 activated **(C)** or IL-7 stimulated **(D)** T cells transduced with MLV- or HIV-based nanoblades co-pseudotyped with BAEV- and VSVG-gps (B + V) in the presence of retronectin. **(C,D)** Representative electrophoresis gels of the PCR products using the WAS2Fw/WAS2Rv primer pair; percentage of edited T cells is indicated under each lane (left) and summarizing graph showing percentage of gene editing (right) (means ± SD, MLV B + V n = 3, HIV B + V n = 3; student t-test, $^{**}p$ < 0.01, n.s, not significant). Survival **(E)** and gene editing **(F)** over time are shown for IL-7 stimulated T cells incubated with MLV nanoblades or not (NT) and continued in culture in the presence of IL-7 (means ± SD, NT n = 3, NB n = 3). Cell survival was determined by DAPI staining and is shown for the nanoblade treated

(Continued)

FIGURE 3 | cells (NB) relative to the not treated cells (NT), for which cell survival was set to 100%. **(F)** The percentage of CD4 and CD8 T cells is shown and a representative electrophoresis and flow cytometry plot are shown for CD45RO and CD45RA phenotyping for day 3 and 10 of IL-7 stimulated T cells incubated with MLV nanoblades or not (NT) and continued in culture in the presence of IL-7 (means ± SD, NT $n = 3$, NB $n = 3$; electrophoresis gel and flow cytometry plot: representative of $n = 3$). **(G)** CD3/CD28 activated purified CD62L$^+$ T cells transduced with MLV- or HIV-derived nanoblades, co-pseudotyped with BaEV- and VSVG-gps (B + V) in the presence of retronectin. Representative electrophoresis gels of the PCR products using the WASFw/WASRv primer pair (see **Figure 2B**); the percentage of edited CD62L$^+$ T cells is indicated under each lane (left) and graph summarizing percentage of gene editing (right) (means ± SD, MLV B + V $n = 3$, HIV B + V $n = 3$; n.s., not significant).

cells) over time (**Figure 3** and **Supplementary Figure 2**). We confirmed that there is no short- nor long-term toxic effect of the nanoblades on cell survival, proliferation and that gene editing is stable over time (**Figures 3E,F** and **Supplementary Figure 2**). Moreover, no difference in CD4/CD8 T cell ratio and in memory vs. naïve T cell proportions was detected in presence or absence of nanoblades (**Figures 3E,F** and **Supplementary Figure 2**).

Another important target cell is the memory T cell, which confers long-term persistence *in vivo* and is characterized by CD62L surface expression. Therefore, we also evaluated gene editing efficiency of nanoblades in sorted CD62L$^+$ T cells. Upon incubation with anti-CD3/anti-CD28-coated beads and nanoblade incubation for 24 h CD62L$^+$ T cells were collected and gene editing was evaluated by PCR. Again, no significant difference in gene editing (10% on average) between the MLV- and HIV-based nanoblades was detected (**Figure 3G**).

Other important immature T-cell targets for gene modification are the T-cell progenitors since they may permit long-term T-cell persistence *in vivo* by assuring a continuous output of modified T cells. It was demonstrated that T-cell progenitors can be generated from CD34$^+$ hematopoietic stem and progenitor cells (HSPCs) in a feeder-cell-free culture system based on Delta-like Ligand 4 coated on culture plates in the presence of a cytokine cocktail (hSCF, hTPO, and hFlt3-L) mimicking the contact with human thymic tissue (Reimann et al., 2012) (**Supplementary Figure 3A**). Additionally, we have recently demonstrated that these *in vitro* generated progenitor T cells (pro T cells) are efficiently transduced by BaEV gp pseudotyped LVs (Bernadin et al., 2019). Moreover, these pro T cells were capable of differentiating into mature T cells *in vitro* and accelerating T-cell reconstitution *in vivo* compared with HSPCs (Bernadin et al., 2019). We therefore evaluated the performance of nanoblades in the pro T cells (**Supplementary Figure 3A**). To distinguish the different T cell populations by flow cytometry, cells were stained with CD7 and CD34 antibodies during differentiation (**Supplementary Figure 3B**). We distinguished between (1) early lymphoid progenitors (ELP; CD34$^+$CD7$^-$) and (2) early thymic progenitors (ETP; CD34$^+$CD7$^+$) and (3) the population of progenitor T cells (Pro T, CD34$^+$ CD7$^+$). We transduced the cells at day 5 of differentiation and collected the cells 24 h later. WAS gene locus showed the expected deletion (19 and 10%) due to concurrent cutting at both gRNA-target sites when using MLV or HIV nanoblades, respectively (**Supplementary Figure 3C**).

As mentioned above, B cells are also valuable targets for genetic engineering including gene editing. Before evaluating gene editing using nanoblades in primary human B cells, we treated the Raji B cell line with nanoblades and observed around

25% deletion with both HIV and MLV nanoblades (**Figure 4A**). Interestingly, when we seeded the Raji cells on Retronectin coated plates and added polybrene a two-fold increase was observed when using both transduction facilitating agents (up to 60% deletion) as compared to using polybrene alone (**Figure 4B**). Therefore, these agents were applied also during nanoblade incubation of primary B cells. It is generally accepted that human B cells are difficult to transduce with classical VSV-G gp pseudotyped vectors (Amirache et al., 2014). In contrast, LVs pseudotyped with BaEV-LVs easily can reach up to 80% B cell transduction. Therefore, we incubated human B cells pre-stimulated through the BCR with Pansorbin A and IL2, with VSV-G and BaEV gp co-pseudotyped MLV and HIV nanoblades for 24 h. We subsequently confirmed by PCR around 12–15% of DSBs at the two different target sites for the gRNA simultaneously resulting in a deletion of the WAS genomic locus (**Figure 4C**).

Nanoblades Allow Efficient Genome Editing in Primary Human HSPCs

Currently, the method of choice to allow efficient gene editing in HSPCs (CD34$^+$ cells) relies on CRISPR/Cas9 RNP electroporation. However, this manipulation affects CD34$^+$ cell viability. For obvious reasons, this should be avoided since CD34$^+$ cells are rare and isolation of sufficient CD34$^+$ cells for gene therapy can be a challenging task, especially in the case of BM failures, a family of genetic diseases that affects directly the HSPCs decreasing their numbers with age in the patients (Verhoeyen et al., 2017).

In contrast to RNP electroporation, nanoblades transfer Cas9/gRNA complexes by a mild intervention, equivalent to enveloped pseudotyped retroviral vectors and might therefore be less toxic. Firstly, we transduced the CD34$^+$ K562 cell line with equivalent amounts of MLV and HIV nanoblades. For K562 cells we obtained up to 65% deletion of the WAS gene using MLV nanoblades and up to 50% with HIV nanoblades (**Figure 5A**). In parallel, the CD34$^+$ cells were pre-stimulated with a cytokine cocktail for 16 h and then incubated with the same doses of nanoblades as used for K562 cells; 24 h later we checked the efficiency of gene editing by PCR using the WASFw and WASRv primer pair (**Figures 2B, 5B**). For primary human CD34$^+$ cells, we observed on average 35% deletion with both nanoblade systems upon a short incubation time (**Figure 5C**). Gene editing efficiency in CD34$^+$ cells is thus only two-fold lower than that obtained in the K562 cell line (**Figure 5B**). Importantly, viability of human CD34$^+$ cells was not at all affected by incubation with nanoblades (**Figure 5D**). Additionally, when the CD34$^+$ cells treated with nanoblades or not were differentiated into myeloid lineages, no differences in CFC frequencies were

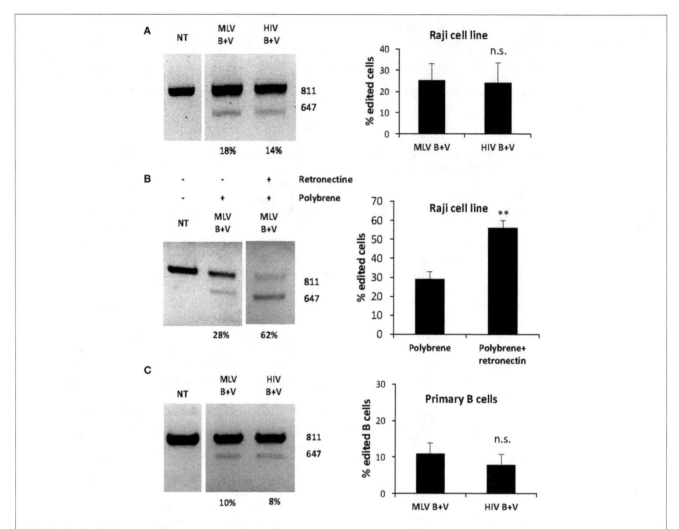

FIGURE 4 | BaEV/VSV-G gp displaying nanoblades allow efficient gene-editing in hB cells. **(A)** Raji cells transduced with MLV- or HIV-based nanoblades co-pseudotyped with BaEV- and VSVG-gps (B + V). Electrophoresis gel of the PCR product using WASFw/WASRv primers with the % gene-editing indicated for each lane (left) and summarizing graph showing percentage of gene editing (right) (means ± SD; MLV B + V n = 4, HIV B + V n = 5), **(B)** Raji cells were treated with polybrene (PB) or with polybrene and Retronectin (PB+R) and then incubated with MLV nanoblades co-pseudotyped with B + V. Electrophoresis gel of the PCR product using WASFw/WASRv primers with the % gene-editing indicated for each lane (left) Graph showing percentage of gene editing (right) (means ± SD; MLV B + V n = 3, HIV B + V n = 3; student t-test, **p < 0.01, n.s., not significant). **(C)** Primary human B cells preactivated with Pansorbin A and IL-2 were incubated with MLV or HIV nanoblades co-pseudotyped with BaEV- and VSVG-gps (B + V). Representative gel of the PCR product using WASFw/WASRv primers with the percentage of gene-editing indicated for each lane (left) and graph showing percentage of gene editing (right) (means ± SD MLV B + V n = 3, HIV B + V n = 3; student t-test, n.s., not significant).

detected (**Figure 5D**). To verify if the editing by nanoblades had an impact on CD34+ cell composition we performed a surface staining for CD34, CD38, and CD90. No differences in the percentage of the most primitive HSCs (CD34$^+$CD38$^-$CD90$^+$) between untreated and nanoblade-treated CD34+ cells were detected. Thus, no skewing of the CD34$^+$ subpopulation was induced (**Figure 5E**). As already mentioned, PCR analysis on genomic DNA only revealed the gene editing when both guide RNAs introduced DSBs simultaneously. However, each gRNA by itself might have induced additional DSBs at their respective target site. These events might also result in frameshift and thus knock-out of the WAS reading frame. Therefore, we separated the 811 bp PCR band from the 647 bp band (cut by both gRNAs)

(**Figure 5C**). The 811 bp PCR product allowed to us to identify the single DSB events that occurred in addition to double DSB at either target site (gRNA 301 and −305). Both gRNA target sequences were separately subjected to Sanger sequencing using adapted primers and the resulting chromatographs were analyzed by ICE and TIDE to estimate the INDEL frequency at each gRNA-target site.

ICE analysis showed INDEL frequencies of up to 27% at the gRNA-301 target site and interestingly the most prevalent deletion consisted of 1 bp insertion (16%) resulting in a frameshift (**Figure 5F**). No additional INDELs were found at the gRNA-305 target site (**Figure 5F**). The same analysis was performed for 293T cells incubated with nanoblades, resulting

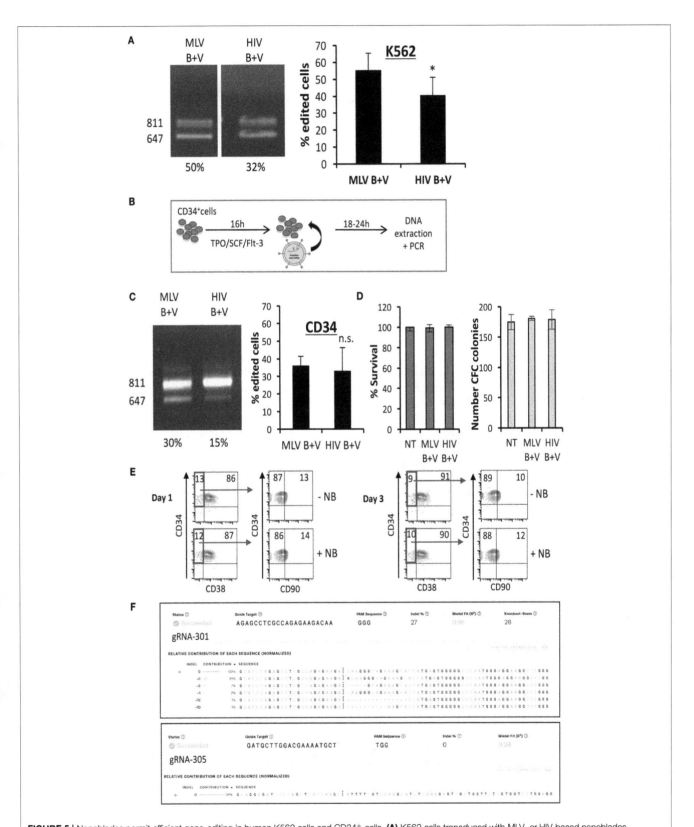

FIGURE 5 | Nanoblades permit efficient gene-editing in human K562 cells and CD34+ cells. **(A)** K562 cells transduced with MLV- or HIV-based nanoblades co-pseudotyped with BaEV- and VSVG-gps (B + V). Electrophoresis gel of the PCR product using WASFw/WASRv primers with the % gene-editing indicated for each lane (left) and summarizing graph showing percentage of gene editing (right) (means ± SD; (MLV B + V n = 7, HIV B + V n = 6; student t-test, $^{*}p$ < 0.05). **(B)** Schematic presentation of protocol used for CD34+ cells. CD34+ cells were activated with cytokines (TPO/SCF/Flt-3) for 16 h, then nanoblades were added and DNA

(Continued)

in 60% DSBs at both gRNA targets simultaneously (**Figure 2C**). ICE analysis of the additional single site INDELs in 293T cells at gRNA-301 target revealed 71% INDEL frequency while at gRNA-305 target INDEL frequencies were much lower reaching only 1% (**Supplementary Figures 4A,B**) in accordance with the differential editing efficiency obtained in CD34$^+$ cells for both gRNA-target sites (**Figure 5F**).

Although cleavage occurs with highest efficiency at on-target sites which are complementary to the gRNA protospacer domain, DSB could occur at loci with one or more mismatched bp compared to the on-target sites (gRNA 301 and 305). These events are called off-target effects and should be reduced to the minimum in gene therapy applications of genome-editing tools. We identified these sites for both gRNAs 301 and 305 (**Supplementary Tables 1, 2**). Firstly, we PCR-amplified some of the off-target sequences and performed the Surveyor assay to reveal possible mismatches that are recognized and cut by the T7 endonuclease. No off-target gene editing was revealed at the analyzed off-target sequences (**Supplementary Figure 5**). Since the Surveyor assay will not detect off-target cleavage < 5% (Sentmanat et al., 2018), we subjected the PCR products of off-target −2, −10 and −12 to Sanger sequencing and ICE analysis no off-target cleavage (INDELs) was detected using ICE analysis. TIDE analysis for the same off-target sites reported 1–3% total editing efficiency, although none of these predicted editing values were significant ($p > 0.001$) (**Supplementary Figure 6**) confirming that no off-target editing occurred.

"Nanoblades" Loaded With Cas9/sgRNA Ribonucleoproteins Combined With AAV6 Encoding for Donor DNA, Allowed Efficient Knock-in in Human CD34$^+$ Cells

MLV nanoblades performed slightly better than HIV nanoblades for gene editing in CD34$^+$ cells (**Figure 5C**), therefore we focused for knock-in experiments on the former ones. For knock-in of an expression cassette into the first exon of the WAS locus, rAAV6 vectors are considered ideal candidates since they allow high-level transduction into CD34$^+$ cells and have been used as tools for donor DNA transfer (Bak et al., 2018; Kuo et al., 2018). We generated an rAAV6 ssDNA vector genome encoding the template for homologous recombination including 3' HR and 5'HR arms of the WAS gene at each side of exon 1 (**Figure 6A**). An expression cassette with GFP under control of the SFFV promoter was inserted between the HR arms. The positions of the gRNAs, associating with Cas9 and loaded into the nanoblades are indicated. The resulting targeted integration cassette in WAS locus is represented and the positions of the primers, which

allow to confirm specific on-target integration are indicated (**Figure 6A**). First, K562 cells were treated with rAAV6 donor vector alone or rAAV6 combined with MLV-based nanoblades. Insertion of the donor template in the WAS locus resulted in a significantly higher percentage of GFP$^+$ K562 cells with high MFI on day 3, 5, 7, and 10 post-treatment as compared to rAAV6 treatment in absence of nanoblades (**Figure 6B**). rAAV6 incubation alone showed a lower percentage GFP$^+$ K562 gradually decreasing over time in agreement with the fact that rAAV6 vectors are not integrative. This was true for rAAV6 used at different MOIs (2E4 to 1E5 vector genomes). K562 genomic DNA was isolated at day 12 post-treatment and integration was confirmed by PCR using the WAS-Fw and GFP-Rv primer pair (**Figure 6A**), confirming genomic integration by homologous recombination when nanoblades were combined with rAAV6 donor vector (**Figure 6C**). As expected, incubation with rAAV6 alones did not lead to detectable on-target integration. Since efficient knock-in was demonstrated into the WAS locus of the K562 cell line, we pre-activated CD34$^+$ cells and treated them with the same combination of nanoblades and rAAV6 as indicated in **Figure 7A**. Addition of increasing amount of rAAV6 in combination with constant amounts of nanoblades resulted in 15% of knock-in for rAAV6 at MOI = 2E4, 20% for MOI = 5E4, and 35% for MOI = 1E5 (**Figure 7B**, day 10). In accordance with results obtained for K562 cells, insertion of the donor template in the WAS locus results in high levels of GFP$^+$ CD34$^+$cells with high MFI on day 3, 6, and 10 post-treatment (**Figure 7B**), while rAAV6 treatment in absence of nanoblades, resulted in decreasing percentages of GFP$^+$ CD34$^+$ cells over time (**Figure 7C**) in accordance with the fact that no integration was detected of the donor cassette at the on-target site (**Figure 7D**). Though not toxic for K562 cells, rAAV6 is known to be toxic at higher MOIs in CD34$^+$ cells. Therefore, CD34$^+$ cells treated with rAAV6 donor + nanoblades or rAAV6 alone were 24 h post-treatment allowed to differentiate into myeloid colony forming cells (CFCs). No significant decrease in number of colonies was detected compared to untransduced CD34$^+$ cells for nanoblades + rAAV6 at MOI 2E4 or 5E4 (**Figure 7E**). In addition, the percentage of GFP$^+$ colonies was equivalent with the initial percentage of GFP$^+$ CD34$^+$ cells from which these vectors were derived (**Figures 7E** vs. **B**).

DISCUSSION

Here we have demonstrated that nanoblades derived from HIV and MLV VLPs can deliver the Cas9-gRNA ribonucleoproteins into human T, B cells and HSPCs in

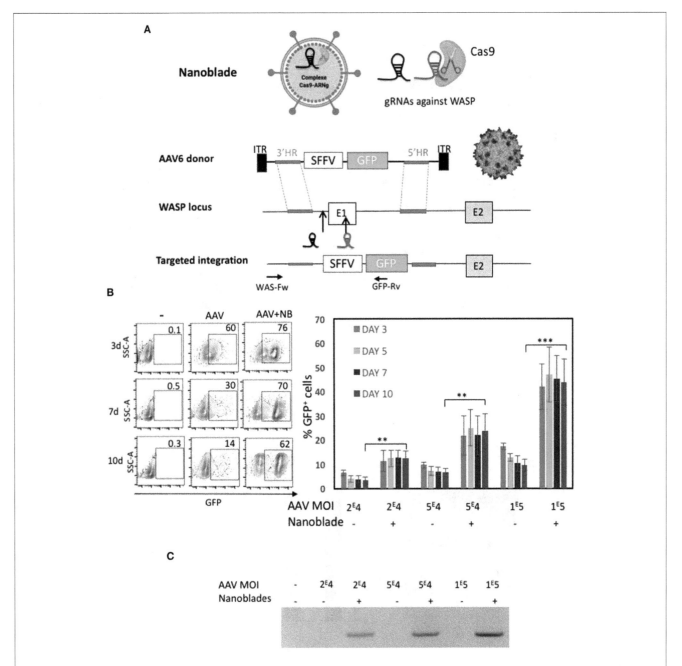

FIGURE 6 | Evaluation of nanoblades combined with rAAV6 encoding donor DNA for WAS gene locus knock-in. **(A)** Schematic representation of the nanoblades loaded with Cas9 and two sgRNA directed to the WAS locus (indicated before and inside the first exon) and the rAAV6 genome carrying the donor DNA for homologous recombination (HR); 3' HR and 5'HR arms are indicated. An expression cassette with GFP under control of the SFFV promoter was inserted between the HR arms. Targeted integration is represented with primer positions indicated used to confirm specific integration (WAS-Fw and GFP-Rv). **(B)** K562 cells were treated with rAAV6 vector alone or rAAV6 combined with MLV based nanoblades. A representative flow cytometry plot for GFP⁺ K562 cells is shown for day 3, 5, 7, and 10 post-treatment (left). A summary of the results is shown in the graph on the right (means ± SD; n = 4; student t-test, **p < 0.01, ***p < 0.001). MOIs for rAAV are indicated. **(C)** K562 genomic DNA at day 12 post-treatment was isolated and integration was determined by PCR using WAS-Fw and GFP-Rv indicated in **A**. The gel is representative of n = 4.

a transient and rapid manner without need for strong activation of these gene therapy targets, conserving thereby their phenotypes. The high-level efficiency achieved in these gene therapy targets relied on combined pseudotyping of the nanoblades with VSV-G and BaEV envelope glycoproteins, assuring high-level incorporation of Cas9 endonuclease associated with gRNA into these VLP-like structures.

Most importantly, like a retroviral transduction of these target cells, no significant toxicity is induced by incubation with the

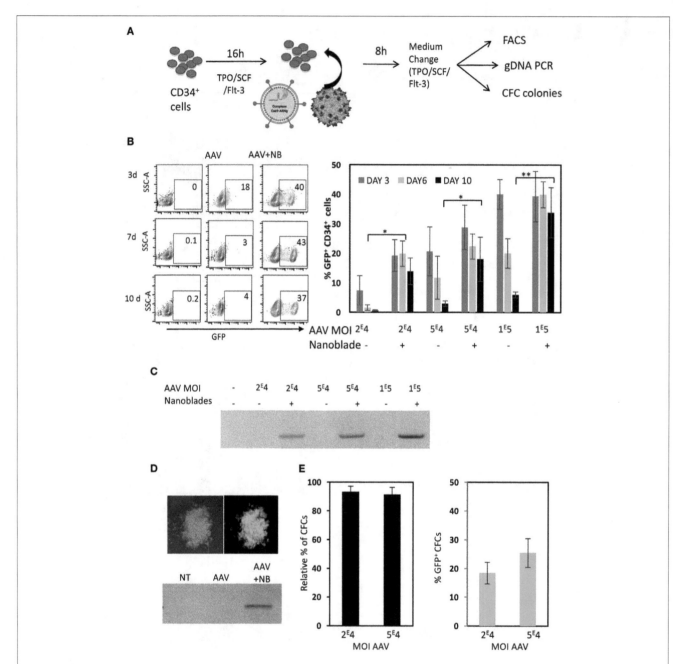

FIGURE 7 | Nanoblades confer knock-in in human CD34⁺ cells when combined with rAAV6 coding for the DNA donor cassette. **(A)** Schematic presentation of protocol used for CD34⁺ cells. CD34⁺ cells were pre-activated for 72 h with cytokines (TPO/SCF/Flt-3), then rAAV6 vector carrying the donor alone or combined with nanoblades were added and DNA extraction was performed after 24 h incubation, while flow cytometry analysis was performed on day 3, 6, and 10. CFC colonies were seeded after 24 h incubation with rAAV6 or rAAV6 + nanoblades and CFC colonies were counted and screened at 14 days for GFP expressing by flow cytometry. **(B)** A representative flow cytometry plot for GFP⁺ CD34⁺ cell is shown for day 3, 6, and 10 post-treatment with rAAV (MOI = 1 × 10⁵) or rAAV+ nanoblades (left). A summary of the results is shown in the graph on the right (means ± SD; $n = 4$; four independent CD34⁺ cell donors; student t-test, *$p < 0.05$, **$p < 0.01$). MOIs for rAAV are indicated. **(C)** Genomic DNA at day 10 post-treatment was isolated and integration was determined by PCR using WAS-Fw and GFP-Rv in **Figure 6A**. Data are representative of $n = 4$. **(D)** At 24 h post-treatment CD34⁺ cells were differentiated into myeloid colonies. At day 14 of differentiation into CFC colonies, colonies were screened for GPF expression and genomic DNA was isolated and integration was determined by PCR using WAS-Fw and GFP-Rv. Data are representative of $n = 3$. **(E)** Relative % of number of colonies for nanoblades + rAAV6 treated CD34⁺ cells compared to untreated CD34⁺ cells and % of GFP⁺ at day 14 of differentiation. MOIs for rAAV6 are indicated.

Cas9/gRNA-loaded nanoblades. This is of utmost importance for gene editing of HSPCs, which are few in number and are not as readily available as T and B cells and easily lose

their "stem cell" character by prolonged cytokine stimulation (Ahmed et al., 2004). We achieved gene editing of up to 40% of the cell revealed DSBs at two different gRNA target sites simultaneously in CD34$^+$ cells upon a brief incubation without toxic effect. This underlines the advantage of the nanoblade technology. Moreover, we revealed that an additional 27% of the CD34$^+$ cells harbored INDELs at a single gRNA target site. Further, HSPCs incubated simultaneously with nanoblades and rAAV6 vector coding for the donor DNA template resulted in up to 30–40 % of stable expression cassette knock-in into the WAS gene locus, levels relevant for clinical HSC-based gene therapy. Indeed, combining nanoblades with rAAV6 has allowed to achieve high level homologous recombination in HSPCs and was dependent on the doses of rAAV6 added. We cannot exclude here that the knock-in is driven mainly by gRNA301 since this guide was more efficient in inserting DSBs than the second gRNA305 in CD34+ cells and 293T cells. However, we cannot distinguish between knock-in upon DSB of gRNA301 or/and gRNA305 since the homologous arms remove both target sites after homologous recombination and insertion into WASP gene locus. Up to now most research groups used Cas9/gRNA RNPs and rAAV6-mediated donor template delivery targeting the CCR5 locus with an efficiency of 11% (Bak et al., 2017). Other authors targeting the IL-2RG locus to correct SCID-X1 achieved 20% HSPCs knock-in without strong toxicity (Pavel-Dinu et al., 2019). For other targeted genomic loci an efficiency of 20–30% was achieved for a monogenic knock-in (De Ravin et al., 2017; Charlesworth et al., 2018; Kuo et al., 2018; Gomez-Ospina et al., 2019; Wagenblast et al., 2019). It is estimated that a minimum gene correction/modification of 10–30% in CD34$^+$ HSPCs is required to obtain a therapeutic benefit in autologous HSC transplantation (Morgan et al., 2017). The nanoblade-mediated gene knock-in in HSPCs achieved an efficiency that becomes clinically relevant opening avenues for multiple genetic diseases and beyond.

Also in human B cells gene editing was achieved using Cas9/gRNA RNPs with high efficiency (Johnson et al., 2018; Wu et al., 2018; Moffett et al., 2019). However, most of these studies though use co-culture of B cells with feeder cells or strong activation cocktails and detailed information on toxicity induced by the electroporation is not clearly evaluated. Moreover, one study reported that immunoglobulin heavy chain locus knock-in using CRISPR/Cas9 in human B cell is quite challenging (Hartweger et al., 2019). Nanoblades provide a tool for mild introduction of the Cas9/gRNA complexes into primary B cells upon brief prestimulation and with little to no effect on B cell survival.

Different platforms are being used to deliver the CRISPR/Cas9-gRNA platform. Lattanzi et al. (Lattanzi et al., 2019) made a side by side comparison between the delivery systems for this gene editing machinery in HSPCs. They concluded that plasmid electroporation, though highly efficient for edited deletions of large genome DNA sequences, was very toxic to the HSPCs revealed by strong reduction of clonogenic potential. RNA-mediated delivery was less efficient for gene editing but associated with high cell toxicity. Delivery via lentiviral transduction was less toxic but gene editing levels in HSPCs were poor. Of importance, lentiviral transduction to deliver Cas9/gRNA will result in stable persistent expression of these components into primary cells such as T cells and

HSCs. This is an interesting approach to knock out genes of interest in primary cells, however, persistent Cas9 expression is not desirable in a therapeutic setting since this might incite an immune response against edited cells and increase off-target editing (Hendel et al., 2015b; Yu et al., 2016; Cameron et al., 2017). Additionally, continued Cas9 expression can lead to cell cycle arrest (Knopp et al., 2018). Finally, RNP-mediated delivery is the method of choice currently for primary cells because it results in high genome editing and much less cytotoxic effect as compared to previous methods above. Gundry et al. (2016) evaluated the impact of Cas9/gRNA RNP electroporation into CD34$^+$ cells. Although this method is less harmful to those previously mentioned and high-level gene editing was detected at 48 h post electroporation, 50% of the cells did not survive. This toxicity level in CD34$^+$ cells was consistent with other reports using the same approach (Genovese et al., 2014; De Ravin et al., 2017; Charlesworth et al., 2018), while higher viability was achieved after optimizing several parameters (Patsali et al., 2019).

Still the aim was to optimize gene editing with minimal cell toxicity. The nanoblades combine actually the low to undetected toxicity of retroviral delivery (VLP) and the transient expression of Cas9/gRNA RNP-mediated gene editing. Indeed, nanoblades confer efficient NHEJ-mediated gene editing in HSPCs but also in T cells but not at expense of significant induced toxicity. Indeed, we demonstrated that gene editing was stable long term in cell lines (293T and K652) treated with nanoblades and did not induce cell death nor effect on proliferation over non-treated cells. In accordance, we did not detect a significant effect on cell survival and proliferation in nanoblade treated vs. untreated primary T cells, nor in their phenotype and gene editing upon long-term culture. We demonstrated this additionally for HSPCs by the fact that they showed equivalent differentiation into myeloid lineages in absence or presence of nanoblades. To evaluate lymphoid differentiation we reconstituted NOD/SCID gammaC–/– (NSG) mice with nanoblades treated CD34$^+$ cells, which were successful in terms of humanization. However, when we isolated CD34$^+$ from the BM and T cells from the spleen of these mice we did not confirm the 30% gene editing that was detected in the initial CD34$^+$ cell population (data not shown). This is not surprising since WASP knock-out CD34+ cells will not engraft in NSG mice if the KNOCK-out is not > 90% since they have a selective disadvantage compared to WASP-positive CD34$^+$ cells (Mani et al., 2009). Moreover, from clinical trials it became clear that the WAS gene therapy conferred selective proliferative advantage for WASP expressing T and B cells and probably also HSCs (Ferrua et al., 2020, JACI).

Another important concern in use of gene editing approaches is the risk of off-target genome editing at loci that are similar in sequence of the on-target site. We have previously shown in the context of a well characterized gRNA targeting the EMX1 locus that plasmid introduction of the different CRISPR/Cas9 components resulted in 6% off-target, while the nanoblades did not reveal off-target genome editing despite of 75% on-target efficiency (Mangeot et al., 2019). In accordance, we confirmed that for two gRNA targeted to different WAS loci loaded into nanoblades no significant cutting could be detected at off-target sequences, although a more extensive off-target analysis is warranted especially when moving forward to the clinic. Equivalent to RNP transfection this is probably due to short and transient expression of the Cas9 complexed with the gRNAs.

Although corrections of β-hemaglobinopaties by gene-editing using HR were achieved in HSCs (Dever et al., 2016; Pavani et al., 2020), NHEJ might offer alternative correction strategies for gene therapy of β-thalassemia and Sickle cell disease. In their most common application, those NHEJ-mediated editing strategies efficiently disrupt disease modifiers or the β-globin locus (Cavazzana et al., 2017), resulting in therapeutic re-activation of fetal γ-globin genes, which is normally shut down in adults. Disruption of disease modifiers, such as of the γ-globin repressor BCL11A, can achieve high-level induction of γ-globin (Wu et al., 2019) in HSPCs by a single CRISPR/Cas9 RNP. Alternatively, disruption of the β-globin locus can be used to remove repressor elements of γ-globin, and in particular mimicking naturally occurring large deletions on the β-globin locus by a double-DSB strategy may achieve efficient γ-globin induction (Antoniani et al., 2018). Here we added to existing functional data for nanoblades by obtaining high-level genomic deletions in the WAS locus with nanoblades carrying two different gRNAs, which taken together validates nanoblades as efficient vectors for both the single- and double-DSB strategies outlined above.

Another monogenic disease that would benefit from nanoblade-mediated correction of HSPCs is the bone marrow failure, Fanconi Anemia (FA). HSPC-based gene therapy is very attractive treatment for FA because corrected stem cells have a selective advantage (Rio et al., 2017). This becomes clear by several different observations. Some FA patients acquired naturally correcting mutations in HSPCs, which led to expansion of these reverted clones and restoration of normal hematopoiesis (Gross et al., 2002; Mankad et al., 2006). Rio et al. achieved the same correction in FA HSPCs using an *ex vivo* lentiviral gene addition approach in a preclinical model recapitulating the expansion of reverted FA HSCs (Rio et al., 2017), which 2 years later was confirmed in the first HSC-LV-based trial for FA conducted without conditioning (Rio et al., 2019). However, since FA patients exhaust their HSCs and are easily induced into apopotosis by *ex vivo* culture and transduction procedures, HSC-based gene therapy is challenging (Verhoeyen et al., 2017). For this particular disease a corrective gene editing strategy would offer huge advantages since: (1) NHEJ repair upon gene-editing is increased in FA cells (Du et al., 2016); (2) NHEJ is the preferred mechanism of repair of DSBs in resting cells (Naka and Hirao, 2011) avoiding pre-stimulation of FA HSCs and avoiding cell death. Though NHEJ normally is used for producing knock-outs in cells by insertions or deletions, the same pathway can be utilized to create an INDEL next to an FA mutation leading to correction of FA phenotype. Roman-Rodriguez et al. (2019) therefore electroporated a pre-selected gRNA associated with Cas9 as RNPs into HSCs from FA patients and achieved correction of FA HSCs confirmed by their proliferative advantage. The introduction of the same Cas9/gRNA complex using nanoblades might allow to correct FA HSCs with even lower toxicity than RNP electroporation.

Three other groups have developed CRISPR/Cas9 vehicles that resemble the nanoblades described here. Knopp et al. (2018) replaced in an MLV retroviral particle, viral components with the MS2 phage packaging machinery to incorporate Cas9 mRNA and sgRNA into these VLPs, which were transiently delivered in multiple cell types. Gee et al. (2020) developed nanovesicles incorporating Cas9 protein and sgRNA, called NanoMedic. Using chemical induced dimerization Cas9 protein and the gRNAs encoding construct carrying a viral packaging signal both were incorporated into these nanovesicles. Indikova and Indik (2020) engineered lentivirus-based nanoparticles to co-package the U6-sgRNA template and the CRISPR/Cas9 fused with a virion-targeted protein Vpr (Vpr.Prot.Cas9), for simultaneous delivery to cells. The three systems were highly efficient for gene editing in cell lines and some in primary cells such as induced pluripotent stem cells. However, these transient CRISPR/Cas9 delivery systems were not evaluated for gene editing in human T, B and HSPCs.

The nanoblades represent a highly flexible platform for gene editing in primary hematopoietic cells and can be established easily in any laboratory. Firstly, only the plasmid coding for the gRNAs needs to be redesigned to target another genomic locus. Moreover, they can harbor two gRNAs as shown here but easily can incorporate multiple gRNAs to permit knock-out of multiple genes at once as we have demonstrated previously (Mangeot et al., 2019). Secondly, continuously, Cas9 proteins are improved to reduce off-target activity or increase efficiency and other targetable nucleases are identified e.g., Cpf1 nucleases, high fidelity Cas9, nickases, hyper-acurate Cas9 (Zetsche et al., 2015; Kleinstiver et al., 2016; Vakulskas et al., 2018). More recently, improved base editors (Webber et al., 2019) are becoming utilized for therapeutic applications (Osborn et al., 2020). All these new components for gene editing can readily be incorporated into nanoblades by fusing them to MLV or HIV gag proteins. Thirdly, since these nanoblades are derived from retroviral vectors, they can benefit from the same surface modifications, a process referred to as pseudotyping. We have previously shown that pseudotyping of HIV-derived vectors with heterologous envelopes such as baboon (BaEV) and measles virus (MV) gps, unlike the VSV-g envelope glycoprotein, allow more efficient fusion of viral membrane with the cell membrane. These BaEV and MV gp pseudotypes improved transduction of human T, B, NK cells, and HSCs (Girard-Gagnepain et al., 2014; Levy et al., 2016; Bernadin et al., 2019; Colamartino et al., 2019). We think that co-pseudotyping with VSV-G and BaEV gps on the nanoblades did not only allow more Cas9 incorporation as demonstrated but that the BaEV gp improved entry into these human blood cells as was true for their LV counterparts. VSV-G on the other hand will help the incorporation of heterologous proteins into the VLPs as it was shown that only VSV-G on its own formed "gesicules" and is able to embark high levels of protein as shown by us and our co-authors (Mangeot et al., 2011; Amirache et al., 2014). Therefore, VSV-G might help Cas9 incorporation into the nanoblades when co-expressed with BAEV gp. We also expect to have a higher incorporation of gRNA into the VSV-G+BAEV gp nanoblades since the incorporation of gRNA is Cas9 dependent as we have shown previously (Mangeot et al., 2019). In the case of MV gp pseudotyping this might even allow to improve nanoblade-mediated gene editing in the most primitive HSCs without stimulation since they allowed high level transduction when pseudotying LVs (Levy et al., 2017). More recently, LVs were engineered to specifically target hCD4$^+$ or hCD8$^+$ T cells through introduction of a scFv or a Designed Ankyrin repeat protein (DARPIN) directed against CD4 or CD8 epitopes into the measles virus glycoprotein H or the Nippa virus (NiV) glycoproteins G (Anliker et al., 2010; Bender et al., 2016). These CD4-MV and CD8-MV retargeted vectors showed, respectively, exclusive transduction into the CD4$^+$ or CD8$^+$ subset of hT cells *in vivo* in humanized NSG mice (Zhou et al., 2012, 2015). Additionally, transductional targeting of B cells and HSCs was achieved by direct inoculation of CD19-MV LVs or CD133-MV LVs, respectively into the bloodstream of humanized NSG mice (Kneissl et al., 2013; Brendel et al., 2015). Importantly, a single administration of CD8NiV-LVs encoding a CD19-CAR in the blood stream of human CD34+ humanized NSG mice generated CD19-CAR expressing CD8 T cells *in vivo*, which led to the depletion of the CD19$^+$ B cells from all hematopoietic tissues (Pfeiffer et al., 2018). Thus, pseudotyping nanoblades with these retargeted envelopes gps might open the way to *in vivo* gene editing avoiding a costly *ex vivo* procedure. Finally, since the nanoblades are derived from retroviral vectors such as MLV or LV, scaling up of nanoblade production for clinical translation will be able to rely on some of the existing facilities and new production processes such as the CliniMACs Prodigy (Miltenyi Biotech, Germany) already available for MLV and LV vectors. Though adaptations will be needed this might speed up clinical translation of these new gene editing tools.

AUTHOR CONTRIBUTIONS

AG-G, MA, OB, FF, SP, GF, and AM-T designed, performed experiments, and analyzed results. FM and KB shared the WAS donor cassette and helped with design of the WAS gRNAs and off-target site identification. PM and CC cloned the HIV-derived nanoblade system. RG and SG performed the analysis for on-target and off-target sequences. EA cloned the donor and produced the rAAV6-donor vector batch. F-LC discussed results and commented the manuscript. ER and PM shared the MLV nanoblade system and co-designed experiments. EV supervised the work, designed, and performed experiments, discussed results and wrote the manuscript. AK made substantial contributions to the acquisition, analysis, or interpretation of data for the work during the revision process. All authors contributed to the article and approved the submitted version.

FUNDING

This work was funded by Labex Ecofect (ANR-11-LABX-0048) of the Université de Lyon, within the program Investissements d'Avenir (ANR-11-IDEX-0007) operated by the French National Research Agency (ANR), Fondation FINOVI. Additionally, funding was received from the CHEMAAV-ANR-19-CE18-0001 grant operated by the French National Research Agency (ANR). RG received support through grants from the KU Leuven C1 funding (C14/17/113) and FWO Vlaanderen (G0B3516N). SG is a doctoral fellow of the Research Foundation–Flanders (FWO-SB 1S23017N). This study was supported by research funding (CRISPR screen Action) from the Canceropôle Provence-Alpes-côte d'Azur, the French National Cancer Institute (INCa) and the Provence -Alpes-côte d'Azur Region.

ACKNOWLEDGMENTS

The authors would like to thank the flow cytometry platform [SFR BioSciences Lyon (UMS3444/US8), Lyon, France] and the lentivector production facility/SFR BioSciences Lyon (UMS3444/US8, Lyon, France).

REFERENCES

Ahmed, F., Ings, S. J., Pizzey, A. R., Blundell, M. P., Thrasher, A. J., Ye, H. T., et al. (2004). Impaired bone marrow homing of cytokine-activated CD34+ cells in the NOD/SCID model. *Blood* 103, 2079–2087. doi: 10.1182/blood-2003-06-1770

Amanna, I. J., and Slifka, M. K. (2010). Mechanisms that determine plasma cell lifespan and the duration of humoral immunity. *Immunol. Rev.* 236, 125–138. doi: 10.1111/j.1600-065X.2010.00912.x

Amirache, F., Levy, C., Costa, C., Mangeot, P. E., Torbett, B. E., Wang, C. X., et al. (2014). Mystery solved: VSV-G-LVs do not allow efficient gene transfer into unstimulated T cells, B cells, and HSCs because they lack the LDL receptor. *Blood* 123, 1422–1424. doi: 10.1182/blood-2013-11-540641

Anliker, B., Abel, T., Kneissl, S., Hlavaty, J., Caputi, A., Brynza, J., et al. (2010). Specific gene transfer to neurons, endothelial cells and hematopoietic progenitors with lentiviral vectors. *Nat. Methods* 7, 929–935. doi: 10.1038/nmeth.1514

Antoniani, C., Meneghini, V., Lattanzi, A., Felix, T., Romano, O., Magrin, E., et al. (2018). Induction of fetal hemoglobin synthesis by CRISPR/Cas9-mediated editing of the human beta-globin locus. *Blood* 131, 1960–1973. doi: 10.1182/blood-2017-10-811505

Antony, J. S., Latifi, N., Haque, A., Lamsfus-Calle, A., Daniel-Moreno, A., Graeter, S., et al. (2018). Gene correction of HBB mutations in CD34(+) hematopoietic stem cells using Cas9 mRNA and ssODN donors. *Mol. Cell Pediatr.* 5:9. doi: 10.1186/s40348-018-0086-1

Ayuso, E., Mingozzi, F., Montane, J., Leon, X., Anguela, X. M., Haurigot, V., et al. (2010). High AAV vector purity results in serotype- and tissue-independent enhancement of transduction efficiency. *Gene Ther.* 17, 503–510. doi: 10.1038/gt.2009.157

Bak, R. O., Dever, D. P., and Porteus, M. H. (2018). CRISPR/Cas9 genome editing in human hematopoietic stem cells. *Nat. Protoc.* 13, 358–376. doi: 10.1038/nprot.2017.143

Bak, R. O., Dever, D. P., Reinisch, A., Cruz Hernandez, D., Majeti, R., and Porteus, M. H. (2017). Multiplexed genetic engineering of human hematopoietic stem and progenitor cells using CRISPR/Cas9 and AAV6. *Elife* 6:e27873. doi: 10.7554/eLife.27873.025

Bender, R. R., Muth, A., Schneider, I. C., Friedel, T., Hartmann, J., Pluckthun, A., et al. (2016). Receptor-targeted Nipah virus glycoproteins improve cell-type selective gene delivery and reveal a preference for membrane-proximal cell attachment. *PLoS Pathog.* 12: e1005641. doi: 10.1371/journal.ppat.1005641

Bernadin, O., Amirache, F., Girard-Gagnepain, A., Moirangthem, R. D., Levy, C., Ma, K., et al. (2019). Baboon envelope LVs efficiently transduced human adult, fetal, and progenitor T cells and corrected SCID-X1 T-cell deficiency. *Blood Adv.* 3, 461–475. doi: 10.1182/bloodadvances.2018027508

Boztug, K., Dewey, R. A., and Klein, C. (2006). Development of hematopoietic stem cell gene therapy for Wiskott-Aldrich syndrome. *Curr. Opin. Mol. Ther.* 8, 390–395. doi: 10.1056/NEJMOa1003548

Brendel, C., Goebel, B., Daniela, A., Brugman, M., Kneissl, S., Schwable, J., et al. (2015). CD133-targeted gene transfer into long-term repopulating hematopoietic stem cells. *Mol. Ther.* 23, 63–70. doi: 10.1038/mt.2014.173

Brinkman, E. K., Chen, T., Amendola, M., and van Steensel, B. (2014). Easy quantitative assessment of genome editing by sequence trace decomposition. *Nucleic Acids Res.* 42:e168. doi: 10.1093/nar/gku936

Cameron, P., Fuller, C. K., Donohoue, P. D., Jones, B. N., Thompson, M. S., Carter, M. M., et al. (2017). Mapping the genomic landscape of CRISPR-Cas9 cleavage. *Nat. Methods* 14, 600–606. doi: 10.1038/nmeth.4284

Canver, M. C., Smith, E. C., Sher, F., Pinello, L., Sanjana, N. E., Shalem, O., et al. (2015). BCL11A enhancer dissection by Cas9-mediated in situ saturating mutagenesis. *Nature* 527, 192–197. doi: 10.1038/nature15521

Cavazzana, M., Antoniani, C., and Miccio, A. (2017). Gene therapy for beta-hemoglobinopathies. *Mol. Ther.* 25, 1142–1154. doi: 10.1016/j.ymthe.2017.03.024

Charlesworth, C. T., Camarena, J., Cromer, M. K., Vaidyanathan, S., Bak, R. O., Carte, J. M., et al. (2018). Priming human repopulating hematopoietic stem and progenitor cells for Cas9/sgRNA gene targeting. *Mol. Ther. Nucleic Acids* 12, 89–104. doi: 10.1016/j.omtn.2018.04.017

Chen, X., Kozhaya, L., Tastan, C., Placek, L., Dogan, M., Horne, M., et al. (2018). Functional interrogation of primary human T cells via CRISPR genetic editing. *J. Immunol.* 201, 1586–1598. doi: 10.4049/jimmunol.1701616

Colamartino, A. B. L., Lemieux, W., Bifsha, P., Nicoletti, S., Chakravarti, N., Sanz, J., et al. (2019). Efficient and robust NK-cell transduction with baboon envelope pseudotyped lentivector. *Front. Immunol.* 10:873. doi: 10.3389/fimmu.2019.02873

Daniel-Moreno, A., Lamsfus-Calle, A., Raju, J., Antony, J. S., Handgretinger, R., and Mezger, M. (2019). CRISPR/Cas9-modified hematopoietic stem cells-present and future perspectives for stem cell transplantation. *Bone Marrow Transplant.* 54, 1940–1950. doi: 10.1038/s41409-019-0510-8

D'Costa, S., Blouin, V., Broucque, F., Penaud-Budloo, M., Francois, A., Perez, I. C., et al. (2016). Practical utilization of recombinant AAV vector reference standards: focus on vector genomes titration by free ITR qPCR. *Mol. Ther. Methods Clin. Dev.* 5:16019. doi: 10.1038/mtm.2016.19

De Ravin, S. S., Li, L., Wu, X., Choi, U., Allen, C., Koontz, S., et al. (2017). CRISPR-Cas9 gene repair of hematopoietic stem cells from patients with X-linked chronic granulomatous disease. *Sci. Transl. Med.* 9:aah3480. doi: 10.1126/scitranslmed.aah3480

Demeulemeester, J., De Rijck, J., Gijsbers, R., and Debyser, Z. (2015). Retroviral integration: site matters: mechanisms and consequences of retroviral integration site selection. *Bioessays* 37, 1202–1214. doi: 10.1002/bies.201500051

Dever, D. P., Bak, R. O., Reinisch, A., Camarena, J., Washington, G., Nicolas, C. E., et al. (2016). CRISPR/Cas9 beta-globin gene targeting in human haematopoietic stem cells. *Nature* 539, 384–389. doi: 10.1038/nature20134

Diez, B., Genovese, P., Roman-Rodriguez, F. J., Alvarez, L., Schiroli, G., Ugalde, L., et al. (2017). Therapeutic gene editing in CD34(+) hematopoietic progenitors from Fanconi anemia patients. *EMBO Mol. Med.* 9, 1574–1588. doi: 10.15252/emmm.201707540

Doudna, J. A., and Charpentier, E. (2014). Genome editing. The new frontier of genome engineering with CRISPR-Cas9. *Science* 346:1258096. doi: 10.1126/science.1258096

Du, W., Amarachintha, S., Wilson, A. F., and Pang, Q. (2016). Hyper-active non-homologous end joining selects for synthetic lethality resistant and pathological Fanconi anemia hematopoietic stem and progenitor cells. *Sci. Rep.* 6:22167. doi: 10.1038/srep22167

Feng, Y. Y., Tang, M., Suzuki, M., Gunasekara, C., Anbe, Y., Hiraoka, Y., et al. (2019). Essential role of NADPH oxidase-dependent production of reactive oxygen species in maintenance of sustained B Cell receptor signaling and B cell proliferation. *J. Immunol.* 202, 2546–2557. doi: 10.4049/jimmunol.1800443

Ferrua, F., Marangoni, F., Aiuti, A., and Grazia Roncarolo, M. (2020). Gene therapy for Wiskott-Aldrich syndrome: history, new vectors, future directions. *JACI* 146, 262–265. doi: 10.1016/j.jaci.2020.06.018

Forthal, D. N. (2014). Functions of antibodies. *Microbiol. Spectr.* 2, 1–17. doi: 10.1128/microbiolsopec.AID.0019.2014

Fusil, F., Calattini, S., Amirache, F., Mancip, J., Costa, C., Robbins, J. B., et al. (2015). A Lentiviral vector allowing physiologically regulated membrane-anchored and secreted antibody expression depending on B-cell maturation status. *Mol. Ther.* 23, 1734–1747. doi: 10.1038/mt.2015.148

Gaj, T., Gersbach, C. A., and Barbas, C. F. III (2013). ZFN, TALEN, and CRISPR/Cas-based methods for genome engineering. *Trends Biotechnol.* 31, 397–405. doi: 10.1016/j.tibtech.2013.04.004

Gaspar, H. B., Cooray, S., Gilmour, K. C., Parsley, K. L., Adams, S., Howe, S. J., et al. (2011). Long-term persistence of a polyclonal T cell repertoire after gene therapy for X-linked severe combined immunodeficiency. *Sci. Transl Med.* 3:97ra79. doi: 10.1126/scitranslmed.3002715

Gee, P., Lung, M. S. Y., Okuzaki, Y., Sasakawa, N., Iguchi, T., Makita, Y., et al. (2020). Extracellular nanovesicles for packaging of CRISPR-Cas9 protein and sgRNA to induce therapeutic exon skipping. *Nat. Commun.* 11:1334. doi: 10.1038/s41467-020-14957-y

Genovese, P., Schiroli, G., Escobar, G., Tomaso, T. D., Firrito, C., Calabria, A., et al. (2014). Targeted genome editing in human repopulating haematopoietic stem cells. *Nature* 510, 235–240. doi: 10.1038/nature13420

Gentner, B., and Naldini, L. (2019). *In vivo* selection for gene-corrected HSPCs advances gene therapy for a rare stem cell disease. *Cell Stem Cell* 25, 592–593. doi: 10.1016/j.stem.2019.10.004

Gilbert, L. A., Horlbeck, M. A., Adamson, B., Villalta, J. E., Chen, Y., Whitehead, E. H., et al. (2014). Genome-scale CRISPR-mediated control of gene repression and activation. *Cell* 159, 647–661. doi: 10.1016/j.cell.2014.09.029

Girard-Gagnepain, A., Amirache, F., Costa, C., Levy, C., Frecha, C., Fusil, F., et al. (2014). Baboon envelope pseudotyped LVs outperform VSV-G-LVs for gene transfer into early-cytokine-stimulated and resting HSCs. *Blood* 124, 1221–1231. doi: 10.1182/blood-2014-02-558163

Gomez-Ospina, N., Scharenberg, S. G., Mostrel, N., Bak, R. O., Mantri, S., Quadros, R. M., et al. (2019). Human genome-edited hematopoietic stem cells phenotypically correct Mucopolysaccharidosis type I. *Nat. Commun.* 10:4045. doi: 10.1038/s41467-019-11962-8

Grez, M., Reichenbach, J., Schwable, J., Seger, R., Dinauer, M. C., and Thrasher, A. J. (2011). Gene therapy of chronic granulomatous disease: the engraftment dilemma. *Mol. Ther.* 19, 28–35. doi: 10.1038/mt.2010.232

Gross, M., Hanenberg, H., Lobitz, S., Friedl, R., Herterich, S., Dietrich, R., et al. (2002). Reverse mosaicism in Fanconi anemia: natural gene therapy via molecular self-correction. *Cytogenet. Genome Res.* 98, 126–135. doi: 10.1159/000069805

Gundry, M. C., Brunetti, L., Lin, A., Mayle, A. E., Kitano, A., Wagner, D., et al. (2016). Highly Efficient genome editing of murine and human hematopoietic progenitor cells by CRISPR/Cas9. *Cell Rep.* 17, 1453–1461. doi: 10.1016/j.celrep.2016.09.092

Gupta, R. M., and Musunuru, K. (2014). Expanding the genetic editing tool kit: ZFNs, TALENs, and CRISPR-Cas9. *J. Clin. Invest.* 124, 4154–4161. doi: 10.1172/JCI72992

Hartweger, H., McGuire, A. T., Horning, M., Taylor, J. J., Dosenovic, P., Yost, D., et al. (2019). HIV-specific humoral immune responses by CRISPR/Cas9-edited B cells. *J. Exp. Med.* 216, 1301–1310. doi: 10.1084/jem.20190287

Heckl, D., Kowalczyk, M. S., Yudovich, D., Belizaire, R., Puram, R. V., McConkey, M. E., et al. (2014). Generation of mouse models of myeloid malignancy with combinatorial genetic lesions using CRISPR-Cas9 genome editing. *Nat. Biotechnol.* 32, 941–946. doi: 10.1038/nbt.2951

Hendel, A., Bak, R. O., Clark, J. T., Kennedy, A. B., Ryan, D. E., Roy, S., et al. (2015a). Chemically modified guide RNAs enhance CRISPR-Cas genome editing in human primary cells. *Nat. Biotechnol.* 33, 985–989. doi: 10.1038/nbt.3290

Hendel, A., Fine, E. J., Bao, G., and Porteus, M. H. (2015b). Quantifying on- and off-target genome editing. *Trends Biotechnol* 33, 132–140. doi: 10.1016/j.tibtech.2014.12.001

Howe, S. J., Mansour, M. R., Schwarzwaelder, K., Bartholomae, C., Hubank, M., Kempski, H., et al. (2008). Insertional mutagenesis combined with acquired somatic mutations causes leukemogenesis following gene therapy of SCID-X1 patients. *J. Clin. Invest.* 118, 3143–3150. doi: 10.1172/JCI35798

Hultquist, J. F., Hiatt, J., Schumann, K., McGregor, M. J., Roth, T. L., Haas, P., et al. (2019). CRISPR-Cas9 genome engineering of primary CD4(+) T cells for the interrogation of HIV-host factor interactions. *Nat. Protoc.* 14, 1–27. doi: 10.1038/s41596-018-0069-7

Hung, K. L., Meitlis, I., Hale, M., Chen, C. Y., Singh, S., Jackson, S. W., et al. (2018). Engineering protein-secreting plasma cells by homology-directed repair in primary human B cells. *Mol. Ther.* 26, 456–467. doi: 10.1016/j.ymthe.2017.11.012

Indikova, I., and Indik, S. (2020). Highly efficient 'hit-and-run' genome editing with unconcentrated lentivectors carrying Vpr.Prot.Cas9 protein produced from RRE-containing transcripts. *Nucleic Acids Res.* 48, 8178–8187. doi: 10.1093/nar/gkaa561

Jinek, M., Chylinski, K., Fonfara, I., Hauer, M., Doudna, J. A., and Charpentier, E. (2012). A programmable dual RNA-guided DNA endonuclease in adaptive bacterial immunity. *Science* 337, 816–882. doi: 10.1126/science.1225829

Johnson, M. J., Laoharawee, K., Lahr, W. S., Webber, B. R., and Moriarity, B. S. (2018). Engineering of primary human B cells with CRISPR/Cas9 targeted nuclease. *Sci. Rep.* 8:12144. doi: 10.1038/s41598-018-30358-0

June, C. H., Riddell, S. R., and Schumacher, T. N. (2015). Adoptive cellular therapy: a race to the finish line. *Sci. Transl. Med.* 7:280ps287. doi: 10.1126/scitranslmed.aaa3643

Kleinstiver, B. P., Pattanayak, V., Prew, M. S., Tsai, S. Q., Nguyen, N. T., Zheng, Z., et al. (2016). High-fidelity CRISPR-Cas9 nucleases with no detectable genome-wide off-target effects. *Nature* 529, 490–495. doi: 10.1038/nature 16526

Kneissl, S., Zhou, Q., Schwenkert, M., Cosset, F. L., Verhoeyen, E., and Buchholz, C. J. (2013). CD19 and CD20 targeted vectors induce minimal activation of resting B lymphocytes. *PLoS ONE* 8:e79047. doi: 10.1371/journal.pone.0079047

Knopp, Y., Geis, F. K., Heckl, D., Horn, S., Neumann, T., Kuehle, J., et al. (2018). Transient retrovirus-based CRISPR/Cas9 all-in-one particles for efficient, targeted gene knockout. *Mol. Ther. Nucleic Acids* 13, 256–274. doi: 10.1016/j.omtn.2018.09.006

Kochenderfer, J. N., Dudley, M. E., Feldman, S. A., Wilson, W. H., Spaner, D. E., Maric, I., et al. (2012). B-cell depletion and remissions of malignancy along with cytokine-associated toxicity in a clinical trial of anti-CD19 chimeric-antigen-receptor-transduced T cells. *Blood* 119, 2709–2720. doi: 10.1182/blood-2011-10-384388

Kuo, C. Y., Long, J. D., Campo-Fernandez, B., de Oliveira, S., Cooper, A. R., Romero, Z., et al. (2018). Site-specific gene editing of human hematopoietic stem cells for X-linked hyper-IgM syndrome. *Cell Rep.* 23, 2606–2616. doi: 10.1016/j.celrep.2018.04.103

Lattanzi, A., Meneghini, V., Pavani, G., Amor, F., Ramadier, S., Felix, T., et al. (2019). Optimization of CRISPR/Cas9 delivery to human hematopoietic stem and progenitor cells for therapeutic genomic rearrangements. *Mol. Ther.* 27, 137–150. doi: 10.1016/j.ymthe.2018.10.008

Levy, C., Amirache, F., Girard-Gagnepain, A., Frecha, C., Roman-Rodriguez, F. J., Bernadin, O., et al. (2017). Measles virus envelope pseudotyped lentiviral vectors transduce quiescent human HSCs at an efficiency without precedent. *Blood Adv.* 1, 2088–2104. doi: 10.1182/bloodadvances.20170 07773

Levy, C., Fusil, F., Amirache, F., Costa, C., Girard-Gagnepain, A., Negre, D., et al. (2016). Baboon envelope pseudotyped lentiviral vectors efficiently transduce human B cells and allow active factor IX B cell secretion in vivo in NOD/SCIDgammac (-/-) mice. *J. Thromb. Haemost.* 14, 2478–2492. doi: 10.1111/jth.13520

Lombardo, A., and Naldini, L. (2014). Genome editing: a tool for research and therapy: targeted genome editing hits the clinic. *Nat. Med.* 20, 1101–1103. doi: 10.1038/nm.3721

Luo, B., Zhan, Y., Luo, M., Dong, H., Liu, J., Lin, Y., et al. (2020). Engineering of α-PD-1 antibody-expressing long-lived plasma cells by CRISPR/Cas9-mediated targeted gene integration. *Cell Death Dis.* 12;11:973. doi: 10.1038/s41419-020-03187-1

Luo, X. M., Maarschalk, E., O'Connell, R. M., Wang, P., Yang, L., and Baltimore, D. (2009). Engineering human hematopoietic stem/progenitor cells to produce a broadly neutralizing anti-HIV antibody after in vitro maturation to human B lymphocytes. *Blood* 113, 1422–1431. doi: 10.1182/blood-2008-09-177139

Mandal, P. K., Ferreira, L. M., Collins, R., Meissner, T. B., Boutwell, C. L., Friesen, M., et al. (2014). Efficient ablation of genes in human hematopoietic stem and effector cells using CRISPR/Cas9. *Cell Stem Cell* 15, 643–652. doi: 10.1016/j.stem.2014.10.004

Mangeot, P. E. (2019). Nanoblades: pseudoviral shuttles for CRISPR-CAS9 delivery. *Virologie (Montrouge)* 23, 3–6. doi: 10.1684/vir.2019.0759

Mangeot, P. E., Dollet, S., Girard, M., Ciancia, C., Joly, S., Peschanski, M., et al. (2011). Protein transfer into human cells by VSV-G-induced nanovesicles. *Mol. Ther.* 19, 1656–1666. doi: 10.1038/mt.2011.138

Mangeot, P. E., Risson, V., Fusil, F., Marnef, A., Laurent, E., Blin, J., et al. (2019). Genome editing in primary cells and in vivo using viral-derived nanoblades loaded with Cas9-sgRNA ribonucleoproteins. *Nat. Commun.* 10:45. doi: 10.1038/s41467-018-07845-z

Mani, M., Venkatasubrahmanyam, S., Sanyal, M., Levy, S., Butte, A., Weinberg, K., and Jahn, T., (2009). Wiskott-Aldrich syndrome protein is an effector of kit signaling. *Blood* 114, 2900–2908. doi: 10.1182/blood-2009-01-200733

Mankad, A., Taniguchi, T., Cox, B., Akkari, Y., Rathbun, R. K., Lucas, L., et al. (2006). Natural gene therapy in monozygotic twins with Fanconi anemia. *Blood* 107, 3084–3090. doi: 10.1182/blood-2005-07-2638

Martyn, G. E., Wienert, B., Yang, L., Shah, M., Norton, L. J., Burdach, J., et al. (2018). Natural regulatory mutations elevate the fetal globin gene via disruption of BCL11A or ZBTB7A binding. *Nat. Genet.* 50, 498–503. doi: 10.1038/s41588-018-0085-0

Maurice, M., Verhoeyen, E., Salmon, P., Trono, D., Russell, S. J., and Cosset, F. L. (2002). Efficient gene transfer into human primary blood lymphocytes by surface-engineered lentiviral vectors that display a T cell-activating polypeptide. *Blood* 99, 2342–2350. doi: 10.1182/blood.V99.7.2342

Mhaidly, R., and Verhoeyen, E. (2020). Humanized mice are precious tools for preclinical evaluation of CAR T and CAR NK cell therapies. *Cancers (Basel)* 12:1915. doi: 10.3390/cancers12071915

Moffett, H. F., Harms, C. K., Fitzpatrick, K. S., Tooley, M. R., Boonyaratanakornkit, J., and Taylor, J. J. (2019). B cells engineered to express pathogen-specific antibodies protect against infection. *Sci. Immunol.* 4:aax0644. doi: 10.1126/sciimmunol.aax0644

Morgan, R. A., Gray, D., Lomova, A., and Kohn, D. B. (2017). Hematopoietic stem cell gene therapy: progress and lessons learned. *Cell Stem Cell* 21, 574–590. doi: 10.1016/j.stem.2017.10.010

Naka, K., and Hirao, A. (2011). Maintenance of genomic integrity in hematopoietic stem cells. *Int. J. Hematol.* 93, 434–439. doi: 10.1007/s12185-011-0793-z

Osborn, M. J., Newby, G. A., McElroy, A. N., Knipping, F., Nielsen, S. C., Riddle, M. J., et al. (2020). Base editor correction of COL7A1 in recessive dystrophic epidermolysis bullosa patient-derived fibroblasts and iPSCs. *J. Invest. Dermatol.* 140, 338–347 e335. doi: 10.1016/j.jid.2019.07.701

Patiroglu, T., Klein, C., Gungor, H. E., Ozdemir, M. A., Witzel, M., Karakukcu, M., et al. (2016). Clinical features and genetic analysis of six patients with Wiskott-Aldrich syndrome reporting two novel mutations: experience of erciyes university, Kayseri, Turkey. *Genet. Couns.* 27, 9–24.

Patsali, P., Turchiano, G., Papasavva, P., Romito, M., Loucari, C. C., Stephanou, C., et al. (2019). Correction of IVS I-110(G>A) β-thalassemia by CRISPR/Cas- and TALEN-mediated disruption of aberrant regulatory elements in human hematopoietic stem and progenitor cells. *Haematologica* 104, e497–e501. doi: 10.3324/haematol.2018.215178

Pavani, G., Laurent, M., Fabiano, A., Cantelli, E., Sakkal, A., Corre, G., et al. (2020). *Ex vivo* editing of human hematopoietic stem cells for erythroid expression of therapeutic proteins. *Nat. Commun.* 11:3778. doi: 10.1038/s41467-020-18036-0

Pavel-Dinu, M., Wiebking, V., Dejene, B. T., Srifa, W., Mantri, S., Nicolas, C. E., et al. (2019). Gene correction for SCID-X1 in long-term hematopoietic stem cells. *Nat. Commun.* 10:1634. doi: 10.1038/s41467-019-09614-y

Pfeiffer, A., Thalheimer, F. B., Hartmann, S., Frank, A. M., Bender, R. R., Danisch, S., et al. (2018). *In vivo* generation of human CD19-CAR T cells results in B-cell depletion and signs of cytokine release syndrome. *EMBO Mol. Med.* 10:e9158. doi: 10.15252/emmm.201809158

Porter, D. L., Levine, B. L., Kalos, M., Bagg, A., and June, C. H. (2011). Chimeric antigen receptor-modified T cells in chronic lymphoid leukemia. *N. Engl. J. Med.* 365, 725–733. doi: 10.1056/NEJMoa1103849

Radbruch, A., Muehlinghaus, G., Luger, E. O., Inamine, A., Smith, K. G., Dorner, T., et al. (2006). Competence and competition: the challenge of becoming a long-lived plasma cell. *Nat. Rev. Immunol.* 6, 741–750. doi: 10.1038/nri1886

Reimann, C., Six, E., Dal-Cortivo, L., Schiavo, A., Appourchaux, K., Lagresle-Peyrou, C., et al. (2012). Human T-lymphoid progenitors generated in a feeder-cell-free delta-like-4 culture system promote T-cell reconstitution in NOD/SCID/gammac(-/-) mice. *Stem Cells* 30, 1771–1780. doi: 10.1002/stem.1145

Ren, J., Liu, X., Fang, C., Jiang, S., June, C. H., and Zhao, Y. (2017). Multiplex genome editing to generate universal CAR T cells resistant to PD1 inhibition. *Clin. Cancer Res.* 23, 2255–2266. doi: 10.1158/1078-0432.CCR-16-1300

Rio, P., Navarro, S., Guenechea, G., Sanchez-Dominguez, R., Lamana, M. L., Yanez, R., et al. (2017). Engraftment and *in vivo* proliferation advantage of gene-corrected mobilized CD34(+) cells from Fanconi anemia patients. *Blood* 130, 1535–1542. doi: 10.1182/blood-2017-03-774174

Rio, P., Navarro, S., Wang, W., Sanchez-Dominguez, R., Pujol, R. M., Segovia, J. C., et al. (2019). Successful engraftment of gene-corrected hematopoietic stem cells in non-conditioned patients with Fanconi anemia. *Nat. Med.* 25, 1396–1401. doi: 10.1038/s41591-019-0550-z

Roman-Rodriguez, F. J., Ugalde, L., Alvarez, L., Diez, B., Ramirez, M. J., Risueno, C., et al. (2019). NHEJ-mediated repair of CRISPR-Cas9-induced DNA breaks efficiently corrects mutations in HSPCs from patients with Fanconi Anemia. *Cell Stem Cell* 25, 607–621 e607. doi: 10.1016/j.stem.2019.08.016

Sander, J. D., and Joung, J. K. (2014). CRISPR-Cas systems for editing, regulating and targeting genomes. *Nat. Biotechnol.* 32, 347–355. doi: 10.1038/nbt.2842

Schiroli, G., Ferrari, S., Conway, A., Jacob, A., Capo, V., Albano, L., et al. (2017). Preclinical modeling highlights the therapeutic potential of hematopoietic stem cell gene editing for correction of SCID-X1. *Sci. Transl. Med.* 9. doi: 10.1126/scitranslmed.aan0820

Sentmanat, M. F., Peters, S. T., Florian, C. P., Connelly, J. P., and Pruett-Miller, S. M. (2018). A survey of validation strategies for CRISPR-Cas9 editing. *Sci. Rep.* doi: 10.1038/s41598-018-19441-8

Shalem, O., Sanjana, N. E., Hartenian, E., Shi, X., Scott, D. A., Mikkelson, T., et al. (2014). Genome-scale CRISPR-Cas9 knockout screening in human cells. *Science* 343, 84–87. doi: 10.1126/science.1247005

Ting, P. Y., Parker, A. E., Lee, J. S., Trussell, C., Sharif, O., Luna, F., et al. (2018). Guide Swap enables genome-scale pooled CRISPR-Cas9 screening in human primary cells. *Nat. Methods* 15, 941–946. doi: 10.1038/s41592-018-0149-1

Tothova, Z., Krill-Burger, J. M., Popova, K. D., Landers, C. C., Sievers, Q. L., Yudovich, D., et al. (2017). Multiplex CRISPR/Cas9-based genome editing in human hematopoietic stem cells models clonal hematopoiesis and myeloid neoplasia. *Cell Stem Cell* 21, 547–555 e548. doi: 10.1016/j.stem.2017.07.015

Townsend, M. H., Shrestha, G., Robison, R. A., and O'Neill, K. L. (2018). The expansion of targetable biomarkers for CAR T cell therapy. *J. Exp. Clin. Cancer Res.* 37:163. doi: 10.1186/s13046-018-0817-0

Vakulskas, C. A., Dever, D. P., Rettig, G. R., Turk, R., Jacobi, A. M., Collingwood, M. A., et al. (2018). A high-fidelity Cas9 mutant delivered as a ribonucleoprotein complex enables efficient gene editing in human hematopoietic stem and progenitor cells. *Nat. Med.* 24, 1216–1224. doi: 10.1038/s41591-018-0137-0

Vasileva, E. A., Shuvalov, O. U., Garabadgiu, A. V., Melino, G., and Barlev, N. A. (2015). Genome-editing tools for stem cell biology. *Cell Death Dis.* 6:e1831. doi: 10.1038/cddis.2015.167

Verhoeyen, E., Roman-Rodriguez, F. J., Cosset, F. L., Levy, C., and Rio, P. (2017). Gene therapy in Fanconi Anemia: a matter of time, safety and gene transfer tool efficiency. *Curr. Gene Ther.* 16, 297–308. doi: 10.2174/1566523217666617010 9114309

Voss, J. E., Gonzalez-Martin, A., Andrabi, R., Fuller, R. P., Murrell, B., McCoy, L. E., et al. (2019). Reprogramming the antigen specificity of B cells using genome-editing technologies. *Elife* 8:42995. doi: 10.7554/eLife.42995

Wagenblast, E., Azkanaz, M., Smith, S. A., Shakib, L., McLeod, J. L., Krivdova, G., et al. (2019). Functional profiling of single CRISPR/Cas9-edited human long-term hematopoietic stem cells. *Nat. Commun.* 10:4730. doi: 10.1038/s41467-019-12726-0

Wang, J., Exline, C. M., DeClercq, J. J., Llewellyn, G. N., Hayward, S. B., Li, P. W., et al. (2015). Homology-driven genome editing in hematopoietic stem and progenitor cells using ZFN mRNA and AAV6 donors. *Nat. Biotechnol.* 33, 1256–1263. doi: 10.1038/nbt.3408

Webber, B. R., Lonetree, C. L., Kluesner, M. G., Johnson, M. J., Pomeroy, E. J., Diers, M. D., et al. (2019). Highly efficient multiplex human T cell engineering without double-strand breaks using Cas9 base editors. *Nat. Commun.* 10:5222. doi: 10.1038/s41467-019-13778-y

Wu, C. M., Roth, T. L., Baglaenko, Y., Ferri, D. M., Brauer, P., Zuniga-Pflucker, J. C., et al. (2018). Genetic engineering in primary human B cells with CRISPR-Cas9 ribonucleoproteins. *J. Immunol. Methods* 457, 33–40. doi: 10.1016/j.jim.2018.03.009

Wu, Y., Zeng, J., Roscoe, B. P., Liu, P., Yao, Q., Lazzarotto, C. R., et al. (2019). Highly efficient therapeutic gene editing of human hematopoietic stem cells. *Nat. Med.* 25, 776–783. doi: 10.1038/s41591-019-0401-y

Yu, K. R., Natanson, H., and Dunbar, C. E. (2016). Gene editing of human hematopoietic stem and progenitor cells: promise and potential hurdles. *Hum. Gene Ther.* 27, 729–740. doi: 10.1089/hum.2016.107

Zetsche, B., Gootenberg, J. S., Abudayyeh, O. O., Slaymaker, I. M., Makarova, K. S., Essletzbichler, P., et al. (2015). Cpf1 is a single RNA-guided endonuclease of a class 2 CRISPR-Cas system. *Cell* 163, 759–771. doi: 10.1016/j.cell.2015.09.038

Zhou, Q., Schneider, I. C., Edes, I., Honegger, A., Bach, P., Schonfeld, K., et al. (2012). T-cell receptor gene transfer exclusively to human CD8(+) cells enhances tumor cell killing. *Blood* 120, 4334–4342. doi: 10.1182/blood-2012-02-412973

Zhou, Q., Uhlig, K. M., Muth, A., Kimpel, J., Levy, C., Munch, R. C., et al. (2015). Exclusive transduction of human CD4+ T cells upon systemic delivery of CD4-targeted lentiviral vectors. *J. Immunol.* 195, 2493–2501. doi: 10.4049/jimmunol.1500956

5

Gene Correction of Point Mutations Using PolyPurine Reverse Hoogsteen Hairpins Technology

Alex J. Félix, Anna Solé, Véronique Noé and Carlos J. Ciudad*

Department of Biochemistry and Physiology, School of Pharmacy and Food Sciences, and Institute for Nanoscience and Nanotechnology (IN2UB), University of Barcelona, Barcelona, Spain

*Correspondence:
Carlos J. Ciudad
cciudad@ub.edu

Monogenic disorders are often the result of single point mutations in specific genes, leading to the production of non-functional proteins. Different blood disorders such as ß-thalassemia, sickle cell disease, hereditary spherocytosis, Fanconi anemia, and Hemophilia A and B are usually caused by point mutations. Gene editing tools including TALENs, ZFNs, or CRISPR/Cas platforms have been developed to correct mutations responsible for different diseases. However, alternative molecular tools such as triplex-forming oligonucleotides and their derivatives (e.g., peptide nucleic acids), not relying on nuclease activity, have also demonstrated their ability to correct mutations in the DNA. Here, we review the Repair-PolyPurine Reverse Hoogsteen hairpins (PPRHs) technology, which can represent an alternative gene editing tool within this field. Repair-PPRHs are non-modified single-stranded DNA molecules formed by two polypurine mirror repeat sequences linked by a five-thymidine bridge, followed by an extended sequence at one end of the molecule which is homologous to the DNA sequence to be repaired but containing the corrected nucleotide. The two polypurine arms of the PPRH are bound by intramolecular reverse-Hoogsteen bonds between the purines, thus forming a hairpin structure. This hairpin core binds to polypyrimidine tracts located relatively near the target mutation in the dsDNA in a sequence-specific manner by Watson-Crick bonds, thus producing a triplex structure which stimulates recombination. This technology has been successfully employed to repair a collection of mutants of the *dhfr* and *aprt* genes within their endogenous *loci* in mammalian cells and could be suitable for the correction of mutations responsible for blood disorders.

Keywords: gene-editing, repair-PPRH, triplex, APRT, DHFR, mutation

Scientists estimate that the global prevalence of all monogenic diseases in the human population is 1%, including over 10,000 different conditions (Control of hereditary diseases. Report of a WHO Scientific Group, 1996). These disorders are often the result of a unique single point mutation in a specific gene that produces a non-functional protein. Recently, nuclease-based gene editing tools such as transcription activator like nucleases, zinc-finger nucleases, or CRISPR/Cas platforms have been extensively used to correct mutations in the DNA (Gaj et al., 2016). Alternatively, molecules such as triplex-forming oligonucleotides (TFOs) (Seidman and Glazer, 2003) or peptide nucleic acids (PNAs) (Ricciardi et al., 2018b) that do not rely on the activity of nucleases to produce the gene correction have been developed. In this instance, the repair event is triggered by the formation of a local triple helix structure near the mutation site that stimulates the cell's own endogenous repair machinery. Here, we will review an alternative triplex-forming molecule named PolyPurine Reverse Hoogsteen (PPRH) hairpin, which has been developed in our laboratory, to correct point mutations in the DNA.

PPRHS

PPRHs are non-modified single-stranded DNA molecules (45–55 nt) formed by two polypurine mirror repeat sequences linked by a five-thymidine bridge (5T). The formation of the hairpin structure is due to the establishment of intramolecular reverse-Hoogsteen bonds between the purines. PPRHs can bind to polypyrimidine tracts in the double-stranded DNA (dsDNA) in a sequence-specific manner via Watson-Crick bonds, thus generating a triple helix in the target site and displacing the polypurine strand of the dsDNA (Coma et al., 2005). This local distortion in the dsDNA interferes with DNA transcription and inhibits the expression of the targeted gene (de Almagro et al., 2009).

During the last decade, we have used PPRHs as gene silencing tools to inhibit genes related to cancer progression such as *dihydrofolate reductase* (*DHFR*) (de Almagro et al., 2009, 2011), *telomerase* (*TERT*) (de Almagro et al., 2009), *BCL2*, *topoisomerase 1* (*TOP1*), *mTOR*, *MDM2*, *C-MYC* (Villalobos et al., 2015), *CHK1*, *WEE1* (Aubets et al., 2020) and *survivin* (*BIRC5*) *in vivo* (Rodríguez et al., 2013). Additionally, we applied the PPRHs technology in immunotherapy approaches by inhibiting the CD47/SIRPα (Bener et al., 2016) and PD-1/PD-L1 pathways (Enríquez et al., 2018; Ciudad et al., 2019). PPRHs and their advantages (low cost of production, stability, and lack of immunogenicity) as gene silencing tools for cancer have been reviewed in Ciudad et al. (2017).

REPAIR-PPRHS

It is known that triplex formation can stimulate repair between a targeted *locus* and a donor DNA sequence by both homology-directed repair (HDR) (Datta et al., 2001; Knauert et al., 2006) and nucleotide excision repair (NER) (Faruqi et al., 2000; Datta et al., 2001; Rogers et al., 2002) pathways. For that reason, we believed that PPRHs could represent an alternative tool for gene correction due to their ability to produce triplex structures and therefore stimulate recombination (between the template and the target site) to correct point mutations in the DNA. To do so, we conceived an advanced design of the PPRH molecules that we called repair-PPRHs. These molecules are PPRH hairpins that bear an extension sequence at one end of the molecule which is homologous to the DNA sequence to be repaired but including the corrected nucleotide instead of the mutated one (**Figure 1A**). In this case, the polypurine hairpin core of the repair-PPRH is designed to bind to a polypyrimidine sequence located near the target mutation, thus producing the PPRH/DNA triplex and stimulating the recombination between the extension sequence of the repair-PPRH and the mutation target site.

In our seminal paper we used repair-PPRHs to correct a point mutation in the *dhfr* gene from Chinese Hamster Ovary (CHO)

cells (Solé et al., 2014). We selected the *dhfr* gene as a model because we could easily identify the repaired clones by applying a DHFR selective culture medium that does not contain glycine, hypoxanthine nor thymidine (-GHT).

First, DNA binding assays were performed to check the capacity of PPRHs to open the target dsDNA for the subsequent binding of a repair oligonucleotide corresponding to the extension sequence of the repair-PPRH. Two PPRHs containing 13 and 23 purines, respectively, directed against polypyrimidine sequences located in exon 6 of the *dhfr* gene were used to perform the binding experiments. We demonstrated that both PPRHs were able to bind and open their target dsDNA sequences ranging from 13 to 25 nt. Moreover, the introduction of an interruption in the duplex to simulate a point mutation did not alter the binding of the PPRH to its target sequence (Solé et al., 2014). The minimum concentration to obtain the binding between the PPRH and its target sequence was 3 nM. Additionally, (Solé et al., 2017) proved that even PPRHs susceptible to fold into stable G4 structures can still bind in a sequence-specific manner to the target DNA and produce triplex formation.

Then, to assess if PPRHs were able to correct a point mutation, we designed a repair-PPRH directed against a non-sense mutation (G>C) located in exon 2 of the *dhfr* minigene contained in the p11Mut expression vector. To do so, a PPRH bearing a polypurine hairpin core of 13 nt was combined with a 25 nt extension sequence homologous to the mutation site but containing the corrected nucleotide. In cells, two different approaches were attempted to repair this mutation in p11Mut. In the first approach, gene correction was achieved by the co-transfection of both p11Mut and the repair-PPRH in *dhfr*-deficient DG44 CHO cells. After incubation, cells were selected in -GHT medium obtaining different repaired clones. The frequency of repair was ~0.15% (Solé et al., 2014). Gene correction was confirmed by DNA sequencing and by determining the levels of DHFR mRNA and protein. In the second approach, we performed the experiment in DG44 cells stably transfected with p11Mut (DG44-p11Mut cell line) since it could resemble to our final aim of correcting a point mutation in the endogenous *locus* of the gene. We confirmed that the repair-PPRH was able to correct the mutation at the same frequency (0.15%) as our first approach (Solé et al., 2014). The levels of DHFR mRNA and protein were recovered compared to the mutant DG44-p11Mut cell line (Solé et al., 2014). In a third approach, we explored the applicability of repair-PPRHs to correct point mutations at the endogenous level. There, a repair-PPRH designed against a mutation in exon 6 (G>-) of the *dhfr* gene was transfected into the DA5 cell line, which contained this specific mutation in the endogenous *locus* of the *dhfr* gene. After selection, surviving cell colonies were acquired at a frequency of 0.01% (Solé et al., 2014). In this case, gene correction frequency was lower than in the previous experiments since the correction was achieved for the first time in the endogenous *locus* of the gene. However, spontaneous corrections were not observed in any of the experiments. The levels of DHFR mRNA and protein were rescued compared to the mutant DA5 cell line. Moreover, we corroborated that the DHFR protein from the repaired clones showed equal or higher DHFR activity levels than the *dhfr*+

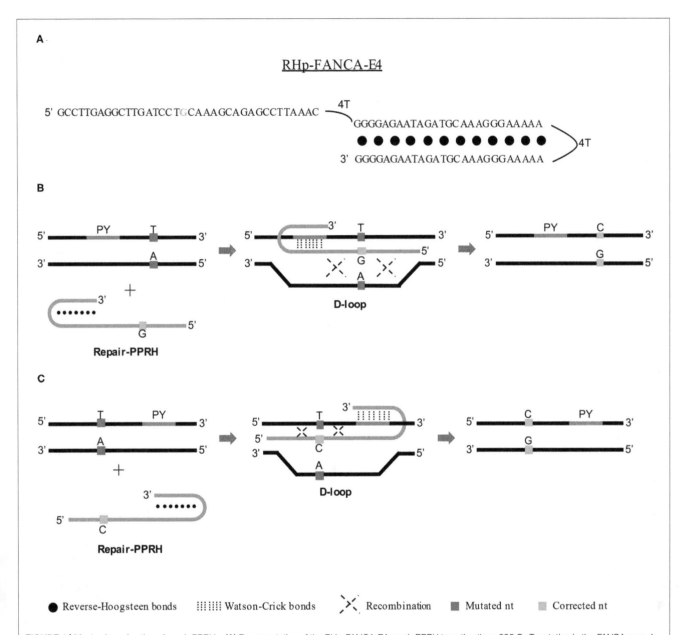

FIGURE 1 | Mechanism of action of repair-PPRHs. **(A)** Representation of the RHp-FANCA-E4 repair-PPRH targeting the c.295 C>T mutation in the *FANCA* gene. In this case, the polypurine hairpin core is bound to the repair domain by an additional four-thymidine bridge following the long-distance repair-PPRH approach. Scheme depicting the mechanism of action of a repair-PPRH when the polypyrimidine target sequence (PY) is located either upstream **(B)** or downstream **(C)** of the mutation.

parental cell line, thus demonstrating that the corrected gene was completely functional (Solé et al., 2014).

FACTORS AFFECTING GENE CORRECTION FREQUENCY

The study of the influence of both hydroxyurea and aphidicolin in the repair frequency was also addressed (Solé et al., 2014). It is known that hydroxyurea inhibits the ribonucleotide reductase enzyme (Bianchi et al., 1986), thus arresting cells in the S phase of the cell cycle by blocking or retarding the movement of the

replication fork caused by the dNTP pools imbalance (Saintigny et al., 2001). In the case of aphidicolin, it is a potent inhibitor of polymerases α, δ and ε, which leads to the blockage of the replication fork and provokes a similar effect to hydroxyurea (Wang, 1991). The effect on replication caused by these agents leads to double-strand DNA breaks (DSBs), which can stimulate both the HDR and the non-homologous end joining (NHEJ) pathways to repair the DNA damage (Lundin et al., 2002). Accordingly, the incubation of both DG44 and DG44-p11Mut cell lines with 5 μg/mL aphidicolin or 2 mM hydroxyurea for 3 h before incubation with the repair-PPRHs increased the repair frequency by 2-fold (Solé et al., 2014). This is in keeping with other studies showing increased gene correction frequencies when incubating repair oligonucleotides after treatment with hydroxyurea or aphidicolin (Parekh-Olmedo et al., 2003; Ferrara et al., 2004; Wu et al., 2005; Chin et al., 2008; Engstrom and Kmiec, 2008).

Finally, since the RAD51 protein plays a central role in homologous recombination (Krejci et al., 2012; Papaioannou et al., 2012) and it is required for triplex-induced recombination (Datta et al., 2001; Gupta et al., 2002), we checked its role in the repair event triggered by repair-PPRHs. Co-transfection of the repair-PPRH with a pRad51 expression vector in DA5 cells led to an increase in gene correction frequency of 10-fold compared to the transfection of the repair-PPRH alone (Solé et al., 2014), thus confirming that homologous recombination is involved in the repair process. Overall, this study represented the proof-of-concept for the usage of PPRHs as gene editing tools.

CORRECTION OF POINT MUTATIONS IN THE ENDOGENOUS *LOCUS*

In the following study, the usage of repair-PPRHs was expanded by correcting a representative compilation of point mutations (insertions, deletions, substitutions, and a double substitution) located in the endogenous *locus* of the *dhfr* gene (Solé et al., 2016). For that purpose, *dhfr*-deficient CHO cell lines derived from the parental cell line UA21 (Urlaub et al., 1983), which carried only one copy of the *dhfr* gene (hemizygous), were selected to perform the repair experiments. DU8 (Urlaub et al., 1989), DF42 (Carothers et al., 1986), DI33A (Chasin et al., 1990; Carothers et al., 1993a), DA5 and DA7 (Carothers et al., 1993b) and DP12B and DP6B (Carothers et al., 1993a) cell lines contained premature STOP codons either in place by a nucleotide substitution or downstream due to frameshift by single deletions, insertions, or by exon skipping, thus producing a non-functional DHFR enzyme (**Table 1**). Repair-PRHs were designed targeting the different mutations and transfected in their corresponding mutant cell lines. After selection in -GHT deficient medium, repaired clones were expanded and analyzed by DNA sequencing of the targeted site, thus demonstrating the correction of the mutation. We also confirmed that the corrected *dhfr* gene was completely functional since the levels of DHFR mRNA and protein were equal or higher than the levels shown by the parental cell line, as well as DHFR enzymatic activity (Solé et al., 2016). In addition, we evaluated the variation in gene correction frequency depending on the number of DF42 cells initially plated to perform the experiment. The maximum frequency value was observed (7.6%) when transfection was carried out with only 1,000 cells (Solé et al., 2016).

One can argue that PPRH molecules present a major limitation since it is necessary to find polypyrimidine stretches relatively close to the target mutation. Despite these polypyrimidine domains are more abundant in the human genome than initially predicted by simple random models (Goñi et al., 2004, 2006), finding a polypyrimidine sequence adjacent to the point mutation can be complicated in some cases. To solve this issue for the DF42 mutant, we designed a long-distance repair-PPRH whose repair domain was targeting the mutation located 662 nt upstream from the polypyrimidine target sequence of the hairpin core. The repair domain of the repair-PPRH was connected to the hairpin core by another 5T loop. This long-distance repair-PPRH was able to correct its targeted mutation showing similar results to the short-distance repair-PPRH used for the correction of the same mutant, thus indicating that adjacency between the target mutation and the polypyrimidine domain was not crucial to achieve the correction.

GENERALITY OF ACTION OF REPAIR-PPRHS

Recently, we demonstrated the generality of action of repair-PPRHs (Félix et al., 2020) by correcting three different mutations in the endogenous *locus* of the *aprt* gene in various *aprt*-deficient CHO cell lines (**Table 1**) named S23, S62, and S1 (Phear et al., 1989). It is worth noting that this gene also served as a disease model in CHO cells, since *aprt* deficiency in humans represents an inherited condition that severely affects the urinary tract and the kidneys (Bollée et al., 2012; Edvardsson et al., 2019). In that study, we designed repair-PPRHs containing polypurine hairpin cores composed of 19–22 nt to assure their specificity and to minimize the off-target effects as much as possible. In all the mutant cell lines we demonstrated the correction of the mutation at the DNA, mRNA and enzymatic levels, showing that the corrected APRT protein was completely functional. Moreover, we used a long-distance repair-PPRH in which the polypyrimidine target sequence was located 24 nt downstream of the S1 mutation site, however, it showed a similar effect to that of the short-distance repair-PPRH (Félix et al., 2020). The influence of the cell cycle phase in the repair event was also studied by performing gene correction experiments either during S phase or in asynchronous conditions. The repair frequency was increased by 2.5-fold in S phase (Félix et al., 2020), which is in accordance with other studies regarding gene correction with repair oligonucleotides (Majumdar et al., 2003; Brachman and Kmiec, 2005; Olsen et al., 2005).

One of our concerns was the possible generation of off-target edits in the repaired genome caused by the treatment with repair-PPRHs. Whole genome sequencing analyses of repaired clones revealed that the repair-PPRH did not produce any random insertions or deletions (indels) in the genome. Moreover, the sequence of the repair-PPRH itself was not detected in any location of the genome (Félix et al., 2020). Finally, we got an insight into the molecular mechanism responsible for the gene correction event. The D-loop structure formation upon binding of the repair-PPRH to its polypyrimidine target sequence was demonstrated by DNA binding assays (Félix et al., 2020), thus serving as a recombination intermediate that stimulates DNA repair (Parekh-Olmedo et al., 2002; Drury and Kmiec, 2003, 2004). The mechanism of action of repair-PPRHs is depicted in **Figures 1B,C**.

Despite the advantages of repair-PPRHs, we would like to state that the main limitations of this technology are the low repair frequency and the delivery. A way to ameliorate the low

TABLE 1 | CHO mutant cell lines corrected by repair-PPRHs.

Cell line	Gene	Mutation	Base change	Coding change	References
DF42	*dhfr*	c.541 Exon 6	Substitution G > T	STOP in place	Solé et al., 2016
DA5		c. 541 Exon 6	Deletion (-G)	STOP at +584 (normal termination is at +562)	
DP12B		c.370 – 2 Intron 4	Substitution A > T	Exon 5 skipped STOP at +504	
DI33A		c. 493 Exon 6	Insertion (+G)	STOP at +505	
DU8		c. 136 + 1 Exon 2/Intron 2	Double substitution GG > AA	Exon 2 skipped STOP at +139	
DA7		c. 235 Exon 3	Substitution G > T	STOP in place	
S23	*aprt*	c. 7 Exon 1	Substitution G > T	STOP in place	Félix et al., 2020
S1		c. 180 Exon 2	Substitution C > G	STOP in place	
S62		c. 505 Exon 5	Substitution G > T	STOP in place	

Position numbers refer to the translational start site (ATG). The correction of the mutant cell lines using repair-PPRHs can be found in the referenced papers.

repair frequency would be to increase the rate of homologous recombination. In this direction, as stated previously, co-transfection of repair-PPRHs with a pRAD51 led to an increase in the correction frequency. Since the rate of homologous recombination is higher in the S phase of the cell cycle, synchronization in the S phase can also increase the correction frequency, as observed for the *dhfr* and *aprt* genes. Regarding the delivery of repair-PPRHs, the development of new liposome formulations (Juliano, 2016) or polymeric nanoparticles (McNeer et al., 2015; Bahal et al., 2016; Ricciardi et al., 2018a) may contribute to improve gene repair. Finally, modification in the backbone of repair-PPRHs including phosphorothioate or locked nucleic acids (LNA) may increase the stability of the molecule and decrease its degradation by nucleases.

To date, we have only tested repair-PPRHs to correct single and double point mutations. Anyhow, most monogenic diseases are just caused by one point mutation in the responsible gene, thus making repair-PPRHs an alternative tool to correct different disorders. In this respect, we constructed **Table 2** to show the versatility for designing repair-PPRHs to correct some of the most common point mutations that affect genes involved in monogenic blood disorders, with the aim of making them available for the scientific community.

CRISPR/CAS SYSTEMS

Nowadays, CRISPR/Cas has become a popular gene editing tool for therapeutic purposes (Osborn et al., 2015; Dever et al., 2016; Sansbury et al., 2019; van de Vrugt et al., 2019; Xiong et al., 2019). Nevertheless, several studies have demonstrated the presence of off-target effects caused by unspecific activity of the CRISPR/Cas system (Cradick et al., 2013; Lin et al., 2014; Schaefer et al., 2017; Anderson et al., 2018; Allen et al., 2019; Cullot et al., 2019).

Unintended on-target effects such as large deletions and complex rearrangements have also been reported (Kosicki et al., 2018). In this regard, Félix et al. showed the absence of off-target effects when using repair-PPRHs to correct point mutations in the *aprt* gene in mammalian cells. Furthermore, since *Staphylococcus pyogenes* and *Staphylococcus aureus* cause infections at high frequencies in human beings, an anti-Cas9 preexisting effector T cell response has been discovered (Charlesworth et al., 2019; Wagner et al., 2019). On the other hand, PPRHs are non-modified (cheap) DNA oligonucleotides that do not activate the innate inflammatory response (Villalobos et al., 2014).

TFOS

The ability of TFOs to stimulate recombination by triple helix formation in mammalian cells was first described in 1996 (Faruqi et al., 1996). Consecutive studies highlighted the potential of TFOs to correct mutations in the DNA by triplex-induced recombination between the target site and a donor DNA molecule (Chan et al., 1999; Culver et al., 1999; Datta et al., 2001). TFO backbone modifications have been developed to increase its binding affinity while reducing nuclease-mediated degradation. Peptide nucleic acids (PNAs) are synthetic DNA analogs composed of N-(2-aminoethyl)-glycine monomers linked by peptide bonds (Nielsen et al., 1991). This neutrally charged backbone allows the PNA to bind with high affinity to DNA, thus forming more stable triplex structures (Kim et al., 1993). Moreover, PNAs are also resistant to nuclease and protease activities (Demidov et al., 1994).

PNAs and their derivatives have been developed to correct mutations responsible for different monogenic diseases. Intranasal delivery of polymeric nanoparticles containing PNAs and donor DNA sequences in cystic fibrosis mice led to the

TABLE 2 | Compendium of repair-PPRHs designed to correct point mutations responsible for 10 different blood disorders.

Blood disorder	Gene	Mutation	Codon change	Name and sequence (5′->3′) of the Repair-PPRH
G6PD deficiency (mediterranean)	G6PD	c.563 C>T Exon 6	TCC>TTC Ser>Phe p.188	RHp-G6PD-E6-C (99 nt) GCCGTCACCAAGAACATTCACGAGTCCTGCATGAGCCAGATGTAAGGC TTGGGCAACGGGAGGGAAGGGCGGAttttAGGCGGGAAGGGAGGGCAACGG
Beta-Thalassemia	HBB	G>A Intron 1 (+110)	TGG>TAG	RHp-HBB-I1-C (91 nt) ACTGACTCTCTCTGCCTATTGGTCTATTTTCCCACCCTTAGttt tAAAAGAAAGGGGAAGAAAAGAttttAGAAAAGAAGGGGAAAGAAAA
Sickle cell disease	HBB	c.70 A>T Exon 1	GAG>GTG Glu>Val p.7	RHp-HBB-E-T (81 nt) CATGGTGCATCTGACTCCTGAGGAGAAGTCTGCCGTTACTGCCCTGT GGGGCAAGGTGAACGttttGCAAGTGGAACGGGG
Porphyria	HMBS	c.33+1 G>A/T Exon 1/ Intron 1	Intron retention 67 bp	RHp-HMBS-E1-T (97 nt) GCAATGCGGCTGCAACGGCCGGTGAGTGCTGAGCCGGTGACCtttt GGAAGGAATGGGGAAATCAGAGAGttttGAGAGACTAAAGGGGTAAGGAAGG
Ferritin Deficiency	FTL	c.310 G>T Exon 3	GAG>TAG Glu>Ter p.104	RHp-FTL-E3-C (93 nt) TGAAAGCTGCCATGGCCCTGGAGAAAAAGCTGAACCAGGCCttt tGGAAAAGAGGGGGAGAGAGCAGttttGGAAAAGAGGGGGAGAGAGCAG
Dyserythropoietic anemia	CODAN1B	c.281 A>G Exon 5	TAT>TGT Tyr>Cys p.94	RHp-C15ORF41-E5-T (102 nt) GAGCCATTAATGAGGGCGCATAGTCCACCTCATTGGCCAGGTCCAGGAGCACTGGGG CAGGAGGTAAAAAGTGGTGAGGttttGGAGTGGTGAAAAATGGAG
Hemophilia A	F8	c.6976 C>T Exon 27	CGA>TGA Arg>Ter p.2326	RHp-F8-E27 (87 nt) CGTTACTGACTCGCTACCTTCGAATTCACCCCCAGAGTTGGtttt GGCAGTGGAGAGGGAGGAGttttGAGGAGGGAGAGGTGACGG
Hemophilia B	F9	c.169 C>T Exon 2	CAA>TAA Gln>Ter p.57	RHp-F9-E2 (100 nt) ATTCTCTCTCAAGGTTCCCTTGAACAAACTCTTCCAATTTACCTtttt AAGAAAAACTGAAATGTAAAAGAAttttAAGAAAATGTAAAGTCAAAAAGAA
Fanconi anemia	FANCA	c.295 C>T Exon 4	CAG>TAG Gln>Ter p.99	RHp-FANCA-E4 (99 nt) GCCTTGAGGCTTGATCCTGCAAAGCAGAGCCTTAAACtttt GGGGAGAATAGATGCAAAGGGAAAAAttttAAAAAGGGAAACGTAGATAAGAGGGG
Von Willebrand	VWF	c.4975 C>T Exon 28	CGA>TGA Arg>Ter p.1659	RHp-VWF-E28 (103 nt) GACGCTCCCCCGAGAGGCTCCTGACCTGGTGCTGCAGAGGTGCTGCTCCGGAGAGG GGCTGCAGAAGGGGTGGGAGAGGGGGAttttAGGGGAGAGGGTGGGGA

The design of the different repair-PPRHs was performed as follows: (i) Finding triplex targeting sites near the mutation using the TFO searching tool (http://utw10685.utweb.utexas. edu/tfo/) (Gaddis et al., 2006); (ii) Devising the corresponding polypurine hairpin core (underlined sequences); (iii) Determining the repair domain of the repair-PPRH corresponding to the homologous sequence of the mutation site but containing the corrected nucleotide (green). In the case of a long-distance repair-PPRH, an additional 4–5 thymidine loop is added between the hairpin core and the repair domain. The abbreviation of the gene responsible for the blood disorder, the position of the mutation and the affected codon are given for each case. The position of the mutation is referred to the translation start site (ATG). TER, termination codon.

correction of the F508del *CFTR* mutation *in vivo* (McNeer et al., 2015). More recently, PNAs delivered by polymeric nanoparticles have been used to correct the *ß-globin* gene both *in vivo* (Bahal et al., 2016) and *in utero* (Ricciardi et al., 2018a) in ß-thalassemic mice with very low off-target activity. The most recent review on PNAs as gene editing tools can be found in Economos et al. (2020).

FINAL REMARKS

It is evident that triplex-mediated repair of mutations in the DNA constitute a powerful gene editing approach that has demonstrated its therapeutic effect *in vivo*. Repair-PPRHs can represent a new tool in this field since they have shown their efficacy to correct different point mutations in the *dhfr* and *aprt loci* in mammalian cells with no detectable off-

target activity. In addition, here we describe a collection of repair-PPRHs designed to correct 10 different blood diseases. A better understanding of the mechanisms by which the repair-PPRH triggers the recombination event may lead to improvements on PPRH design, thus increasing the frequency of correction.

AUTHOR CONTRIBUTIONS

AF, AS, and CC wrote the original draft and VN revised the manuscript. All authors contributed to the article and approved the submitted version.

REFERENCES

Allen, F., Crepaldi, L., Alsinet, C., and Parts, L. (2019). Predicting the mutations generated by repair of Cas9-induced double-strand breaks. *Nat. Biotechnol.* 37, 64–82. doi: 10.1038/nbt.4317

Anderson, K. R., Haeussler, M., Watanabe, C., and Warming, S. (2018). CRISPR off-target analysis in genetically engineered rats and mice. *Nat. Methods* 15, 512–514. doi: 10.1038/s41592-018-0011-5

Aubets, E., Noé, V., and Ciudad, C. J. (2020). Targeting replication stress response using polypurine reverse hoogsteen hairpins directed against WEE1 and CHK1 genes in human cancer cells. *Biochem. Pharmacol.* 175:113911. doi: 10.1016/j.bcp.2020.113911

Bahal, R., Ali McNeer, N., Quijano, E., and Glazer, P. M. (2016). In vivo correction of anaemia in β-thalassemic mice by γ3PNA-mediated gene editing with nanoparticle delivery. *Nat. Commun.* 7:13304. doi: 10.1038/ncomms13304

Bener, G., J., Félix, A., Sánchez de Diego, C., Pascual Fabregat, I., and Ciudad, C. J. (2016). Silencing of CD47 and SIRPα by Polypurine reverse Hoogsteen hairpins to promote MCF-7 breast cancer cells death by PMA-differentiated THP-1 cells. *BMC Immunol.* 17:32. doi: 10.1186/s12865-016-0170-z

Bianchi, V., Pontis, E., and Reichard, P. (1986). Changes of deoxyribonucleoside triphosphate pools induced by hydroxyurea and their relation to DNA synthesis. *J. Biol. Chem.* 261, 16037–16042.

Bollée, G., Harambat, J., Bensman, A., Knebelmann, B., Daudon, M., and Ceballos-Picot, I. (2012). Adenine phosphoribosyltransferase deficiency. *Clin. J. Am. Soc. Nephrol.* 7, 1521–1527. doi: 10.2215/CJN.02320312

Brachman, E. E., and Kmiec, E. B. (2005). Gene repair in mammalian cells is stimulated by the elongation of S phase and transient stalling of replication forks. *DNA Repair* 4, 445–457. doi: 10.1016/j.dnarep.2004.11.007

Carothers, A. M., Urlaub, G., Grunberger, D., and Chasin, L. A. (1993a). Splicing mutants and their second-site suppressors at the dihydrofolate reductase locus in Chinese hamster ovary cells. *Mol. Cell. Biol.* 13, 5085–5098. doi: 10.1128/MCB.13.8.5085

Carothers, A. M., Urlaub, G., Mucha, J., Yuan, W., Chasin, L. A., and Grunberger, D. (1993b). A mutational hot spot induced by N-hydroxy-aminofluorene in dihydrofolate reductase mutants of Chinese hamster ovary cells. *Carcinogenesis* 14, 2181–2184. doi: 10.1093/carcin/14.10.2181

Carothers, A. M., Urlaub, G., Steigerwalt, R. W., Chasin, L. A., and Grunberger, D. (1986). Characterization of mutations induced by 2-(N-acetoxy-N-acetyl)aminofluorene in the dihydrofolate reductase gene of cultured hamster cells. *Proc. Natl. Acad. Sci. U.S.A.* 83, 6519–6523. doi: 10.1073/pnas.83.17.6519

Chan, P. P., Lin, M., Fawad Faruqi, A., Powell, J., Seidman, M. M., and Glazer, P. M. (1999). Targeted correction of an episomal gene in mammalian cells by a short DNA fragment tethered to a triplex-forming oligonucleotide. *J. Biol. Chem.* 274, 11541–11548. doi: 10.1074/jbc.274.17.11541

Charlesworth, C. T., Deshpande, P. S., Dever, D. P., and Porteus, M. H. (2019). Identification of preexisting adaptive immunity to Cas9 proteins in humans. *Nat. Med.* 25, 249–254. doi: 10.1038/s41591-018-0326-x

Chasin, L. A., Urlaub, G., Mitchell, P., and Grunberger, D. (1990). RNA processing mutants at the dihydrofolate reductase locus in Chinese hamster ovary cells. *Progr. Clin. Biol. Res.* 340A, 295–304.

Chin, J. Y., Kuan, J. Y., Lonkar, P. S., and Glazer, P. M. (2008). Correction of a splice-site mutation in the beta-globin gene stimulated by triplex-forming peptide nucleic acids. *Proc. Natl. Acad. Sci. U.S.A.* 105, 13514–13519. doi: 10.1073/pnas.0711793105

Ciudad, C. J., Medina Enriquez, M. M., Félix, A. J., Bener, G., and Noé, V. (2019). Silencing PD-1 and PD-L1: the potential of PolyPurine reverse hoogsteen hairpins for the elimination of tumor cells. *Immunotherapy* 11, 369–372. doi: 10.2217/imt-2018-0215

Ciudad, C. J., Rodríguez, L., Villalobos, X., Félix, A. J., and Noé, V. (2017). Polypurine reverse hoogsteen hairpins as a gene silencing tool for cancer. *Curr. Med. Chem.* 24, 2809–2826. doi: 10.2174/0929867324666170301114127

Coma, S., Noé, V., Eritja, R., and Ciudad, C. J. (2005). Strand displacement of double-stranded DNA by triplex-forming antiparallel purine-hairpins. *Oligonucleotides* 15, 269–283. doi: 10.1089/oli.2005.15.269

Control of hereditary diseases. Report of a WHO and Scientific Group (1996). World Health Organization Technical Report Series, 865, 1–84.

Cradick, T. J., Fine, E. J., Antico, C. J., and Bao, G. (2013). CRISPR/Cas9 systems targeting β-globin and CCR5 genes have substantial off-target activity. *Nucleic Acids Res.* 41, 9584–9592. doi: 10.1093/nar/gkt714

Cullot, G., Boutin, J., Toutain, J., and Bedel, A. (2019). CRISPR-Cas9 genome editing induces megabase-scale chromosomal truncations. *Nat. Commun.* 10:1136. doi: 10.1038/s41467-019-09006-2

Culver, K. W., Hsieh, W.-T., Huyen, Y., and Khorlin, A. (1999). The goal of correcting point mutations in living human correction of chromosomal point mutations in human cells with bifunctional oligonucleotides. *Nat. Biotechnol.* 17:13684.

Datta, H. J., Chan, P. P., Vasquez, K. M., Gupta, R. C., and Glazer, P. M. (2001). Triplex-induced recombination in human cell-free extracts. *J. Biol. Chem.* 276, 18018–18023. doi: 10.1074/jbc.M011646200

de Almagro, M. C., Coma, S., Noe, V., and Ciudad, C. J. (2009). Polypurine hairpins directed against the template strand of DNA knock down the expression of mammalian genes. *J. Biol. Chem.* 284, 11579–11589. doi: 10.1074/jbc.M900981200

de Almagro, M. C., Mencia, N., Noé, V., and Ciudad, C. J. (2011). Coding polypurine hairpins cause target-induced cell death in breast cancer cells. *Human Gene Therapy* 22, 451–463. doi: 10.1089/hum.2010.102

Demidov, V. V., Potaman, V. N., Frank-Kamenetskil, M. D., and Nlelsen, P. E. (1994). Stability of peptide nucleic acids in human serum and cellular extracts. *Biochem. Pharmacol.* 48, 1310–1313. doi: 10.1016/0006-2952(94)90171-6

Dever, D. P., Bak, R. O., Reinisch, A., and Porteus, M. H. (2016). CRISPR/Cas9 β-globin gene targeting in human haematopoietic stem cells. *Nature* 539, 384–389. doi: 10.1038/nature20134

Drury, M. D., and Kmiec, E. B. (2003). DNA pairing is an important step in the process of targeted nucleotide exchange. *Nucleic Acids Res.* 31, 899–910. doi: 10.1093/nar/gkg171

Drury, M. D., and Kmiec, E. B. (2004). Double displacement loops (double d-loops) are templates for oligonucleotide-directed mutagenesis and gene repair. *Oligonucleotides* 14, 274–286. doi: 10.1089/oli.2004.14.274

Economos, N. G., Oyaghire, S., Quijano, E., Ricciardi, A. S., Mark Saltzman, W., and Glazer, P. M. (2020). Peptide nucleic acids and gene editing: perspectives on structure and repair. *Molecules* 25:E735. doi: 10.3390/molecules25030735

Edvardsson, V. O., Sahota, A., and Palsson, R. (2019). Adenine phosphoribosyltransferase deficiency. In: GeneReviews, 1–19.

Engstrom, J. U., and Kmiec, E. B. (2008). DNA replication, cell cycle progression and the targeted gene repair reaction. *Cell Cycle* 7, 1402–1414. doi: 10.4161/cc.7.10.5826

Enríquez, M. M. M., J., Félix, A., Ciudad, C. J., Noé, V., and Ahmad, A. (2018). Cancer immunotherapy using PolyPurine Reverse Hoogsteen hairpins targeting the PD-1/PD-L1 pathway in human tumor cells. *PLoS ONE.* 13:e0206818. doi: 10.1371/journal.pone.0206818

Faruqi, A. F., Datta, H. J., Carroll, D., Seidman, M. M., and Glazer, P. M. (2000). Triple-helix formation induces recombination in mammalian cells via a nucleotide excision repair-dependent pathway. *Mol. Cell. Biol.* 20, 990–1000. doi: 10.1128/MCB.20.3.990-1000.2000

Faruqi, A. F., Seidman, M. M., Segal, D. J., Carroll, D., and Glazer, P. M. (1996). Recombination induced by triple-helix-targeted DNA damage in mammalian cells. *Mol. Cell. Biol.* 16, 6820–6828. doi: 10.1128/MCB.16.12.6820

Félix, A. J., Ciudad, C. J., and Noé, V. (2020). Correction of the aprt gene using repair-polypurine reverse hoogsteen hairpins in mammalian cells. *Mol. Ther. Nucleic Acids* 19, 683–695. doi: 10.1016/j.omtn.2019.12.015

Ferrara, L., Parekh-Olmedo, H., and Kmiec, E. B. (2004). Enhanced oligonucleotide-directed gene targeting in mammalian cells following treatment with DNA damaging agents. *Exp. Cell Res.* 300, 170–179. doi: 10.1016/j.yexcr.2004.06.021

Gaddis, S. S., Wu, Q., Thames, H. D., and Vasquez, K. M. (2006). A web-based search engine for triplex-forming oligonucleotide target sequences. *Oligonucleotides* 16, 196–201. doi: 10.1089/oli.2006.16.196

Gaj, T., Sirk, S. J., Shui, S. L., and Liu, J. (2016). Genome-editing technologies: Principles and applications. *Cold Spring Harbor Perspectives in Biol.* 8:12. doi: 10.1101/cshperspect.a023754

Goñi, J. R., de la Cruz, X., and Orozco, M. (2004). Triplex-forming oligonucleotide target sequences in the human genome. *Nucleic Acids Res.* 32, 354–360. doi: 10.1093/nar/gkh188

Goñi, J. R., Vaquerizas, J. M., Dopazo, J., and Orozco, M. (2006). Exploring the reasons for the large density of triplex-forming oligonucleotide target sequences in the human regulatory regions. *BMC Genom.* 7:63. doi: 10.1186/1471-2164-7-63

Gupta, R. C., Bazemore, L. R., Golub, E. I., and Radding, C. M. (2002). Activities of human recombination protein Rad51. *Proc. Natl. Acad. Sci. U.S.A.* 94, 463–468. doi: 10.1073/pnas.94.2.463

Juliano, R. L. (2016). The delivery of therapeutic oligonucleotides. *Nucleic Acids Res.* 44, 6518–6548. doi: 10.1093/nar/gkw236

Kim, S. K., Nordén, B., Nielsen, P. E., Egholm, M., Buchardt, O., and Berg, R. H. (1993). Right-handed triplex formed between peptide nucleic acid PNA-T8 and Poly(dA) shown by linear and circular dichroism spectroscopy. *J. Am. Chem. Soc.* 115, 6477–6481. doi: 10.1021/ja00068a001

Knauert, M. P., Kalish, J. M., Hegan, D. C., and Glazer, P. M. (2006). Triplex-stimulated intermolecular recombination at a single-copy genomic target. *Mol. Ther.* 14, 392–400. doi: 10.1016/j.ymthe.2006.03.020

Kosicki, M., Tomberg, K., and Bradley, A. (2018). Repair of double-strand breaks induced by CRISPR-Cas9 leads to large deletions and complex rearrangements. *Nat. Biotechnol.* 36:4192. doi: 10.1038/nbt.4192

Krejci, L., Altmannova, V., Spirek, M., and Zhao, X. (2012). Homologous recombination and its regulation. *Nucleic Acids Res.* 40, 5795–5818. doi: 10.1093/nar/gks270

Lin, Y., Cradick, T. J., Brown, M. T., and Bao, G. (2014). CRISPR/Cas9 systems have off-target activity with insertions or deletions between target DNA and guide RNA sequences. *Nucleic Acids Res.* 42, 7473–7485. doi: 10.1093/nar/gku402

Lundin, C., Erixon, K., Arnaudeau, C., and Helleday, T. (2002). Different roles for nonhomologous end joining and homologous recombination following replication arrest in mammalian cells. *Mol. Cell. Biol.* 22, 5869–5878. doi: 10.1128/MCB.22.16.5869-5878.2002

Majumdar, A., Puri, N., Cuenoud, B., and Seidman, M. M. (2003). Cell cycle modulation of gene targeting by a triple helix-forming oligonucleotide. *J. Biol. Chem.* 278, 11072–11077. doi: 10.1074/jbc.M211837200

McNeer, N. A., Anandalingam, K., Fields, R. J., and Egan, M. E. (2015). Nanoparticles that deliver triplex-forming peptide nucleic acid molecules correct F508del CFTR in airway epithelium. *Nat. Commun.* 6:7952. doi: 10.1038/ncomms7952

Nielsen, P. E., Egholm, M., Berg, R. H., and Buchardt, O. (1991). Sequence-selective recognition of DNA by strand displacement with a thymine-substituted polyamide. *Science* 254, 1497–1500. doi: 10.1126/science.1962210

Olsen, P., Randol, M., and Krauss, S. (2005). Implications of cell cycle progression on functional sequence correction by short single-stranded DNA oligonucleotides. *Gene Therapy* 12, 546–551. doi: 10.1038/sj.gt.3302454

Osborn, M. J., Gabriel, R., Webber, B. R., and Tolar, J. (2015). Fanconi anemia gene editing by the CRISPR/Cas9 system. *Human Gene Therapy* 26, 114–126. doi: 10.1089/hum.2014.111

Papaioannou, I., Simons, J. P., and Owen, J. S. (2012). Oligonucleotide-directed gene-editing technology: mechanisms and future prospects. *Exp. Opin. Biol. Ther.* 12, 329–342. doi: 10.1517/14712598.2012.660522

Parekh-Olmedo, H., Drury, M., and Kmiec, E. B. (2002). Targeted nucleotide exchange in Saccharomyces cerevisiae directed by short oligonucleotides containing locked nucleic acids. *Chem. Biol.* 9, 1073–1084. doi: 10.1016/S1074-5521(02)00236-3

Parekh-Olmedo, H., Engstrom, J. U., and Kmiec, E. B. (2003). The effect of hydroxyurea and trichostatin a on targeted nucleotide exchange in yeast and mammalian cells. *Annals N. Y. Acad. Sci.* 1002, 43–55. doi: 10.1196/annals.1281.006

Phear, G., Armstrong, W., and Meuth, M. (1989). Molecular basis of spontaneous mutation at the aprt locus of hamster cells. *J. Mol. Biol.* 209, 577–582. doi: 10.1016/0022-2836(89)90595-0

Ricciardi, A. S., Bahal, R., Farrelly, J. S., and Saltzman, W. M. (2018a). *In utero* nanoparticle delivery for site-specific genome editing. *Nat. Commun.* 9:2481. doi: 10.1038/s41467-018-04894-2

Ricciardi, A. S., Quijano, E., Putman, R., Saltzman, W. M., and Glazer, P. M. (2018b). Peptide nucleic acids as a tool for site-specific gene editing. *Molecules* 23, 1–15. doi: 10.3390/molecules23030632

Rodríguez, L., Villalobos, X., Dakhel, S., and Noé, V. (2013). Polypurine reverse Hoogsteen hairpins as a gene therapy tool against survivin in human prostate cancer PC3 cells *in vitro* and *in vivo*. *Biochem. Pharmacol.* 86, 1541–1554. doi: 10.1016/j.bcp.2013.09.013

Rogers, F. A., Vasquez, K. M., Egholm, M., and Glazer, P. M. (2002). Site-directed recombination via bifunctional PNA-DNA conjugates. *Proc. Natl. Acad. Sci. U.S.A.* 99, 16695–16700. doi: 10.1073/pnas.262556899

Saintigny, Y., Delacôte, F., Varès, G., and Lopez, B. S. (2001). Characterization of homologous recombination induced by replication inhibition in mammalian cells. *EMBO J.* 20, 3861–3870. doi: 10.1093/emboj/20.14.3861

Sansbury, B. M., Hewes, A. M., and Kmiec, E. B. (2019). Understanding the diversity of genetic outcomes from CRISPR-Cas generated homology-directed repair. *Commun. Biol.* 2:458. doi: 10.1038/s42003-019-0705-y

Schaefer, K. A., Wu, W. H., Colgan, D. F., Tsang, S. H., Bassuk, A. G., and Mahajan, V. B. (2017). Unexpected mutations after CRISPR-Cas9 editing *in vivo*. *Nat. Methods* 14, 547–548. doi: 10.1038/nmeth.4293

Seidman, M. M., and Glazer, P. M. (2003). The potential for gene repair via triple helix formation. *J. Clin. Invest.* 112, 487–552. doi: 10.1172/JCI19552

Solé, A., Ciudad, C. J., Chasin, L. A., and Noé, V. (2016). Correction of point mutations at the endogenous locus of the dihydrofolate reductase gene using repair-PolyPurine Reverse Hoogsteen hairpins in mammalian cells. *Biochem. Pharmacol.* 110–111, 16–24. doi: 10.1016/j.bcp.2016.04.002

Solé, A., Delagoutte, E., Ciudad, C. J., Noé, V., and Alberti, P. (2017). Polypurine reverse-Hoogsteen (PPRH) oligonucleotides can form triplexes with their target sequences even under conditions where they fold into G-quadruplexes. *Sci. Rep.* 7:39898. doi: 10.1038/srep39898

Solé, A., Villalobos, X., Ciudad, C. J., and No,é, V. (2014). Repair of single-point mutations by polypurine reverse hoogsteen hairpins. *Human Gene Therapy Methods* 25, 288–302. doi: 10.1089/hgtb.2014.049

Urlaub, G., Kands, E., Carothers, A. M., and Chasin, L. A. (1983). Deletion of the diploid dihydrofolate reductase locus from cultured mammalian cells. *Cell* 33, 9–10. doi: 10.1016/0092-8674(83)90422-1

Urlaub, G., Mitchell, P. J., Ciudad, C. J., and Chasin, L. A. (1989). Nonsense mutations in the dihydrofolate reductase gene affect RNA processing. *Mol. Cell. Biol.* 9, 2868–2880. doi: 10.1128/MCB.9.7.2868

van de Vrugt, H. J., Harmsen, T., Riepsaame, J., and te Riele, H. (2019). Effective CRISPR/Cas9-mediated correction of a Fanconi anemia defect by error-prone end joining or templated repair. *Sci. Rep.* 9:768. doi: 10.1038/s41598-018-36506-w

Villalobos, X., Rodríguez, L., Prévot, J., Oleaga, C., Ciudad, C. J., and Noé, V. (2014). Stability and immunogenicity properties of the gene-silencing polypurine reverse hoogsteen hairpins. *Mol. Pharmaceut.* 11, 254–264. doi: 10.1021/mp400431f

Villalobos, X., Rodríguez, L., Sol,é, A., and No,é, V. (2015). Effect of polypurine reverse hoogsteen hairpins on relevant cancer target genes in different human cell lines. *Nucleic Acid Therapeut.* 25, 198–208. doi: 10.1089/nat.2015.0531

Wagner, D. L., Amini, L., Wendering, D. J., and Schmueck-Henneresse, M. (2019). High prevalence of Streptococcus pyogenes Cas9-reactive T cells within the adult human population. *Nat. Med.* 25, 242–248. doi: 10.1038/s41591-018-0204-6

Wang, T. S. (1991). Eukaryotic DNA polymerases. *Annual Rev. Biochem.* 60, 513–52. doi: 10.1146/annurev.bi.60.070191.002501

Wu, X. S., Xin, L., Yin, W. X., and Liang, C. C. (2005). Increased efficiency of oligonucleotide-mediated gene repair through slowing replication fork progression. *Proc. Natl. Acad. Sci. U.S.A.* 102, 2508–2513. doi: 10.1073/pnas.0406991102

Xiong, Z., Xie, Y., Yang, Y., and Sun, X. (2019). Efficient gene correction of an aberrant splice site in β-thalassaemia iPSCs by CRISPR/Cas9 and single-strand oligodeoxynucleotides. *J. Cell. Mol. Med.* 23, 8046–8057. doi: 10.1111/jcmm.14669

6

Genomic Engineering in Human Hematopoietic Stem Cells: Hype or Hope?

Stefanie Klaver-Flores[1], Hidde A. Zittersteijn[2], Kirsten Canté-Barrett[1], Arjan Lankester[3], Rob C. Hoeben[2], Manuel A. F. V. Gonçalves[2], Karin Pike-Overzet[1] and Frank J. T. Staal[1]*

[1] Department of Immunology, Leiden University Medical Center, Leiden, Netherlands, [2] Department of Cell and Chemical Biology, Leiden University Medical Center, Leiden, Netherlands, [3] Department of Pediatrics, Willem-Alexander Children's Hospital, Leiden University Medical Center, Leiden, Netherlands

*Correspondence:
Frank J. T. Staal
f.j.t.staal@lumc.nl

Many gene editing techniques are developed and tested, yet, most of these are optimized for transformed cell lines, which differ from their primary cell counterparts in terms of transfectability, cell death propensity, differentiation capability, and chromatin accessibility to gene editing tools. Researchers are working to overcome the challenges associated with gene editing of primary cells, namely, at the level of improving the gene editing tool components, e.g., the use of modified single guide RNAs, more efficient delivery of Cas9 and RNA in the ribonucleoprotein of these cells. Despite these efforts, the low efficiency of proper gene editing in true primary cells is an obstacle that needs to be overcome in order to generate sufficiently high numbers of corrected cells for therapeutic use. In addition, many of the therapeutic candidate genes for gene editing are expressed in more mature blood cell lineages but not in the hematopoietic stem cells (HSCs), where they are tightly packed in heterochromatin, making them less accessible to gene editing enzymes. Bringing HSCs in proliferation is sometimes seen as a solution to overcome lack of chromatin access, but the induction of proliferation in HSCs often is associated with loss of stemness. The documented occurrences of off-target effects and, importantly, on-target side effects also raise important safety issues. In conclusion, many obstacles still remain to be overcome before gene editing in HSCs for gene correction purposes can be applied clinically. In this review, in a perspective way, we will discuss the challenges of researching and developing a novel genetic engineering therapy for monogenic blood and immune system disorders.

Keywords: CRISPR-Cas9, gene editing, hematopoietic stem cells, stem cell biology, genomic engineering, therapeutic, clinic

INTRODUCTION

During the last decade, a wide range of scientific advances have emerged in the field of genomic engineering. Those advances vary from γ-retroviruses to self-inactivating lentiviruses, and from designed meganucleases to the more versatile, hence more powerful, CRISPR/Cas-based systems. What makes gene editing technologies interesting for researchers and clinicians, but also for the general public is their potential for therapeutic application in a range of genetic and acquired diseases, such as inborn errors of immunity (IEI) (Gatti et al., 1968), hemoglobinopathies including sickle cell disease (SCD) (Johnson et al., 1984; Lucarelli et al., 1984), cystic fibrosis, certain types of cancers, and viral diseases such as AIDS (White and Khalili, 2016; Shim et al., 2017; Porteus, 2019; Shahryari et al., 2019). However, these promising state-of-the-art technologies face a number of obstacles that prompt questions regarding their safety and efficiency especially when considering clinical applications. Preeminent amongst these obstacles are the generation of off-target effects with associated potential tumorigenicity, and immune responses triggered by the delivery vehicles and/or the gene editing reagents themselves (Doudna and Charpentier, 2014; Shim et al., 2017). In this perspective, we provide a brief overview of hematopoietic stem cell (HSC) biology and *ex vivo* expansion protocols, followed by a critical discussion about the scientific basis for the development of novel HSC gene editing therapies for blood and immune disorders.

HEMATOPOIETIC STEM CELLS

Stem cells are cells of embryonic, fetal or adult origin, capable of dividing indefinitely (Staal et al., 2011). All stem cells, regardless of their origin, have three characteristics that distinguish them from other cell types: (i) they are undifferentiated and non-specialized cells; (ii) are able to divide and renew themselves indefinitely; and (iii) are able to differentiate into specialized cells when subjected to certain physiological or experimental conditions. Those cells can be classified, according to their origin or their differentiation capacity, into embryonic and non-embryonic stem cells that can be pluripotent or multipotent, respectively.

Hematopoietic stem cells (HSC) comprise a heterogeneous and relatively small group of cells that have the ability to self-renew and differentiate into specialized cells of the blood tissue and the immune system. Those cells are characterized by being the most immature in the differentiation hierarchy for blood cells.

In the classic model of hematopoiesis, the most primitive HSC progenitor cells (phenotypically defined as CD34$^+$ CD38$^-$ CD90$^+$ CD45RA$^-$ and CD49f$^-$), differentiate into progenitors that further give rise to other blood cells (Notta et al., 2011). The recently identified Junction adhesion molecule-2 (Jam2) is highly expressed in HSCs and can generate T cells, have been suggested as novel surface markers in HSCs (Radulovic et al., 2019). Also, recently other two molecules have been identified as a relatively robust surface marker in human HSCs. The Endothelial protein C receptor (EPCR) is highly conserved in LT-HSCs (Fares et al., 2017), and the Endothelial cell-selective adhesion molecule (ESAM) is highly expressed in HSCs and MPPs, in a long-term lifetime. Thus, the ESAM seems to have a big influence in HSC differentiation path in different studies (Ooi et al., 2009; Yokota et al., 2009; Ishibashi et al., 2016; Roch et al., 2017).

For clinical applications, the interest of using HSCs has been increasing over the years. Among the difficulties faced by the researchers are the number of cells extracted from the patient, and also the fact that those cells undergo symmetrical and asymmetrical cell divisions when cultured. In an *ex vivo*

expansion approach, the symmetrical cell division leads to an increase in the number of cells (Morrison and Kimble, 2006), achieved by the use of different combinations of growth factors and cytokines, such as SCF, TPO, Flt3-L, IL-3, and IL-6 (Sauvageau et al., 2004; Buza-Vidas et al., 2006; Hofmeister et al., 2007; Metcalf, 2008). Aside from that, other compounds are screened and tested for their potential for *in vitro* HSC expansion, including Stemregenin1 (SR1) and UM171 molecules (Boitano et al., 2010; Fares et al., 2014). The SR1 molecule was the first identified with the property of supporting the expansion of human and murine HSCs *in vitro* (Boitano et al., 2010), and has clinical benefit when cultured with the aforementioned cytokines cocktail (Wagner et al., 2016). The UM171 has been shown to be a good and promising candidate for *ex vivo* expansion of human cord blood HSCs (Fares et al., 2014). A recent clinical trial is using the UM171 with the purpose of *ex vivo* expansion of HSCs for allogeneic transplantation and gene therapy (NCT02668315), which suggests the potential use in *ex vivo* gene therapy. An interesting recently identified compound is CPI203, which acts at the epigenetic level to expand human CD34$^+$ cells in NSG mouse models and may support *ex vivo* expansion of human HSCs (Hua et al., 2020; Staal and Fibbe, 2020).

STATE-OF-THE-ART GENOME ENGINEERING OF HSCs

Allogeneic-hematopoietic stem cell transplants (allo-HSCT) have been used since the late 1960's to offer a potential lifetime cure for a variety of monogenic hematological diseases (Thomas et al., 1975). The main benefit of successful allo-HSCT is that the patient is cured for life, highlighting the concept that transplantation of healthy donor-derived HSCs containing the correct gene variant can reconstitute a functional hematopoietic system. While allo-HSCT can cure multiple blood and immune system disorders, clinical problems remain due to the challenge of finding a suitable HLA-matched bone marrow donor together with need for strong conditioning regimens for HSC engraftment, potentially resulting in subsequent complications such as graft-vs.-host disease (GvHD) or incomplete reconstitution of blood cell lineages. Moreover, chemotherapeutic conditioning regimens may result in infertility or development of lymphomas later in life. In patient genotype-specific cases when a suitable HLA-matched donor is not available, mismatched related donors are often used, however at the cost of increased morbidity and incomplete immune recovery leading to lower quality of life. To overcome these limitations of allo-HSCT, researchers initially have developed retroviral vectors that carry a recombinant version of the correct gene for permanent transfer into autologous CD34$^+$ cell-enriched HSCs that. The *ex vivo*, genetically modified CD34$^+$ cells that include HSCs are infused back into the patient and the genetically modified cells engraft and subsequently produce hematopoietic cells expressing the therapeutic gene (**Figure 1**). This *ex vivo* gene therapy principle has been shown to be efficacious in diseases such as severe combined immunodeficiency due to adenosine deaminase deficiency (ADA-SCID) (Aiuti et al., 2009), X-linked severe combined immunodeficiency (Hacein-Bey-Abina et al., 2002, 2010; Pavel-Dinu et al., 2019) and more recently for hemoglobinopathies including SCD, conditions that require high levels of therapeutic gene expression to attain phenotypic rescue (Woods et al., 2006; Badat and Davies, 2017). Currently, departing from "classic" gene therapy, gene editing technology based on programmable nucleases is offering the perspective for changing the genome of HSCs with unprecedented specificity and accuracy. Together with increased knowledge of the mechanisms that regulate human hematopoiesis, this has created the possibility to further developing cell and gene therapies for inherited diseases of the blood cell compartment. Backed by many years of fundamental research and, at times serendipity, the discovery of restriction enzymes was followed by that of other classes of DNA-modifying tools, including site-specific recombinases and programmable nucleases, such as meganucleases (MGN), zinc-finger nucleases (ZNFs), transcription activator-like effector (TALE) nucleases (TALENs), and more recently, powerful RNA-guided nucleases based on clustered regularly interspaced short palindromic repeats (CRISPR)-CRISPR-associated endonuclease (Cas) systems (Chandrasegaran and Carroll, 2016; Chen and Goncalves, 2018). In this context, the non-integrating adeno-associated vector (AVV) has become a widely exploited vehicle of donor DNA template that is required for homology directed repair (HDR) in HSCs (Bak et al., 2018). Single-strand and double-strand oligodeoxynucleotides (ODN) are also emerging as effective means to deliver donor template for HDR in many clinical relevant settings (Chen et al., 2015). The engineering of meganucleases with new DNA-binding specificities has been challenging in large part due to the fact that the DNA recognition and cleavage sites are located in the same domain. In contrast to the meganucleases, the DNA binding domains of ZFNs and TALENs are distinct from that of their FokI cleavage domains whose (catalytic) activation depends on target DNA binding of a working ZFN or TALEN pair resulting in local dimerization (Urnov et al., 2010). The ZFNs and TALENs DNA-binding domain consist of zing-finger motif and TALE repeat arrays, respectively, with each zinc-finger motif binding to specific nucleotide triplets and each TALE repeat recognizing individual single nucleotides. The changes of the zinc-finger motifs can be done by the nucleotides that are surrounding its triple target. As a consequence of this sequence context dependency, generating robust and highly specific ZFNs often requires complex protein engineering methods involving reiterative optimization cycles and/or screening of large zinc-finger libraries (Cathomen and Keith Joung, 2008). The straightforward TALE repeat-to-nucleotide one-to-one recognition code together with the fact that binding of a TALE repeat to its target nucleotide is not substantially altered by neighboring nucleotides (Mussolino and Cathomen, 2012), makes the assembly of functional and highly specific TALENs easier and more flexible than that of ZFNs (Jinek et al., 2013). While each programmable nuclease platform is at different stages of clinical development, RNA-guided CRISPR/Cas-based systems are becoming the tools of

choice for pursuing genetic therapies based on genome editing principles and technologies. This principally stems from their high efficiency and increasingly improving specificity, as well as from their versatile RNA-dependent programmability and easy-to-use versatile design.

CRISPR sequences together with CRISPR-associated (Cas) protein genes form CRISPR/Cas loci as part of the adaptive immune systems in prokaryotes organisms, evolved as a strategy to fend off infectious agents, e.g., bacteriophages and foreign plasmids (Horvath and Barrangou, 2010; Wiedenheft et al., 2012; Rath et al., 2015). Scientists have been investigating the properties of these exquisite defense mechanisms encoded in various CRISPR loci for over 20 years. Crucially, in 2012, the real potential of CRISPR/Cas systems for genomic engineering purposes was uncovered in seminal studies by Gasiunas et al. (2012) and Jinek et al. (2012). In particular, through these eminent *in vitro* biochemical studies, these teams found that Cas9 proteins from *Streptococcus thermophilus* and *Streptococcus pyogenes*, respectively, are RNA-programmable site-specific endonucleases. Later, the CRISPR system was readily adapted by independent research groups that had the aim of turning the technique into a powerful genome editing platform for genome editing purposes in mammalian cells (Cho et al., 2013; Cong et al., 2013; Jinek et al., 2013; Mali et al., 2013).

Key adaptations involved codon-optimization of Cas9 reading frames encoding nuclease localization motifs and fusion of native trans-activating CRISPR RNA and CRISPR RNA moieties to form a so-called single-guide gRNA (sgRNA). The latter component binds to the Cas9 protein and address it to a target sequence consisting of a protospacer adjacent motif (NGG; in the case of *S. pyogenes* Cas9) and a typically 20 nucleotide-long sequence complementary to the $5'$ end of the sgRNA (spacer). Upon target site binding and sgRNA-DNA hybridization, the HNH and RuvC-like nuclease domains of Cas9 become active resulting in site-specific DNA cleavage, of inducing double-stranded DNA (dsDNA) breaks at a specific genomic target region, homologous to the crRNA spacer sequence.

Two major DNA repair pathways exist in humans. The endogenous non-homologous end-joining (NHEJ) and homology-directed repair (HDR) pathways are responsible for repair of the double-stranded chromosomal breaks made by programmable nucleases allowing for the removal or insertion of new genetic information at specific genomic loci (Jinek et al., 2012). Typically, NHEJ processes are exploited for knocking-out preexisting genetic information after the exclusive transfer of programmable nucleases, whilst the HDR mechanism is mostly used for knocking-in new genetic information after the delivery of programmable nucleases together with exogenous (donor) DNA templates.

The prokaryotic-CRISPR/Cas9 genome editing tool has changed our ability to change and manipulate specific sequences of DNA and RNA in living cells from diverse species, including mammalian cells. The CRISPR/Cas9 system for genetic engineering is an exciting advancement for HSC gene therapy, although it potentially comes with safety risks,

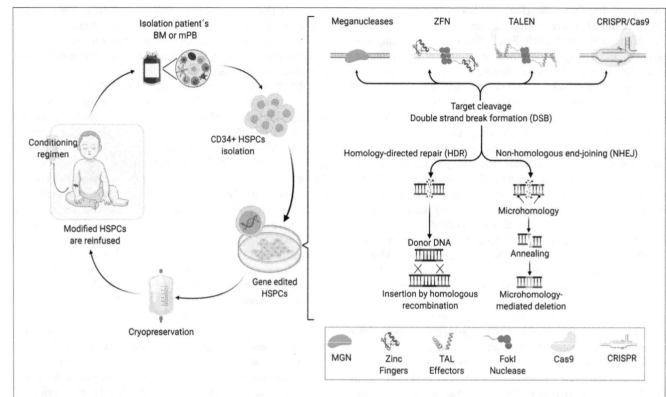

FIGURE 1 | Representation of *ex vivo* HSCs gene editing, showing the crucial steps of the process. After harvesting the hematopoietic stem and progenitor cells (HSPCs) from mobilized peripheral blood or bone marrow, the CD34+ cells are enriched and cultured *ex vivo* in the presence of growth factors, which allows the maintenance and expansion of self-renewing stem cells, and are then subjected to gene editing tool transfer (e.g., meganucleases, ZFNs, TALENs, or CRISPR/Cas-derived nucleases). When the nuclease induces a standard DNA double-strand break (DSB) at the desired genomic *loci*, the homology-directed repair (HDR) machinery are recruited in order to repair the DNA, where a template donor DNA is supplied for the homologous recombination between the template and chromosomal DNA, or by non-homologous end-joining (NHEJ) without a homologous template DNA, resulting in small indels generation (insertions and deletions) if there is only one cut, or triggers large DNA deletions if two cuts. After the treatment, the patient receives a specific conditioning regimen that depletes endogenous HSPCs from the bone marrow and makes space for the *ex vivo* engineered cells to engraft. The gene-corrected cells are then reinfused intravenously and engraft in the bone marrow.

such as suboptimal specificity correlated with off-target effects and on-target but unwanted mutations, immunogenicity, and unfavorable bio-distribution.

THE CHALLENGES OF GENOME ENGINEERING IN HSCs

Genome-editing tools in the form of the aforementioned programmable nucleases and their derivatives can, in principle, be projected for correcting or disrupting any disease-causing gene typically via knocking-in and knocking-out exogenous and endogenous DNA sequences, respectively, or via the introduction of specific point mutations (Byrne et al., 2014). HSCs are optimal target cells for therapeutic genome editing technologies owing to their self-renewal and differentiation capabilities (Hoke et al., 2012; Liu et al., 2012; Lee et al., 2019). However, these genome editing tools and strategies are initially mostly developed and tested in transformed cell lines that differ from their primary cell counterparts in key aspects, such as transfectability, cell death propensity, loss of differentiation capabilities, ploidy, and chromatin accessibility (**Figure 2**). Primary cells, unlike

immortalized or full-fledged transformed cells, for the most part maintain their biological identity in proper culture systems, yet, they can only be propagated for a few generations *in vitro* before reaching senescence and, in the case of true HSCs, they are difficult to expand *in vitro*.

Hence, when thinking about applying these genome editing tools and strategies to primary cells, and in particular HSCs, one faces numerous challenges associated with the aforementioned intrinsic characteristics of these target cells and the sub-optimal performance of gene editing procedures, such as on-target and off-target side effects, as well as insertional mutagenesis risks and unregulated transgene expression resulting from random chromosomal integration of exogenous (donor) DNA templates (Crisostomo et al., 2006). In order to meet the safety requirements and other important criteria such as a high efficacy, high quality and good reproducibility, it is crucial that the genome-editing tool is proper developed and tested in appropriate cell types.

One of the most challenging issues of *ex vivo* genome-editing of HSCs, besides the low viability and the decreased differentiation potential of these cells upon prolonged culture,

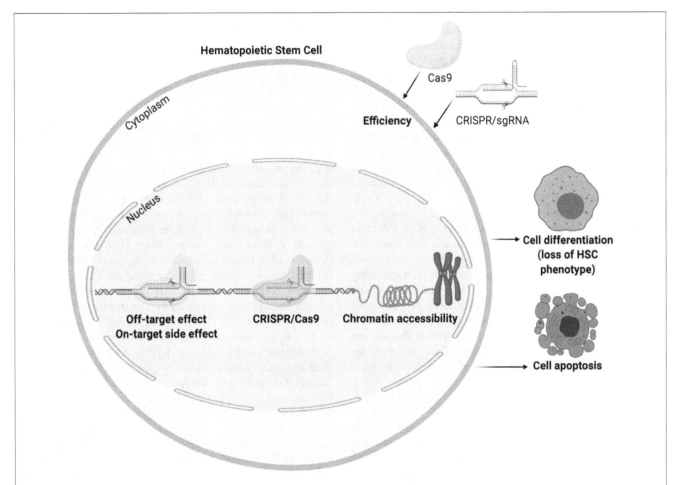

FIGURE 2 | Points of improvement in CRISPR mediated gene correction in HSCs. Efficiency of delivery, off-target effects (targeting the wrong locus), side effects on the target sites (unwanted indels, translocations, and mutations), lack of accessible chromatin, apoptosis due to the harsh procedures, and loss of stemness are all problems that need to be tackled before obtaining clinically relevant HSC numbers that can be transplanted in patients.

is the difficulty in achieving high gene delivery efficiencies. Part of the difficulty is the absence of methods that permit the *in vitro* identification and, thus, selection of *bona fide* HSCs (gene-modified or otherwise) from cultured hematopoietic cells. Another component of the difficulty concerns the gene transfer into HSCs. Because the existing protocols do not employ drug selection, the gene transduction methods need to yield enough functionally reconstituted cells for a good therapeutic response. Another limitation when applying genome-editing in HSCs is the low transplanted cell engraftment capacity due to their poor viability after gene-editing, especially when high percentages of non-edited cells are present after the *ex vivo* modification (Naldini, 2019). For those cases, the enrichment of the CD34$^+$ fraction using a combination of additional hematopoietic surface markers may be important for the improvement of cell engraftment and repopulation, although these additional cell manipulations might lead to loss of stemness and cell death. Along these lines, it is necessary to identify which specific gene-editing tools and strategies are the most appropriate for each disease, and consider whether, on the basis

of the disease phenotype, the modified cells present a selective advantage that might reduce conditioning regimens and increase the cell engraftment capacity.

GENOME EDITING TECHNIQUES: TRANSITION TO THE CLINIC

The introduction of gene-editing tools in the form of engineered nucleases has provided strong support to the idea that targeted genetic therapies for treating monogenetic diseases of the hematopoietic system is achievable. Yet, there are multi-tier bottlenecks on the path to transitioning from applying HSC-directed gene-editing laboratory technologies to the clinic. To overcome these bottlenecks it will be crucial to develop and combine delivery agents and gene-editing reagents that allow for efficient and precise gene-editing at the HSCs level. Further, these integrated gene editing procedures need to be scalable under good manufacturing practice conditions, and, clearly, neither cytotoxic, or genotoxic. Moreover, there are other points that should have important improvements, such as the delivery of the homologous donor templates and the nuclease of choice.

Regardless of their class, programmable nucleases are capable of achieving high specificity, especially once individual reagents are identified and optimized for cleaving target sequences and not off-target sites (Akcakaya et al., 2018), but it is important to know that none of them are perfect. However, even when using the highly specific nucleases, when making changes at the desired target site, unintentional changes can be induced elsewhere in the genome due to, for instance, differences in nuclease amounts and chromosomal accessibility in different cell types. Indeed, these parameters might influence DNA cleavage and NHEJ-mediated repair (profiles) at secondary sites (White et al., 2017). These unwanted genome-modifying events present a modest hazard in experimental systems, where conclusions can be validated by (i) comparing independent gene-edited cells and organisms, (ii) "cleaning-up" the genetic background by out-breeding/cross-breeding and (ii) complementing gene knockouts via introducing wild-type gene sequences. However, for therapeutic applications off-target effects are more problematic. Methods have been developed for detecting, locating and quantifying those off-target effects (Koo et al., 2015). When applied in human therapy, we need to be assured that the adverse effects of the treatment are as minimal as possible while the one originally addressed gene is repaired.

Besides off-target effects, adverse effects caused by cleavage at the desired side of modification have also been reported (Kosicki et al., 2018; Chen et al., 2020). These unwarranted on-target effects can affect not only the genotype but also the phenotype of gene-edited cells (Chen et al., 2020) and are more difficult to assess, but clearly are undesired. In addition, as aforementioned, the efficiency of gene modification can be reduced due to the limited accessibly of target sequences tightly packed in heterochromatic regions (Chen et al., 2016; Daer et al., 2017), resulting in a lack of efficient delivery of the Cas enzyme or the DNA template needed for repair via homologous recombination. The limited access of gene editing reagents to the DNA can perhaps be overcome at some target loci by forcing the HSCs to enter into the S and M phases. However, ex vivo proliferation of HSCs without losing their stemness properties is still a daunting task (Tajer et al., 2019).

Despite these problems, researchers have reported significant advances in gene editing of HSCs for SCID. For instance, Genovese et al. have shown that gene editing for X-SCID is in principle possible (Genovese et al., 2014). In this report, ZFNs were used and the efficacy was relatively low, but some correction was obtained in human long-term repopulating HSCs transplanted in immune-deficient mice. The next improvement consisted of using RGN nucleofection for introducing an IL2RG transgene delivered via an adeno-associated viral vector pseudo-type (i.e., AAV6) into the first exon of the IL2RG gene that is deficient in X-SCID (Pavel-Dinu et al., 2019). The reported gene correction efficiencies were much higher but the phenotypic differences between corrected and uncorrected HSCs transplanted were only minor, with modest increases in T and NK cells, the two lineages affected in this type

of SCID (Pavel-Dinu et al., 2019). This indicated that even for a relatively easy target such as an X-linked gene which only requires correction in one allele, efficacies need to be significantly improved for clinical application. Gene editing is particularly attractive for diseases where the expression of affected gene normally is strictly regulated. While gene addition approaches work well for X-linked SCID (Hacein-Bey-Abina et al., 2002; Pavel-Dinu et al., 2019), ADA-SCID (Aiuti et al., 2009), Wiskott–Aldrich syndrome (WAS) (Braun et al., 2014), RAG1-SCID (Garcia-Perez et al., 2020), and b-globin disease (Dong and Rivella, 2017), for IL7Rα-SCID and for the Hyper IgM syndrome (caused by mutations in the CD40L gene), gene addition with constitutively expressing vectors will cause severe side effects (Kuo et al., 2018). However, also for diseases caused by defects in such genes significant progress is being made. Indeed, Kohn et al. reported specific insertion of a recombinant CD40L sequence downstream of the endogenous CD40L promoter using RGNs and an AAV-delivered donor template (Kuo et al., 2018). Relevant levels of gene modification were achieved in primary HSCs and in patient-derived T cells. Therefore, significant progress is made to clinical implementation of these techniques. Nevertheless, clinical trials using CRISPR and HSCs have been confined to gene deletion strategies rather than editing of mutant genes. Examples include a gene disruption approach to delete the CCR5 HIV coreceptor and the disruption of erythroid lineage-specific enhancer of the BCL11A suppressor protein in the g-globin gene to induce re-expression of fetal g-globin in thalassemia patients (NCT03745287) (Psatha et al., 2018). Indeed, for bona fide gene editing in Hyper IgM syndrome due to CD40L mutations, T cells rather than HSCs are being proposed as target cells in clinical trials.

REGULATORY AUTHORITIES

In the last three decades, the ex vivo gene therapy in HSCs has been progressing substantially from the pre-clinical stage to clinical trials (Thrasher and Williams, 2017; Staal et al., 2019). With the FDA-approved first clinical trial gene-editing of HSCs for the treatment of HIV using the ZFNs CCR5 (Tebas et al., 2014), a new paradigm treatment in cell and gene therapy had been started. Before wide-spread clinical approval, however, there are several regulatory hurdles. Regulation may be complex and vary across countries and continents because gene-editing medicine entails the unprecedented introduction of designed alterations in the genetic make-up of some of the patient's cells. As a minimum, regulators will focus on whether the gene disruption/restoration is based on robust preclinical evidence, as illustrated by the US FDA approval of multiple clinical trials.

Although there is a great promise for gene-editing in the future of medicine, the regulatory approval by the competent authorities will not be granted in the short term. One of the reasons is because the authorities strictly guard safety and well-being of patients (White et al., 2017). One of the major obstacles is that there is no clear consensus regarding the occurrence of on-target and off-target alterations by the gene-editing tools, and also it is not clear when and how these effects should be monitored in the clinical applications (Joung, 2015). Regulatory authorities and the pharmaceutical industry of Europe, Japan, and the USA have developed some consideration documents regarding gene therapy (Coppens et al., 2018; de Wilde et al., 2018), indicating that more regulatory harmonization is indispensable in order to realize the therapeutic benefits of genome editing worldwide.

The versatility and robustness of gene-editing approaches are expected to positively contribute to the development of novel somatic disease treatments. However, the technology could also lead to some unfavorable social phenomena due to high prices and public misconceptions. The general public should understand that so far only a few gene therapy products have been approved by health regulators worldwide. Moreover, scientists have the obligation to provide the public with accurate and realistic information regarding the prospects, as well as the problems associated with the use of somatic gene-editing therapy. In addition, good communication between researchers and the regulatory authorities are key to fulfill the promises and to achieve the medical benefits of genome editing. Communication and cooperation should foster an increase in worldwide regulatory harmonization. This should eventually lead to clinical benefit for those affected with inborn diseases.

FINAL REMARKS

Tremendous progress has been made in the field of gene editing over the last few years. However, no clinical trials using this technology have been used so far to treat immune deficiencies via gene editing for reasons of efficiency and safety. To have HSC gene editing working safely at the scale needed for clinical application remains challenging and will require carefully designed protocols using the correct target cells, assays to detect potential side effects, and comparisons with more conventional allo-HSCT and gene addition therapy methods. Such efforts will hopefully lead to the clinical application of gene editing techniques to cure monogenetic diseases of the hematopoietic system.

AUTHOR CONTRIBUTIONS

All authors listed have made a substantial, direct and intellectual contribution to the work, and approved it for publication.

REFERENCES

Aiuti, A., Cattaneo, F., Galimberti, S., Benninghoff, U., Cassani, B., Callegaro, L., et al. (2009). Gene therapy for immunodeficiency due to adenosine deaminase deficiency. *N. Engl. J. Med.* 360, 447–458. doi: 10.1056/NEJMoa0805817

Akcakaya, P., Bobbin, M. L., Guo, J. A., Malagon-Lopez, J., Clement, K., Garcia, S. P., et al. (2018). *In vivo* CRISPR editing with no detectable genome-wide off-target mutations. *Nature* 561, 416–419. doi: 10.1038/s41586-018-0500-9

Badat, M., and Davies, J. (2017). Gene therapy in a patient with sickle cell disease. *N. Engl. J. Med.* 376, 2093–2094. doi: 10.1056/NEJMc1704009

Bak, R. O., Dever, D. P., and Porteus, M. H. (2018). CRISPR/Cas9 genome editing in human hematopoietic stem cells. *Nat. Protoc.* 13, 358–376. doi: 10.1038/nprot.2017.143

Boitano, A. E., Wang, J., Romeo, R., Bouchez, L. C., Parker, A. E., Sutton, S. E., et al. (2010). Aryl hydrocarbon receptor antagonists promote the expansion of human hematopoietic stem cells. *Science* 329, 1345–1348. doi: 10.1126/science.1191536

Braun, C. J., Boztug, K., Paruzynski, A., Witzel, M., Schwarzer, A., Rothe, M., et al. (2014). Gene therapy for wiskott-aldrich syndrome–long-term efficacy and genotoxicity. *Sci. Transl. Med.* 6:227ra33. doi: 10.1126/scitranslmed.3007280

Buza-Vidas, N., Antonchuk, J., Qian, H., Mansson, R., Luc, S., Zandi, S., et al. (2006). Cytokines regulate postnatal hematopoietic stem cell expansion: opposing roles of thrombopoietin and LNK. *Genes Dev.* 20, 2018–2023. doi: 10.1101/gad.385606

Byrne, S. M., Mali, P., and Church, G. M. (2014). Genome editing in human stem cells. *Meth. Enzymol.* 546, 119–138. doi: 10.1016/B978-0-12-801185-0.00006-4

Cathomen, T., and Keith Joung, J. (2008). Zinc-finger nucleases: the next generation emerges. *Mol. Ther.* 16, 1200–1207. doi: 10.1038/mt.2008.114

Chandrasegaran, S., and Carroll, D. (2016). Origins of programmable nucleases for genome engineering. *J. Mol. Biol.* 428(5 Pt B), 963–89. doi: 10.1016/j.jmb.2015.10.014

Chen, F., Pruett-Miller, S. M., and Davis, G. D. (2015). Gene editing using ssODNs with engineered endonucleases. *Methods Mol. Biol.* 1239, 251–265. doi: 10.1007/978-1-4939-1862-1_14

Chen, X., and Goncalves, M. (2018). DNA, RNA, and protein tools for editing the genetic information in human cells. *iScience* 6, 247–263. doi: 10.1016/j.isci.2018.08.001

Chen, X., Rinsma, M., Janssen, J. M., Liu, J., Maggio, I., and Goncalves, M. A. (2016). Probing the impact of chromatin conformation on genome editing tools. *Nucleic Acids Res.* 44, 6482–6492. doi: 10.1093/nar/gkw524

Chen, X., Tasca, F., Wang, Q., Liu, J., Janssen, J. M., Brescia, M. D., et al. (2020). Expanding the editable genome and CRISPR-Cas9 versatility using DNA cutting-free gene targeting based on in trans paired nicking. *Nucleic Acids Res.* 48, 974–995. doi: 10.1093/nar/gkz1121

Cho, S. W., Kim, S., Kim, J. M., and Kim, J. S. (2013). Targeted genome engineering in human cells with the Cas9 RNA-guided endonuclease. *Nat. Biotechnol.* 31, 230–232. doi: 10.1038/nbt.2507

Cong, L., Ran, F. A., Cox, D., Lin, S., Barretto, R., Habib, N., et al. (2013). Multiplex genome engineering using CRISPR/Cas systems. *Science* 339, 819–823. doi: 10.1126/science.1231143

Coppens, D. G. M., de Wilde, S., Guchelaar, H. J., De Bruin, M. L., Leufkens, H. G. M., Meij, P., et al. (2018). A decade of marketing approval of gene and cell-based therapies in the united states, European union and Japan: an evaluation of regulatory decision-making. *Cytotherapy* 20, 769–778. doi: 10.1016/j.jcyt.2018.03.038

Crisostomo, P. R., Wang, M., Wairiuko, G. M., Morrell, E. D., Terrell, A. M., Seshadri, P., et al. (2006). High passage number of stem cells adversely affects stem cell activation and myocardial protection. *Shock* 26, 575–580. doi: 10.1097/01.shk.0000235087.45798.93

Daer, R. M., Cutts, J. P., Brafman, D. A., and Haynes, K. A. (2017). The impact of chromatin dynamics on cas9-mediated genome editing in human cells. *ACS Synth. Biol.* 6, 428–438. doi: 10.1021/acssynbio.5b00299

de Wilde, S., Coppens, D. G. M., Hoekman, J., de Bruin, M. L., Leufkens, H. G. M., Guchelaar, H. J., et al. (2018). EU decision-making for marketing authorization of advanced therapy medicinal products: a case study. *Drug Discov. Today* 23, 1328–1333. doi: 10.1016/j.drudis.2018.03.008

Dong, A. C., and Rivella, S. (2017). Gene addition strategies for beta-thalassemia and sickle cell anemia. *Adv. Exp. Med. Biol.* 1013, 155–176. doi: 10.1007/978-1-4939-7299-9_6

Doudna, J. A., and Charpentier, E. (2014). Genome editing. The new frontier of genome engineering with CRISPR-Cas9. *Science* 346:1258096. doi: 10.1126/science.1258096

Fares, I., Chagraoui, J., Gareau, Y., Gingras, S., Ruel, R., Mayotte, N., et al. (2014). Cord blood expansion. Pyrimidoindole derivatives are agonists of human hematopoietic stem cell self-renewal. *Science* 345, 1509–1512. doi: 10.1126/science.1256337

Fares, I., Chagraoui, J., Lehnertz, B., MacRae, T., Mayotte, N., Tomellini, E., et al. (2017). EPCR expression marks UM171-expanded CD34(+) cord blood stem cells. *Blood* 129, 3344–3351. doi: 10.1182/blood-2016-11-750729

Garcia-Perez, L., van Eggermond, M., van Roon, L., Vloemans, S. A., Cordes, M., Schambach, A., et al. (2020). Successful preclinical development of gene therapy for recombinase-activating gene-1-Deficient SCID. *Mol. Ther. Methods Clin. Dev.* 17, 666–682. doi: 10.1016/j.omtm.2020.03.016

Gasiunas, G., Barrangou, R., Horvath, P., and Siksnys, V. (2012). Cas9-crRNA ribonucleoprotein complex mediates specific DNA cleavage for adaptive immunity in bacteria. *Proc. Natl. Acad. Sci. U.S.A.* 109, E2579–E2586. doi: 10.1073/pnas.1208507109

Gatti, R. A., Meuwissen, H. J., Allen, H. D., Hong, R., and Good, R. A. (1968). Immunological reconstitution of sex-linked lymphopenic immunological deficiency. *Lancet* 2, 1366–1369. doi: 10.1016/S0140-6736(68)92673-1

Genovese, P., Schiroli, G., Escobar, G., Tomaso, T. D., Firrito, C., Calabria, A., et al. (2014). Targeted genome editing in human repopulating haematopoietic stem cells. *Nature* 510, 235–240. doi: 10.1038/nature13420

Hacein-Bey-Abina, S., Hauer, J., Lim, A., Picard, C., Wang, G. P., Berry, C. C., et al. (2010). Efficacy of gene therapy for X-linked severe combined immunodeficiency. *N. Engl. J. Med.* 363, 355–364. doi: 10.1056/NEJMoa1000164

Hacein-Bey-Abina, S., Le Deist, F., Carlier, F., Bouneaud, C., Hue, C., De Villartay, J. P., et al. (2002). Sustained correction of X-linked severe combined immunodeficiency by *ex vivo* gene therapy. *N. Engl. J. Med.* 346, 1185–1193. doi: 10.1056/NEJMoa012616

Hofmeister, C. C., Zhang, J., Knight, K. L., and Le P, Stiff, P. J. (2007). *Ex vivo* expansion of umbilical cord blood stem cells for transplantation: growing knowledge from the hematopoietic niche. *Bone Marrow Transplant.* 39, 11–23. doi: 10.1038/sj.bmt.1705538

Hoke, N. N., Salloum, F. N., Kass, D. A., Das, A., and Kukreja, R. C. (2012). Preconditioning by phosphodiesterase-5 inhibition improves therapeutic efficacy of adipose-derived stem cells following myocardial infarction in mice. *Stem Cells* 30, 326–335. doi: 10.1002/stem.789

Horvath, P., and Barrangou, R. (2010). CRISPR/Cas, the immune system of bacteria and archaea. *Science* 327, 167–170. doi: 10.1126/science.1179555

Hua, P., Hester, J., Adigbli, G., Li, R., Psaila, B., Roy, A., et al. (2020). The BET inhibitor CPI203 promotes *ex vivo* expansion of cord blood long-term repopulating HSCs and megakaryocytes. *Blood* 136, 2410–2415. doi: 10.1182/blood.2020005357

Ishibashi, T., Yokota, T., Tanaka, H., Ichii, M., Sudo, T., Satoh, Y., et al. (2016). ESAM is a novel human hematopoietic stem cell marker associated with a subset of human leukemias. *Exp. Hematol.* 44, 269.e1–81.e1. doi: 10.1016/j.exphem.2015.12.010

Jinek, M., Chylinski, K., Fonfara, I., Hauer, M., Doudna, J. A., and Charpentier, E. (2012). A programmable dual-RNA-guided DNA endonuclease in adaptive bacterial immunity. *Science* 337, 816–821. doi: 10.1126/science.1225829

Jinek, M., East, A., Cheng, A., Lin, S., Ma, E., and Doudna, J. (2013). RNA-programmed genome editing in human cells. *Elife* 2:e00471. doi: 10.7554/eLife.00471

Johnson, F. L., Look, A. T., Gockerman, J., Ruggiero, M. R., Dalla-Pozza, L., and Billings, F. T. III. (1984). Bone-marrow transplantation in a patient with sickle-cell anemia. *N. Engl. J. Med.* 311, 780–783. doi: 10.1056/NEJM198409203111207

Joung, J. K. (2015). Unwanted mutations: standards needed for gene-editing errors. *Nature* 523:158. doi: 10.1038/523158a

Koo, T., Lee, J., and Kim, J. S. (2015). Measuring and reducing off-target activities of programmable nucleases including CRISPR-Cas9. *Mol. Cells* 38, 475–481. doi: 10.14348/molcells.2015.0103

Kosicki, M., Tomberg, K., and Bradley, A. (2018). Repair of double-strand breaks induced by CRISPR-Cas9 leads to large deletions and complex rearrangements. *Nat. Biotechnol.* 36, 765–771. doi: 10.1038/nbt.4192

Kuo, C. Y., Long, J. D., Campo-Fernandez, B., de Oliveira, S., Cooper, A. R., Romero, Z., et al. (2018). Site-specific gene editing of human hematopoietic stem cells for X-linked hyper-IgM syndrome. *Cell Rep.* 23, 2606–2616. doi: 10.1016/j.celrep.2018.04.103

Lee, J., Bayarsaikhan, D., Arivazhagan, R., Park, H., Lim, B., Gwak, P., et al. (2019). CRISPR/Cas9 edited sRAGE-MSCs protect neuronal death in parkinsons disease model. *Int. J. Stem Cells* 12, 114–124. doi: 10.15283/ijsc18110

Liu, X., Wu, Y., Li, Z., Yang, J., Xue, J., Hu, Y., et al. (2012). Targeting of the human coagulation factor IX gene at rDNA locus of human embryonic stem cells. *PLoS ONE* 7:e37071. doi: 10.1371/journal.pone.0037071

Lucarelli, G., Polchi, P., Izzi, T., Manna, M., Agostinelli, F., Delfini, C., et al. (1984). Allogeneic marrow transplantation for thalassemia. *Exp. Hematol.* 12, 676–681.

Mali, P., Yang, L., Esvelt, K. M., Aach, J., Guell, M., DiCarlo, J. E., et al. (2013). RNA-guided human genome engineering via Cas9. *Science* 339, 823–826. doi: 10.1126/science.1232033

Metcalf, D. (2008). Hematopoietic cytokines. *Blood* 111, 485–491. doi: 10.1182/blood-2007-03-079681

Morrison, S. J., and Kimble, J. (2006). Asymmetric and symmetric stem-cell divisions in development and cancer. *Nature* 441, 1068–1074. doi: 10.1038/nature04956

Mussolino, C., and Cathomen, T. (2012). TALE nucleases: tailored genome engineering made easy. *Curr. Opin. Biotechnol.* 23, 644–650. doi: 10.1016/j.copbio.2012.01.013

Naldini, L. (2019). Genetic engineering of hematopoiesis: current stage of clinical translation and future perspectives. *EMBO Mol. Med.* 11:e9958. doi: 10.15252/emmm.201809958

Notta, F., Doulatov, S., Laurenti, E., Poeppl, A., Jurisica, I., and Dick, J. E. (2011). Isolation of single human hematopoietic stem cells capable of long-term multilineage engraftment. *Science* 333, 218–221. doi: 10.1126/science.1201219

Ooi, A. G., Karsunky, H., Majeti, R., Butz, S., Vestweber, D., Ishida, T., et al. (2009). The adhesion molecule esam1 is a novel hematopoietic stem cell marker. *Stem Cells* 27, 653–661. doi: 10.1634/stemcells.2008-0824

Pavel-Dinu, M., Wiebking, V., Dejene, B. T., Srifa, W., Mantri, S., Nicolas, C. E., et al. (2019). Author correction: gene correction for SCID-X1 in long-term hematopoietic stem cells. *Nat. Commun.* 10:5624. doi: 10.1038/s41467-019-13620-5

Porteus, M. H. (2019). A new class of medicines through DNA editing. *N. Engl. J. Med.* 380, 947–959. doi: 10.1056/NEJMra1800729

Psatha, N., Reik, A., Phelps, S., Zhou, Y., Dalas, D., Yannaki, E., et al. (2018). Disruption of the BCL11A erythroid enhancer reactivates fetal hemoglobin in erythroid cells of patients with beta-thalassemia major. *Mol. Ther. Methods Clin. Dev.* 10, 313–326. doi: 10.1016/j.omtm.2018.08.003

Radulovic, V., van der Garde, M., Koide, S., Sigurdsson, V., Lang, S., Kaneko, S., et al. (2019). Junctional adhesion molecule 2 represents a subset of hematopoietic stem cells with enhanced potential for T lymphopoiesis. *Cell Rep.* 27, 2826–36.e5. doi: 10.1016/j.celrep.2019.05.028

Rath, D., Amlinger, L., Rath, A., and Lundgren, M. (2015). The CRISPR-Cas immune system: biology, mechanisms and applications. *Biochimie* 117, 119–128. doi: 10.1016/j.biochi.2015.03.025

Roch, A., Giger, S., Girotra, M., Campos, V., Vannini, N., Naveiras, O., et al. (2017). Single-cell analyses identify bioengineered niches for enhanced maintenance of hematopoietic stem cells. *Nat. Commun.* 8:221. doi: 10.1038/s41467-017-00291-3

Sauvageau, G., Iscove, N. N., and Humphries, R. K. (2004). *In vitro* and *in vivo* expansion of hematopoietic stem cells. *Oncogene* 23, 7223–7232. doi: 10.1038/sj.onc.1207942

Shahryari, A., Saghaeian Jazi, M., Mohammadi, S., Razavi Nikoo, H., Nazari, Z., Hosseini, E. S., et al. (2019). Development and clinical translation of approved gene therapy products for genetic disorders. *Front. Genet.* 10:868. doi: 10.3389/fgene.2019.00868

Shim, G., Kim, D., Park, G. T., Jin, H., Suh, S. K., and Oh, Y. K. (2017). Therapeutic gene editing: delivery and regulatory perspectives. *Acta Pharmacol. Sin.* 38, 738–753. doi: 10.1038/aps.2017.2

Staal, F. J., Baum, C., Cowan, C., Dzierzak, E., Hacein-Bey-Abina, S., Karlsson, S., et al. (2011). Stem cell self-renewal: lessons from bone marrow, gut and iPS toward clinical applications. *Leukemia* 25, 1095–1102. doi: 10.1038/leu.2011.52

Staal, F. J. T., Aiuti, A., and Cavazzana, M. (2019). Autologous stem-cell-based gene therapy for inherited disorders: state of the art and perspectives. *Front. Pediatr.* 7:443. doi: 10.3389/fped.2019.00443

Staal, F. J. T., and Fibbe, W. E. (2020). BETting on stem cell expansion. *Blood* 136, 2364–2365. doi: 10.1182/blood.2020007759

Tajer, P., Pike-Overzet, K., Arias, S., Havenga, M., and Staal, F. J. T. (2019). *Ex vivo* expansion of hematopoietic stem cells for therapeutic purposes: lessons from development and the niche. *Cells* 8:169. doi: 10.3390/cells8020169

Tebas, P., Stein, D., Tang, W. W., Frank, I., Wang, S. Q., Lee, G., et al. (2014). Gene editing of CCR5 in autologous CD4 T cells of persons infected with HIV. *N. Engl. J. Med.* 370, 901–910. doi: 10.1056/NEJMoa1300662

Thomas, E. D., Storb, R., Clift, R. A., Fefer, A., Johnson, L., Neiman, P. E., et al. (1975). Bone-marrow transplantation (second of two parts). *N. Engl. J. Med.* 292, 895–902. doi: 10.1056/NEJM197504242921706

Thrasher, A. J., and Williams, D. A. (2017). Evolving gene therapy in primary immunodeficiency. *Mol. Ther.* 25, 1132–1141. doi: 10.1016/j.ymthe.2017.03.018

Urnov, F. D., Rebar, E. J., Holmes, M. C., Zhang, H. S., and Gregory, P. D. (2010). Genome editing with engineered zinc finger nucleases. *Nat. Rev. Genet.* 11, 636–646. doi: 10.1038/nrg2842

Wagner, J. E. Jr., Brunstein, C. G., Boitano, A. E., DeFor, T. E., McKenna, D., Sumstad, D., et al. (2016). Phase I/II trial of StemRegenin-1 expanded umbilical cord blood hematopoietic stem cells supports testing as a stand-alone graft. *Cell Stem Cell* 18, 144–155. doi: 10.1016/j.stem.2015.10.004

White, M., Whittaker, R., Gandara, C., and Stoll, E. A. (2017). A guide to approaching regulatory considerations for lentiviral-mediated gene therapies. *Hum. Gene Ther. Methods* 28, 163–176. doi: 10.1089/hgtb.2017.096

White, M. K., and Khalili, K. (2016). CRISPR/Cas9 and cancer targets: future possibilities and present challenges. *Oncotarget* 7, 12305–12317. doi: 10.18632/oncotarget.7104

Wiedenheft, B., Sternberg, S. H., and Doudna, J. A. (2012). RNA-guided genetic silencing systems in bacteria and archaea. *Nature* 482, 331–338. doi: 10.1038/nature10886

Woods, N. B., Bottero, V., Schmidt, M., von Kalle, C., and Verma, I. M. (2006). Gene therapy: therapeutic gene causing lymphoma. *Nature* 440:1123. doi: 10.1038/4401123a

Yokota, T., Oritani, K., Butz, S., Kokame, K., Kincade, P. W., Miyata, T., et al. (2009). The endothelial antigen ESAM marks primitive hematopoietic progenitors throughout life in mice. *Blood* 113, 2914–2923. doi: 10.1182/blood-2008-07-167106

7

A Small Key for a Heavy Door: Genetic Therapies for the Treatment of Hemoglobinopathies

Hidde A. Zittersteijn[1]*, Cornelis L. Harteveld[2], Stefanie Klaver-Flores[3],
Arjan C. Lankester[4], Rob C. Hoeben[1], Frank J. T. Staal[3] and Manuel A. F. V. Gonçalves[1]

[1] Department of Cell and Chemical Biology, Leiden University Medical Center, Leiden, Netherlands, [2] Department of Human and Clinical Genetics, The Hemoglobinopathies Laboratory, Leiden University Medical Center, Leiden, Netherlands, [3] Department of Immunology, Leiden University Medical Center, Leiden, Netherlands, [4] Department of Pediatrics, Stem Cell Transplantation Program, Willem-Alexander Children's Hospital, Leiden University Medical Center, Leiden, Netherlands

*Correspondence:
Hidde A. Zittersteijn
h.a.zittersteijn@lumc.nl

Throughout the past decades, the search for a treatment for severe hemoglobinopathies has gained increased interest within the scientific community. The discovery that ɣ-globin expression from intact *HBG* alleles complements defective *HBB* alleles underlying β-thalassemia and sickle cell disease, has provided a promising opening for research directed at relieving ɣ-globin repression mechanisms and, thereby, improve clinical outcomes for patients. Various gene editing strategies aim to reverse the fetal-to-adult hemoglobin switch to up-regulate ɣ-globin expression through disabling either *HBG* repressor genes or repressor binding sites in the *HBG* promoter regions. In addition to these *HBB* mutation-independent strategies involving fetal hemoglobin (HbF) synthesis de-repression, the expanding genome editing toolkit is providing increased accuracy to *HBB* mutation-specific strategies encompassing adult hemoglobin (HbA) restoration for a personalized treatment of hemoglobinopathies. Moreover, besides genome editing, more conventional gene addition strategies continue under investigation to restore HbA expression. Together, this research makes hemoglobinopathies a fertile ground for testing various innovative genetic therapies with high translational potential. Indeed, the progressive understanding of the molecular clockwork underlying the hemoglobin switch together with the ongoing optimization of genome editing tools heightens the prospect for the development of effective and safe treatments for hemoglobinopathies. In this context, clinical genetics plays an equally crucial role by shedding light on the complexity of the disease and the role of ameliorating genetic modifiers. Here, we cover the most recent insights on the molecular mechanisms underlying hemoglobin biology and hemoglobinopathies while providing an overview of state-of-the-art gene editing platforms. Additionally, current genetic therapies under development, are equally discussed.

Keywords: gene therapy, genome editing, hemoglobinopathies, fetal globin induction, thalasseamia, sickle-cell disease (SCD), hemoglobin switch, gamma-globin

INTRODUCTION

Hemoglobinopathies are the world's most common group of monogenic disorders with an estimated 7% of the global population carrying these diseases (Piel, 2016). Particularly prevalent in Africa, Asia and the Mediterranean, hemoglobinopathies are presently distributed globally due to increased migration rates (Williams and Weatherall, 2012; Piel, 2016). The clinical presentation of hemoglobinopathies varies from mild to severe, depending on the type of inherited mutation, the zygosity of the mutation and the co-inheritance status of ameliorating genetic modifiers, such as hereditary persistence of fetal hemoglobin (HPFH).

By applying X-ray crystallography to hemoglobin, Max Perutz pioneered the use of structural information to uncover how mutations lead to disease at the molecular and atomic levels (Perutz, 1962). These and subsequent fundamental insights on hemoglobin biology formed the basis for the development of conventional treatments sustaining the clinical management of hemoglobinopathies, in particular, blood transfusion, iron chelation and pharmaceutical induction of fetal hemoglobin (HbF) (Kohne, 2011). Yet, for severe clinical cases requiring regular blood transfusions, the only curable option is allogeneic hematopoietic stem cell transplantation (allo-HSCT). New insights in pre-transplant evaluation, donor selection, stem cell source and post-transplant management, together with the implementation of reduced-intensity conditioning (RIC) regimens and pre-transplant immunosuppressive therapy, have all greatly improved treatment outcomes. However, allo-HSCT still suffers from limited donor availability issues as well as morbidity and mortality risks associated with suboptimal donor matching (Angelucci et al., 2014; Baronciani et al., 2016; Zaidman et al., 2016; Anurathapan et al., 2020). Moreover, allo-HSCT protocols for sickle-cell disease (SCD) are more difficult to define than those for β-thalassemia major due to their more complex prognostic disease-severity criteria. This makes it more difficult to optimize allo-HSCT protocols for each patient (Angelucci et al., 2014).

The ongoing development of various candidate genetic therapies raises the possibility that autologous hematopoietic stem cell transplantation (auto-HSCT) will complement, or perhaps even replace, allo-HSCT as a preferable treatment modality. Importantly, the efficient and safe collection of long-term repopulating hematopoietic stem cells (HSCs) from patients with severe hemoglobinopathies is crucial for the success of genetic therapies. The development of plerixafor-based mobilization regimens has resulted in an efficient and safe manner of collecting long-term engrafting HSCs from both SCD and β-thalassemia patients (Yannaki et al., 2013; Baiamonte et al., 2015; Boulad et al., 2018; Esrick et al., 2018; Uchida et al., 2020). Of notice, considering the relative high prevalence of hemoglobinopathies in low- to middle-income regions, spanning over sub-Saharan Africa, the Mediterranean, the Middle East and South-east Asia, bottlenecks for a world-wide implementation of both allo- and auto-HSCT are the costs and requirements for specialized centers. For this reason, considerable efforts continue to be directed toward the improvement of standard and easy-to-implement palliative treatments and diagnostics (Taher et al., 2018; Ikawa et al., 2019; Iolascon et al., 2019).

With regard to candidate curative genetic therapies, one can consider three main aspects driving their progression toward clinical application. Firstly, the fundamental understanding of hemoglobin biology, in which knowledge on genetics, cell biology and human development is combined to obtain a comprehensive understanding of the molecular clockwork underlying hemoglobin-linked phenotypes under homeostatic and disease states. Secondly, clinical genetics play a crucial role in allocating the cause for specific hemoglobinopathies and in identifying any disease modifying genetic traits. Lastly, research on innovative genetic techniques, e.g., lentiviral vector (LV)-mediated gene addition, or gene editing based on programmable nucleases, e.g., zinc-finger nucleases (ZFNs), transcription activator-like effector nucleases (TALENs) and RNA-guided nucleases (RGNs) based on clustered regularly interspaced short palindromic repeats (CRISPR)-associated (Cas) proteins (CRISPR-Cas), is required to permanently rescue pathological phenotypes through the transplantation of genetically modified HSCs.

As mentioned before, knowledge on the molecular, cellular and developmental processes underlying hemoglobinopathies is extensive. As such, it provides a rich foundation on which novel genetic therapy concepts can be built upon and tested. Currently, there are two main categories of genetic therapies being developed for treating hemoglobinopathies, i.e., gene therapy and gene editing involving exogenous gene addition and direct modification of endogenous DNA, respectively. Backed by decades of fundamental and pre-clinical research, gene therapy is the first modality of genetic therapy entering clinical trials targeting diseases of the hematopoietic system (Cavazzana et al., 2019).

In this review, we provide an overview of the current understanding of the molecular mechanisms governing hemoglobin biology in homeostasis and disease states. Subsequently, building on this knowledge, we cover the ongoing efforts aiming at the development of gene-centered treatments for hemoglobinopathies and, in the process, discuss the underlying state-of-the-art genetic technologies.

THE MOLECULAR HEMOGLOBIN CLOCKWORK UNDERLYING HEALTH AND DISEASE

The fundamentals of hemoglobin biology entail an intricate clockwork of molecular mechanisms that enable a balanced expression of various globin subunits during human development (Cao and Moi, 2002). Hemoglobin is a tetrameric protein present in red blood cells (RBCs) specialized in the transport of oxygen and carbon dioxide throughout the body. It consists of two sets of two identical globin chains, categorized as two α- and two non-α globin chains, each of which forming a heme pocket containing a heme-group with

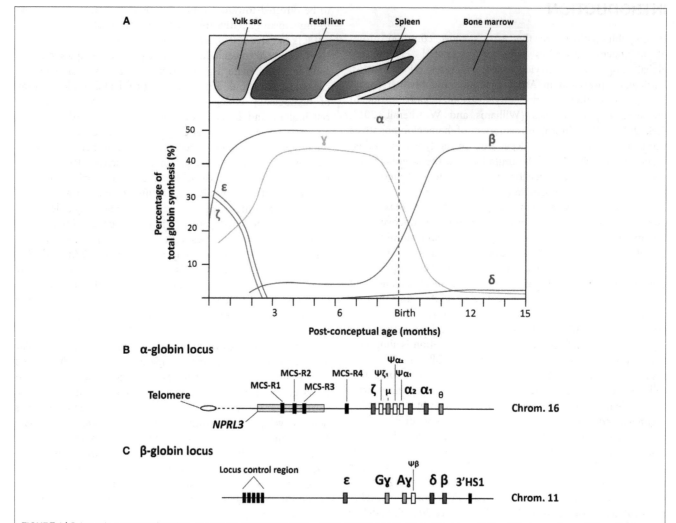

FIGURE 1 | Schematic representation of the hemoglobin switches and the α- and β-globin loci. **(A)** Schematic representation of the human hemoglobin switches before and after birth displaying each globin chain expression levels as the percentage of total globin synthesis. **(B)** Detailed schematic representation of the α-globin locus containing the *NPRL3* gene in which three of the four multispecies conserved regions (MCS-R1-4) lie. The chronological order of ζ-, α2-, and α1-globin expression follows the genomic order of the respective α-like globin genes, i.e., *HBZ, HBA2,* and *HBA1,* respectively along the cluster. Furthermore, the three inactive globin pseudogenes (Ψ) are depicted together with the theta-gene. **(C)** Schematic representation of the β-globin locus containing the locus control region (LCR), the genes coding functional ε-, Gγ-, Aγ-, δ-, and β-globin proteins (i.e., *HBE, HBG2, HBG1, HBD,* and *HBB,* respectively), the β-pseudogene, also known as *HBBP1,* and the 3'HS1 enhancer element.

a central iron ion that gives hemoglobin its oxygen carrying capacity and distinctive red color. During human development, the composition of hemoglobin molecules changes in that different pairs of globin subunits assemble in a process called hemoglobin switching. During the first 3 months of gestation, the hemoglobin tetramer starts as embryonic hemoglobin ($\zeta_2\varepsilon_2$, $\alpha_2\varepsilon_2$, and $\zeta_2\gamma_2$), then as fetal hemoglobin ($\alpha_2\gamma_2$) and, finally, shortly after birth, acquires the composition of adult hemoglobin ($\alpha_2\delta_2$ and $\alpha_2\beta_2$). These hemoglobin variants are expressed in the embryonic yolk sac, fetal liver, spleen (albeit to a much lower extent compared to the bone marrow) and bone marrow, respectively (**Figure 1A**). To regulate high expression levels of the various globin genes through the different developmental stages and tissues, besides the canonical *cis*-acting regulatory sequences, a complex, yet robust, regulatory mechanism has

evolved (Chada et al., 1985; Townes et al., 1985; Kollias et al., 1986). In the following sections, we provide an overview of the current understanding of this mechanism for both α- and β-like globin expression by discussing the α- and β-globin loci and their regulatory elements (**Figures 1B,C**).

Regulation of the α-globin Genes

The ~26 kb α-globin locus contains the ζ-globin gene (ζ or *HBZ*), the duplicated α-globin genes (α_2 and α_1, *HBA2* and *HBA1*, respectively), two transcriptionally active genes with unknown function (μ and θ) and 3 pseudogenes (ψζ1, ψα2, and ψα1). This cluster is located near the telomeric end of the short arm of chromosome 16 (Higgs et al., 1989) (**Figure 1B**) While the ζ- and α-globin genes contribute to the hemoglobin formation during human development, the three pseudogenes are non-functional

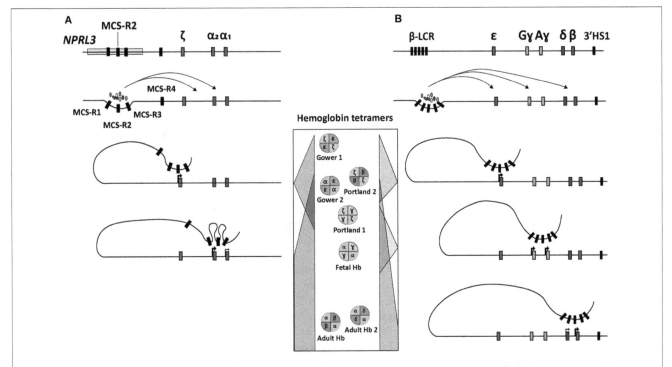

FIGURE 2 | Schematic representation of hemoglobin regulation. **(A)** Structure of the α-globin locus showing the recruitment of tissue-specific transcription factors at the distal regulatory regions (MCS-R1-4) and subsequent sequential chromosomal looping directing the orderly expression of ζ-, α2-, and α1-globin. **(B)** Structure of the β-globin locus depicting the recruitment of tissue-specific transcription factors at the distal regulatory elements (LCR) and ensuing sequential chromosomal looping governing orderly expression of ε, Gγ, Aγ, δ, and β-globin. In the center, the concomittant hemoglobin tetramer variants are displayed according to the chronological order of human development (top-to-bottom).

due to the presence of inactivating mutations. Interestingly, the μ and θ genes show high homology to the α-globin genes and, albeit at much lower rates than ζ, α2, and α1, they are actively transcribed in erythroid cells, yet, without yielding detectable protein products (Marks et al., 1986; Clegg, 1987; Hsu et al., 1988; Albitar et al., 1992a). It is hypothesized that the μ and θ genes are in transition toward becoming completely inactive pseudogenes, or that the globin-like gene products function sufficiently at very low levels (Goh et al., 2005).

Concerning the ζ- and α-globin differential expression process, an interesting observation was made through clinical genetics in which a family with α-thalassemia had an intact α-globin locus but carried a large (∼62 kb) deletion upstream of the α-globin locus (Hatton et al., 1990; Higgs et al., 1990). In particular, in an ∼10–50 kb range upstream of the α-globin cluster four so-called multispecies conserved sequences (MCS-R1-4) were identified as crucial regulatory regions for the expression of the α-globin genes (Hughes et al., 2005) (**Figure 1B**). From these four MCS regions, MCS-R2, formerly known as DNase I hypersensitivity (HS) site HS-40, is considered the major enhancer since it is the only regulatory element capable of driving α-globin expression by itself (Sharpe et al., 1992; Higgs and Wood, 2008). By using humanized mouse models in which the MCS-R2 element was dissected (Wallace et al., 2007), several studies elucidated key functions of this enhancer in α-globin regulation, i.e., binding of tissue-specific transcription factors,

long-range chromatin looping and transcription initiation (De Gobbi et al., 2007; Vernimmen et al., 2009, 2011). More specifically, owing to the presence of multiple conserved binding sites for erythroid-specific transcription factors, such as GATA1, GATA2, NF-E2, and SCL/TAL1 (De Gobbi et al., 2007; Vernimmen et al., 2009), MCS-R2, in concert with the other MCS elements, enhances α-globin gene expression by fostering the recruitment of the transcription preinitiation complex and the formation of long-range intra-chromosomal loops (Vernimmen, 2014) (**Figure 2A**). Additionally, through the recruitment of JMJD3, the MCS-R2 plays an important role in the eviction of the polycomb repressive complex 2 from the CpG-islands at the α-globin genes, thereby removing the repressive H3K27me3 epigenetic chromatin modification (Garrick et al., 2008; Vernimmen et al., 2011). The importance of the interplay between the α-globin gene cluster and the distal enhancers is also supported by the conservation of the latter elements, spanning an ∼135 kb region, in various mammalian species (Tufarelli et al., 2004; Hughes et al., 2005; Philipsen and Hardison, 2018). Interestingly, after the switch from embryonic to fetal hemoglobin, the identical α1- and α2-globin genes are differentially expressed in that the expression level of the latter is 2-3 fold higher than that of the former (Liebhaber and Kan, 1981; Albitar et al., 1992b). This is presumably due to its positioning closer to the upstream MCS-R1-4 enhancer region (Higgs et al., 1989).

α-thalassemia

Depending on the number of α-globin genes affected, there are four clinically distinguishable forms of α-thalassemia (MIM # 604131), namely, silent carrier, carrier with symptoms, Hemoglobin H disease and α-thalassemia major. These forms range in severity from no symptomology to a lethal condition named Bart's hydrops fetalis (Farashi and Harteveld, 2018). The causes for α-thalassemia can be found in a variety of mutations that results in compromised α-globin expression and, ultimately, in α- vs. non-α-chain imbalances. The clinical severity of the disease is mainly determined by the number of α-globin genes that are disrupted or deleted. During the adult and fetal developmental stages, the relative excess in β-like globin chains, due to a reduction in α-globin chains, leads to the accumulation of non-functional tetramers called HbH (β_4) and Hb Bart's (γ_4), respectively. These insoluble tetramers precipitate intracellularly and cause the disruption of the RBC membrane leading to hemolytic anemia. In the case of Bart's hydrops fetalis syndrome, the fetus lacks hemoglobin tetramers containing α-globin altogether making it dependent on the expression of Hb Portland ($\zeta_2\gamma_2$) (King and Higgs, 2018) (**Figure 2**). This temporally delimited gene complementation phenomenon allows the fetus to survive until the 23rd to 38th week of gestation (King and Higgs, 2018).

There are two distinct α-thalassemia-causing genotypes. The first entails the disruption or deletion of one of the two α-globin genes either in one or both alleles and is annotated as α^+-thalassemia. The second comprises the absence, usually through a large deletion, of both α-genes in *cis*, i.e., on the same chromosomal locus, and is annotated as α^0-thalassemia. The most frequent type of mutations affecting the expression of the α-globin genes are α^+-thalassemic deletions of one or both of the α-globin genes (~80%), of which the most common deletions are -$\alpha^{3.7}$ and -$\alpha^{4.2}$ (Farashi and Harteveld, 2018). These small deletions occur through misalignment of the respective Z- and X-homology boxes during meiosis, causing the loss of one of the α-globin genes (Farashi and Harteveld, 2018). The fact that the majority of α-thalassemia-causing mutations are small deletions is attributed to the relatively open chromatin structure at α-globin loci, combined with the high density of homologous sequences in this region in the form of gene duplications and *Alu* repeats (Harteveld et al., 1997; Farashi and Harteveld, 2018). Although less common, a wide range of point mutations causing α^+-thalassemia have also been documented. These mutations affect a plethora of processes, e.g., α-globin gene transcription, mRNA processing, globin chain stability as well as interactions with α-hemoglobin stabilizing protein (AHSP), internal heme-pocket sites and α-b-globin helix-structures (Farashi and Harteveld, 2018).

An interesting rare syndrome that is associated with α-thalassemia is the X-linked mental retardation syndrome ATR-X (OMIM:301040). Characterized by severe mental retardation and dysmorphic features this syndrome shows striking similarities among patients. The molecular cause of ATR-X are point mutations in the *ATRX* gene (Xq13.3) encoding a chromatin-associated protein belonging to the SNF2 family of helicase/adenosine triphosphatases (Gibbons, 2006). Although the connection between ATRX mutations and α-thalassemia is not completely clear, the ATRX protein was found to be a transcriptional regulator affecting α-globin gene expression (Gibbons et al., 2003, 2008; De La Fuente et al., 2011).

The larger deletions, encompassing both α-globin genes in a single chromosomal locus, causing α^0-thalassemia, occur less frequently than the smaller deletions found in α^+-thalassemia. Homozygosity for such an α^0-deletion causes the development of the aforementioned Hb Bart's hydrops fetalis syndrome. In cases where the ζ-globin gene is also deleted, homozygotes will not survive past the earliest stages of development (Farashi and Harteveld, 2018).

Regulation of the β-globin Genes

The β-globin locus spans over ~70 kb and expresses five functional globins, in particular, ε, Gγ, Aγ, δ, and β from the *HBE*, *HBG2*, *HBG1*, *HBD*, and *HBB* alleles, respectively. The expression from the various β-globin gene cluster members takes place sequentially throughout human development (Cao and Moi, 2002; Stamatoyannopoulos, 2005) (**Figures 1A,C and 2B**). In addition, the β-globin locus contains a single pseudogene, i.e., *HBBP1* ($\psi\beta$), which is inactive (Harris et al., 1984). During the first 6 weeks of gestation, ε-globin is expressed in the embryonic yolk sac and forms embryonic hemoglobin tetramers, i.e., $\zeta_2\varepsilon_2$ and $\alpha_2\varepsilon_2$. Next, ε-globin expression is switched off whilst the expression of the two γ-globin genes *HBG2* and *HBG1* starts in the fetal liver forming $\alpha_2\gamma_2$ hemoglobin tetramers. Around birth, during the gradual transition of the main tissue of expression from fetal liver to bone marrow, the synthesis of γ-globin in erythroid cells is repressed whilst that of β-globin is activated forming adult $\alpha_2\beta_2$ hemoglobin tetramers (**Figures 1A, 2B**). This sequential activation and repression of globin genes, in specific hematopoietic tissues, requires complex mechanisms ensuring proper spatiotemporal control over gene product synthesis. Therefore, similar to the α-globin genes, the expression patterns of β-globin genes is regulated through canonical *cis*-acting elements within or proximal to individual genes that function in concert with a series of distal upstream enhancer elements present at the 5'-end of the locus in a chromosomal segment called the locus control region (LCR) (Crossley and Orkin, 1993; Cao and Moi, 2002).

The functional importance of the LCR was first identified through the observation of β-globin silencing in individuals with deletions in this region causing γδβ-thalassemia (Van der Ploeg et al., 1980; Kioussis et al., 1983). The LCR contains four erythroid-specific DNase I HS sites, i.e., HS 1 through 4 (HS1-4), and one constitutive HS site (HS-5) further upstream. Together, these *cis*-acting elements enhance globin gene expression (Cao and Moi, 2002). The enhancer elements HS1-4 contain sequences that interact with various proteins, such as, transcription factors GATA1, TAL1, E2A, LMO2, LDB1 and NF-E2 that, together, cooperate in the recruitment of the RNA polymerase II holoenzyme (Lowrey et al., 1992; Zhou et al., 2004; Liang et al., 2008; Borg et al., 2010; Stadhouders et al., 2014; Cavazzana et al., 2017). Indeed, these DNA-protein interactions facilitate the assembly of structural regulatory conformations, such as loop formation, that ultimately favor transcription initiation

(Noordermeer and de Laat, 2008) (**Figure 2B**). According to their sequential location along the β-globin locus, and hence depending on their relative distance to the LCR, the β-globin genes are differentially regulated during development (Hanscombe et al., 1991).

In the context of recent research aiming at the development of genetic therapies for hemoglobinopathies, a crucial aspect of β-globin gene regulation concerns the fetal-to-adult hemoglobin switch. Owing to the ameliorating effects of HPFH in patients with either β-thalassemia or SCD, there is an increasing number of investigations focused on this particular fetal-to-adult hemoglobin switch. The resulting insights are guiding molecular strategies that aim at relieving the ɣ-globin repressing mechanisms. The most recent insights and therapeutic efforts are discussed later.

β-thalassemia and Sickle Cell Disease

β-thalassemia

β-thalassemia (MIM # 613985) is an autosomal recessive disorder caused by a large spectrum of mutations (>300 known) that reduce or abolish the production of the β-globin chain expressed from the *HBB* gene (Thein, 2013; Kountouris et al., 2014). When a mutation causes a complete or partial reduction of β-globin, it is referred to as a β^0- or β^+-thalassemia mutation, respectively. Due to the compromised expression of β-globin, excessive free α-globin chains builds-up intracellularly. This excess forms inclusion bodies that lead to RBC loss due to hemolysis and ineffective erythropoiesis. Hence, the degree to which the β-globin expression is affected by a specific mutation together with the co-inheritance status of genetic modifying traits, such as those conferring elevated ɣ-globin (i.e., HPFH) or reduced α-globin expression, can have a major influence on the clinical presentation of β-thalassemia (Thein, 2018). Additionally, genetic modifiers that ameliorate any secondary complications resulting from the disease pathophysiology (e.g., anemia) or from treatment regimens (e.g., excessive iron loads due to repeated transfusions), are also important parameters determining disease progression and severity (Thein, 2018). Interestingly, in contrast to α-thalassemia, the most common type of mutations in β-thalassemia are non-deletional mutations (Thein, 2013). These non-deletional mutations can affect gene transcription (e.g., promoter disruption), RNA processing (e.g., abnormal splicing due to the creation of cryptic splice sites) and mRNA translation (e.g., generation of premature stop codons) (Thein, 2018). The rarer deletional mutations causing β-thalassemia consist of both small and large deletions encompassing the *HBB* gene itself, the LCR or both (Thein, 2013, 2018).

By virtue of the in-depth knowledge about the complex genetics of β-thalassemia and advanced DNA sequencing technologies, it is currently possible to guide clinical management on the basis of the patient's genotype, i.e., causative mutations and genetic modifiers (Badens et al., 2011; Danjou et al., 2011).

Sickle Cell Disease

Similar to β-thalassemia, SCD (a.k.a. sickle cell anemia; MIM #603903) is an autosomal recessive disease affecting normal β-globin function. However, in contrast to β-thalassemia, SCD is caused by a single T→A substitution leading to the translation of valine instead of glutamic acid at position 6 of the β-globin chain (Ingram, 1956; Murayama, 1967). Due to this cell sickling (S) mutation, HbS tetramers carrying the abnormal β^S globin chains polymerize through hydrophobic valine interactions that form large HbS polymers (Sundd et al., 2019). As a consequence, RBCs become more rigid and distorted, acquire a sickled shape and suffer from cellular stress, dehydration and hemolysis (Kato et al., 2018; Sundd et al., 2019). The severity of SCD mostly depends on the zygosity underlying the sickle cell trait and on the co-inheritance of other *HBB* mutations, such as, the structural HbC or β-thalassemic mutations (β^+ or β^0) (Kato et al., 2018). The most common form of SCD is caused by the Hemoglobin SS genotype (Hb SS) in which a patient inherits HbS alleles from both parents. Together with the co-inheritance of HbS and β^0 alleles, Hb SS is the most clinically severe form of SCD. Interestingly, co-inheritance of SCD and α-thalassemia occurs frequently, which can have an ameliorating effect on disease severity (Rumaney et al., 2014; Saraf et al., 2014). However, this is not always the case as in these HbS/α-thalassemic patients the occurrence of complications, such as aseptic necrosis and retinal disease, seems to be higher (Saraf et al., 2014). Another important genetic modifier is the co-inheritance of HPFH. In this case, the presence of increased numbers of HbF RBCs (F-cells) dilutes the amount of HbS RBCs thereby reducing their contribution to SCD severity. Moreover, heterologous HbF/HbS tetramers ($\alpha_2\beta^S\gamma$) do not favor pathologic HbS polymerization (Akinsheye et al., 2011). Interestingly, the most important ameliorating effect of fetal globin on the SCD phenotype is its enhanced oxygen affinity which leads to increased oxygen tension in the RBCs carrying HbS. This prevents sickling as low intracellular oxygen levels are usually required for pathologic HbS polymerization to occur (Henry et al., 2020). Indeed, for instance, polymorphisms in important ɣ-globin-regulating loci (e.g., *BCL11A* and *HBS1L-MYB*) leading to ɣ-globin persistence into adulthood can ameliorate the clinical severity of SCD (Lettre et al., 2008; Creary et al., 2009; Makani et al., 2011; Sokolova et al., 2019). For this reason, the investigation of both conventional and genetic approaches that lead to the up-regulation of ɣ-globin synthesis post-birth has acquired particular interest in the search for better SCD treatments.

The Role of Clinical Genetics and Family Studies

Diagnostics of affected patients as well as asymptomatic carriers of novel genetic variants provide insights into the expression and regulation of the globin genes. A paradigmatic example of this was the discovery in a Dutch family with β^0-thalassemia that the LCR regulates β-globin expression over a long distance (Van der Ploeg et al., 1980). Indeed, in addition to cell and mouse models, the processes by which distal *cis*-acting elements regulate α- and β-globin gene expression have been investigated extensively through genotyping and phenotyping studies of patients and their families. Sometimes, through these studies, unexpected differences between humans and mice are observed.

As mentioned before, the major conserved sequences of the HS-40 region of the α-globin gene cluster consists of four important elements MCS-R1-4 of which MCS-R2 was found to be most essential for α-globin gene expression in mice (Higgs and Wood, 2008). With the introduction of multiplex ligation-dependent probe amplification (MLPA) to screen for copy number variation in the globin gene clusters (Harteveld et al., 2005), deletions and duplications influencing globin expression patterns readily uncovered homozygosity for MCS-R2 deletions in patients suffering from HbH disease (Coelho et al., 2010; Sollaino et al., 2010). This finding suggests a complex role of the MCS-R1-4 elements in α-globin gene regulation.

A major advantage of the hemoglobinopathies as disease models for unraveling gene control processes is the availability of large amounts of diagnostic data from patients and carriers alike. In contrast to many other human recessive diseases, carriers are relatively easy to detect by hematologic and biochemical analyses of their RBCs (Traeger-Synodinos et al., 2015). Moreover, as the globin genes are relatively small they are readily covered by Sanger sequencing, which permits establishing clear genotype-phenotype correlations in an easy and straightforward manner.

Families with unexplained α- or β-thalassemia or with elevated expression of HbF were crucial in the discovery of *trans*-acting factors involved in ɣ-globin gene regulation, such as those encoded by *BCL11A*, *MYB,* and *KLF1* (Thein, 2018). More recently, for families with unexplained microcytic hypochromic anemia and elevated HbA₂, or with unexplained β-thalassemia intermedia phenotypes, whole genome sequencing (WGS) analysis revealed the involvement of a hitherto unsuspected trans-acting factor (Spt5) encoded by *SUPT5H*, which, when haplo-insufficient, reduced β-globin gene expression (Achour et al., 2020). Although the exact relationship between SUPT5H and β-globin expression remains to be elucidated, zebrafish studies showed a downregulation of the erythroid transcription factor gata1 as a result of foggy/Spt5 knockdown with a subsequent decrease in embryonic erythropoiesis observed (Taneda et al., 2011). It has been hypothesized that the interaction of foggy/Spt5 with gata1 in zebrafish is comparable to that in humans in which FOG1 and GATA1 cooperate in up-regulating *HBB* expression (Achour et al., 2020). Analyses of these families may provide additional information about how β-globin gene expression is regulated and, in doing so, aid in identifying new targets for treatments based on genetic interventions.

As the field of molecular genetics continues to grow, additional genetic variants in families with rare and unexplained thalassemia phenotypes are expected to be found even before diagnosis are established at the hematological level. For instance, through next generation sequencing (NGS) techniques such as whole exome sequencing (WES) and WGS.

GENETIC THERAPIES FOR HEMOGLOBINOPATHIES

Although the outcomes of allo-HSCT have significantly improved in recent decades, the treatment remains suboptimal due to limited donor availability and associated risks, such

as, graft-versus-host disease. Therefore, numerous efforts are being directed to treatments based on auto-HSCT in which the patient's own stem cells are harvested, genetically modified *ex vivo* and reinfused back to the patient. In order to appreciate the full potential of genetic therapies for the treatment of hemoglobinopathies, it is important to understand the wide range of genetic toolsets that are under development. Therefore, in the following sections, we briefly cover the currently available genetic techniques and discuss their testing for the treatment of β-thalassemia and SCD.

Lentiviral Vector-Mediated Gene Therapy

Initially, realistic prospects for gene therapy of hematological disorders arose with the introduction of ɣ-retroviral vectors (ɣ-RVs), such as those based on the Moloney murine leukemia virus, owing to their ability to stably integrate exogenous DNA into target-cell chromosomes. After the emergence of serious adverse events caused by insertional oncogenesis in a few clinical trials using ɣ-RVs, self-inactivating (SIN) lentiviral vectors (LVs) based on the human immunodeficiency virus type 1 (HIV-1), were introduced (Naldini et al., 1996; Nowrouzi et al., 2011). SIN ɣ-RVs and SIN LVs have viral enhancer sequences present in their long terminal repeats (LTRs) deleted so that, upon chromosomal integration, there is a reduced chance for deregulating cellular genes, e.g., proto-oncogenes (Yu et al., 1986; Zufferey et al., 1998). LVs are especially effective at transducing non-dividing cells as their karyophilic pre-integration complexes do not require mitosis-dependent breakdown of the nuclear envelope to access chromosomal DNA (Naldini et al., 1996). Moreover, LVs have a preference for integrating their reverse transcribed complementary DNA (cDNA) genomes into coding sequences of active genes, whereas ɣ-RVs preferentially integrate near regulatory regions and transcription start sites (Schröder et al., 2002; Wu et al., 2003). Therefore, SIN LVs have become more widely investigated for treating primary immune deficiencies (PIDs), such as, X-linked severe combined immunodeficiency (X-SCID), adenosine deaminase severe combined immunodeficiency (ADA-SCID) and Wiskott-Aldrich syndrome (WAS) (Fischer et al., 2015), as well as for treating metabolic disorders, such as, adrenoleukodystrophy and metachromatic leukodystrophy (Cartier et al., 2009; Biffi et al., 2013).

LVs are currently being tested for treating hemoglobinopathies as well. The main strategies can be categorized in (i) transgene addition (**Figure 3A**), (ii) short hairpin RNA (shRNA)-mediated *BCL11A* knockdown (**Figure 3B**) and (iii) forced chromatin looping (**Figure 3C**) (Breda et al., 2016; Cavazzana et al., 2017; Sii-Felice et al., 2020). The first strategy preceded the other two and is currently the most common and advanced in terms of clinical translation. Indeed, there are a variety of efforts directed at generating LVs carrying recombinant β-like globin gene sequences with the goal of achieving therapeutic levels of transgene expression in RBCs derived from LV-transduced HSCs. To this end, the combined optimization of LCR elements, transgenes and vector genomes is permitting the achievement of efficient transduction of HSCs and subsequent therapeutic protein

LV-mediated strategies

A Gene addition

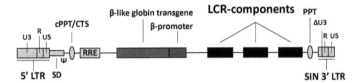

B BCL11A knock-down

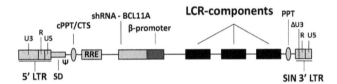

C Forced chromatin looping

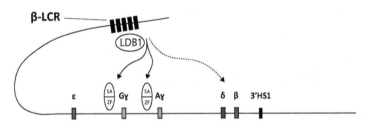

FIGURE 3 | Overview of LV-based gene therapy strategies currently under investigation for the genetic correction of β-hemoglobinopathies. **(A)** Gene addition. Structure of a LV construct for transgene addition relying on the expression of β-like globin chains to rebalance α-chain to non-α-chain ratios. **(B)** BCL11A knock-down. Structure of a LV construct for relieving ɣ-globin repression through shRNA-BCL11A-mediated BCL11A knockdown. **(C)** Forced chromatin looping. Directed loop-formation by LV-mediated delivery of fusion products between LDB1 self-association (SA) domains and zinc-finger (ZF) arrays targeting the *HBG2* and *HBG1* promoter sequences to up-regulate Gɣ- and Aɣ-globin synthesis, respectively. LCR, locus control region; LTR, HIV-1 long terminal repeat; Ψ, HIV-1 packaging signal; RRE, Rev response element; cPPT/CTS, central polypurine tract and central termination sequence; ΔU3, 3' LTR with U3 deletion for self-inactivation of HIV-1 regulatory sequences upon chromosomal integration of recombinant LV genomes.

levels in RBCs (May et al., 2000; Negre et al., 2015; Cavazzana et al., 2017; Sii-Felice et al., 2020). For instance, concerning the optimization of LCR elements in particular, it was demonstrated that incorporating in LV genomes large sequences spanning the HS2, HS3 and HS4 elements, instead of the respective minimal core sequences, yielded sustained and high amounts of recombinant β-globin in RBCs of transplanted mice (May et al., 2000). An initial β-thalassemia gene therapy course was tested in a transfusion-dependent β^E/β^0 patient using the Lentiglobin HPV569 vector (Malik et al., 2005; Cavazzana-Calvo et al., 2010) (**Table 1**). This HPV569 vector carries a cassette encoding a β-globin chain containing an amino acid substitution (β^{T87Q}) found in the ɣ-globin chain. Of note, this mutation prevents the polymerization of this recombinant β-globin chain with residual HbS hemoglobin molecules in SCD patients, making the treatment applicable to treat both β-thalassemia and SCD

(Adachi et al., 1994; Pawliuk et al., 2001; Negre et al., 2016). Importantly, to achieve high levels of β^{T87Q} globin chain synthesis, the LV genome harbors a minimal β-globin gene promoter together with three LCR elements, i.e., HS2, HS3, and HS4. Finally, upon reverse transcription of the incoming vector RNA genomes and ensuing cDNA chromosomal integration, the β^{T87Q} globin transgene becomes flanked by two copies of the chicken β-globin HS4 chromatin insulator (cHS4) located in the vector LTRs. The enhancer-blocking properties of the cHS4 insulator aims at reducing the chance for insertional oncogenesis due to spurious LCR-driven activation of nearby proto-oncogenes (Emery et al., 2000; Arumugam et al., 2007). Yet, despite achieving high-level βT87Q-globin expression, the HPV569 vector had to be redesigned due to low functional titers and transcriptional activation of the cellular *HMGA2* gene resulting in clonal expansion (Cavazzana-Calvo et al., 2010;

Negre et al., 2016). More specifically, chromosomal integration of the vector cDNA in a few cells originated aberrant *HMGA2* transcripts whose origins were mapped to a cryptic splice site in the cHS4 insulator core present in the 5' LTR (Negre et al., 2016). The newly designed vector, named BB305, lacks the cHS4 insulator and contains a hybrid 5'-LTR with cytomegalovirus *immediate-early* gene regulatory elements (CMV) to increase vector RNA synthesis during its production yielding, as a result, higher titers of functional vector particles (Negre et al., 2016).

Since the initial development of the aforementioned Lentiglobin vectors HPV569 and BB305, other LV-based β-thalassemia and SCD gene therapy products have emerged and entered clinical trials, namely GLOBE, OTL-300, ARU-1801, Lenti-βAS3-FB, and DREPAGLOBE (Sii-Felice et al., 2020) (**Table 1**). The genomes of these LVs differ among each other in several aspects, namely: (i) LCR HS site composition (HS2-4), (ii) type of transgene (i.e., wildtype β-globin, β^{T87Q}-globin or hybrid βγ-globin), (iii) absence or presence of insulators (i.e., cHS4 or FII/BEAD-A; Ramezani et al., 2008); and (iv) vector promoter sequences (i.e., hybrid CMV/5'LTR or wildtype 5'LTR; Cavazzana et al., 2017; Sii-Felice et al., 2020).

Interestingly, intra-femoral injection of HSCs into immunodeficient NOD/SCID recipient mice was shown to increase the frequency of long-term repopulating cells when compared to intravenous injection and, at the same time, reduce the trapping of HSCs in non-target organs (Yahata et al., 2003; Feng et al., 2008). Based on these findings, a clinical trial with the GLOBE vector included the intra-bone infusion of genetically modified HSCs, which, so far, has yielded promising clinical results in terms of rapid HSC engraftment and ensuing hematopoietic system reconstitution (Marktel et al., 2019).

Moreover, a recent study has employed a "forward-oriented" SIN LV design, in which the therapeutic β-globin transgene is transcribed in the "forward" instead of the "reverse" orientation relative to the vector backbone, which is used in the previously mentioned LVs (Uchida et al., 2019). In this specific vector design, the *HBB* intron 2 is not spliced out during vector production owing to the incorporation of the HIV-1 Rev response element (RRE) within this intron. This redesigned vector can be produced at 6-fold higher titers and transduces HSCs at 4- to 10-fold higher rates than their "reverse-oriented" counterparts (Uchida et al., 2019). Importantly, the transduced HSCs showed robust long-term engraftment and β-globin expression in Rhesus macaques up to 3 years post-transplantation (Uchida et al., 2019).

Besides gene addition strategies, a LV expressing a microRNA-adapted shRNA (shRNA^miR), constructed for inducing fetal γ-globin synthesis, has also progressed to a clinical trial stage (**Table 1**; Brendel et al., 2020). Before its application in a clinical setting, this LV was optimized to minimize the cytotoxicity of shRNA expression and BCL11A knock-down in HSCs (Brendel et al., 2016). In particular, by implementing erythroid lineage-specific expression of the shRNA^miR directed to *BCL11A* transcripts, a 90% reduction of BCL11A protein levels led to a 60–70% increase in γ-globin expression. Importantly, the genetically modified HSCs were capable of long-term engraftment in mice (Brendel et al., 2016). This optimized LV vector, named BCH-BB694, achieved efficient transduction of healthy and SCD

CD34$^+$ donor cells as determined by quantification of vector copy numbers (VCNs) resulting in a 3- to 5-fold increase in HbF amounts when compared to mock-transduced cells (Brendel et al., 2020). The demonstration of high CD34$^+$ cell transduction efficiencies, without compromising HSC function, together with the ability to produce the BCH-BB694 vector at high titers under good manufacturing practices (GMP) conditions, has permitted the initiation of a phase 1/2 clinical trial (**Table 1**).

Another LV-based experimental gene therapy aiming at enhancing γ-globin expression involves forcing the looping of the LCR toward the γ-globin promoter region (Deng et al., 2012, 2014; Breda et al., 2016; Krivega and Dean, 2016) (**Figure 3C**). In this strategy, the regular role of the transcription factor LDB1 in loop-formation is exploited by expressing a fusion product consisting of the LDB1 Self-Association (SA) domain linked to zinc-finger motifs that recognize the β-globin gene promoter (Deng et al., 2012). After the demonstration of the effectiveness of this elegant forced-looping approach bringing the LCR in close vicinity of the β-globin gene promoter in GATA1 null erythroblasts, a similar strategy was tested for inducing γ-globin expression in primary human adult erythroblasts. This resulted in an impressive 85% increase in LCR/γ-globin gene contacts and a corresponding up-regulation of γ-globin expression (Deng et al., 2014).

Genome Editing: Basic Principles and Platforms

In this section we focus on gene editing applications for the treatment of hemoglobinopathies. A brief summary is provided on common gene editing platforms, including ZFNs, TALENs and RGNs, as well as on recent gene editing approaches comprising RGNs with high-fidelity Cas9 variants and Cas9 nickase-based techniques, such as base editing and prime editing.

Programmable nucleases can modify specific genomic sequences in eukaryotic cells in a highly precise and efficient manner to, for instance, study the function of genes or correct genes associated with human disorders, both acquired and inborn (Zittersteijn et al., 2020). With the increasing number of candidate genetic therapies entering clinical trials such as those discussed in the previous section, it is clear that the application of advanced therapy medicinal products (ATMPs) is gaining momentum (Hirakawa et al., 2020). Interestingly, feeding the progression of safer and more targeted ATMPs, innovative genome editing techniques are under development, including those directed at treating hemoglobinopathies (Cornu et al., 2017; Li H. et al., 2020).

Typically, programmable nuclease-assisted gene editing consists in inducing targeted chromosomal DSBs in living cells to trigger endogenous DNA repair pathways in bringing about specific genetic changes. There are two main processes by which a DSB can be repaired in mammalian cells, namely, (i) end-to-end ligation of chromosomal termini, involving non-homologous end joining (NHEJ) pathways, e.g., classical NHEJ and microhomology-mediated end joining (MMEJ), and (ii) exogenous (donor) DNA-templated repair, involving homology-directed repair (HDR) (Chandrasegaran and Carroll,

TABLE 1 | Genetic therapies in development based on SIN LVs.

Phase	Product name	Clinical trial	Vector	Therapeutic element	Disorder	Sponsor	Status	Results
I/II	Lentiglobin (HPV569)	LG001	SIN LV	β(T87Q)	TM	Bluebird Bio	Completed	1 patient (β0/βE): 1/1 TI
I	TNS9.3.55	NCT01639690	SIN LV	Wildtype β-globin	TM	Memorial Sloan-Kettering Cancer Center	Active/Not recruiting	Insufficient engraftment and clinical benefit
I/II	Lentiglobin (BB305)	NCT01745120 (HGB-204)	SIN LV	β(T87Q)	TM	Bluebird Bio	Completed	Total: 16/18 reached primary endpoint. Non-β0/β0: 8/10 TI; 2/10 73% and 43% reduction of ATV. β0/β0: 3/8 TI; 1/8 TI for 13 months; 4/8 53% reduction of ATV
I/II	Lentiglobin (BB305)	NCT02151526 (HGB-205)	SIN LV	β(T87Q)	TM & SCD	Bluebird Bio	Completed	TM: 3/4 TI. SCD: three patients had HbAβ(T87Q) contribution of 47.9%, 7.9% and 25.8%
I/II	ZYNTEGLO (Lentiglobin BB305)	NCT02140554 (HGB-206)	SIN LV	β(T87Q)	SCD	Bluebird Bio	Active/Not recruiting	Group A (BMH; n = 7): HbAb(T87Q) 0.5-1.2 g/dl. Group B (BMH & MA; n = 2): 3.2-7.2 g/dl. Group C (MA; n = 32): 22/32 >40% of HbAb(T87Q) contribution (total Hb 9.6-15.1 g/dL; HbAb(T87Q) 2.7-8.9 g/dL). 19/32: Complete elimination of VOCs at 24 months after treatment
III	ZYNTEGLO (Lentiglobin BB305)	NCT02906202 (HGB-207)	SIN LV	β(T87Q)	TM	Bluebird Bio	Active/Not recruiting	HbAβ(T87Q) contribution of: 79.8% (6 months; n = 11); 74.2% (12 months; n = 8); 77.2% (18 months; n = 2)
III	ZYNTEGLO (Lentiglobin BB305)	NCT03207009 (HGB-212)	SIN LV	β(T87Q)	TM	Bluebird Bio	Active/Recruiting	15 TDT patients. 6/8 evaluable patients TI for median 13.6 MPT (Median Hb: 11.5 g/dl). 11/13 patients TI >7 MPT with HbAβ(T87Q) 8.8-14.0 g/dl
Long-term follow-up	ZYNTEGLO (Lentiglobin BB305)	NCT02633943	SIN LV	β(T87Q)	TM & SCD	Bluebird Bio	Enrolling by invitation	32 patients (22 phase I/II; 10 phase III): 14/22 and 9/10 TI (TI patients remained TI for median 39.4 months (min-max:19.4-69.4 months)
I/II	OTL-300 (GLOBE)	NCT02453477	SIN LV	Wildtype β-globin	TM	IRCCS San Raffaele - Telethon	Closed	7 patients (β0 or severe β+). Adults: 3/3 reduced transfusion requirement. Children: 3/4 pediatric patients TI
Long-term follow-up	OTL-300 (GLOBE)	NCT03275051	SIN LV	Wildtype β-globin	TM	Orchard Therapeutics	Active/Not recruiting	8/9 patients (β0 or severe β+) reached primary endpoint after 1 year. Adults: 3/3 reduced transfusion requirement. Children: 4/6 TI; 1/6 reduced transfusion requirement; 1/6 no reduced transfusion requirement due to poor engraftment
I/II	ARU-1801 (RVT-1801)	NCT02186418	SIN LV	γ (G16D)	SCD	Aruvant	Active/Recruiting	2 βS/β0 patients with RIC: Excellent safety, feasibility, minimal post-transplant toxicity, and sustained genetically modified cells in PB and BM over 1 year after treatment
I/II	Lenti-βAS3-FB	NCT02247843	SIN LV	β(T87Q/E2 2A/G16D)	SCD	Donald Kohn (University of California)	Active/Recruiting	No results published yet
I/II	DREPAGLOBE (GLOBE1-βAS3)	NCT03964792	SIN LV	β(T87Q/E2 2A/G16D)	SCD	Assistance Publique - Hôpitaux de Paris	Active/Recruiting	No results published yet

(Continued)

TABLE 1 | Continued

Phase	Product name	Clinical trial	Vector	Therapeutic element	Disorder	Sponsor	Status	Results
I	BCH-BB694	NCT03282656	SIN LV	miRNA - BCL11A	SCD	David Williams (Boston Children's Hospital)	Active/Recruiting	6 patients treated. 6/6: Stable HbF induction (20.4-41.3%). Robust increase in F-cells among RBCs (58.9-93.6%).
I	CSL200	NCT04091737	SIN LV	ɣ (G16D) + shRNA734 (BCL11A)	SCD	CSL Behring	Active/Recruiting	No results published yet

TM, β-thalassemia major; SCD, Sickle cell disease; TI, Transfusion independent; ATV, Annual transfusion volume; BMH, Bone marrow harvest; MA, Mobilization/apheresis; MPT, Months post-treatment; RIC, Reduced-intensity conditioning regimen; VOC, Vaso-occlusive crises; PB, Peripheral blood; BM, bone marrow.

2016; Chang H. H. Y. et al., 2017; **Figure 4**). By building on this knowledge, programmable nucleases are designed to target specific genomic sequences and establish desired gene editing outcomes (e.g., gene knock-ins or knock-outs) (Maggio and Gonçalves, 2015). In mammalian cells, the most active DNA repair pathway is the classic NHEJ which usually results in the precise re-ligation of the chromosomal ends. However, multiple cycles of cleavage and re-ligation caused by the presence of a programmable nuclease, can eventually lead to small insertions or deletions (indels) that, by disrupting the nuclease recognition sequence, become permanently installed in the target cell population (Chandrasegaran and Carroll, 2016; Chang H. H. Y. et al., 2017) (**Figure 4**). When established at gene coding sequences, these indels lead to frameshifts that effectively result in target gene knock-outs (Chandrasegaran and Carroll, 2016). NHEJ and MMEJ can also be exploited to knock-in exogenous donor DNA into a programable nuclease target site. Often, however, the resulting junctions between donor and target DNA harbor indels. More predictable and precise DNA edits are accomplished via HDR after introducing into target cells an exogenous donor DNA template containing sequences homologous to the target site region together with a cognate programmable nuclease (Chandrasegaran and Carroll, 2016). HDR-mediated gene editing is, however, restricted to the S and late G2 phases of the cell cycle and, as a consequence, has its utility limited to dividing cells.

Genome Editing Platforms

Clearly, genome editing based on ZFNs, TALENs and RGNs allows for a more precise genetic engineering of cells and organisms than that offered by retroviral vector systems, which suffer from heterogeneous transgene expression levels and insertional mutagenesis risks inherent to their semi-random integrative nature (Schröder et al., 2002; Wu et al., 2003; Maldarelli et al., 2014). Programmable nucleases should, ideally, act in a temporally limited "hit-and-run" fashion, especially when applied in a translational setting to minimizing off-target effects. Regardless, these gene editing tools bear the risk of inducing unwanted genome-modifying events, in the form of off-target indels, chromosomal translocations and, most pervasively, on-target indels and large rearrangements (Cradick et al., 2013; Fu et al., 2013; Hsu et al., 2013; Zhang et al., 2015; Kosicki et al., 2018; Carroll, 2019; Chen et al., 2020). To monitor off-target effects in particular and assess their potential risks, an increasing number of genome-wide screening methods is building up (Zischewski et al., 2017; Kim et al., 2019), and include, GUIDE-seq (Tsai et al., 2015), LAM-HTGTS (Frock et al., 2015; Chen et al., 2020) and, more recently, DISCOVER-seq (Wienert et al., 2019). Insights from applying these methodologies are guiding the optimization of genome editing tools, focusing on improving their specificity without compromising their targeted DSB formation efficiencies.

Zinc-Finger Nucleases

ZFNs were the first broadly used programmable nuclease platform (Kim et al., 1996; Chandrasegaran and Carroll, 2016)

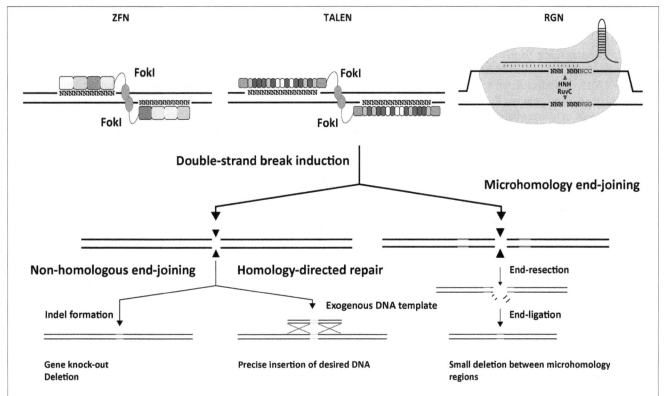

FIGURE 4 | Schematic representation of the three main classes of programmable nucleases (i.e., ZFNs, TALENs, and RGNs based on the prototypic *S. pyogenes* CRISPR-Cas9 system) and the DNA repair pathways underlying different gene editing outcomes resulting from the induction of targeted double-strand breaks. See text for details.

(**Figure 4**). These artificial modular proteins consist of an array of Cys_2His_2 zinc-finger motifs (typically 4 to 6), each designed to recognize a DNA triplet, fused to a catalytic domain derived from the FokI restriction enzyme. Each ZFN monomer recognizes a specific sequence of 12 to 18 nucleotides with the induction of a DSB requiring the dimerization of two FokI catalytic domains brought together by target DNA binding of a working pair of ZFN monomers (Rahman et al., 2011; Chandrasegaran and Carroll, 2016). The assembly of functional ZFNs with high specificity is complicated due to context-dependent effects. In particular, the fact that individual zinc-fingers can alter the orientation of adjacent motifs or interact with triplets recognized by neighboring motifs (Rahman et al., 2011; Chandrasegaran and Carroll, 2016).

Transcription Activator-Like Effector Nucleases

TALENs were developed on the basis of the discovery that TALE proteins found in certain phytopathogenic bacteria (e.g., *Xanthomonas* sp.), are capable of recognizing specific DNA sequences through their DNA-binding units called TALE repeats (Christian et al., 2010; Miller et al., 2011; Chandrasegaran and Carroll, 2016) (**Figure 4**). In particular, the finding that individual TALE repeats bind via their, so-called, repeat variable di-residues (RVDs) to specific nucleotides on the DNA (Boch et al., 2009; Moscou and Bogdanove, 2009). Hence, customizing

TALE DNA-binding domains to a predefined target sequence simply requires the assembly of an array of TALE repeats in which each repeat is predicted to interact with its cognate nucleotide. Similarly to ZFNs, TALENs are artificial modular proteins consisting of a DNA-binding domain fused to the FokI nuclease domain that, through target DNA binding of a working TALEN pair, dimerizes and induces a site-specific DSB (Christian et al., 2010; Miller et al., 2011; Chandrasegaran and Carroll, 2016). Equally similar to ZFNs, once optimized, TALENs exhibit high specificities and efficiencies. Yet, the process of producing and validating TALENs is typically less complex and laborious than that of ZFNs as, in contrast to the binding of individual zinc-finger motifs to target DNA triplets, the binding of TALE repeats to their target nucleotides is substantially less altered by the type of context-dependent effects that zinc-fingers suffer from (Mussolino and Cathomen, 2012).

RNA-Guided Nucleases

Shortly after the introduction of TALENs, a genome editing platform derived from prokaryotic class 2 type II CRISPR-Cas9 adaptive immune systems emerged (Cho et al., 2013; Cong et al., 2013; Jinek et al., 2013; Mali et al., 2013) (**Figures 4, 5**). This platform was built on plenty of fundamental insights culminating on the finding that Cas9 proteins from *Streptococcus thermophilus* and *Streptococcus pyogenes* are in fact RNA-guided site-specific endonucleases (Gasiunas et al., 2012; Jinek et al., 2012). Hence, as RGNs rely on RNA-DNA hybridizations for target DNA cleavage, they have a protein engineering-free mode of construction making them more easily customizable than ZFNs or TALENs (Doudna and Charpentier, 2014; Maggio and Gonçalves, 2015; Chandrasegaran and Carroll, 2016).

The adaptation of native RGNs into engineered RGNs designed to work in mammalian cells consisted of (i) assembling single-guide RNAs (gRNAs) by fusing sequence-tailored CRISPR RNAs (crRNAs) to a common scaffolding *trans*-activating CRISPR RNA (tracrRNA), (ii) codon-optimization of the Cas9 open reading frame; and (iii) addition of nuclear localization signals to the Cas9 protein (Cho et al., 2013; Cong et al., 2013; Jinek et al., 2013; Mali et al., 2013; Maggio et al., 2020). Once in target cells, Cas9:gRNA ribonucleoprotein complexes scan the genome for protospacer-adjacent motifs (PAMs), that read NGG in the case of *S. pyogenes* RGNs. This short DNA motif is recognized by the PAM-interacting domain (PID) of Cas9 (Anders et al., 2014). If next to the PAM lies a typically 18-21 nucleotide-long sequence (protospacer) complementary to the 5'-end of the crRNA (spacer), gRNA:DNA hybridization ensues leading to the activation of the two Cas9 nuclease domains (i.e., HNH and RuvC-like). The subsequent cleavage of the double-stranded DNA substrate occurs within the protospacer sequence typically three base-pairs away from the PAM.

Similarly to ZFNs and TALENs, RGNs can induce DSBs at off-target sequences (Cradick et al., 2013; Fu et al., 2013; Hsu et al., 2013; Frock et al., 2015; Chen et al., 2020). Therefore, to minimize deleterious effects caused by off-target DNA cleavage, considerable efforts are ongoing devoted to improve the precision of gene editing tools and strategies such as, by developing high-fidelity Cas9 nucleases and developing Cas9 nickase-based approaches which do not rely on the catalytic induction of DSBs. These precise gene editing technologies are briefly reviewed next.

Precision Gene Editing Based on High-Fidelity Nucleases, Nickases, Base Editors and Prime Editors

The generation and isolation of Cas9 variants with various point mutations through rational protein design and directed evolution approaches, respectively, have led to an array of high-fidelity Cas9 nucleases that next to greatly reduced off-target activities retain, for the most part, on-target efficiencies (Kim et al., 2019). Moreover, RGNs containing Cas9 nickases (Doudna and Charpentier, 2014) (**Figure 5**), developed through the disruption of one of the two aforementioned catalytic domains of the Cas9 nuclease, show interesting safety enhancements owing to the fact that the single-stranded DNA breaks (nicks) that they generate are intrinsically less disruptive than DSBs. Indeed, in the context of HDR-based gene editing experiments, researchers have found that coordinated nicking of target and donor DNA by Cas9 nickases can yield high gene knock-in frequencies while minimizing the characteristic by-products of Cas9 nucleases, i.e., NHEJ-derived indels at target and off-target sequences (Chen et al., 2017, 2020; Nakajima et al., 2018; Hyodo et al., 2020).

With the arrival of base editors, it is also now possible to introduce specific point mutations in living cells without the necessity for inducing DSBs or delivering donor DNA templates

(Komor et al., 2016; Gaudelli et al., 2017) (**Figure 5**). Base editors consist of a Cas9 nickase (i.e., Cas9^{D10A}) covalently linked to either a cytidine or adenine deaminase capable of inducing C→T or A→G transitions, respectively (Komor et al., 2016; Gaudelli et al., 2017). Typically, base editors induce these transitions within a 4-base pair (bp) base editing window. Similar to the growing number of nucleases derived from CRISPR systems evolved in different prokaryotes (Chen and Gonçalves, 2018), base editors are continuously being optimized to, for example, expand their PAM-recognition capabilities and reduce their off-target activities at both the genomic and transcriptomic levels (Koblan et al., 2018; Grunewald et al., 2019; Park and Beal, 2019; Zuo et al., 2019; Anzalone et al., 2020).

The most recent addition to the DSB-free gene editing toolkit independent of donor DNA delivery comes in the form of prime editors (Anzalone et al., 2019) (**Figure 5**). Although prime editing is a recent technique, so far mostly investigated in cell lines, it shows substantial potential including for the treatment of genetic disorders. In comparison with base editing, prime editing offers a broader range of targeted genomic edits in that it permits installing not only transitions but also transversions and small indels. Prime editors consist of a Cas9 nickase (i.e., Cas9^{H840A}) covalently linked to an engineered Molony murine leukemia virus reverse transcriptase (RT) optimized owing to five point mutations enhancing its stability and processivity (Anzalone et al., 2019). Besides a Cas9^{H840A}::RT complex, prime editing requires a 3'-end extended gRNA, named prime editor gRNA (pegRNA), that simultaneously provides a primer and a template for the RT. Specifically, the pegRNA consists of a conventional sequence-tailored gRNA linked to a primer binding site (PBS) and a RT template encoding the edit of interest. Via the PAM-interacting domain of the Cas9 nickase, the prime editor recognizes the PAM and, after hybridization between the crRNA portion of the pegRNA and the target sequence, the PAM-containing DNA strand is nicked. The resulting single-stranded genomic DNA anneals to the PBS of the pegRNA providing a primer for RT-mediated cDNA synthesis. The resulting DNA copy containing the edit eventually hybridizes to the complementary chromosomal target sequence with non-hybridizing DNA flap removal leading to edit installation at the target site presumably following DNA replication or mismatch repair (Anzalone et al., 2019).

CRISPR-Cas12a

The Cas12a nuclease, formally known as Cpf1, belongs to the class 2 type V CRISPR system found in, amongst other bacterial species, *Francisella novicida* (Makarova et al., 2020). In contrast to the *S. pyogenes* Cas9 nuclease, Cas12a from *F. novicida* (i) recognizes a T-rich PAM (i.e., TTTV), (ii) requires a crRNA and no tracrRNA and (iii) seems to have a single RuvC-like domain mediating the staggered cleavage of double-stranded DNA strands with 4-5 nt overhangs distal from the PAM (Zetsche et al., 2015) (**Figure 5E**). Optimization of the Cas12a nuclease is ongoing, mainly focusing on broadening their PAM recognition sites and further improving their intrinsically high target site

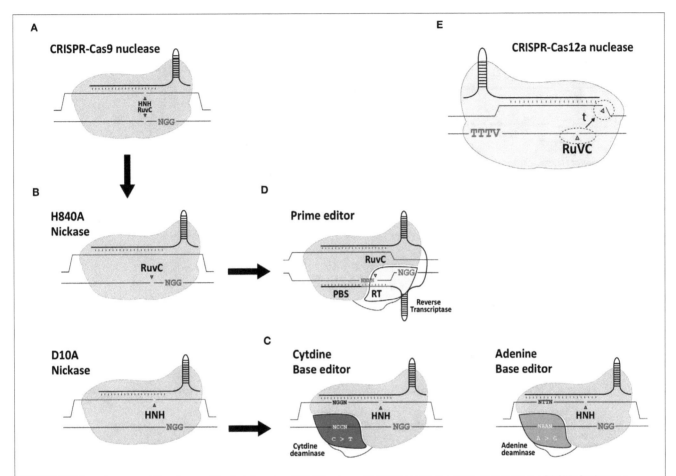

FIGURE 5 | Schematic representation of gene editing tools based on CRISPR systems. **(A)** RGN based on the prototypic *S. pyogenes* CRISPR-Cas9 system. **(B)** RGNs containing the sequence- and strand-specific nuclease (nickase) Cas9^H840A or Cas9^D10A. **(C)** Base editors. The basic components of base editors consist of a nickase (typically *S. pyogenes* Cas9^D10A) fused to a cytidine deaminase or engineered adenine deaminase. **(D)** Prime editors. The basic components of prime editors consist of a nickase (typically *S. pyogenes* Cas9^H840A) linked to an engineered reverse transcriptase. **(E)** RGN based on a CRISPR-Cas12a system. Cas12a has a single RuvC-like domain responsible for staggered DNA end formation from the sequential cleavage of both target site strands (dashed circles: location of cleavage; t: time). Red letters; protospacer adjacent motifs.

specificities (Kleinstiver et al., 2016, 2019; Gao et al., 2017; Tóth et al., 2020).

Genome Editing Strategies for the Treatment of Hemoglobinopathies

The tailoring of genome editing strategies for the genetic correction of hemoglobinopathies is progressing rapidly. These strategies can be divided in two main categories: (i) *HBB* mutation-independent; and (ii) *HBB* mutation-specific.

The mutation-independent approaches encompass the majority of these gene editing efforts in part owing to their compatibility with treating most patients regardless of their genotypes. Generically, mutation-independent strategies depend on the de-repression of HbF synthesis through the disruption of molecular mechanisms underlying ɣ-globin gene repression by, for instance, knocking-out repressor protein binding sites or the repressor genes themselves (Wienert et al., 2018; Demirci et al., 2020). Alternatively, instead of activating HbF synthesis, to complement the lack

of β-globin, HDR-mediated gene editing is being exploited to directly correct the *HBB* gene itself via the introduction of programmable nucleases and donor DNA templates into HSCs (Dever et al., 2016; Antony et al., 2018; Pattabhi et al., 2019). The mutation-specific strategies are so far mostly based on targeted DSB formation for ablating aberrant splicing sites causing β-thalassemia (Patsali et al., 2019a). Although most gene editing efforts are directed toward the correction of β-hemoglobinopathies, i.e., β-thalassemia major and SCD, there are also studies focusing on the correction of α-thalassemia (Chang and Bouhassira, 2012; Yingjun et al., 2019).

HBB Mutation-Independent Genome Editing Strategies

As discussed previously, insights into the fetal-to-adult hemoglobin switch continue being amassed in part owing to their importance for the development of mutation-independent gene complementation strategies for treating β-hemoglobinopathies, the world's most common group of monogenic disorders

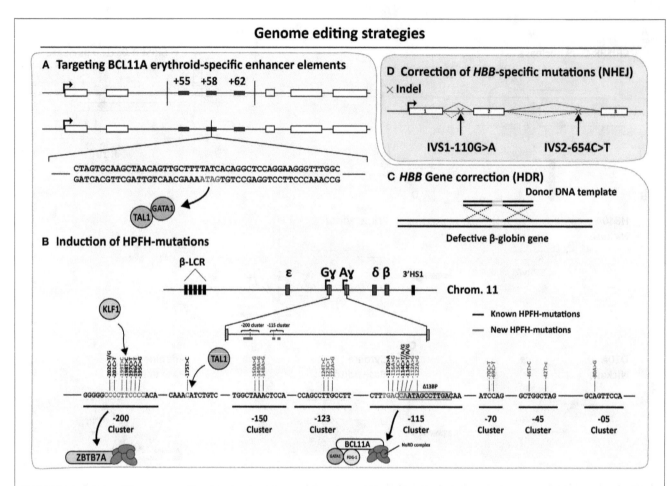

FIGURE 6 | An overview of the genome editing strategies directed at correcting β-hemoglobinopathies. **(A–C)** Mutation-independent gene editing strategies.
(A) Disruption of erythroid-specific *BCL11A* expression through the disablement of enhancer elements based on, targeted deletions or GATA1-binding site disruption.
(B) Introduction of HPFH or HPFH-like mutations near the *HBG* transcriptional start sites. **(C)** HDR-dependent *HBB* correction. **(D)** Mutation-specific
NHEJ-dependent strategies targeting aberrant splice motifs for the correction of β-thalassemia.

(Sankaran and Orkin, 2013; Vinjamur et al., 2018; Wienert et al., 2018). During the fetal-to-adult hemoglobin switch, ɤ-globin expression is repressed by molecular mechanisms involving key transcription factors, such as, BCL11A, LRF/ZBTB7A, SOX6, and KLF1 (Sankaran et al., 2008; Masuda et al., 2016; Li et al., 2017). Indeed, initial genome-wide association studies (GWAS) focused on identifying loci involved in fetal γ-globin repression, such as, *HBS1L-MYB* and *BCL11A* (Menzel et al., 2007; Uda et al., 2008). Furthermore, SNPs found in the β-globin locus of SCD patients with elevated HbF levels uncovered *cis*-acting elements controlling fetal γ-globin repression (Lettre et al., 2008). Since then, the regulation of *HBS1L-MYB* and *BCL11A*, underwent extensive investigations to confirm and further elucidate the nodal role of these genes in the control of fetal γ-globin gene expression (Lettre et al., 2008; Fanis et al., 2014). For instance, the BCL11A-mediated control of γ-globin gene expression was confirmed through shRNA-mediated knockdown experiments (Sankaran et al., 2008). Importantly, besides its role in the erythrocytic lineage, the DNA-binding protein BCL11A is also involved in other key hematopoietic processes, such as, in the control of HSC differentiation and quiescence as well as lymphoid development (Liu et al., 2003; Tsang et al., 2015; Luc et al., 2016). Thus, to prevent systemic ablation of BCL11A in all hematopoietic lineages, it is important to restrict BCL11A-disrupting genetic interventions to the erythrocytic compartment. Crucially, three DNase I HS sites located in the intron 2 of *BCL11A* were identified and confirmed to represent erythroid-specific *BCL11A* enhancers (Bauer et al., 2013) (**Figure 6**). The first gene editing experiments targeting these erythroid-specific enhancer elements were done by using CRISPR-Cas9-based RGNs to dissect their individual and combined roles through targeted DNA deletions (Canver et al., 2015) (**Figure 6**). This study, besides confirming the importance of the three *BCL11A* enhancer elements in repressing ɤ-globin expression, has also identified the particularly significant contribution of the so-called +58 enhancer element in this process (Canver et al., 2015). The reason for this heightened contribution in ɤ-globin repression was hypothesized to result from the binding of transcription-activating GATA1/TAL1 complexes to a GATA1 binding site present within the +58 enhancer (Bauer et al., 2013; Bauer and Orkin, 2015) (**Figure 6A**). Recent gene editing experiments, using both ZFNs and CRISPR-Cas9-based RGNs, targeting this specific GATA1 binding site confirmed its crucial function in controlling *BCL11A* expression within the erythrocytic lineage. As a result, these experiments further support increasing fetal γ-globin levels through NHEJ-mediated disruption of the GATA1/TAL1-binding sequence in the +58 enhancer (Chang K. H. et al., 2017; Psatha et al., 2018; Wu et al., 2019) (**Figure 6A**). Moreover, a more exquisite ablation of the GATA1-binding site in the *BCL11A* +58 erythroid enhancer was recently achieved by using base editing (Zeng et al., 2020). In this study, high editing efficiencies led to the up-regulation of γ-globin synthesis in RBCs differentiated from SCD patient-derived CD34+ cells. This data indicates that base editing is a promising approach for treating SCD and β-thalassemia (Zeng et al., 2020). Although the relevance of BCL11A in fetal γ-globin repression has been clearly established through the abovementioned *BCL11A*-targeting genetic studies, additional and potentially complementary gene editing strategies are evolving. Amongst these are those based on targeting the binding sites of repressor proteins located within the regulatory regions of the γ-globin-encoding *HBG* genes themselves. Inspired by naturally occurring HPFH-conferring mutations, two regions upstream of the *HBG* promoter sequences were identified as LRF/ZBTB7A and BCL11A binding sites, i.e.,−200 bp and −115 bp distal from the *HBG* transcription start sites (Martyn et al., 2018) (**Figure 6B**: −115 and −200 clusters). A similar contemporary study on the interactions between BCL11A and regulatory DNA near the *HBG* promoters revealed a distal TGACCA motif that proved to be essential for BCL11A binding (Liu et al., 2018). The functional importance of LRF/ZBTB7A and BCL11A binding sites on the control of *HBG* expression, was further confirmed through their targeted disruption by CRISPR-Cas9-based RGNs (Liu et al., 2018; Martyn et al., 2018).

Based on these findings, and the knowledge on naturally occurring mutations conferring HPFH phenotypes, gene editing strategies are being developed aiming at disrupting or removing these specific *HBG* repressor binding sites and mimicking other HPFH-conferring mutations (Wienert et al., 2015; Traxler et al., 2016; Ye et al., 2016; Antoniani et al., 2018; Humbert et al., 2019; Lux et al., 2019; Métais et al., 2019; Wang et al., 2020; Weber et al., 2020) (**Figure 6B**). Moreover, several *ex vivo* genetic therapy experiments in animal models using gene editing tools designed for the de-repression of ɤ-globin expression achieved promising results without compromising the functionality of the transplanted stem cells (Humbert et al., 2019; Lux et al., 2019; Métais et al., 2019; Weber et al., 2020). Interestingly, by using CRISPR-Cas12a-based RGNs, researchers were able to mimic an HPFH-causing 13-bp deletion within the CCAAT-box of the *HBG* promoter in CD34+ cells (De Dreuzy et al., 2019). In these experiments, high editing frequencies were measured (80–90%) resulting in a 40% increase in HbF levels. Importantly, cell engraftment followed by long-term polyclonal

multilineage repopulation was achieved upon transplantation of the treated CD34+ cell populations into NBSGW mice (De Dreuzy et al., 2019).

Currently, two strategies targeting the GATA1 binding site in the *BCL11A* +58 erythroid-specific enhancer have entered clinical trials for both β-thalassemia and SCD (**Table 2**). The *ex vivo* genetic therapy strategy utilizing the CRISPR-Cas9-based RGN platform to treat SCD (clinical trial NCT03745287), so far resulted in 6 patients treated of which 3 patients remained vaso-occlusive crisis free (VOC-free) with fetal hemoglobin levels up to 48% (**Table 2**). When applied in β-thalassemia patients (clinical trial NCT03655678), this strategy led to elevated HbF levels (ranging from 40.9% to 97.7%) and, importantly, blood transfusion independency for 7 out of 13 patients infused with CTX001 (**Table 2**). Another strategy makes use of ZFNs to disrupt the GATA1 binding site of the +58 erythroid-specific enhancer of *BCL11A* in cells from SCD and β-thalassemia patients (clinical trials NCT03653247 and NCT03432364, respectively) (**Table 2**). Other clinical trials involving the *ex vivo* gene editing and subsequent transplantation of autologous CD34+ cells for treating patients with SCD and β-thalassemia, are ongoing (**Table 2**).

Although the current focus is on installing mutations known to confer a naturally occurring HPFH phenotype, eight *de novo*-created mutations yielding a HPFH-like phenotype have recently been presented in yet to be peer reviewed data (Ravi et al., 2020). These mutations have been identified by the systematic induction of point mutations by base editors at *HBG* distal regulatory regions or at sequences near the *HBG* transcription start site (**Figure 6B**). These recent findings broaden the range of candidate *HBG* target sites and in doing so, increase the options for therapeutic gene editing based on the de-repression of ɤ-globin protein synthesis.

Besides creating a HPFH-like phenotype through the installation of NHEJ-derived indels and point mutations at *BCL11A* and *HBG* alleles through the delivery of programmable nucleases and base editors, respectively, other gene editing strategies under investigation comprise instead HDR-mediated *HBB* correction (**Figure 6C**). However, achieving HDR-mediated gene editing in *bona fide* HSCs is challenging due to their mostly quiescent nature and poor amenability to transfection and transduction methods needed to deliver the necessary gene editing tools (i.e., donor DNA templates and RGNs). Exposing HSCs *ex vivo* to small-molecule drugs and growth factors favoring survival and limited cell cycle entry can improve gene editing frequencies (Genovese et al., 2014) but not without, at least in part, impacting their basic properties of life-long self-renewal and multi-lineage differentiation capacities.

Despite this, there are studies providing proof-of-principles for the targeted integration of exogenous DNA sequences in HSCs by using ZFNs, TALENs and RGNs (DeWitt et al., 2016; Antony et al., 2018; Pattabhi et al., 2019). Of notice, direct comparison of these three programmable nuclease platforms showed particularly high NHEJ-derived indel frequencies when using the CRISPR-Cas9-based RGN platform (Antony et al., 2018). Furthermore, Pattabhi and coworkers compared HDR-mediated *HBB* editing in HSCs using AAV9 vs. single-stranded

TABLE 2 | Genetic therapies in development based on gene editing.

Phase	Product name	Clinical trial	Target cell	Delivery	Nuclease	Target gene & effect	Disorder	Status	Sponsor	Results
I/II	ST-400	NCT03432364	CD34+	Electroporated mRNA	ZFN	Disruption of erythroid enhancer of BCL11A gene	TM	Active/Not recruiting	Sangamo	**Five patients (3/5 prelim. data): 1/3**—23% on-target indels 2.7 g/dl HbF (0.9 g/dl at baseline); **2/3**—73% on-target indels <1 g/dl HbF; **3/3**—54% on-target indels 2.8 g/dl HbF
I/II	BIVV003	NCT03653247	CD34+	Electroporated mRNA	ZFN	Disruption of erythroid enhancer of BCL11A gene	SCD	Recruiting	Bioverativ (Sanofi)	No results published yet
I/II	CTX001 (CLIMB-111)	NCT03655678	CD34+	Electroporated RNP	CRISPR-Cas9	Disruption of erythroid enhancer of BCL11A gene	TM	Recruiting	Vertex pharmaceuticals inc.	13 patients treated. TM: 7/13 TI with 3-18 months of follow-up. Total Hb from 9.7 - 14.1 g/dL and fetal Hb levels from 40.9 - 97.7%
I/II	CTX001 (CLIMB-121)	NCT03745287	CD34+	Electroporated RNP	CRISPR-Cas9	Disruption of erythroid enhancer of BCL11A gene	SCD	Recruiting	Vertex pharmaceuticals inc.	6 patients treated. VOC-free: 3/3; 3-15 months after CTX001 infusion. Total Hb from 11.5 - 13.2 g/dL and fetal Hb levels from 31.3 - 48%.
I/II	-	NCT04211480	CD34+	Electroporated RNP	CRISPR-Cas9	BCL11A binding site disruption HBG promoter	TM	Recruiting	Shanghai Bioray Laboratory Inc.	2 patients: 1 MPT HbF levels increased to 76 and 97 g/L HbF (total Hb 129 and 115 g/L, resp.) TI at 75 DPT
Long-term follow-up	CTX001	NCT04208529	CD34+	Electroporated RNP	CRISPR-Cas9	Disruption of erythroid enhancer of BCL11A gene	TM & SCD	-	Vertex pharmaceuticals inc.	-

TM, beta thalassemia major; TI, Transfusion independent; DPT, Days post-treatment; MPT, Months post-treatment; VOC, Vaso-occlusive crises.

oligodeoxyribonucleotide (ssODN) donors (Pattabhi et al., 2019). Moreover, Shinn and colleagues have been able to demonstrate that controlled proliferation and quiescence of HSCs can yield up to a 6-fold increase in HDR/NHEJ ratios in human CD34$^+$ cells *in vitro* and *in vivo* (Shin et al., 2020). Although various research efforts have been improving HDR efficiencies in HSCs, additional tools and/or protocol modifications are likely to be required in order to achieve gene editing frequencies clinically meaningful to the sustained rescue of SCD and β-thalassemia phenotypes.

Another mutation-independent gene editing strategy, albeit less pursued, consists of down-regulating α-globin expression and, therefore, establishing a more balanced proportion amongst the hemoglobin chains. Amongst the first *HBA1*-targeting approaches were those based on RNA interference encompassing the delivery of small interfering RNA (siRNA) or shRNA molecules into murine β-thalassemic primary erythrocytes (Voon et al., 2008), β-thalassemia heterozygous single-cell mouse embryos (Xie et al., 2007) and a β-thalassemia mouse model after tail vein injection (Xie et al., 2011; Mettananda et al., 2015). More recently, a study based on the delivery of RGN multiplexes designed for the targeted deletion of the aforementioned MCS-R2 regulatory element resulted in a reduced α-globin synthesis with a corresponding reduction in hemoglobin chain imbalances in primary human HSCs (Mettananda et al., 2017).

HBB Mutation-Specific Genome Editing Strategies

Concerning the *HBB* mutation-specific gene editing strategies for hemoglobinopathies, these have hitherto mostly targeted mutations that create cryptic splice sites that, via aberrant splicing and ensuing coding sequence frameshifts, cause β-thalassemia (Patsali et al., 2019b; Xu et al., 2019). By relying on the installation of indels after NHEJ-mediated repair of DSBs induced by Cas9 or Cas12a nucleases, higher *HBB* correction efficiencies are achieved than those involving HDR-mediated gene editing. Since these type of mutations (e.g., IVS1-110G>A and IVS2-654C>T) are particularly common (Kountouris et al., 2014), disruption of aberrant regulatory elements (DARE) approaches might become highly relevant for the correction of the disease in the β-thalassemia patient population (Patsali et al., 2019a) (**Figure 6D**). However, it is worth mentioning that the high sequence identity between *HBB* and other genes in the β-globin locus cluster heightens the risk for adverse events stemming from intra- and inter-chromosomal rearrangements in the form of, for instance, large deletions and translocations, respectively (Long et al., 2018). Hence, concerning this issue, it should be valuable investigating the efficiency and accuracy of DARE via DSB-free base editing and prime editing as alternative approaches to programmable nuclease-induced indel formation.

CONCLUSIONS AND PROSPECTS

The development of genetic therapies for treating hemoglobinopathies is progressing at a sustained pace. Gene therapy technologies based on LV-mediated *HBB* gene supplementation have in fact reached advanced clinical trial stages (**Table 1**). Although improved LV designs present reduced safety concerns associated with insertional oncogenesis (e.g., HIV-1 SIN constructs with miniaturized *HBB* enhancer/promoter elements), life-long monitoring for the emergence of potentially hazardous monoclonal expansions of HSC progenies, is warranted. Importantly, LV-based gene therapies are showing promising results in terms of achieving clinically relevant β-like globin expression levels in initial and ongoing clinical trials (**Table 1**) (Sii-Felice et al., 2020).

The gathering of fundamental insights on developmentally regulated ɤ-globin repression and chromatin looping mechanisms, constitute additional significant developments as they guide the search for novel genetic therapies (Krivega and Dean, 2016; Wienert et al., 2018; Brendel et al., 2020). Moreover, one should equally stress the crucial contribution of clinical genetics to the unraveling of such fundamental mechanisms of hemoglobin biology. Indeed, by learning from and leveraging upon distinct natural mutations causing pathology or phenotype amelioration, it is now possible to pursue *HBB* mutation-independent and *HBB* mutation-specific genetic therapies. Indeed, gene editing platforms with increasing accuracy are offering the prospect for modifying genomic sequences underlying severe hemoglobinopathies through either mutation-dependent or independent strategies. Promising results from pre-clinical models and early-stage clinical trials point to a role for gene editing in the treatment of hemoglobinopathies (**Table 2**). Despite these developments, further improvements are clearly in demand to establish genome editing as a broadly applicable and safe therapeutic option for hemoglobinopathies. The need for high corrective-gene expression levels and high frequencies of gene edited cells means that improving gene editing tools must go hand-in-hand with implementing systems for their delivery into *bona fide* HSCs.

In this context, episomal (i.e., non-integrating) viral vectors, such as adenoviral (AdV) vectors and adeno-associated viral (AAV) vectors, are promising agents for introducing gene editing components into HSCs, in particular, certain capsid pseudo-typed variants (Chen and Gonçalves, 2016; Li and Lieber, 2019; Li C. et al., 2020; Tasca et al., 2020; Yang et al., 2020). For instance, AAV serotype 6 (AAV6) seems to be particularly effective in transducing HSCs when compared to other AAV serotypes, making it a valuable platform to test, amongst others, HDR-mediated *HBB* gene correction strategies (Pattabhi et al., 2019; Yang et al., 2020). It is also possible that, in addition to their efficient HSC transduction, the peculiar structure of AAV vector genomes, consisting of single-stranded DNA ended by palindromic inverted terminal repeats, contributes to donor-target DNA recombination (Holkers et al., 2012). On the other hand, recent experiments indicate that AAV vector genomes trigger a p53-dependent DNA damage response in HSPCs and, through non-homologous recombination processes, integrate at significant rates at RGN target sites in murine tissues (Hanlon et al., 2019; Nelson et al., 2019; Schiroli et al., 2019). The latter data are consistent with earlier results disclosing that a measurable fraction of AAV donor DNA becomes "captured" at ZFN-induced DSBs in murine livers (Li et al., 2011; Anguela et al., 2013). These events might be most problematic in cases where

AAV vector genomes encode programmable nucleases as they directly raise issues concerning the permanency of these tools in transduced cells.

Collectively, these findings stress the need to (i) closely monitoring the impact and precision of gene repair procedures in target cells regardless of their type and replication status (Maggio and Gonçalves, 2015); and (ii) expand the range of delivery agents that, like AAVs, are devoid of viral genes but that, in contrast to these vectors, permit transferring recombinant DNA larger than ~4.7 kb; which is the packaging capacity of AAV capsids. Concerning the latter aspect, high-capacity AdV vectors endowed with the cell tropism of species B adenoviruses (e.g., serotypes 35 and 50) are valuable candidates owing to their efficient transduction of HSCs and high genetic payload (i.e., up to 36 kb) (Li and Lieber, 2019; Tasca et al., 2020).

Equally regarding the ultimate performance of gene editing interventions, it is worth mentioning that various types of stem and progenitor cells, including HSPCs, are particularly susceptible to p53-dependent cell cycle arrest and apoptosis, even when subjected to a limited number of targeted DSBs (Haapaniemi et al., 2018; Ihry et al., 2018; Schiroli et al., 2019). Moreover, besides triggering intended gene editing outcomes, targeted DSBs can negatively impact the genotype and phenotype of gene edited cells by installing potentially hazardous allelic and non-allelic chromosomal rearrangements and decreasing cell fitness, respectively (Frock et al., 2015; Kosicki et al., 2018; Chen et al., 2020).

Hence, looking ahead, besides seeking to enhance absolute gene editing efficiencies, an equally important priority will be continuing to improve the safety profile of gene editing procedures as a whole. To this end, macromolecular enzymatic complexes that bring about targeted and precise genomic modifications without catalytic induction of DSBs might become particularly valuable and include, nicking RGNs and their derivative base and prime editor proteins as well as engineered or molecularly evolved site-specific recombinases and CRISPR-based transposases and recombinases (Komor et al., 2016; Chen et al., 2017; Gaudelli et al., 2017; Nakajima et al., 2018; Anzalone et al., 2019, 2020; Klompe et al., 2019; Strecker et al., 2019; Hyodo et al., 2020).

In conclusion, knowledge from hemoglobin biology and clinical genetics studies, together with the herein covered rapid expansion of gene editing techniques, are accelerating the development of genetic therapies for treating hemoglobinopathies. These advances are in turn expected to capitalize and build upon gene transfer and stem cell technologies underlying *ex vivo* transduction and autologous transplantation of HSCs into afflicted patients. This being said, in addition to regulatory requirements, robust and affordable GMP-grade platforms for up-scaling and downstream processing of AMTPs will be crucial before genetic therapies for hemoglobinopathies become broadly available to those in need (Staal et al., 2019).

AUTHOR CONTRIBUTIONS

HZ wrote the manuscript with the contributions from the other authors. All authors have reviewed and edited the work.

REFERENCES

Achour, A., Koopmann, T., Castel, R., Santen, G. W. E., Hollander den, N., Knijnenburg, J., et al. (2020). A new gene associated with a beta-thalassemia phenotype: the observation of variants in SUPT5H. *Blood* 136, 1789–1793. doi: 10.1182/blood.2020005934

Adachi, K., Konitzer, P., and Surrey, S. (1994). Role of gamma 87 Gln in the inhibition of hemoglobin S polymerization by hemoglobin F. *J. Biol. Chem.* 269, 9562–9567.

Akinsheye, I., Alsultan, A., Solovieff, N., Ngo, D., Baldwin, C. T., Sebastiani, P., et al. (2011). Fetal hemoglobin in sickle cell anemia. *Blood* 118, 19–27. doi: 10.1182/blood-2011-03-325258

Albitar, M., Care, A., Peschle, C., and Liebhaber, S. A. (1992a). Developmental switching of messenger RNA expression from the human alpha-globin cluster: fetal/adult pattern of theta-globin gene expression. *Blood* 80, 1586–1591. doi: 10.1182/blood.V80.6.1586.1586

Albitar, M., Cash, F. E., Peschle, C., and Liebhaber, S. A. (1992b). Developmental switch in the relative expression of the alpha 1- and alpha 2-globin genes in humans and in transgenic mice. *Blood* 79, 2471–2474. doi: 10.1182/blood.V79.9.2471.2471

Anders, C., Niewoehner, O., Duerst, A., and Jinek, M. (2014). Structural basis of PAM-dependent target DNA recognition by the Cas9 endonuclease. *Nature* 513, 569–573. doi: 10.1038/nature13579

Angelucci, E., Matthes-Martin, S., Baronciani, D., Bernaudin, F., Bonanomi, S., Cappellini, M. D., et al. (2014). Hematopoietic stem cell transplantation in thalassemia major and sickle cell disease: indications and management recommendations from an international expert panel. *Haematologica* 99, 811–820. doi: 10.3324/haematol.2013.099747

Anguela, X. M., Sharma, R., Doyon, Y., Miller, J. C., Li, H., Haurigot, V., et al. (2013). Robust ZFN-mediated genome editing in adult hemophilic mice. *Blood* 122, 3283–3287. doi: 10.1182/blood-2013-04-497354

Antoniani, C., Meneghini, V., Lattanzi, A., Felix, T., Romano, O., Magrin, E., et al. (2018). Induction of fetal hemoglobin synthesis by CRISPR/Cas9-mediated editing of the human β-globin locus. *Blood* 131, 1960–1973. doi: 10.1182/blood-2017-10-811505

Antony, J. S., Latifi, N., Akma, H., Lamsfus-Calle, A., Daniel-Moreno, A., Graeter, S., et al. (2018). Gene correction of HBB mutations in CD34+ hematopoietic stem cells using Cas9 mRNA and ssODN donors. *Mol. Cell Pediatr.* 5:9. doi: 10.1186/s40348-018-0086-1

Anurathapan, U., Hongeng, S., Pakakasama, S., Songdej, D., Sirachainan, N., Pongphitcha, P., et al. (2020). Hematopoietic stem cell transplantation for severe thalassemia patients from haploidentical donors using a novel conditioning regimen. *Biol. Blood Marrow Transplant.* 26, 1106–1112. doi: 10.1016/j.bbmt.2020.01.002

Anzalone, A. V., Koblan, L. W., and Liu, D. R. (2020). Genome editing with CRISPR-Cas nucleases, base editors, transposases and prime editors. *Nat. Biotechnol.* 38, 824–844. doi: 10.1038/s41587-020-0561-9

Anzalone, A. V., Randolph, P. B., Davis, J. R., Sousa, A. A., Koblan, L. W., Levy, J. M., et al. (2019). Search-and-replace genome editing without double-strand breaks or donor DNA. *Nature* 576, 149–157. doi: 10.1038/s41586-019-1711-4

Arumugam, P. I., Scholes, J., Perelman, N., Xia, P., Yee, J. K., and Malik, P. (2007). Improved human beta-globin expression from self-inactivating lentiviral vectors carrying the chicken hypersensitive site-4 (cHS4) insulator element. *Mol. Ther.* 15, 1863–1871. doi: 10.1038/sj.mt.6300259

Badens, C., Joly, P., Agouti, I., Thuret, I., Gonnet, K., Fattoum, S., et al. (2011). Variants in genetic modifiers of β-thalassemia can help to predict the major or intermedia type of the disease. *Haematologica* 96, 1712–1714. doi: 10.3324/haematol.2011.046748

Baiamonte, E., Rita, B., Rosalia Di, S., Melania Lo, I., Barbara, S., Flavia, C., et al. (2015). Hematopoietic stem cell mobilization for gene therapy: the combination of G-CSF+plerixafor in patients with beta-thalassemia major provides high yields of CD34+ cells with primitive signatures. *Blood* 126:4412. doi: 10.1182/blood.V126.23.4412.4412

Baronciani, D., Angelucci, E., Potschger, U., Gaziev, J., Yesilipek, A., Zecca, M., et al. (2016). Hemopoietic stem cell transplantation in thalassemia: a report from the European society for blood and bone marrow transplantation hemoglobinopathy registry, 2000-2010. *Bone Marrow Transplant.* 51, 536–541. doi: 10.1038/bmt.2015.293

Bauer, D. E., Kamran, S. C., Lessard, S., Xu, J., Fujiwara, Y., Lin, C., et al. (2013). An erythroid enhancer of BCL11A subject to genetic variation determines fetal hemoglobin level. *Science* 342, 253–257. doi: 10.1126/science.1242088

Bauer, D. E., and Orkin, S. H. (2015). Hemoglobin switching's surprise: the versatile transcription factor BCL11A is a master repressor of fetal hemoglobin. *Curr. Opin. Genet. Dev.* 33, 62–70. doi: 10.1016/j.gde.2015.08.001

Biffi, A., Montini, E., Lorioli, L., Cesani, M., Fumagalli, F., Plati, T., et al. (2013). Lentiviral hematopoietic stem cell gene therapy benefits metachromatic leukodystrophy. *Science* 341:1233158. doi: 10.1126/science.1233158

Boch, J., Scholze, H., Schornack, S., Landgraf, A., Hahn, S., Kay, S., et al. (2009). Breaking the code of DNA binding specificity of TAL-type III effectors. *Science* 326, 1509–1512. doi: 10.1126/science.1178811

Borg, J., Papadopoulos, P., Georgitsi, M., Gutiérrez, L., Grech, G., Fanis, P., et al. (2010). Haploinsufficiency for the erythroid transcription factor KLF1 causes hereditary persistence of fetal hemoglobin. *Nat. Genet.* 42, 801–805. doi: 10.1038/ng.630

Boulad, F., Shore, T., van Besien, K., Minniti, C., Barbu-Stevanovic, M., Fedus, S. W., et al. (2018). Safety and efficacy of plerixafor dose escalation for the mobilization of CD34^{+} hematopoietic progenitor cells in patients with sickle cell disease: interim results. *Haematologica* 103, 770–777. doi: 10.3324/haematol.2017.187047

Breda, L., Motta, I., Lourenco, S., Gemmo, C., Deng, W., Rupon, J. W., et al. (2016). Forced chromatin looping raises fetal hemoglobin in adult sickle cells to higher levels than pharmacologic inducers. *Blood* 128, 1139–1143. doi: 10.1182/blood-2016-01-691089

Brendel, C., Guda, S., Renella, R., Bauer, D. E., Canver, M. C., Kim, Y. J., et al. (2016). Lineage-specific BCL11A knockdown circumvents toxicities and reverses sickle phenotype. *J. Clin. Invest.* 126, 3868–3878. doi: 10.1172/JCI87885

Brendel, C., Negre, O., Rothe, M., Guda, S., Parsons, G., Harris, C., et al. (2020). Preclinical evaluation of a novel lentiviral vector driving lineage-specific BCL11A knockdown for sickle cell gene therapy. *Mol. Ther. Methods Clin. Dev.* 17, 589–600. doi: 10.1016/j.omtm.2020.03.015

Canver, M. C., Smith, E. C., Sher, F., Pinello, L., Sanjana, N. E., Shalem, O., et al. (2015). BCL11A enhancer dissection by Cas9-mediated *in situ* saturating mutagenesis. *Nature* 527, 192–197. doi: 10.1038/nature15521

Cao, A., and Moi, P. (2002). Regulation of the globin genes. *Pediatr. Res.* 51, 415–421. doi: 10.1203/00006450-200204000-00003

Carroll, D. (2019). Collateral damage: benchmarking off-target effects in genome editing. *Genome Biol.* 20:114. doi: 10.1186/s13059-019-1725-0

Cartier, N., Hacein-Bey-Abina, S., Bartholomae, C. C., Veres, G., Schmidt, M., Kutschera, I., et al. (2009). Hematopoietic stem cell gene therapy with a lentiviral vector in X-linked adrenoleukodystrophy. *Science* 326, 818–823. doi: 10.1126/science.1171242

Cavazzana, M., Antoniani, C., and Miccio, A. (2017). Gene therapy for β-hemoglobinopathies. *Mol. Ther.* 25, 1142–1154. doi: 10.1016/j.ymthe.2017.03.024

Cavazzana, M., Bushman, F. D., Miccio, A., André-Schmutz, I., and Six, E. (2019). Gene therapy targeting haematopoietic stem cells for inherited diseases: progress and challenges. *Nat. Rev. Drug Discov.* 18, 447–462. doi: 10.1038/s41573-019-0020-9

Cavazzana-Calvo, M., Payen, E., Negre, O., Wang, G., Hehir, K., Fusil, F., et al. (2010). Transfusion independence and HMGA2 activation after gene therapy of human β-thalassaemia. *Nature* 467, 318–322. doi: 10.1038/nature09328

Chada, K., Magram, J., Raphael, K., Radice, G., Lacy, E., and Costantini, F. (1985). Specific expression of a foreign β-globin gene in erythroid cells of transgenic mice. *Nature* 314, 377–380. doi: 10.1038/314377a0

Chandrasegaran, S., and Carroll, D. (2016). Origins of programmable nucleases for genome engineering. *J. Mol. Biol.* 428, 963–989. doi: 10.1016/j.jmb.2015.10.014

Chang, C. J., and Bouhassira, E. E. (2012). Zinc-finger nuclease-mediated correction of α-thalassemia in iPS cells. *Blood* 120, 3906–3914. doi: 10.1182/blood-2012-03-420703

Chang, H. H. Y., Pannunzio, N. R., Adachi, N., and Lieber, M. R. (2017). Non-homologous DNA end joining and alternative pathways to double-strand break repair. *Nat. Rev. Mol. Cell Biol.* 18, 495–506. doi: 10.1038/nrm.2017.48

Chang, K. H., Smith, S. E., Sullivan, T., Chen, K., Zhou, Q., West, J. A., et al. (2017). Long-term engraftment and fetal globin induction upon BCL11A gene editing in bone-marrow-derived CD34^{+} hematopoietic stem and progenitor cells. *Mol. Ther. Methods Clin. Dev.* 4, 137–148. doi: 10.1016/j.omtm.2016.12.009

Chen, X., and Gonçalves, M. A. F. V. (2016). Engineered viruses as genome editing devices. *Mol. Ther.* 24, 447–457. doi: 10.1038/mt.2015.164

Chen, X., and Gonçalves, M. A. F. V. (2018). DNA, RNA, and protein tools for editing the genetic information in human cells. *iScience* 6, 247–263. doi: 10.1016/j.isci.2018.08.001

Chen, X., Janssen, J. M., Liu, J., Maggio, I., 't Jong, A. E. J., Mikkers, H. M. M., et al. (2017). In trans paired nicking triggers seamless genome editing without double-stranded DNA cutting. *Nat. Commun.* 8:657. doi: 10.1038/s41467-017-00687-1

Chen, X., Tasca, F., Wang, Q., Liu, J., Janssen, J. M., Brescia, M. D., et al. (2020). Expanding the editable genome and CRISPR-Cas9 versatility using DNA cutting-free gene targeting based on in trans paired nicking. *Nucleic Acids Res.* 48, 974–995. doi: 10.1093/nar/gkz1121

Cho, S. W., Kim, S., Kim, J. M., and Kim, J. S. (2013). Targeted genome engineering in human cells with the Cas9 RNA-guided endonuclease. *Nat. Biotechnol.* 31, 230–232. doi: 10.1038/nbt.2507

Christian, M., Cermak, T., Doyle, E. L., Schmidt, C., Zhang, F., Hummel, A., et al. (2010). Targeting DNA double-strand breaks with TAL effector nucleases. *Genetics* 186, 757–761. doi: 10.1534/genetics.110.120717

Clegg, J. B. (1987). Can the product of the theta gene be a real globin? *Nature* 329, 465–466. doi: 10.1038/329465a0

Coelho, A., Picanço, I., Seuanes, F., Seixas, M. T., and Faustino, P. (2010). Novel large deletions in the human alpha-globin gene cluster: clarifying the HS-40 long-range regulatory role in the native chromosome environment. *Blood Cells Mol. Dis.* 45, 147–153. doi: 10.1016/j.bcmd.2010.05.010

Cong, L., Ran, F. A., Cox, D., Lin, S., Barretto, R., Habib, N., et al. (2013). Multiplex genome engineering using CRISPR/Cas systems. *Science* 339, 819–823. doi: 10.1126/science.1231143

Cornu, T. I., Mussolino, C., and Cathomen, T. (2017). Refining strategies to translate genome editing to the clinic. *Nat. Med.* 23, 415–423. doi: 10.1038/nm.4313

Cradick, T. J., Fine, E. J., Antico, C. J., and Bao, G. (2013). CRISPR/Cas9 systems targeting beta-globin and CCR5 genes have substantial off-target activity. *Nucleic Acids Res.* 41, 9584–9592. doi: 10.1093/nar/gkt714

Creary, L. E., Ulug, P., Menzel, S., McKenzie, C. A., Hanchard, N. A., Taylor, V., et al. (2009). Genetic variation on chromosome 6 influences F cell levels in healthy individuals of African descent and HbF levels in sickle cell patients. *PLoS ONE* 4:e4218. doi: 10.1371/journal.pone.0004218

Crossley, M., and Orkin, S. H. (1993). Regulation of the beta-globin locus. *Curr. Opin. Genet. Dev.* 3, 232–237. doi: 10.1016/0959-437X(93)90028-N

Danjou, F., Anni, F., and Galanello, R. (2011). Beta-thalassemia: from genotype to phenotype. *Haematologica* 96, 1573–1575. doi: 10.3324/haematol.2011.055962

De Dreuzy, E., Heath, J., Zuris, J. A., Sousa, P., Viswanathan, R., Scott, S., et al. (2019). EDIT-301: an experimental autologous cell therapy comprising Cas12a-RNP modified mPB-CD34+ cells for the potential treatment of SCD. *Blood* 134:4636. doi: 10.1182/blood-2019-130256

De Gobbi, M., Anguita, E., Hughes, J., Sloane-Stanley, J. A., Sharpe, J. A., Koch, C. M., et al. (2007). Tissue-specific histone modification and transcription factor binding in alpha globin gene expression. *Blood* 110, 4503–4510. doi: 10.1182/blood-2007-06-097964

De La Fuente, R., Baumann, C., and Viveiros, M. M. (2011). Role of ATRX in chromatin structure and function: implications for chromosome instability and human disease. *Reproduction* 142, 221–234. doi: 10.1530/REP-10-0380

Demirci, S., Leonard, A., and Tisdale, J. F. (2020). Genome editing strategies for fetal hemoglobin induction in beta-hemoglobinopathies. *Hum. Mol. Genet.* 29, R100–R106. doi: 10.1093/hmg/ddaa088

Deng, W., Lee, J., Wang, H., Miller, J., Reik, A., Gregory, P. D., et al. (2012). Controlling long-range genomic interactions at a native locus by targeted tethering of a looping factor. *Cell* 149, 1233–1244. doi: 10.1016/j.cell.2012.03.051

Deng, W., Rupon, J. W., Krivega, I., Breda, L., Motta, I., Jahn, K. S., et al. (2014). Reactivation of developmentally silenced globin genes by forced chromatin looping. *Cell* 158, 849–860. doi: 10.1016/j.cell.2014.05.050

Dever, D. P., Bak, R. O., Reinisch, A., Camarena, J., Washington, G., Nicolas, C. E., et al. (2016). CRISPR/Cas9 β-globin gene targeting in human haematopoietic stem cells. *Nature* 539, 384–389. doi: 10.1038/nature20134

DeWitt, M. A., Magis, W., Bray, N. L., Wang, T., Berman, J. R., Urbinati, F., et al. (2016). Selection-free genome editing of the sickle mutation in human adult hematopoietic stem/progenitor cells. *Sci. Transl. Med.* 8:360ra134. doi: 10.1126/scitranslmed.aaf9336

Doudna, J. A., and Charpentier, E. (2014). Genome editing. The new frontier of genome engineering with CRISPR-Cas9. *Science* 346:1258096. doi: 10.1126/science.1258096

Emery, D. W., Yannaki, E., Tubb, J., and Stamatoyannopoulos, G. (2000). A chromatin insulator protects retrovirus vectors from chromosomal position effects. *Proc. Natl. Acad. Sci. U.S.A.* 97, 9150–9155. doi: 10.1073/pnas.160159597

Esrick, E. B., Manis, J. P., Daley, H., Baricordi, C., Trébéden-Negre, H., Pierciey, F. J., et al. (2018). Successful hematopoietic stem cell mobilization and apheresis collection using plerixafor alone in sickle cell patients. *Blood Adv.* 2, 2505–2512. doi: 10.1182/bloodadvances.2018016725

Fanis, P., Kousiappa, I., Phylactides, M., and Kleanthous, M. (2014). Genotyping of BCL11A and HBS1L-MYB SNPs associated with fetal haemoglobin levels: a SNaPshot minisequencing approach. *BMC Genomics* 15:108. doi: 10.1186/1471-2164-15-108

Farashi, S., and Harteveld, C. L. (2018). Molecular basis of α-thalassemia. *Blood Cells Mol. Dis.* 70, 43–53. doi: 10.1016/j.bcmd.2017.09.004

Feng, Q., Chow, P. K., Frassoni, F., Phua, C. M., Tan, P. K., Prasath, A., et al. (2008). Nonhuman primate allogeneic hematopoietic stem cell transplantation by intraosseus vs intravenous injection: engraftment, donor cell distribution, and mechanistic basis. *Exp. Hematol.* 36, 1556–1566. doi: 10.1016/j.exphem.2008.06.010

Fischer, A. S., Abina, H. B., Touzot, F., and Cavazzana, M. (2015). Gene therapy for primary immunodeficiencies. *Clin. Genet.* 88, 507–515. doi: 10.1111/cge.12576

Frock, R. L., Hu, J., Meyers, R. M., Ho, Y. J., Kii, E., and Alt, F. W. (2015). Genome-wide detection of DNA double-stranded breaks induced by engineered nucleases. *Nat. Biotechnol.* 33, 179–186. doi: 10.1038/nbt.3101

Fu, Y., Foden, J. A., Khayter, C., Maeder, M. L., Reyon, D., Joung, J. K., et al. (2013). High-frequency off-target mutagenesis induced by CRISPR-Cas nucleases in human cells. *Nat. Biotechnol.* 31, 822–826. doi: 10.1038/nbt.2623

Gao, L., Cox, D. B. T., Yan, W. X., Manteiga, J. C., Schneider, M. W., Yamano, T., et al. (2017). Engineered Cpf1 variants with altered PAM specificities. *Nat. Biotechnol.* 35, 789–792. doi: 10.1038/nbt.3900

Garrick, D., De Gobbi, M., Samara, V., Rugless, M., Holland, M., Ayyub, H., et al. (2008). The role of the polycomb complex in silencing alpha-globin gene expression in nonerythroid cells. *Blood* 112, 3889–3899. doi: 10.1182/blood-2008-06-161901

Gasiunas, G., Barrangou, R., Horvath, P., and Siksnys, V. (2012). Cas9-crRNA ribonucleoprotein complex mediates specific DNA cleavage for adaptive immunity in bacteria. *Proc. Natl. Acad. Sci. U.S.A.* 109, E2579–E2586. doi: 10.1073/pnas.1208507109

Gaudelli, N. M., Komor, A. C., Rees, H. A., Packer, M. S., Badran, A. H., Bryson, D. I., et al. (2017). Programmable base editing of A*T to G*C in genomic DNA without DNA cleavage. *Nature* 551, 464–471. doi: 10.1038/nature24644

Genovese, P., Schiroli, G., Escobar, G., Tomaso, T. D., Firrito, C., Calabria, A., et al. (2014). Targeted genome editing in human repopulating haematopoietic stem cells. *Nature* 510, 235–240. doi: 10.1038/nature13420

Gibbons, R. (2006). Alpha thalassaemia-mental retardation, X linked. *Orphanet J. Rare Dis.* 1:15. doi: 10.1186/1750-1172-1-15

Gibbons, R. J., Pellagatti, A., Garrick, D., Wood, W. G., Malik, N., Ayyub, H., et al. (2003). Identification of acquired somatic mutations in the gene encoding chromatin-remodeling factor ATRX in the alpha-thalassemia myelodysplasia syndrome (ATMDS). *Nat. Genet.* 34, 446–449. doi: 10.1038/ng1213

Gibbons, R. J., Wada, T., Fisher, C. A., Malik, N., Mitson, M. J., Steensma, D. P., et al. (2008). Mutations in the chromatin-associated protein ATRX. *Hum. Mutat.* 29, 796–802. doi: 10.1002/humu.20734

Goh, S. H., Lee, Y. T., Bhanu, N. V., Cam, M. C., Desper, R., Martin, B. M. (2005). A newly discovered human α-globin gene. *Blood* 106, 1466–1472. doi: 10.1182/blood-2005-03-0948

Grunewald, J., Zhou, R., Iyer, S., Lareau, C. A., Garcia, S. P., Aryee, M. J., et al. (2019). CRISPR DNA base editors with reduced RNA off-target and self-editing activities. *Nat. Biotechnol.* 37, 1041–1048. doi: 10.1038/s41587-019-0236-6

Haapaniemi, E., Botla, S., Persson, J., Schmierer, B., and Taipale, J. (2018). CRISPR-Cas9 genome editing induces a p53-mediated DNA damage response. *Nat. Med.* 24, 927–930. doi: 10.1038/s41591-018-0049-z

Hanlon, K. S., Kleinstiver, B. P., Garcia, S. P., Zaborowski, M. P., Volak, A., Spirig, S. E., et al. (2019). High levels of AAV vector integration into CRISPR-induced DNA breaks. *Nat. Commun.* 10:4439. doi: 10.1038/s41467-019-12449-2

Hanscombe, O., Whyatt, D., Fraser, P., Yannoutsos, N., Greaves, D., Dillon, N., et al. (1991). Importance of globin gene order for correct developmental expression. *Genes Dev.* 5, 1387–1394. doi: 10.1101/gad.5.8.1387

Harris, S., Barrie, P. A., Weiss, M. L., and Jeffreys, A. J. (1984). The primate psi beta 1 gene. An ancient beta-globin pseudogene. *J. Mol. Biol.* 180, 785–801. doi: 10.1016/0022-2836(84)90257-2

Harteveld, C. L., Voskamp, A., Phylipsen, M., Akkermans, N., den Dunnen, J. T., White, S. J., et al. (2005). Nine unknown rearrangements in 16p13.3 and 11p15.4 causing alpha- and beta-thalassaemia characterised by high resolution multiplex ligation-dependent probe amplification. *J. Med. Genet.* 42, 922–931. doi: 10.1136/jmg.2005.033597

Harteveld, K. L., Losekoot, M., Fodde, R., Giordano, P. C., and Bernini, L. F. (1997). The involvement of Alu repeats in recombination events at the alpha-globin gene cluster: characterization of two alphazero-thalassaemia deletion breakpoints. *Hum. Genet.* 99, 528–534. doi: 10.1007/s004390050401

Hatton, C. S., Wilkie, A. O., Drysdale, H. C., Wood, W. G., Vickers, M. A., Sharpe, J., et al. (1990). Alpha-thalassemia caused by a large (62 kb) deletion upstream of the human alpha globin gene cluster. *Blood* 76, 221–227. doi: 10.1182/blood.V76.1.221.221

Henry, E. R., Cellmer, T., Dunkelberger, E. B., Metaferia, B., Hofrichter, J., Li, Q., et al. (2020). Allosteric control of hemoglobin S fiber formation by oxygen and its relation to the pathophysiology of sickle cell disease. *Proc. Natl. Acad. Sci. U.S.A.* 117, 15018–15027. doi: 10.1073/pnas.1922004117

Higgs, D. R., Vickers, M. A., Wilkie, A. O., Pretorius, I. M., Jarman, A. P., and Weatherall, D. J. (1989). A review of the molecular genetics of the human alpha-globin gene cluster. *Blood* 73, 1081–1104. doi: 10.1182/blood.V73.5.1081.1081

Higgs, D. R., and Wood, W. G. (2008). Long-range regulation of alpha globin gene expression during erythropoiesis. *Curr. Opin. Hematol.* 15, 176–183. doi: 10.1097/MOH.0b013e3282f734c4

Higgs, D. R., Wood, W. G., Jarman, A. P., Sharpe, J., Lida, J., Pretorius, I. M., et al. (1990). A major positive regulatory region located far upstream of the human alpha-globin gene locus. *Genes Dev.* 4, 1588–1601. doi: 10.1101/gad.4.9.1588

Hirakawa, M. P., Krishnakumar, R., Timlin, J. A., Carney, J. P., and Butler, K. S. (2020). Gene editing and CRISPR in the clinic: current and future perspectives. *Biosci. Rep.* 40:BSR20200127. doi: 10.1042/BSR20200127

Holkers, M., de Vries, A. A., and Gonçalves, M. A. F. V. (2012). Nonspaced inverted DNA repeats are preferential targets for homology-directed gene repair in mammalian cells. *Nucleic Acids Res.* 40, 1984–1999. doi: 10.1093/nar/gkr976

Hsu, P. D., Scott, D. A., Weinstein, J. A., Ran, F. A., Konermann, S., Agarwala, V., et al. (2013). DNA targeting specificity of RNA-guided Cas9 nucleases. *Nat. Biotechnol.* 31, 827–832. doi: 10.1038/nbt.2647

Hsu, S. L., Marks, J., Shaw, J. P., Tam, M., Higgs, D. R., Shen, C. C., et al. (1988). Structure and expression of the human θl globin gene. *Nature* 331, 94–96. doi: 10.1038/331094a0

Hughes, J. R., Cheng, J. F., Ventress, N., Prabhakar, S., Clark, K., Anguita, E., et al. (2005). Annotation of cis-regulatory elements by identification, subclassification, and functional assessment of multispecies conserved sequences. *Proc. Natl. Acad. Sci. U.S.A.* 102, 9830–9835. doi: 10.1073/pnas.0503401102

Humbert, O., Radtke, S., Samuelson, C., Carrillo, R. R., Perez, A. M., Reddy, S. S., et al. (2019). Therapeutically relevant engraftment of a CRISPR-Cas9-edited HSC-enriched population with HbF reactivation in nonhuman primates. *Sci. Transl. Med.* 11:eaaw3768. doi: 10.1126/scitranslmed.aaw3768

Hyodo, T., Rahman, M. L., Karnan, S., Ito, T., Toyoda, A., Ota, A., et al. (2020). Tandem paired nicking promotes precise genome editing with scarce interference by p53. *Cell Rep.* 30, 1195–207.e7. doi: 10.1016/j.celrep.2019.12.064

Ihry, R. J., Worringer, K. A., Salick, M. R., Frias, E., Ho, D., Theriault, K., et al. (2018). p53 inhibits CRISPR-Cas9 engineering in human pluripotent stem cells. *Nat. Med.* 24, 939–946. doi: 10.1038/s41591-018-0050-6

Ikawa, Y., Miccio, A., Magrin, E., Kwiatkowski, J. L., Rivella, S., and Cavazzana, M. (2019). Gene therapy of hemoglobinopathies: progress and future challenges. *Hum. Mol. Genet.* 28, R24–R30. doi: 10.1093/hmg/ddz172

Ingram, V. M. (1956). A specific chemical difference between the globins of normal human and sickle-cell anaemia haemoglobin. *Nature* 178, 792–794. doi: 10.1038/178792a0

Iolascon, A., De Franceschi, L., Muckenthaler, M., Taher, A., Rees, D., de Montalembert, M., et al. (2019). EHA research roadmap on hemoglobinopathies and thalassemia: an update. *Hemasphere* 3:e208. doi: 10.1097/HS9.0000000000000208

Jinek, M., Chylinski, K., Fonfara, I., Hauer, M., Doudna, J. A., and Charpentier, E. (2012). A programmable dual-RNA-guided DNA endonuclease in adaptive bacterial immunity. *Science* 337, 816–821. doi: 10.1126/science.1225829

Jinek, M., East, A., Cheng, A., Lin, S., Ma, E., and Doudna, J. (2013). RNA-programmed genome editing in human cells. *Elife* 2:e00471. doi: 10.7554/eLife.00471.009

Kato, G. J., Piel, F. B., Reid, C. D., Gaston, M. H., Ohene-Frempong, K., Krishnamurti, L., et al. (2018). Sickle cell disease. *Nat. Rev. Dis. Primers* 4:18010. doi: 10.1038/nrdp.2018.10

Kim, D., Luk, K., Wolfe, S. A., and Kim, J. S. (2019). Evaluating and enhancing target specificity of gene-editing nucleases and deaminases. *Annu. Rev. Biochem.* 88, 191–220. doi: 10.1146/annurev-biochem-013118-111730

Kim, Y. G., Cha, J., and Chandrasegaran, S. (1996). Hybrid restriction enzymes: zinc finger fusions to Fok I cleavage domain. *Proc. Natl. Acad. Sci. U.S.A.* 93, 1156–1160. doi: 10.1073/pnas.93.3.1156

King, A. J., and Higgs, D. R. (2018). Potential new approaches to the management of the Hb Bart's hydrops fetalis syndrome: the most severe form of α-thalassemia. *Hematol. Am. Soc. Hematol. Educ. Program* 2018, 353–360. doi: 10.1182/asheducation-2018.1.353

Kioussis, D., Vanin, E., de Lange, T., Flavell, R. A., and Grosveld, F. G. (1983). Beta-globin gene inactivation by DNA translocation in gamma beta-thalassaemia. *Nature* 306, 662–666. doi: 10.1038/306662a0

Kleinstiver, B. P., Sousa, A. A., Walton, R. T., Tak, Y. E., Hsu, J. Y., Clement, K., et al. (2019). Engineered CRISPR-Cas12a variants with increased activities and improved targeting ranges for gene, epigenetic and base editing. *Nat. Biotechnol.* 37, 276–282. doi: 10.1038/s41587-018-0011-0

Kleinstiver, B. P., Tsai, S. Q., Prew, M. S., Nguyen, N. T., Welch, M. M., Lopez, J. M., et al. (2016). Genome-wide specificities of CRISPR-Cas Cpf1 nucleases in human cells, *Nat. Biotechnol.* 34, 869–874. doi: 10.1038/nbt.3620

Klompe, S. E., Vo, P. L. H., Halpin-Healy, T. S., and Sternberg, S. H. (2019). Transposon-encoded CRISPR-Cas systems direct RNA-guided DNA integration. *Nature* 571, 219–225. doi: 10.1038/s41586-019-1323-z

Koblan, L. W., Doman, J. L., Wilson, C., Levy, J. M., Tay, T., Newby, G. A., et al. (2018). Improving cytidine and adenine base editors by expression optimization and ancestral reconstruction. *Nat. Biotechnol.* 36, 843–846. doi: 10.1038/nbt.4172

Kohne, E. (2011). Hemoglobinopathies: clinical manifestations, diagnosis, and treatment. *Dtsch. Arztebl. Int.* 108, 532–540. doi: 10.3238/arztebl.2011.0532

Kollias, G., Wrighton, N., Hurst, J., and Grosveld, F. (1986). Regulated expression of human A gamma-, beta-, and hybrid gamma beta-globin genes in transgenic mice: manipulation of the developmental expression patterns. *Cell* 46, 89–94. doi: 10.1016/0092-8674(86)90862-7

Komor, A. C., Kim, Y. B., Packer, M. S., Zuris, J. A., and Liu, D. R. (2016). Programmable editing of a target base in genomic DNA without double-stranded DNA cleavage. *Nature* 533, 420–424. doi: 10.1038/nature17946

Kosicki, M., Tomberg, K., and Bradley, A. (2018). Repair of double-strand breaks induced by CRISPR-Cas9 leads to large deletions and complex rearrangements. *Nat. Biotechnol.* 36, 765–771. doi: 10.1038/nbt.4192

Kountouris, P., Lederer, C. W., Fanis, P., Feleki, X., Old, J., and Kleanthous, M. (2014). IthaGenes: an interactive database for haemoglobin variations and epidemiology. *PLoS ONE* 9:e103020. doi: 10.1371/journal.pone.0103020

Krivega, I., and Dean, A. (2016). Chromatin looping as a target for altering erythroid gene expression. *Ann. N. Y. Acad. Sci.* 1368, 31–39. doi: 10.1111/nyas.13012

Lettre, G., Sankaran, V. G., Bezerra, M. A., Araújo, A. S., Uda, M., Sanna, S., et al. (2008). DNA polymorphisms at the BCL11A, HBS1L-MYB, and beta-globin loci associate with fetal hemoglobin levels and pain crises in sickle cell disease. *Proc. Natl. Acad. Sci. U.S.A.* 105, 11869–11874. doi: 10.1073/pnas.0804799105

Li, C., and Lieber, A. (2019). Adenovirus vectors in hematopoietic stem cell genome editing. *FEBS Lett.* 593, 3623–3648. doi: 10.1002/1873-3468.13668

Li, C., Wang, H., Georgakopoulou, A., Gil, S., Yannaki, E., and Lieber, A. (2020). *In vivo* HSC gene therapy using a Bi-modular HDAd5/35++ vector cures sickle cell disease in a mouse model. *Mol. Ther.* 29, 1–16. doi: 10.1016/j.ymthe.2020.09.001

Li, H., Haurigot, V., Doyon, Y., Li, T., Wong, S. Y., Bhagwat, A. S., et al. (2011). *In vivo* genome editing restores haemostasis in a mouse model of haemophilia. *Nature* 475, 217–221. doi: 10.1038/nature10177

Li, H., Yang, Y., Hong, W., Huang, M., Wu, M., and Zhao, X. (2020). Applications of genome editing technology in the targeted therapy of human diseases: mechanisms, advances and prospects. *Signal Transduction Targeted Ther.* 5:1. doi: 10.1038/s41392-019-0089-y

Li, J., Lai, Y., Luo, J., Luo, L., Liu, R., Liu, Z., et al. (2017). SOX6 downregulation induces γ-globin in human β-thalassemia major erythroid cells. *Biomed Res. Int.* 2017:9496058. doi: 10.1155/2017/9496058

Liang, S., Moghimi, B., Yang, T. P., Strouboulis, J., and Bungert, J. (2008). Locus control region mediated regulation of adult beta-globin gene expression. *J. Cell. Biochem.* 105, 9–16. doi: 10.1002/jcb.21820

Liebhaber, S. A., and Kan, Y. W. (1981). Differentiation of the mRNA transcripts originating from the alpha 1- and alpha 2-globin loci in normals and alpha-thalassemics. *J. Clin. Invest.* 68, 439–446. doi: 10.1172/JCI110273

Liu, N., Hargreaves, V. V., Zhu, Q., Kurland, J. V., Hong, J., Kim, W., et al. (2018). direct promoter repression by BCL11A controls the fetal to adult hemoglobin switch. *Cell* 173, 430–42.e17. doi: 10.1016/j.cell.2018.03.016

Liu, P., Keller, J. R., Ortiz, M., Tessarollo, L., Rachel, R. A., Nakamura, T., et al. (2003). Bcl11a is essential for normal lymphoid development. *Nat. Immunol.* 4, 525–532. doi: 10.1038/ni925

Long, J., Hoban, M. D., Cooper, A. R., Kaufman, M. L., Kuo, C. Y., Campo-Fernandez, B., et al. (2018). Characterization of gene alterations following editing of the β-globin gene locus in hematopoietic stem/progenitor cells. *Mol. Ther.* 26, 468–479. doi: 10.1016/j.ymthe.2017.11.001

Lowrey, C. H., Bodine, D. M., and Nienhuis, A. W. (1992). Mechanism of DNase I hypersensitive site formation within the human globin locus control region. *Proc. Natl. Acad. Sci. U.S.A.* 89, 1143–1147. doi: 10.1073/pnas.89.3.1143

Luc, S., Huang, J., McEldoon, J. L., Somuncular, E., Li, D., Rhodes, C., et al. (2016). Bcl11a Deficiency leads to hematopoietic stem cell defects with an aging-like phenotype. *Cell Rep.* 16, 3181–3194. doi: 10.1016/j.celrep.2016.08.064

Lux, C. T., Pattabhi, S., Berger, M., Nourigat, C., Flowers, D. A., Negre, O., et al. (2019). TALEN-mediated gene editing of HBG in human hematopoietic stem cells leads to therapeutic fetal hemoglobin induction. *Mol. Ther. Methods Clin. Dev.* 12, 175–183. doi: 10.1016/j.omtm.2018.12.008

Maggio, I., and Gonçalves, M. A. F. V. (2015). Genome editing at the crossroads of delivery, specificity, and fidelity. *Trends Biotechnol.* 33, 280–291. doi: 10.1016/j.tibtech.2015.02.011

Maggio, I., Zittersteijn, H. A., Wang, Q., Liu, J., Janssen, J. M., Ojeda, I. T., et al. (2020). Integrating gene delivery and gene-editing technologies by adenoviral vector transfer of optimized CRISPR-Cas9 components. *Gene Ther.* 27, 209–225. doi: 10.1038/s41434-019-0119-y

Makani, J., Menzel, S., Nkya, S., Cox, S. E., Drasar, E., Soka, D., et al. (2011). Genetics of fetal hemoglobin in tanzanian and British patients with sickle cell anemia. *Blood* 117, 1390–1392. doi: 10.1182/blood-2010-08-302703

Makarova, K. S., Wolf, Y. I., Iranzo, J., Shmakov, S. A., Alkhnbashi, O. S., Brouns, S. J. J., et al. (2020). Evolutionary classification of CRISPR-Cas systems: a burst of class 2 and derived variants. *Nat. Rev. Microbiol.* 18, 67–83. doi: 10.1038/s41579-019-0299-x

Maldarelli, F., Wu, X., Su, L., Simonetti, F. R., Shao, W., Hill, S., et al. (2014). HIV latency. Specific HIV integration sites are linked to clonal expansion and persistence of infected cells. *Science* 345, 179–183. doi: 10.1126/science.1254194

Mali, P., Yang, L., Esvelt, K. M., Aach, J., Guell, M., DiCarlo, J. E., et al. (2013). RNA-guided human genome engineering via Cas9. *Science* 339, 823–826. doi: 10.1126/science.1232033

Malik, P., Arumugam, P. I., Yee, J. K., and Puthenveetil, G. (2005). Successful correction of the human cooley's anemia beta-thalassemia major phenotype using a lentiviral vector flanked by the chicken hypersensitive site 4 chromatin insulator. *Ann. N. Y. Acad. Sci.* 1054, 238–249. doi: 10.1196/annals. 1345.030

Marks, J., Shaw, J. P., and Shen, C. K. (1986). Sequence organization and genomic complexity of primate theta 1 globin gene, a novel alpha-globin-like gene. *Nature* 321, 785–788. doi: 10.1038/321785a0

Marktel, S., Scaramuzza, S., Cicalese, M. P., Giglio, F., Galimberti, S., Lidonnici, M. R., et al. (2019). Intrabone hematopoietic stem cell gene therapy for adult and pediatric patients affected by transfusion-dependent ß-thalassemia. *Nat. Med.* 25, 234–241. doi: 10.1038/s41591-018-0301-6

Martyn, G. E., Wienert, B., Yang, L., Shah, M., Norton, L. J., Burdach, J., et al. (2018). Natural regulatory mutations elevate the fetal globin gene via disruption of BCL11A or ZBTB7A binding. *Nat. Genet.* 50, 498–503. doi: 10.1038/s41588-018-0085-0

Masuda, T., Wang, X., Maeda, M., Canver, M. C., Sher, F., Funnell, A. P., et al. (2016). Transcription factors LRF and BCL11A independently repress expression of fetal hemoglobin. *Science* 351, 285–289. doi: 10.1126/science.aad3312

May, C., Rivella, S., Callegari, J., Heller, G., Gaensler, K. M., Luzzatto, L., et al. (2000). Therapeutic haemoglobin synthesis in beta-thalassaemic mice expressing lentivirus-encoded human beta-globin. *Nature* 406, 82–86. doi: 10.1038/35017565

Menzel, S., Garner, C., Gut, I., Matsuda, F., Yamaguchi, M., Heath, S., et al. (2007). A QTL influencing F cell production maps to a gene encoding a zinc-finger protein on chromosome 2p15. *Nat. Genet.* 39, 1197–1199. doi: 10.1038/ng2108

Métais, J. Y., Doerfler, P. A., Mayuranathan, T., Bauer, D. E., Fowler, S. C., Hsieh, M. M., et al. (2019). Genome editing of HBG1 and HBG2 to induce fetal hemoglobin. *Blood Adv.* 3, 3379–3392. doi: 10.1182/bloodadvances.2019000820

Mettananda, S., Fisher, C. A., Hay, D., Badat, M., Quek, L., Clark, K., et al. (2017). Editing an α-globin enhancer in primary human hematopoietic stem cells as a treatment for β-thalassemia. *Nat. Commun.* 8:424. doi: 10.1038/s41467-017-00479-7

Mettananda, S., Gibbons, R. J., and Higgs, D. R. (2015). α-Globin as a molecular target in the treatment of β-thalassemia. *Blood* 125, 3694–3701. doi: 10.1182/blood-2015-03-633594

Miller, J. C., Tan, S., Qiao, G., Barlow, K. A., Wang, J., Xia, D. F., et al. (2011). A TALE nuclease architecture for efficient genome editing. *Nat. Biotechnol.* 29, 143–148. doi: 10.1038/nbt.1755

Moscou, M. J., and Bogdanove, A. J. (2009). A simple cipher governs DNA recognition by TAL effectors. *Science* 326:1501. doi: 10.1126/science.1178817

Murayama, M. (1967). Structure of sickle cell hemoglobin and molecular mechanism of the sickling phenomenon. *Clin. Chem.* 13, 578–588. doi: 10.1093/clinchem/13.7.578

Mussolino, C., and Cathomen, T. (2012). TALE nucleases: tailored genome engineering made easy. *Curr. Opin. Biotechnol.* 23, 644–650. doi: 10.1016/j.copbio.2012.01.013

Nakajima, K., Zhou, Y., Tomita, A., Hirade, Y., Gurumurthy, C. B., and Nakada, S. (2018). Precise and efficient nucleotide substitution near genomic nick via noncanonical homology-directed repair. *Genome Res.* 28, 223–230. doi: 10.1101/gr.226027.117

Naldini, L., Blomer, U., Gallay, P., Ory, D., Mulligan, R., Gage, F. H., et al. (1996). *In vivo* gene delivery and stable transduction of nondividing cells by a lentiviral vector. *Science* 272, 263–267. doi: 10.1126/science.272.5259.263

Negre, O., Bartholomae, C., Beuzard, Y., Cavazzana, M., Christiansen, L., Courne, C., et al. (2015). Preclinical evaluation of efficacy and safety of an improved lentiviral vector for the treatment of β-thalassemia and sickle cell disease. *Curr. Gene Ther.* 15, 64–81. doi: 10.2174/1566523214666141127095336

Negre, O., Eggimann, A. V., Beuzard, Y., Ribeil, J. A., Bourget, P., Borwornpinyo, S., et al. (2016). Gene Therapy of the β-hemoglobinopathies by lentiviral transfer of the β(A(T87Q))-globin gene. *Hum. Gene Ther.* 27, 148–165. doi: 10.1089/hum.2016.007

Nelson, C. E., Wu, Y., Gemberling, M. P., Oliver, M. L., Waller, M. A., Bohning, J. D., et al. (2019). Long-term evaluation of AAV-CRISPR genome editing for duchenne muscular dystrophy. *Nat. Med.* 25, 427–432. doi: 10.1038/s41591-019-0344-3

Noordermeer, D., and de Laat, W. (2008). Joining the loops: beta-globin gene regulation. *IUBMB Life* 60, 824–833. doi: 10.1002/iub.129

Nowrouzi, A., Glimm, H., von Kalle, C., and Schmidt, M. (2011). Retroviral vectors: post entry events and genomic alterations. *Viruses* 3, 429–455. doi: 10.3390/v3050429

Park, S., and Beal, P. A. (2019). Off-target editing by CRISPR-guided DNA base editors. *Biochemistry* 58, 3727–3734. doi: 10.1021/acs.biochem.9b00573

Patsali, P., Mussolino, C., Ladas, P., Floga, A., Kolnagou, A., Christou, S., et al. (2019a). The scope for thalassemia gene therapy by disruption of aberrant regulatory elements. *J. Clin. Med.* 8:1959. doi: 10.3390/jcm8111959

Patsali, P., Turchiano, G., Papasavva, P., Romito, M., Loucari, C. C., Stephanou, C., et al. (2019b). Correction of IVS I-110(G>A) β-thalassemia by CRISPR/Cas- and TALEN-mediated disruption of aberrant regulatory elements in human hematopoietic stem and progenitor cells. *Haematologica* 104, e497–e501. doi: 10.3324/haematol.2018.215178

Pattabhi, S., Lotti, S. N., Berger, M. P., Singh, S., Lux, C. T., Jacoby, K., et al. (2019). *In vivo* outcome of homology-directed repair at the HBB gene in HSC using alternative donor template delivery methods. *Mol. Ther. Nucleic Acids* 17, 277–288. doi: 10.1016/j.omtn.2019.05.025

Pawliuk, R., Westerman, K. A., Fabry, M. E., Payen, E., Tighe, R., Bouhassira, E. E., et al. (2001). Correction of sickle cell disease in transgenic mouse models by gene therapy. *Science* 294, 2368–2371. doi: 10.1126/science.1065806

Perutz, M. F. (1962). Relation between structure and sequence of hæmoglobin. *Nature* 194, 914–917. doi: 10.1038/194914a0

Philipsen, S., and Hardison, R. C. (2018). Evolution of hemoglobin loci and their regulatory elements. *Blood Cells Mol. Dis.* 70, 2–12. doi: 10.1016/j.bcmd.2017.08.001

Piel, F. B. (2016). The present and future global burden of the inherited disorders of hemoglobin. *Hematol. Oncol. Clin. North Am.* 30, 327–341. doi: 10.1016/j.hoc.2015.11.004

Psatha, N., Reik, A., Phelps, S., Zhou, Y., Dalas, D., Yannaki, E., et al. (2018). Disruption of the BCL11A erythroid enhancer reactivates fetal hemoglobin in erythroid cells of patients with β-thalassemia major. *Mol. Ther. Methods Clin. Dev.* 10, 313–326. doi: 10.1016/j.omtm.2018.08.003

Rahman, S. H., Maeder, M. L., Joung, J. K., and Cathomen, T. (2011). Zinc-finger nucleases for somatic gene therapy: the next frontier. *Hum. Gene Ther.* 22, 925–933. doi: 10.1089/hum.2011.087

Ramezani, A., Hawley, T. S., and Hawley, R. G. (2008). Combinatorial incorporation of enhancer-blocking components of the chicken beta-globin 5′HS4 and human T-cell receptor alpha/delta BEAD-1 insulators in self-inactivating retroviral vectors reduces their genotoxic potential. *Stem Cells.* 26, 3257–3266. doi: 10.1634/stemcells.2008-0258

Ravi, N. S., Wienert, B., Wyman, S. K., Vu, J., Pai, A. A., Balasubramanian, P., et al. (2020). Identification of novel HPFH-like mutations by CRISPR base editing that elevates the expression of fetal hemoglobin. *bioRxiv* doi: 10.1101/2020.06.30.178715

Rumaney, M. B., Ngo Bitoungui, V. J., Vorster, A. A., Ramesar, R., Kengne, A. P., Ngogang, J., et al. (2014). The co-inheritance of alpha-thalassemia and sickle cell anemia is associated with better hematological indices and lower consultations rate in Cameroonian patients and could improve their survival. *PLoS ONE* 9:e100516. doi: 10.1371/journal.pone.0100516

Sankaran, V. G., Menne, T. F., Xu, J., Akie, T. E., Lettre, G., Van Handel, B., et al. (2008). Human fetal hemoglobin expression is regulated by the developmental stage-specific repressor BCL11A. *Science* 322, 1839–1842. doi: 10.1126/science.1165409

Sankaran, V. G., and Orkin, S. H. (2013). The switch from fetal to adult hemoglobin. *Cold Spring Harb. Perspect. Med.* 3:a011643. doi: 10.1101/cshperspect.a011643

Saraf, S. L., Molokie, R. E., Nouraie, M., Sable, C. A., Luchtman-Jones, L., Ensing, G. J., et al. (2014). Differences in the clinical and genotypic presentation of sickle cell disease around the world. *Paediatr. Respir. Rev.* 15, 4–12. doi: 10.1016/j.prrv.2013.11.003

Schiroli, G., Conti, A., Ferrari, S., Della Volpe, L., Jacob, A., Albano, L., et al. (2019). Precise gene editing preserves hematopoietic stem cell function following transient p53-mediated DNA damage response. *Cell Stem Cell* 24, 551–65.e8. doi: 10.1016/j.stem.2019.02.019

Schröder, A. R., Shinn, P., Chen, H., Berry, C., Ecker, J. R., and Bushman, F. (2002). HIV-1 integration in the human genome favors active genes and local hotspots. *Cell* 110, 521–529. doi: 10.1016/S0092-8674(02)00864-4

Sharpe, J. A., Chan-Thomas, P. S., Lida, J., Ayyub, H., Wood, W. G., and Higgs, D. R. (1992). Analysis of the human alpha globin upstream regulatory element (HS-40) in transgenic mice. *EMBO J.* 11, 4565–4572. doi: 10.1002/j.1460-2075.1992.tb05558.x

Shin, J. J., Schröder, M. S., Caiado, F., Wyman, S. K., Bray, N. L., Bordi, M., et al. (2020). Controlled cycling and quiescence enables efficient HDR in engraftment-enriched adult hematopoietic stem and progenitor cells. *Cell Rep.* 32:108093. doi: 10.1016/j.celrep.2020.108093

Sii-Felice, K., Negre, O., Brendel, C., Tubsuwan, A., Morel,-À.-l'Huissier, E., Filardo, C., et al. (2020). Innovative therapies for hemoglobin disorders. *BioDrugs* 34, 625–647. doi: 10.1007/s40259-020-00439-6

Sokolova, A., Mararenko, A., Rozin, A., Podrumar, A., and Gotlieb, V. (2019). Hereditary persistence of hemoglobin F is protective against red cell sickling. A case report and brief review. *Hematol. Oncol. Stem Cell Ther.* 12, 215–219. doi: 10.1016/j.hemonc.2017.09.003

Sollaino, M. C., Paglietti, M. E., Loi, D., Congiu, R., Podda, R., and Galanello, R. (2010). Homozygous deletion of the major alpha-globin regulatory element (MCS-R2) responsible for a severe case of hemoglobin H disease. *Blood* 116, 2193–2194. doi: 10.1182/blood-2010-04-281345

Staal, F. J. T., Aiuti, A., and Cavazzana, M. (2019). Autologous stem-cell-based gene therapy for inherited disorders: state of the art and perspectives. *Front. Pediatr.* 7:443. doi: 10.3389/fped.2019.00443

Stadhouders, R., Aktuna, S., Thongjuea, S., Aghajanirefah, A., Pourfarzad, F., van Ijcken, W., et al. (2014). HBS1L-MYB intergenic variants modulate fetal hemoglobin via long-range MYB enhancers. *J. Clin. Invest.* 124, 1699–1710. doi: 10.1172/JCI71520

Stamatoyannopoulos, G. (2005). Control of globin gene expression during development and erythroid differentiation. *Exp. Hematol.* 33, 259–271. doi: 10.1016/j.exphem.2004.11.007

Strecker, J., Ladha, A., Gardner, Z., Schmid-Burgk, J. L., Makarova, K. S., Koonin, E. V., et al. (2019). RNA-guided DNA insertion with CRISPR-associated transposases. *Science* 365, 48–53. doi: 10.1126/science.aax9181

Sundd, P., Gladwin, M. T., and Novelli, E. M. (2019). Pathophysiology of sickle cell disease. *Annu. Rev. Pathol.* 14, 263–292. doi: 10.1146/annurev-pathmechdis-012418-012838

Taher, A. T., Weatherall, D. J., and Cappellini, M. D. (2018). Thalassaemia. *Lancet* 391, 155–167. doi: 10.1016/S0140-6736(17)31822-6

Taneda, T., Zhu, W., Cao, Q., Watanabe, H., Yamaguchi, Y., Handa, H., et al. (2011). Erythropoiesis is regulated by the transcription elongation factor Foggy/Spt5 through gata1 gene regulation. *Genes Cells* 16, 231–242. doi: 10.1111/j.1365-2443.2010.01481.x

Tasca, F., Wang, Q., and Gonçalves, M. A. F. V. (2020). Adenoviral vectors meet gene editing: a rising partnership for the genomic engineering of human stem cells and their progeny. *Cells* 9:953. doi: 10.3390/cells9040953

Thein, S. L. (2013). The molecular basis of β-thalassemia. *Cold Spring Harb. Perspect. Med.* 3:a011700. doi: 10.1101/cshperspect.a011700

Thein, S. L. (2018). Molecular basis of β thalassemia and potential therapeutic targets. *Blood Cells Mol. Dis.* 70, 54–65. doi: 10.1016/j.bcmd.2017.06.001

Tóth, E., Varga, É., Kulcsár, P. I., Kocsis-Jutka, V., Krausz, S. L., Nyeste, A., et al. (2020). Improved LbCas12a variants with altered PAM specificities further

broaden the genome targeting range of Cas12a nucleases. *Nucleic Acids Res.* 48, 3722–3733. doi: 10.1093/nar/gkaa110

Townes, T. M., Lingrel, J. B., Chen, H. Y., Brinster, R. L., and Palmiter, R. D. (1985). Erythroid-specific expression of human beta-globin genes in transgenic mice. *EMBO J.* 4, 1715–1723. doi: 10.1002/j.1460-2075.1985.tb03841.x

Traeger-Synodinos, J., Harteveld, C. L., Old, J. M., Petrou, M., Galanello, R., Giordano, P., et al. (2015). EMQN best practice guidelines for molecular and haematology methods for carrier identification and prenatal diagnosis of the haemoglobinopathies. *Eur. J. Hum. Genet.* 23, 426–437. doi: 10.1038/ejhg.2014.131

Traxler, E. A., Yao, Y., Wang, Y. D., Woodard, K. J., Kurita, R., Nakamura, Y., et al. (2016). A genome-editing strategy to treat β-hemoglobinopathies that recapitulates a mutation associated with a benign genetic condition. *Nat. Med.* 22, 987–990. doi: 10.1038/nm.4170

Tsai, S. Q., Zheng, Z., Nguyen, N. T., Liebers, M., Topkar, V. V., Thapar, V., et al. (2015). GUIDE-seq enables genome-wide profiling of off-target cleavage by CRISPR-Cas nucleases. *Nat. Biotechnol.* 33, 187–197. doi: 10.1038/nbt.3117

Tsang, J. C., Yu, Y., Burke, S., Buettner, F., Wang, C., Kolodziejczyk, A. A., et al. (2015). Single-cell transcriptomic reconstruction reveals cell cycle and multi-lineage differentiation defects in Bcl11a-deficient hematopoietic stem cells. *Genome Biol.* 16:178. doi: 10.1186/s13059-015-0739-5

Tufarelli, C., Hardison, R., Miller, W., Hughes, J., Clark, K., Ventress, N., et al. (2004). Comparative analysis of the alpha-like globin clusters in mouse, rat, and human chromosomes indicates a mechanism underlying breaks in conserved synteny. *Genome Res.* 14, 623–630. doi: 10.1101/gr.2143604

Uchida, N., Hsieh, M. M., Raines, L., Haro-Mora, J. J., Demirci, S., Bonifacino, A. C., et al. (2019). Development of a forward-oriented therapeutic lentiviral vector for hemoglobin disorders. *Nat. Commun.* 10:4479. doi: 10.1038/s41467-019-12456-3

Uchida, N., Leonard, A., Stroncek, D., Panch, S. R., West, K., Molloy, E., et al. (2020). Safe and efficient peripheral blood stem cell collection in patients with sickle cell disease using plerixafor. *Haematologica* 105:236182. doi: 10.3324/haematol.2019.236182

Uda, M., Galanello, R., Sanna, S., Lettre, G., Sankaran, V. G., Chen, W., et al. (2008). Genome-wide association study shows BCL11A associated with persistent fetal hemoglobin and amelioration of the phenotype of beta-thalassemia. *Proc. Natl. Acad. Sci. U.S.A.* 105, 1620–1625. doi: 10.1073/pnas.0711566105

Van der Ploeg, L. H., Konings, A., Oort, M., Roos, D., Bernini, L., and Flavell, R. A. (1980). gamma-beta-Thalassaemia studies showing that deletion of the gamma- and delta-genes influences beta-globin gene expression in man. *Nature* 283, 637–642. doi: 10.1038/283637a0

Vernimmen, D. (2014). Uncovering enhancer functions using the α-globin locus. *PLoS Genet.* 10:e1004668. doi: 10.1371/journal.pgen.1004668

Vernimmen, D., Lynch, M. D., De Gobbi, M., Garrick, D., Sharpe, J. A., Sloane-Stanley, J. A., et al. (2011). Polycomb eviction as a new distant enhancer function. *Genes Dev.* 25, 1583–1588. doi: 10.1101/gad.16985411

Vernimmen, D., Marques-Kranc, F., Sharpe, J. A., Sloane-Stanley, J. A., Wood, W. G., Wallace, H. A., et al. (2009). Chromosome looping at the human alpha-globin locus is mediated via the major upstream regulatory element (HS−40). *Blood* 114, 4253–4260. doi: 10.1182/blood-2009-03-213439

Vinjamur, D. S., Bauer, D. E., and Orkin, S. H. (2018). Recent progress in understanding and manipulating haemoglobin switching for the haemoglobinopathies. *Br. J. Haematol.* 180, 630–643. doi: 10.1111/bjh.15038

Voon, H. P., Wardan, H., and Vadolas, J. (2008). siRNA-mediated reduction of alpha-globin results in phenotypic improvements in beta-thalassemic cells. *Haematologica* 93, 1238–1242. doi: 10.3324/haematol.12555

Wallace, H. A., Marques-Kranc, F., Richardson, M., Luna-Crespo, F., Sharpe, J. A., Hughes, J., et al. (2007). Manipulating the mouse genome to engineer precise functional syntenic replacements with human sequence. *Cell* 128, 197–209. doi: 10.1016/j.cell.2006.11.044

Wang, L., Li, L., Ma, Y., Hu, H., Li, Q., Yang, Y., et al. (2020). Reactivation of γ-globin expression through Cas9 or base editor to treat β-hemoglobinopathies. *Cell Res.* 30, 276–278. doi: 10.1038/s41422-019-0267-z

Weber, L., Frati, G., Felix, T., Hardouin, G., Casini, A., Wollenschlaeger, C., et al. (2020). Editing a γ-globin repressor binding site restores fetal hemoglobin synthesis and corrects the sickle cell disease phenotype. *Sci. Adv.* 6:eaay9392. doi: 10.1126/sciadv.aay9392

Wienert, B., Funnell, A. P., Norton, L. J., Pearson, R. C., Wilkinson-White, L. E., Lester, K., et al. (2015). Editing the genome to introduce a beneficial naturally occurring mutation associated with increased fetal globin. *Nat. Commun.* 6:7085. doi: 10.1038/ncomms8085

Wienert, B., Martyn, G. E., Funnell, A. P. W., Quinlan, K. G. R., and Crossley, M. (2018). Wake-up sleepy gene: reactivating fetal globin for β-hemoglobinopathies. *Trends Genet.* 34, 927–940. doi: 10.1016/j.tig.2018.09.004

Wienert, B., Wyman, S. K., Richardson, C. D., Yeh, C. D., Akcakaya, P., Porritt, M. J., et al. (2019). Unbiased detection of CRISPR off-targets *in vivo* using DISCOVER-Seq. *Science* 364, 286–289. doi: 10.1101/469635

Williams, T. N., and Weatherall, D. J. (2012). World distribution, population genetics, and health burden of the hemoglobinopathies. *Cold Spring Harb. Perspect. Med.* 2:a011692. doi: 10.1101/cshperspect.a011692

Wu, X., Li, Y., Crise, B., and Burgess, S. M. (2003). Transcription start regions in the human genome are favored targets for MLV integration. *Science* 300, 1749–1751. doi: 10.1126/science.1083413

Wu, Y., Zeng, J., Roscoe, B. P., Liu, P., Yao, Q., Lazzarotto, C. R., et al. (2019). Highly efficient therapeutic gene editing of human hematopoietic stem cells. *Nat. Med.* 25, 776–783. doi: 10.1038/s41591-019-0401-y

Xie, S. Y., Li, W., Ren, Z. R., Huang, S. Z., Zeng, F., and Zeng, Y. T. (2011). Correction of β654-thalassaemia mice using direct intravenous injection of siRNA and antisense RNA vectors. *Int. J. Hematol.* 93, 301–310. doi: 10.1007/s12185-010-0727-1

Xie, S. Y., Ren, Z. R., Zhang, J. Z., Guo, X. B., Wang, Q. X., Wang, S., et al. (2007). Restoration of the balanced alpha/beta-globin gene expression in beta654-thalassemia mice using combined RNAi and antisense RNA approach. *Hum. Mol. Genet.* 16, 2616–2625. doi: 10.1093/hmg/ddm218

Xu, S., Luk, K., Yao, Q., Shen, A. H., Zeng, J., Wu, Y., et al. (2019). Editing aberrant splice sites efficiently restores β-globin expression in β-thalassemia. *Blood* 133, 2255–2262. doi: 10.1182/blood-2019-01-895094

Yahata, T., Ando, K., Sato, T., Miyatake, H., Nakamura, Y., Muguruma, Y., et al. (2003). A highly sensitive strategy for SCID-repopulating cell assay by direct injection of primitive human hematopoietic cells into NOD/SCID mice bone marrow. *Blood* 101, 2905–2913. doi: 10.1182/blood-2002-07-1995

Yang, H., Qing, K., Keeler, G. D., Yin, L., Mietzsch, M., Ling, C., et al. (2020). Enhanced transduction of human hematopoietic stem cells by AAV6 vectors: implications in gene therapy and genome editing. *Mol. Ther. Nucleic Acids* 20, 451–458. doi: 10.1016/j.omtn.2020.03.009

Yannaki, E., Karponi, G., Zervou, F., Constantinou, V., Bouinta, A., Tachynopoulou, V., et al. (2013). Hematopoietic stem cell mobilization for gene therapy: superior mobilization by the combination of granulocyte-colony stimulating factor plus plerixafor in patients with β-thalassemia major. *Hum. Gene Ther.* 24, 852–860. doi: 10.1089/hum.2013.163

Ye, L., Wang, J., Tan, Y., Beyer, A. I., Xie, F., Muench, M. O., et al. (2016). Genome editing using CRISPR-Cas9 to create the HPFH genotype in HSPCs: an approach for treating sickle cell disease and β-thalassemia. *Proc. Natl. Acad. Sci. U.S.A.* 113, 10661–10665. doi: 10.1073/pnas.1612075113

Yingjun, X., Yuhuan, X., Yuchang, C., Dongzhi, L., Ding, W., Bing, S., et al. (2019). CRISPR/Cas9 gene correction of HbH-CS thalassemia-induced pluripotent stem cells. *Ann. Hematol.* 98, 2661–2671. doi: 10.1007/s00277-019-03763-2

Yu, S. F., von Rüden, T., Kantoff, P. W., Garber, C., Seiberg, M., Rüther, U., et al. (1986). Self-inactivating retroviral vectors designed for transfer of whole genes into mammalian cells. *Proc. Natl. Acad. Sci. U.S.A.* 83, 3194–3198. doi: 10.1073/pnas.83.10.3194

Zaidman, I., Rowe, J. M., Khalil, A., Ben-Arush, M., and Elhasid, R. (2016). Allogeneic stem cell transplantation in congenital hemoglobinopathies using a tailored busulfan-based conditioning regimen: single-center experience. *Biol. Blood Marrow Transplant.* 22, 1043–1048. doi: 10.1016/j.bbmt.2016.03.003

Zeng, J., Wu, Y., Ren, C., Bonanno, J., Shen, A. H., Shea, D., et al. (2020). Therapeutic base editing of human hematopoietic stem cells. *Nat. Med.* 26, 535–541. doi: 10.1038/s41591-020-0790-y

Zetsche, B., Gootenberg, J. S., Abudayyeh, O. O., Slaymaker, I. M., Makarova, K. S., Essletzbichler, P., et al. (2015). Cpf1 is a single RNA-guided endonuclease of a class 2 CRISPR-Cas system. *Cell* 163, 759–771. doi: 10.1016/j.cell.2015.09.038

Zhang, X. H., Tee, L. Y., Wang, X. G., Huang, Q. S., and Yang, S. H. (2015). Off-target effects in CRISPR/Cas9-mediated genome engineering. *Mol. Ther. Nucleic Acids* 4:e264. doi: 10.1038/mtna.2015.37

Zhou, W., Zhao, Q., Sutton, R., Cumming, H., Wang, X., Cerruti, L., et al. (2004). The role of p22 NF-E4 in human globin gene switching. *J. Biol. Chem.* 279, 26227–26232. doi: 10.1074/jbc.M402191200

Zischewski, J., Fischer, R., and Bortesi, L. (2017). Detection of on-target and off-target mutations generated by CRISPR/Cas9 and other sequence-specific nucleases. *Biotechnol. Adv.* 35, 95–104. doi: 10.1016/j.biotechadv.2016.12.003

Zittersteijn, H. A., Gonçalves, M. A. F. V., and Hoeben, R. C. (2020). A primer to gene therapy: progress, prospects, and problems. *J. Inherit. Metab. Dis.* 1–20. doi: 10.1002/jimd.12270

Zufferey, R., Dull, T., Mandel, R. J., Bukovsky, A., Quiroz, D., Naldini, L., et al. (1998). Self-inactivating lentivirus vector for safe and efficient *in vivo* gene delivery. *J. Virol.* 72, 9873–9880. doi: 10.1128/JVI.72.12.9873-9880.1998

Zuo, E., Sun, Y., Wei, W., Yuan, T., Ying, W., Sun, H., et al. (2019). Cytosine base editor generates substantial off-target single-nucleotide variants in mouse embryos. *Science* 364, 289–292. doi: 10.1126/science.aav9973

8

Gene Editing of Hematopoietic Stem Cells: Hopes and Hurdles Toward Clinical Translation

Samuele Ferrari [1,2†], Valentina Vavassori [1,2†], Daniele Canarutto [1,2,3†], Aurelien Jacob [1,4], Maria Carmina Castiello [1,5], Attya Omer Javed [1] and Pietro Genovese [6,7,8,9*]

[1] San Raffaele Telethon Institute for Gene Therapy (SR-Tiget), Istituto di Ricovero e Cura a Carattere Scientifico San Raffaele Scientific Institute, Milan, Italy, [2] PhD course in Molecular Medicine, Vita-Salute San Raffele University, Milan, Italy, [3] Pediatric Immunohematology and Bone Marrow Transplantation Unit, Istituto di Ricovero e Cura a Carattere Scientifico Ospedale San Raffaele, Milan, Italy, [4] PhD Program in Translational and Molecular Medicine (DIMET), Milano-Bicocca University, Monza, Italy, [5] Institute of Genetic and Biomedical Research Milan Unit, National Research Council, Milan, Italy, [6] Division of Hematology/Oncology, Boston Children's Hospital, Boston, MA, United States, [7] Department of Pediatric Oncology, Dana-Farber Cancer Institute, Boston, MA, United States, [8] Harvard Stem Cell Institute, Cambridge, MA, United States, [9] Department of Pediatrics, Harvard Medical School, Boston, MA, United States

*Correspondence:
Pietro Genovese
pietro_genovese@dfci.harvard.edu

[†] These authors have contributed equally to this work

In the field of hematology, gene therapies based on integrating vectors have reached outstanding results for a number of human diseases. With the advent of novel programmable nucleases, such as CRISPR/Cas9, it has been possible to expand the applications of gene therapy beyond semi-random gene addition to site-specific modification of the genome, holding the promise for safer genetic manipulation. Here we review the state of the art of *ex vivo* gene editing with programmable nucleases in human hematopoietic stem and progenitor cells (HSPCs). We highlight the potential advantages and the current challenges toward safe and effective clinical translation of gene editing for the treatment of hematological diseases.

Keywords: gene editing, hematopoietic stem cell, CRISPR/Cas, gene therapy, hematological diseases

INTRODUCTION

Gene therapy aims to treat human diseases by modifying the cell genome e.g., by replacing a defective gene or providing a novel cellular function. In most cases, gene therapy exploits the knowledge on viral biology to generate recombinant vectors able to carry and transfer an exogenous coding cassette into patients' cells. The remarkable progresses in collection and *in vitro* manipulation of HSPCs have enabled the development of *ex vivo* gene therapy strategies, which confine the manipulation to a defined cell subset, thus diminishing the risk of off-target effects and bystander toxicity spillover. *Ex vivo* gene therapy based on semi-randomly integrating retro- (RV) or lenti-viral (LV) vectors has demonstrated an outstanding potential for the treatment of several inherited and acquired hematological diseases (Ghosh et al., 2015; Naldini, 2019). To this goal, autologous HSPCs are harvested, transduced *in vitro* by viral vectors and ultimately infused into the patient. A conditioning regimen is usually administered prior to infusion to deplete host cells and maximize engraftment of the engineered product (Bernardo and Aiuti, 2016).

The discovery and repurposing of programmable molecules, such as nucleases, base editors and prime editors have opened the door to targeted genome editing, i.e., site-specific nucleotide(s) deletion, insertion and substitution, or integration of a therapeutic transgene cassette at a pre-determined genomic locus (Doudna, 2020). These new technologies may be exploited to deliver a wide spectrum of genetic manipulations, with potential applications for several hematological diseases. Indeed, targeted genome editing by programmable nucleases has already entered the clinic and is currently being tested with encouraging results (Xu et al., 2019; Frangoul et al., 2021). While blossoming, gene editing is still in its infancy, and both knowledge and technological gaps await to be filled to broaden its clinical applicability. Furthermore, safety and efficacy, both in the short and long term, are still unknown.

In this Review, we highlight the therapeutic potential and the current challenges toward clinical translation of targeted genome editing by programmable nucleases in human HSPCs for the treatment of blood diseases.

PROGRAMMABLE NUCLEASES FOR TARGETED GENOME EDITING

Programmable nucleases are chimeric molecules composed by (i) a protein- or an RNA-based DNA binding structure, which dictates nuclease specificity, and (ii) an effector domain with catalytic nuclease activity, which induces a DNA double strand break (DSB) nearby or within the binding site. Zinc Finger Nucleases (ZFNs), Transcription Activator-Like Effector Nucleases (TALENs), and Clustered Regularly Interspaced Short Palindromic Repeats (CRISPR)/Cas systems are the most exploited nuclease platforms for targeted genome editing (Carroll, 2014).

ZFNs are composed by an array of three to six zinc-finger (ZF) DNA binding domains, linked by a flexible peptide linker to a non-specific FokI cleavage domain. Each ZF domain is composed by 30 amino acids and recognizes nucleotide triplets in the major groove of the DNA double helix; in total each ZFN recognizes 9–18 nucleotides (Gaj et al., 2013). Sequence and structure of the aforementioned flexible peptide linker is fundamental to achieve efficient cleavage and targeting specificity (Handel and Cathomen, 2011). Mechanistically, a pair of ZFN monomers must bind the DNA, typically in a head-to-head configuration, by associating with DNA strands of opposite polarity and leaving a 5–7 bp gap. This leads to dimerization of the two FokI domains that catalyze the DNA DSB (Urnov et al., 2010).

TALENs consist of a DNA-binding domain composed by modular TALE repeats, fused with a FokI nuclease domain. Each TALE repeat is composed by 33–35 amino acids and recognizes a single nucleotide; specificity is determined by two hypervariable residues, known as Repeated Variable Diresidues (RVDs) (Gaj et al., 2013). Indeed, TALE repeats can be assembled together in a rather straightforward way to pair the desired DNA sequence, nucleotide by nucleotide. As for ZFNs, a pair of TALEN monomers is necessary to introduce a DSB.

Finally, CRISPR/Cas is an RNA-based DNA targeting-system found in bacteria as an acquired immune system against transmissible genetic elements, such as viruses and plasmids (Barrangou et al., 2007; Brouns et al., 2008; Garneau et al., 2010). *Streptococcus pyogenes* (Sp) Cas9 protein (SpCas9) (Nozawa et al., 2011), which belongs to type II family of CRISPR/Cas systems, is the most widely used platform for CRISPR-based targeted genome editing. Mechanistically, the CRISPR/Cas9 system is composed by a single-stranded guide RNA (sgRNA) and the Cas9 endonuclease, which is the enzyme required to mediate target DNA cleavage. The sgRNA contains a unique 20 base-pair sequence which complements the target DNA site, and can

be easily customized to bind the desired genomic sequence by Watson-Crick base-pairing (Jinek et al., 2012). The presence of a protospacer adjacent motif (PAM), immediately downstream the target DNA site, is necessary to efficiently bind and cut the DNA, e.g. 5′-NGG-3′ for SpCas9, although some cleavage activity has also been observed with the 5′-NAG-3′ motif (Hsu et al., 2013; Sternberg et al., 2014).

All these platforms have intrinsic advantages and disadvantages (Gaj et al., 2013). TALENs can be easily assembled in arbitrarily large arrays to bind the sequence of interest, but their intrinsic repetitiveness and large size impair efficient cloning and limit delivery by viral vectors. ZFNs are relatively smaller in size and easier to clone, but difficult to design and optimize, due to the lack of a stringent recognition code and the interdependence of each module with the surrounding ones. Both tools have a limited range of targetable DNA sequences as ZFNs prefer G-rich sequences (Isalan, 2012), while TALENs typically bind low G content sites strictly beginning with a T base (Bogdanove and Voytas, 2011). Instead, the CRISPR/Cas9 system is more flexible, and targeting is usually easier and faster, as it suffices to design and synthetize a sgRNA complementary to the sequence(s) of interest. Multiple sequences may be targeted simultaneously, and no protein optimization is required. Because of its features, the popularity of CRISPR/Cas technology rapidly surpassed that of ZFNs and TALENs.

Still, CRISPR/Cas9 is not free from limitations, the main being the distribution of PAM sequences, that constrains the set of targetable sequences. Indeed, huge efforts have been made to expand the repertoire of potential targets. Cas9 homologs (e.g., Cas12a/Cpf1) (Zetsche et al., 2015a) and Cas9 proteins requiring different PAM sequences have been identified in other bacteria species (Ran et al., 2015; Xu et al., 2015; Lee et al., 2016; Müller et al., 2016); Cas9 variants with relaxed PAM preferences (Cas-NG and xCas) (Hu et al., 2018; Nishimasu et al., 2018) or unconventional PAM profiles (SpCas9-VQR, VRQR and VRER) (Kleinstiver et al., 2015, 2016) have been developed by directed evolution or structure-guided engineering. Recently, a SpCas9 variant (SpRY), requiring a 5′-NRN-3' PAM, has been generated to edit previously inaccessible genetic sites, significantly overcoming most PAM-related limitations (Walton et al., 2020). To date, little data has been generated in primary blood cell types with the aforementioned tools (Wang et al., 2017; Xiao et al., 2019), which would thus require further validation to be employed for hematological diseases.

THERAPEUTIC OPPORTUNITIES FOR TARGETED GENOME EDITING IN HSPCs

Induction of one or multiple DNA DSB(s) by programmable nucleases triggers the DNA damage response (DDR), which mediates DNA repair and ultimately defines cell fate. DNA DSB repair mainly occurs by the non-homologous end joining (NHEJ) pathway or the homology-directed repair (HDR) pathway (Chapman et al., 2012), although alternative pathways have also been described (Yeh et al., 2019). The NHEJ machinery stitches the broken DNA ends in an error prone way, often by deleting or inserting random bases (indels). Instead, the HDR pathway exploits a homologous DNA template, like the sister chromatid, to faithfully repair the DNA breaks. While NHEJ is active throughout the cell cycle, HDR is confined to S/G2 phases (Branzei and Foiani, 2008; Heyer et al., 2010). Both NHEJ- and HDR-mediated repair of nuclease-induced DNA DSBs have been explored for therapeutic purposes in HSPCs (**Figure 1**).

NHEJ-based genome editing finds the following applications: **(i) targeted gene knock-out**: NHEJ-mediated indels directed to a coding sequence may result in frameshift mutations and generation of premature stop codons, which can render the targeted gene non-functional. This strategy can be used to silence a pathogenic gene or induce resistance against a pathogen by knocking out genes that facilitate infections, e.g., the disruption of the *CCR5* open reading frame in hematopoietic cells to confer resistance to HIV infection (Wang and Cannon, 2016; Xu et al., 2019); **(ii) restoration of the correct reading frame**: NHEJ-mediated indels can be exploited to restore the normal reading frame of a gene and thus correct frame-shift mutations. This strategy may be suitable to correct some Fanconi Anemia disease-causing mutations on *FANCA* gene in HSPCs (Román-Rodríguez et al., 2019); **(iii) introduction of a targeted deletion**: programmable nucleases can be used to create two DBSs flanking a region of interest, which is excised and deleted as the gap is repaired by NHEJ (Lee et al., 2010). This strategy can be exploited to remove one or more pathogenic exons, to cut dominant triplet expansion or to delete a regulatory region that alters protein expression. Deletion of the erythroid specific enhancer of *BCL11A* (Bauer et al., 2013), a transcriptional repressor that inhibits fetal hemoglobin (Hb-F) expression, can enhance the levels of Hb-F, resulting in phenotype alleviation of sickle cell disease (SCD) and β-thalassemia.

HDR-mediated genome editing requires the supply of a DNA donor template, harboring homologous sequences with the nuclease target site, and may be exploited for the following applications: **(i) targeted correction of point mutations**: delivery of a nuclease that cleaves close to the mutation site and of a donor template containing the wild-type sequence (Urnov et al., 2005) can be exploited to correct single nucleotide mutations. This approach may be suitable for SCD, which is caused by a single amino acid substitution (Glu to Val) in the sixth position of the *HBB* gene (Dever et al., 2016; DeWitt et al., 2016; Park et al., 2019; Pattabhi et al., 2019; Romero et al., 2019), and for X-linked chronic granulomatous disease (CGD), often caused by mutations in the *CYBB* gene (De Ravin et al., 2017, 2021); **(ii) *in situ* gene correction by targeted insertion of a cDNA**: many monogenetic diseases are not caused by a recurrent single nucleotide mutation, but rather different mutations affecting the same gene. Integration of a functional cDNA, spanning the mutation hotspots, in the intended region of the target gene (e.g., endogenous start codon, intronic region), can simultaneously bypass all downstream mutations (Voit et al., 2014). Proof-of-principle of this approach has been demonstrated for several hematological diseases, including X-linked severe combined immunodeficiency (SCID-X1) (Schiroli et al., 2017; Pavel-Dinu et al., 2019), CGD (Sweeney et al., 2017), Hyper-IgM 1 syndrome (Hubbard et al., 2016; Kuo et al., 2018; Vavassori et al., 2021)

and Wiskott-Aldrich syndrome (WAS) (Rai et al., 2020); **(iii) targeted gene addition into a safe harbor locus**: integration of a therapeutic cassette in a specific region of the genome might represent a valuable strategy when constitutive overexpression of the transgene is required in order to obtain a therapeutic effect (Moehle et al., 2007). The best locations for gene addition in the genome are genomic safe harbors, categorized as genomic locations that are tolerant to homozygous gene inactivation, support robust transgene expression, and tolerate integration of the transgene and its regulatory elements without causing any adverse effects, such as malignant transformation or altered cellular function (Sadelain et al., 2012). One representative application is the targeted integration of corrective *gp91phox* transgene in *AAVS1* locus for treating CGD (De Ravin et al., 2016); **(iv) transgene expression using endogenous regulatory elements**: control of transgene expression by endogenous regulatory elements can provide high, robust and cell specific expression of proteins. Examples are α-L-iduronidase (Hurler syndrome, OMIM #607014), α-galactosidase (Fabry disease, OMIM #301500), lysosomal acid lipase (Wolman disease, OMIM #278000), and factor IX (Hemophilia B, OMIM #306900), that under the transcriptional control of the endogenous α-globin promoter resulted in erythroid-specific expression (Pavani et al., 2020).

CHALLENGES AND ADVANCES TOWARD CLINICAL APPLICATION OF HSPC GENE EDITING

Preliminary results encourage clinical translation of HSPC gene editing for blood disorders. However, a number of issues must be addressed, ranging from sourcing and culturing of the cells, delivery of the nucleases and the corrective template, nuclease activity, and efficiency of gene correction, particularly in the long-term repopulating HSC fraction. Depending on the disease setting, each of these aspects must be accounted for comprehensive risk/benefit evaluation of the therapeutic strategy. Several studies in the last years were focused on the optimization of the editing protocol and the development of novel tools and strategies to maximize editing efficiency and specificity for its safe and successful empowerment.

Tailoring *ex vivo* Cell Culture Conditions

Cell culture protocols must strike a balance between permissiveness to editing manipulation, cell expansion and maintenance of the stemness potential (**Figure 2**). Fine-tuning of culture conditions and editing timing have been pursued to promote HSPC cell cycle progression and activation, and to achieve sustained editing, while preserving long-term persistence of engineered cells. Indeed, HDR-mediated gene editing is constrained in slowly cycling and quiescent primitive HSCs. Generally, the expression level of the DNA repair machinery correlates with the cell proliferation activity and stemness; therefore, long-term repopulating HSCs show lower permissiveness to HDR than committed progenitors (Beerman et al., 2014; Biechonski et al., 2018; Schiroli et al., 2019). *Ex vivo*

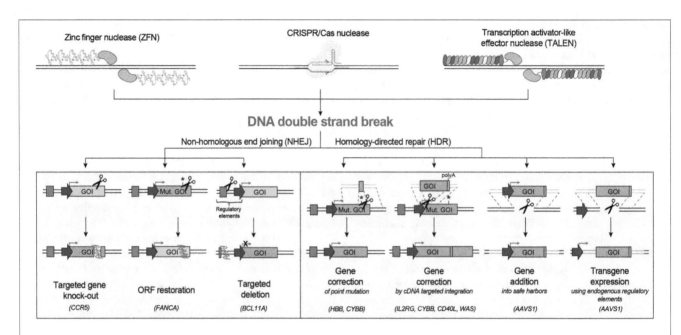

FIGURE 1 | Schematic of the main DNA double strand break repair mechanisms in human cells and their possible applications for targeted genome editing. NHEJ pathway engagement may be exploited for knocking-out a gene, correcting a gene by restoring its open reading frame (ORF), inserting a targeted deletion. HDR pathway engagement may be exploited for gene correction of point or multiple mutations, gene addition in a safe harbor locus or targeted transgene expression using endogenous regulatory elements. Mut. GOI, Mutated Gene Of Interest.

culture of HSPCs for 48 or 72 h before editing, in presence of cytokine mixtures containing at least SCF, FLT-3L, and TPO (Walasek et al., 2012), pushes repopulating cells to exit from quiescence and transit through S/G_2 phases, thus increasing HDR efficiency (Genovese et al., 2014; Zonari et al., 2017; Bak et al., 2018). However, prolonged culture times lead to cell differentiation and multipotency loss. Supplementation of the culture medium with stemness preserving compounds, such as Stem Regenin-1 (Boitano et al., 2010), UM171 (Fares et al., 2014) and 16,16-dimethyl prostaglandin E2 (dmPGE$_2$) (Hoggatt et al., 2009), helps to maintain the long-term multilineage repopulation capacity of human edited HSPCs transplanted in immunodeficient mouse models, partially overcoming the drawbacks of prolonged culture (Charlesworth et al., 2018; Ferrari et al., 2020).

Delivery Vehicles for Programmable Nucleases and DNA Template for HDR-Mediated Editing

Several platforms have been tested to deliver the programmable nucleases and the HDR template in hematopoietic cells with the ultimate goals of maximizing editing efficiency and minimizing treatment toxicity. The proof-of-concept for *in vitro* HDR-mediated integration has been made by delivering both the nuclease and the donor cassette with viral vectors in human HSPCs (Lombardo et al., 2007). Later electroporation became the method of choice to efficiently deliver programmable nucleases in *ex vivo* cultured HSPCs (Genovese et al., 2014). *In vitro* transcribed mRNA encoding for the nucleases (Genovese et al., 2014; Wang et al., 2015; Schiroli et al., 2017) or

ribonucleoprotein (RNP) assembled with recombinant Cas protein and sgRNA (Hendel et al., 2015; Dever et al., 2016) have become the gold standard to achieve a high but transient nuclease activity in HSPCs and other target cells (Hubbard et al., 2016; Eyquem et al., 2017). Transduction with viral vectors as integrase-defective LVs (IDLVs) or adeno-associated vectors serotype 6 (AAV6) (Genovese et al., 2014; Wang et al., 2015; Dever et al., 2016; Schiroli et al., 2017; Kuo et al., 2018; Pavel-Dinu et al., 2019; Rai et al., 2020), as well as the electroporation of single-stranded phosphorothioate-modified oligodeoxynucleotides (ssODNs) (DeWitt et al., 2016; De Ravin et al., 2017, 2021; Park et al., 2019; Pattabhi et al., 2019; Romero et al., 2019), are the vehicles currently preferred to deliver the DNA template for HDR in HSPCs. Overall, these platforms offer a broad spectrum of cargo capacities and may be suitable for different editing strategies. Short ssODN are limited in length and may be applied for *in situ* gene correction of small disease-causing mutations. Conversely, AAV6 and IDLV welcome larger payloads (approximately up to 4.7 and 8 kb, respectively), suitable for targeted integration of long therapeutic cassettes. Instead, adenoviral vectors and other non-viral vehicles, such as plasmids and double-stranded DNA templates, found limited applications in primary hematopoietic cells due to poor efficiency and tolerability, albeit with some exceptions (Roth et al., 2018).

Maximizing HDR Editing Efficiency

The absolute and relative numbers of cells that need to be edited depend on the disease and on the therapeutic strategy. For instance, as the absence of IL2RG is lethal for developing lymphocytes, the strong selective advantage of functional T cell progenitors over affected ones may compensate for relatively low

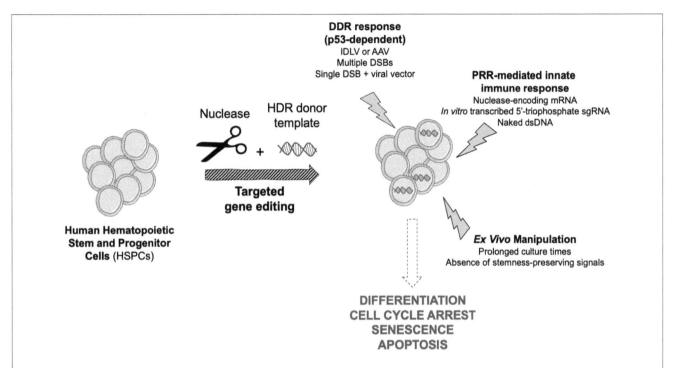

FIGURE 2 | Schematic of cellular responses triggered by targeted genome editing in human HSPCs. Gene editing reagents, procedure and *ex vivo* manipulation may trigger complex cellular responses in HSPCs, ultimately leading to differentiation, cell cycle arrest, senescence, and apoptosis. DDR, DNA Damage Response; PRR, Pattern Recognition Receptor.

editing efficiencies, and <10% of functional HSPCs are predicted to be sufficient to rescue the SCID-X1 phenotype (Schiroli et al., 2017). Conversely, the minimal proportion of edited cells must be substantially higher to fully rescue the pathological features of patients affected by other blood disorders, such as hemoglobinopathies or Hyper-IgM1 (Abraham et al., 2017; Marktel et al., 2019; Vavassori et al., 2021; Wilkinson et al., 2021). Indeed, suboptimal HDR editing efficiency remains a major constrain for broader application of this technology, as opposed to the high efficiency of NHEJ-mediated editing (Humbert et al., 2019; Frangoul et al., 2021).

In pioneering gene editing studies on human HSPCs, IDLV transduction combined with ZFNs mRNA electroporation led to 5–10% HDR editing in the bulk CD34+ population and 2–5% in the primitive CD34+CD133+CD90+ HSPC fraction, which entails cells with long-term engraftment capacity in immunodeficient mice (Genovese et al., 2014). Instead, switching to AAV6 vectors for HDR DNA template delivery has allowed increasing up to 5-fold the HDR editing efficiency in primitive HSPCs compared to the IDLV-based protocol, regardless of the nuclease platforms employed (Wang et al., 2015; Dever et al., 2016; Schiroli et al., 2017; Kuo et al., 2018; Pavel-Dinu et al., 2019; Rai et al., 2020). Of note, IDLV transduction in presence of cyclosporin H enhanced HDR efficiency up to 15–20% in the long-term progeny of human engrafting HSPCs by relieving interferon-induced transmembrane protein 3 (IFTM3)-mediated entry restriction (Petrillo et al., 2018; Soldi et al., 2020), thus suggesting that the total DNA load into the nucleus of transduced cells is still a limiting step for HDR engagement. Nevertheless,

other molecular mechanisms enhancing HDR efficiency with AAV6 still remain partially elusive. Recruitment of HDR factors by AAV inverted terminal repeats (Hirsch, 2015) and engagement of alternative pathways exploiting single-stranded templates for DNA DSB repair may contribute to the enhancement of HDR editing (Yeh et al., 2019). Of note, ssODNs allow for gene correction efficiencies similar to those obtained with AAV6 in primitive HSPCs long term after xenotransplantation (De Ravin et al., 2017; Pattabhi et al., 2019; Romero et al., 2019). ssODNs likely engage DNA DSB repair mechanisms distinct from those of IDLV and possibly AAV6, preferring the single-stranded template repair (SSTR) pathway rather than the conventional HDR (Richardson et al., 2018).

Despite these substantial steps forward, HDR editing efficiency is still limited for some applications. Several strategies were proposed to enhance HDR efficiency in mammalian cells by transiently manipulating the DNA repair pathways or the cell cycle status. NHEJ inhibition by small molecules or proteins, tethering of HDR-promoting factors to Cas9 nuclease, or S/G2 cell synchronization, favored HDR engagement upon nuclease-induced DNA DSB in cell lines and pluripotent cells (Chu et al., 2015; Maruyama et al., 2015; Gutschner et al., 2016; Charpentier et al., 2018; Jayavaradhan et al., 2019). However, the efficacy of these approaches in long-term repopulating HSCs has been limited (Kuo et al., 2018; De Ravin et al., 2021) or unproven. Recently, promoting cell cycle progression, either by maintaining low cell concentration during *ex vivo* manipulation (Charlesworth et al., 2018) or with cell-cycle modulators (Ferrari et al., 2020; Shin et al., 2020), has been reported as the most efficient strategy to enhance HDR editing in human long-term repopulating HSCs.

Enrichment for cells undergoing the intended genome modification may be an alternative (or even complementary) strategy to increase the proportion, but not the number, of edited cells in the graft and reduce the competition with the unedited counterpart. Gene correction may be amenable to sort for edited cells by exploiting endogenous markers expressed on the cellular membrane. As a paradigmatic example, selection of *HBB*-edited HSPCs was achieved by embedding a reporter cassette in the HDR template, reaching up to 90% HDR-edited cells in the long-term graft (Dever et al., 2016). In another study, simultaneous editing of the locus of interest and of an unrelated gene providing drug-resistance to chemical compounds allowed to efficiently enrich for human edited HSPCs in marker-free settings (Agudelo et al., 2017).

Tolerability of the Gene Editing Procedure

To counter the constant threat of DNA damaging agents, cells have evolved a panel of repair mechanisms, as well as senescence and programmed cell death pathways. Indeed, both the DSB and the delivery of an exogenous donor template that are instrumental to gene editing may trigger complex cellular responses potentially leading to harmful outcomes (**Figure 2**). However, the consequences of gene editing on cell fitness, as well as NHEJ/HDR proficiency, may vary across different cell types and strongly depend on cell biology. Likely due to their fundamental role in blood homeostasis, human HSPCs are evolutionarily more sensitive than cell lines and other cell types to extensive manipulation; therefore, the gene editing procedures have to be substantially tailored to maximize tolerability.

As a first line of host defense, human immune cells exhibit pattern recognition receptors (PRRs), which sense pathogen-associated molecular patterns (PAMPs), such as exogenous nucleic acids, and promote the release of type I interferons (IFNs) and other cytokines (Piras and Kajaste-Rudnitski, 2020). Activation of PRRs in HSPCs and overexpression of IFN-stimulated genes (ISGs) can induce a variety of outcomes, including exit from quiescence, differentiation and apoptosis (Essers et al., 2009; Sato et al., 2009; Liu et al., 2012). *In vitro* transcribed 5′-triphosphate sgRNAs and mRNAs encoding for nucleases may strongly activate ISGs via PRRs, decreasing cell viability and clonogenic potential (Mu et al., 2019). Dampening of these responses has been obtained by switching to chemically synthetized sgRNAs or high-pressure liquid chromatography (HPLC)-purified mRNAs incorporating base analogs (Hendel et al., 2015; Schiroli et al., 2017). Furthermore, electroporation of CRISPR/Cas9 machinery as RNP, rather than mRNA, is reported to be stealthier in human HSPCs (Cromer et al., 2018). Of note, IFN induction may also affect concomitant viral transduction, thus constraining HDR template delivery for some vectors (Petrillo et al., 2018). Moreover, secondary structures or nucleic acid hybrids present in viral vector genomes may be recognized by the host and activate transient cellular responses (Piras and Kajaste-Rudnitski, 2020).

Cell sensors are triggered not only by the presence of exogenous proteins and nucleic acid, but also by the DNA damage evoked by their action. Nuclease toxicity mediated by p53 was in fact observed in: (i) induced pluripotent stem cells (iPSCs) (Ihry et al., 2018) and cell lines (Haapaniemi et al., 2018; Enache et al., 2020), leading to apoptosis or cell cycle arrest; (ii) HSPCs with a remarkable impact on clonogenic capacity (Schiroli et al., 2019). Accordingly, multiple DSBs resulted in a higher p53-dependent DDR in HSPCs, up to the establishment of pro-inflammatory transcriptional programs, with corresponding higher impact on the clonogenic potential (Schiroli et al., 2019).

Both AAV6- and IDLV-mediated template delivery are sensed by HSPCs (Piras et al., 2017; Schiroli et al., 2019). In particular, AAV6 transduction per se triggers a robust p53 response, which cumulates with the one elicited from concomitant exposure to nucleases. These convergent inputs lead to substantial HSPC proliferation slowdown, shrinkage of the human graft size and oligoclonal reconstitution by edited cells upon xenotransplantation in immunodeficient mice (Ferrari et al., 2020). The molecular cascade leading to p53 activation has not been fully elucidated yet. Interestingly, however, transient p53 inhibition confined in the first 24 h of the editing process enhanced tolerability of the procedure and restored polyclonal composition of the human graft, preserving HSPC multilineage potential (Schiroli et al., 2019; Ferrari et al., 2020). Moreover, p53 inhibition may mitigate the theoretical risk of increasing the proportion of p53$^{-/-}$ mutant clones with high oncogenic potential, which are typically rare in a HSPC population from healthy donors but could be more frequent in patients with specific genetic diseases, such as Fanconi anemia or Diamond-Blackfan anemia (Lipton and Ellis, 2009; Ceccaldi et al., 2011). While a transient p53 inhibition raises the theoretical concern of inappropriately rescuing cells with chromosomal aberrations and high mutational burden, no increase in the mutational load was reported by its incomplete and transitory inhibition (Garaycoechea et al., 2018; Schiroli et al., 2019). Moreover, even if some rare genotoxic event occurred, prompt restoration of the p53 pathway may be expected to counter-select cells that have acquired them before the occurrence of the subsequent hits necessary for oncogenic transformation (Di Micco et al., 2006; Bondar and Medzhitov, 2010).

Conversely, the use of ssODN instead of viral vectors as HDR template does not cumulatively elicit p53 activation and is well-tolerated by HSPCs, with no impact on their repopulation capacity (Pattabhi et al., 2019; Romero et al., 2019).

Assessment of Editing Genotoxicity and Optimization of Nuclease Specificity

Specificity of programmable nucleases is defined as the ratio between on-target and off-target activity, i.e., the DNA DSB frequency at the intended target site and at unintended genomic loci. Although genome editing offers higher level of specificity than genetic engineering platforms based on semi-randomly integrating vectors, off-target generation of DNA DSBs could be a major source of genotoxicity. Nuclease off-target activity may have no biological consequences, or instead be cytotoxic, knock-out tumor suppressor genes, induce off-target incorporation of the donor DNA, or trigger chromosomal rearrangements. Its burden may vary depending on the nuclease platform, donor DNA and the targeted DNA sequence. Moreover, unintended on-target events, such as excision or insertion of arbitrary DNA fragments, have been reported upon gene editing in non-hematopoietic cell types (Kosicki et al., 2018; Hanlon et al., 2019; Nelson et al., 2019). The consequences of unintended on- or off-target events are expected to differ depending on the overall editing strategy and disease setting, and thus require case-by-case evaluation. Furthermore, off-target events may be presumed to be more tolerated in fully differentiated and short-lived cell types. Hence, careful assessment of nuclease specificity is mandatory when aiming to clinical translation of engineered HSPCs because these cells will have to support life-long hematopoiesis by performing several cycles of self-renewal and differentiation in the patient.

Given the hit and run nature of the programmable nucleases, comprehensive detection of off-target activity requires the development of innovative and specific tools. To this goal, a panel of *in silico* prediction algorithms (Haeussler et al., 2016; Labun et al., 2019) as well as *in vitro* (e.g., DIGENOME-seq, CIRCLE-seq) (Kim et al., 2015; Tsai et al., 2017) and *in cellulo* assays (e.g., IDLV trapping, GUIDE-seq) (Gabriel et al., 2011; Tsai et al., 2015) have been developed. All these methods show considerable sensitivity and specificity issues and none of them alone allows to comprehensively and precisely identify nuclease off-target sites, even because no gold standard exists. Indeed, bioinformatic tools and *in vitro* assays typically return a large number of putative off-target sites, but many of them do not overlap with those either found by *in cellulo* assays or validated by targeted next generation sequencing (NGS). The combination of more than one assay is generally advised in order to collect a broader panel of putative off-target sites that can be then validated by targeted NGS in the cell type of interest. On the other hand, it is debatable whether nuclease off-target sites revealed by *in silico* or *in vitro* assays but not confirmed by *in cellulo* assays or during the validation phase should be considered as false-positive events. The NGS detection limit (0.1–0.01%) is likely a major limitation toward comprehensive assessment of the off-target nuclease activity in view of clinical translation. For instance, up to 10^5 cells in the drug product might have unmeasurable nuclease activity at an off-target site considering the dose of edited HSPCs commonly administered in gene therapy settings (from 10^7 to 10^9) (Gaspar et al., 2011; Sessa et al., 2016; Eichler et al., 2017; Thompson et al., 2018; Ferrua et al., 2019; Marktel et al., 2019; Esrick et al., 2021). Furthermore, specificity analyses usually do not take into account the wide spectrum of genomic polymorphism in the human population, thus likely dropping out potentially relevant individual- and population-specific off-target sites. *Ad hoc* assays to stringently and comprehensively assess the genotoxicity profile of programmable nucleases, on top and beyond the off-target events, are currently lacking and would be of relevance to address any safety concern at preclinical stage. Although no guidelines currently exist, previously validated unintended on- and off-target events should be strictly monitored after infusion in patients, similarly to longitudinal integration site analyses that are considered a standard in current gene addition clinical protocols (Aiuti et al., 2013; Thompson et al., 2018).

Off-target activity depends on: (i) the sequence homology between on- and off- target sites; (ii) the DNA affinity of the nuclease; (iii) the duration of exposure. To minimize off-target events, several strategies have been pursued, leveraging the last two aspects, as well as sgRNA screening to identify those predicted being more specific for targeting the intended region. Indeed, prolonged nuclease activity and high nuclease concentration decrease editing specificity (Hsu et al., 2013; Pattanayak et al., 2013; Kim et al., 2014; Shapiro et al., 2020), which instead can be improved by transient nuclease expression, e.g. via mRNA or RNP (Dever et al., 2016), or the use of split or inducible Cas9 mutants (Davis et al., 2015; Nihongaki et al., 2015; Zetsche et al., 2015b).

In the last years, extensive engineering improved CRISPR/Cas9 specificity and efficiency by modifying sgRNA and Cas9 architecture. The use of 5′-truncated sgRNAs (tru-gRNA) resulted in similar on-target activity as standard ones but several-fold lower off-target activity (Fu et al., 2014), likely reducing the interaction energy at the RNA–DNA heteroduplex level (Lim et al., 2016). The addition of two guanines at the 5′ end of the sgRNA also reduced off-target activity, albeit also decreasing on-target editing in some cases (Cho et al., 2014). Instead, chemical modifications (2′-O-methyl-3′phosphorothiorate or 2′-O-methyl-3′thiophosphonoacetate) of the three terminal nucleotides at the 5′ and 3′ ends improved the specificity profile and enhanced tolerability compared to unmodified sgRNA in hematopoietic cells (Hendel et al., 2015). As for what concerns Cas9, novel variants [eSpCas9(1.1) and SpCas9-HF1] with higher fidelity resulting from dampened interaction strength with the DNA (Kleinstiver et al., 2016; Slaymaker et al., 2016), have been identified by structure-guided mutagenesis. However, these variants showed lower on-target activity than wild-type SpCas9 in human HSPCs when delivered as RNP (DeWitt et al., 2016; Vakulskas et al., 2018). Recently, other highly specific SpCas9 variants, such as EvoCas9 (Casini et al., 2018), SniperCas9 (Lee et al., 2018) and HiFi-Cas (Vakulskas et al., 2018) were discovered by directed evolution approaches. The latter showed improved fidelity and high on-target editing over wild-type SpCas9 in human HSPCs. Similar approaches have been also pursued for other gene editing tools, including ZFNs and TALENs (Miller et al., 2007; Hubbard et al., 2015).

Although detailed analyses and considerations on nuclease specificity are imperative, the presence of some unwanted genomic events does not necessarily preclude gene editing from proceeding toward safe clinical applications. Precaution dictates that efforts should be made toward minimizing their incidence, but their actual consequences may depend on the specific context. An unintended genomic event may in theory contribute to cancer, contingently with its genomic location and its nature. However, since oncogenic transformation is multifaceted and multistep, the same mutations may or not give rise to tumors also depending on genetic background and the subsequent exposure to other genotoxic events. For reference, pathogenic mutations may remain silent for many years, and result in overt disease in a small fraction of individuals who endure another genomic "hit" (Greaves, 2018). Moreover, healthy individuals may harbor clonal hematopoiesis due to oncogenic mutations which can persist for years without evidence of pathogenicity despite increasing the risk of malignant transformation (Takahashi et al., 2017; Zink et al., 2017). On the contrary, in disease settings in which clonal expansion of the edited cells is already triggered by a strong selective advantage conferred by gene correction, the same genotoxic events might promote oncogenic transformation.

Manufacturing for Therapeutic Gene Editing Protocol

In the last decades, the gene and cell therapy field faced an exponential expansion thanks to the accumulation of several clinical successes of both *ex vivo* and *in vivo* gene transfer approaches. The results of these studies are also providing important information about cell manufacturing, vector development and therapeutic efficacy, which represent a solid background and increase the expectation for the development of more precise gene editing approaches. Despite several similarities between the manufacturing of gene transferred and gene edited HSPCs (e.g., conditioning regimens for HSPC collection and transplantation, protocols for *in vitro* CD34+ cell selection, activation, culture, and transduction), the editing procedure requires additional and peculiar manipulation steps that only now will encounter their first clinical validation (**Figure 3**). Among these, the electroporation process used for the delivery of the editing components and the transduction of HSPCs with AAV6 vectors represent the innovations linked to major unknowns. In fact, there is still no direct evidence that these procedures will actually allow long-term engraftment of edited HSCs in a human subject. While state-of-the-art xenotransplantation studies on immunodeficient mice are showing promising results, critical species-specific differences in the procedure for the gene editing of murine and non-human primates (NHP) HSPCs significantly affect the yield, fitness, and potential immunogenicity of the cellular product, thus limiting the predictive value of such pre-clinical models (Schiroli et al., 2017; Kim et al., 2018; Humbert et al., 2019; Wilkinson et al., 2021). Moreover, the scaling-up of lab-grade to clinical-grade processes requires implementation of adequate manufacturing facility that support scalability of the procedures while encompassing the complex requirements to meet current good manufacturing practices (cGMP). The ideal cell manufacturing process needs to be robust, reproducible and cost-effective to be extended to multiple therapeutic applications. Finally, the safety, purity, and potency for the end-of-process cellular products need to be carefully defined to meet quality-control standards and regulatory agencies guidelines, which however still need to be tailored, based on accumulation of additional scientific knowledge. Indeed, manufacturing of edited HSPCs is still at the very beginning of clinical testing and regulatory agencies have to closely collaborate with scientists to identify the critical requirements that would better fit the needs of these advanced therapy medicinal products (ATMPs). Some clinical studies implying gene disruption in HSPCs with CRISPR-Cas9 (Frangoul et al., 2021) (NCT03745287/NCT03655678) are currently revealing precious information to prepare this transition. As light is shed on the effective and potential safety issues, it will become easier to define the appropriate framework of safety standards for subsequent applications.

Tracking Edited HSPCs to Assess Safety, Efficacy, and Persistence of the Therapeutic Gene Edited Product

The study design of phase I/II HSPC gene editing clinical trials cannot exempt by the identification of a panel of adequate safety and efficacy endpoints, which would allow investigators to assess whether the proposed treatment meet the therapeutic expectations with a favorable risk/benefit ratio. However, clinical readouts must be complemented by *ad hoc* molecular analyses aimed at assessing long-term engraftment, persistence and multilineage differentiation potential of edited HSPCs, e.g., by the quantification of the editing efficiency at the on-target locus over time and across hematopoietic cell lineages during patients' follow up. Moreover, the assessment of genomic integrity as well as nuclease activity at validated off-target sites (if any) both in the manufactured cell product and within the patients' graft would comprehensively characterize the engineered cell product and early identify clonal drifts driven by the expansion of hematopoietic clones harboring structural genomic abnormalities or unintended editing outcomes.

In this framework, monitoring the clonal composition of the edited cell graft would provide precious additional information about the efficiency of the manufacturing process, the long-term multilineage repopulating potential of human edited HSPCs and the safety profile of the therapeutic approach. Quantification of the indel diversity within gene-edited alleles can function as a surrogate readout of clonal complexity of the edited cell population to track the dynamics of edited clones (McKenna et al., 2016; Kalhor et al., 2018; Román-Rodríguez et al., 2019; Ferrari et al., 2020). Recent studies in NHP models have shown a remarkable reduction of clonal complexity from the infused cell product to the graft with a direct correlation between the number of multilineage repopulating clones and the infused dose of edited cells (Demirci et al., 2020). Still, the preferential generation of specific edits by NHEJ repair (van Overbeek et al., 2016) and the occurrence of biallelic modifications might not provide sufficient complexity of the gene-edited allele population to exhaustively investigate clonal composition. The use of unique molecular identifier (e.g., random DNA sequences used as surrogate barcodes) embedded in the HDR template would enable tracking of HDR-edited clones, which would be otherwise indistinguishable from each other due to the high-fidelity nature of the HDR. HSPC editing with barcoded templates have uncovered the oligoclonal composition of the human HDR-edited xenograft in immunodeficient mice (Ferrari et al., 2020; Sharma et al., 2021) mainly attributable to the biological impact of the editing procedure, although most of the engrafting clones still retained multilineage and self-renewal potential. While the generation and the use of barcoded HDR template libraries with suitable complexity for clinical application would be extremely challenging and may rise theoretical safety concerns due to the random generation and integration of potentially functional/regulatory DNA sequences

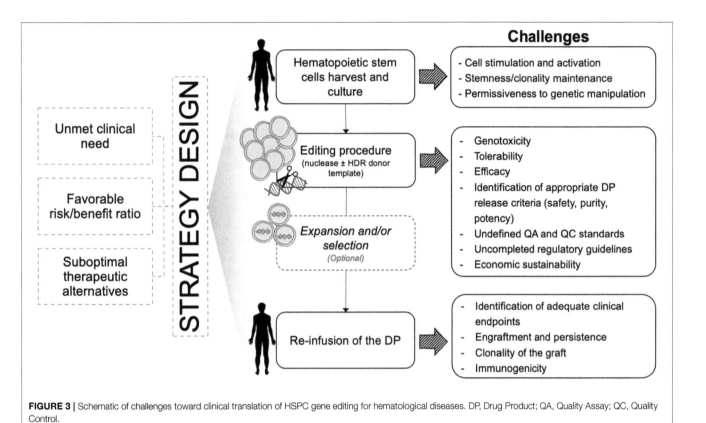

FIGURE 3 | Schematic of challenges toward clinical translation of HSPC gene editing for hematological diseases. DP, Drug Product; QA, Quality Assay; QC, Quality Control.

(e.g., transcription factor binding sites), this tool may be useful to validate the manufacturing process and the use of improved editing protocols.

Overall, preclinical observations of clonal dynamics reassure about long-term persistence of edited HSPCs after transplantation, even though the aforementioned loss of clonal complexity from the infused product to the edited cell graft prompts implementation and optimization of low-burden manufacturing processes, as well as monitoring clonal composition of the graft in first-in-man HSPC gene editing clinical trials.

Economic Sustainability of ATMPs Based on Edited HSPCs

HSPC gene editing is a form of personalized medicine currently entailing complex and costly procedures, especially regarding the manufacturing and delivery processes, which are rising prices of such ATMPs to millions of US dollars. As occurred with gene replacement therapies, some of which have already reached Food and Drug Administration (FDA) and European Medicines Agency (EMA) approval for commercialization (Touchot and Flume, 2017), such high costs might be sustainable for the development of better treatments for ultra-rare and rare disorders, particularly in some countries. Indeed, (i) a single administration of the therapy may establish stable benefits with a substantial saving on the cost of repeated life-long administration of conventional therapies and (ii) the limited numbers of treated

patients will not significantly impact the refunding system, except for the likely need to split the payment of a one-time treatment and distribute the credit along multiple years, thus mimicking the burden of a life-long therapy. Yet, now that the bar of these advanced therapeutic approaches has been elevated to reach more frequent diseases affecting a large number of people, such as hemoglobinopathies, this business model might result to be inadequate. The risk is that such high costs for ATMP production might impose socio-economic limits that could impair access to these new therapies and/or constrain their sustainable commercialization, thus ultimately affecting their availability for the patients (Wilson and Carroll, 2019). Nevertheless, the rapidly expanding technological advances in the gene therapy field are broadly considered a bottomless source of solutions for the aforementioned problems. The development of more efficient vector production systems, such advanced packaging cell lines or improved purification strategies (Grieger et al., 2016; Kotin and Snyder, 2017) as well as the implementation of small, automated, closed systems for cell manufacturing, which enable the de-centralized "point-of-care" generation of cellular therapies, will further ease the clinical testing of gene edited ATMPs and will soon significantly reduce their manufacturing costs. Indeed, the potential for an economically sustainable marketing of *ex vivo* gene therapies is well-supported by the exploding interest of big pharma's and venture capitals in the field, which foresee a favorable financial balance for these advanced therapies in the near future.

GENE ADDITION VS. GENE EDITING: OVERLAPPING OR DIVERGENT POTENTIAL?

Gene transfer by RVs constituted a milestone in the history of gene therapy. Unfortunately, early enthusiasm following the therapeutic potential for congenital immunodeficiencies was suddenly quenched by the frequent malignant transformation of transduced cells (Cavazzana-Calvo et al., 2000; Hacein-Bey-Abina et al., 2003a,b, 2008; Howe et al., 2008; Stein et al., 2010; Braun et al., 2014), due to the overexpression of proto-oncogenes triggered by enhancer sequences within the U3 region of the 5′ long terminal repeat (LTR) of the nearby integrated vector. The transition from the RV to the LV platform and the generation of self-inactivating vectors by deletion of the LTR enhancer sequences resulted in a safer integration profile (Montini et al., 2006) and led to widespread use of modern LV for a number of diseases, such as hemoglobinopathies, enzymopathies and congenital immunodeficiencies (Sessa et al., 2016; Fraldi et al., 2018; Thompson et al., 2018; Mamcarz et al., 2019; Marktel et al., 2019; Kohn et al., 2020).

Insofar as variability in inter-cellular vector copy number, semi-random integration pattern, and gross regulation of cassette expression are not a priori an issue, LVs are arguably the best available platform for gene addition. However, some genotoxicity events might still occur upon LV integration, such as the vector-mediated disruption of relevant genomic elements or tumor suppressor genes and/or the generation of aberrant splicing variants of endogenous genes fused to the transgene cassette (Cavazzana-Calvo et al., 2010). Furthermore, the restoration of a complex physiological regulation of the transgene in the limiting size of the vector cassette may represent an additional problem in some disease contexts. The semi-random integration pattern of RVs and LVs discourages their discourages their use for those diseases where unregulated expression of the corrective gene might have potentially dangerous consequences, such as the case of genes that have a direct impact on cell proliferation and/or differentiation or genes that need a high expression level to restore their physiologic function. These disease categories include several primary immunodeficiencies, such as Hyper IgM 1 syndrome (Brown et al., 1998; Sacco et al., 2000; Hubbard et al., 2016; Kuo et al., 2018; Vavassori et al., 2021), RAG1/RAG2 deficiency (Villa et al., 2020) and, possibly, Fanconi anemia (Román-Rodríguez et al., 2019; van de Vrugt et al., 2019) for which the presumed increased risk of cell transformation or inadequate expression currently limit the development of competitive gene addition approaches and that can thus represent a suitable setting for a first in human testing of site-specific gene editing approaches. Moreover, therapeutic genome editing also extends the possible applications of precise DNA surgery to several vacant clinical contexts that cannot be efficiently addressed by conventional gene therapy strategies. Among others, the generation of HIV-resistant CCR5 knock-out cells (Xu et al., 2017, 2019), the deletion of regulatory regions (Bauer et al., 2013) or the correction of dominant negative mutations (Nasri et al., 2020)

are applications that require exquisitely site-specific action of programmable enzymes.

Beyond the aforementioned examples, the potential applications of gene addition and gene editing overlap to a significant extent. Indeed, some degree of competition may arise for specific diseases whereby on-site restoration of gene function is expected to confer benefits in terms of expression. For instance, LV-based gene therapy for WAS reduced bleeding events but did not fully restore platelet levels (Ferrua et al., 2019). While the culprit is not entirely clear (Fischer, 2019), it has been postulated that full reconstitution of *in situ* physiological expression is required to fully correct the phenotype, thus opening the door to gene editing strategies (Rai et al., 2020). Another paradigmatic case is that of hemoglobinopathies, whereby clinical benefit may theoretically be achieved by (i) *HBB* gene addition/correction, or (ii) restoration of Hb-F expression by inactivating *BCL11A* (Sankaran et al., 2008; Basak et al., 2015). On one hand, *HBB* gene addition has proven to be feasible for both SCD and β-thalassemia (Thompson et al., 2018; Marktel et al., 2019), apparently leaving less room for HDR-based *HBB* editing (Dever et al., 2016; DeWitt et al., 2016; Kuo et al., 2018; Park et al., 2019; Pattabhi et al., 2019). On the other hand, suppression of *BCL11A* has been successfully achieved both with a LV encoding for a *BCL11A*-specific short hairpin RNA (Esrick et al., 2021), as well as by CRISPR-mediated knockout (Frangoul et al., 2021). Safety, efficacy and market success of these novel therapies, irrespectively of the platform, are anyhow expected to be benchmarked against betibeglogene autotemcel (Zynteglo), which has recently been approved by the FDA for the treatment of β-thalassemia (while the approval for SCD is still pending). As hemoglobinopathies are relatively frequent, it is possible that both gene addition and gene editing therapies with the same indication will be granted market approval, both in the USA and in other countries. This will allow for real-life side-by-side comparison of the different technologies in a not-so-distant future, which will highlight their respective advantages and disadvantages despite likely leaving space for more than a single winner, as normally occurs with other more conventional therapies (Fernandes et al., 2020).

Overall, the current efficiency of HDR-mediated gene correction is significantly lower than that achievable with LVs, thus diminishing its competitive advantage for a number of applications whereby high fraction of corrected cells is required. Still, the sword of Damocles of genotoxicity is hanging on both LV and gene editing platforms, either due to integration and inactivation of cancer suppressor genes, or to genomic rearrangements and off-target effects.

CONCLUSIONS

The outstanding advantages and the current technological limitations of targeted genome editing are the main weights in the two sides of the scale when considering the opportunity of translating intriguing new therapeutic approaches into clinics.

However, their "weight" might remarkably change depending on the target disease. Therefore, the decision to move gene editing toward human testing requires a case-by-case assessment and must be balanced against clinical need. In this scenario, the presence of competing treatments, either as standard of care or under clinical evaluation, and the costs of developing and commercializing ATMPs, might further restrict the space for the application of HSPC gene editing in blood disorders (Wilson and Carroll, 2019).

Ultimately, the rationale of testing novel gene editing-based strategies depends on the presumed benefit offered to the patient with respect to his prognosis with the best available therapy. It is reasonable to offer HSPC gene editing based products at first to patients with no alternative options and a dismal prognosis or to those for who the standard of care is presumed to be more toxic, such as those affected by severe congenital immunodeficiencies or DNA repair defects. Clinical testing of gene editing approaches in these applications would provide a first detailed characterization of their safety profile. This would also allow to define the appropriate assays to follow the dynamics of unwanted genomic events in time and establish their clinical relevance, setting the thresholds to manage the genotoxic risk. These data would then pave the way for their application to other diseases with a less dismal prognosis and alternative therapies, such as HIV and enzymopathies.

AUTHOR CONTRIBUTIONS

SF, VV, and DC conceived and wrote the manuscript. AJac, MC, and AJav contributed with ideas and discussion and wrote the manuscript. PG organized, supervised, and wrote the manuscript. All authors contributed to the article and approved the submitted version.

FUNDING

This work was supported by grants to: PG from the Gene Therapy Program of Dana-Farber/Boston Children's Cancer and Blood Disorders Center, the Immune deficiency Foundation, the Telethon Foundation (TIGET grant E3) and the Italian Ministry of Health (GR-2016-02364847). MC was supported by grants to Anna Villa from Telethon (TIGET grant E2) and the Italian Ministry of University and Research (PRIN 2017 Prot. 20175XHBPN). DC and AJav were supported by grants to Luigi Naldini from Telethon (TIGET grant E4), the Italian Ministry of Health (PE-2016-02363691; E-Rare-3 JTC 2017), the Italian Ministry of University and Research (PRIN 2017 Prot. 20175XHBPN), the EU Horizon2020 Program (UPGRADE), and the Louis-Jeantet Foundation through the 2019 Jeantet-Collen Prize for Translational Medicine.

REFERENCES

Abraham, A., Hsieh, M., Eapen, M., Fitzhugh, C., Carreras, J., Keesler, D., et al. (2017). Relationship between mixed donor–recipient chimerism and disease recurrence after hematopoietic cell transplantation for sickle cell disease. *Biol. Blood Marrow Transplant.* 23, 2178–2183. doi: 10.1016/j.bbmt.2017.08.038

Agudelo, D., Duringer, A., Bozoyan, L., Huard, C. C., Carter, S., Loehr, J., et al. (2017). Marker-free coselection for CRISPR-driven genome editing in human cells. *Nat. Methods* 14, 615–620. doi: 10.1038/nmeth.4265

Aiuti, A., Biasco, L., Scaramuzza, S., Ferrua, F., Cicalese, M. P., Baricordi, C., et al. (2013). Lentiviral hematopoietic stem cell gene therapy in patients with wiskott-aldrich syndrome. *Science* 341:1233151. doi: 10.1126/science.1233151

Bak, R. O., Dever, D. P., and Porteus, M. H. (2018). CRISPR/Cas9 genome editing in human hematopoietic stem cells. *Nat. Protoc.* 13, 358–376. doi: 10.1038/nprot.2017.143

Barrangou, R., Fremaux, C., Deveau, H., Richards, M., Boyaval, P., Moineau, S., et al. (2007). CRISPR provides acquired resistance against viruses in prokaryotes. *Science* 315, 1709–1712. doi: 10.1126/science.1138140

Basak, A., Hancarova, M., Ulirsch, J. C., Balci, T. B., Trkova, M., Pelisek, M., et al. (2015). BCL11A deletions result in fetal hemoglobin persistence and neurodevelopmental alterations. *J. Clin. Invest.* 125, 2363–2368. doi: 10.1172/JCI81163

Bauer, D. E., Kamran, S. C., Lessard, S., Xu, J., Fujiwara, Y., Lin, C., et al. (2013). An erythroid enhancer of BCL11A subject to genetic variation determines fetal hemoglobin level. *Science* 342, 253–257. doi: 10.1126/science.12 42088

Beerman, I., Seita, J., Inlay, M. A., Weissman, I. L., and Rossi, D. J. (2014). Quiescent hematopoietic stem cells accumulate DNA damage during aging that is repaired upon entry into cell cycle. *Cell Stem Cell* 15, 37–50. doi: 10.1016/j.stem.2014.04.016

Bernardo, M. E., and Aiuti, A. (2016). The role of conditioning in hematopoietic stem-cell gene therapy. *Hum. Gene Ther.* 27, 741–748. doi: 10.1089/hum.2016.103

Biechonski, S., Olender, L., Zipin-Roitman, A., Yassin, M., Aqaqe, N., Marcu-Malina, V., et al. (2018). Attenuated DNA damage responses and increased apoptosis characterize human hematopoietic stem cells exposed to irradiation. *Sci. Rep.* 8:6071. doi: 10.1038/s41598-018-24440-w

Bogdanove, A. J., and Voytas, D. F. (2011). TAL effectors: customizable proteins for DNA targeting. *Science* 333, 1843–1846. doi: 10.1126/science.1204094

Boitano, A. E., Wang, J., Romeo, R., Bouchez, L. C., Parker, A. E., Sutton, S. E., et al. (2010). Aryl hydrocarbon receptor antagonists promote the expansion of human hematopoietic stem cells. *Science* 329, 1345–1348. doi: 10.1126/science.1191536

Bondar, T., and Medzhitov, R. (2010). p53-Mediated hematopoietic stem and progenitor cell competition. *Cell Stem Cell* 6, 309–322. doi: 10.1016/j.stem.2010.03.002

Branzei, D., and Foiani, M. (2008). Regulation of DNA repair throughout the cell cycle. *Nat. Rev. Mol. Cell Biol.* 9, 297–308. doi: 10.1038/nrm2351

Braun, C. J., Boztug, K., Paruzynski, A., Witzel, M., Schwarzer, A., Rothe, M., et al. (2014). Gene therapy for Wiskott-Aldrich syndrome-long-term efficacy and genotoxicity. *Sci. Transl. Med.* 6:227ra33. doi: 10.1126/scitranslmed. 3007280

Brouns, S. J. J., Jore, M. M., Lundgren, M., Westra, E. R., Slijkhuis, R. J. H., Snijders, A. P. L., et al. (2008). Small CRISPR RNAs guide antiviral defense in prokaryotes. *Science* 321, 960–964. doi: 10.1126/science.1159689

Brown, M. P., Topham, D. J., Sangster, M. Y., Zhao, J., Flynn, K. J., Surman, S. L., et al. (1998). Thymic lymphoproliferative disease after successful correction of CD40 ligand deficiency by gene transfer in mice. *Nat. Med.* 4, 1253–1260. doi: 10.1038/3233

Carroll, D. (2014). Genome engineering with targetable nucleases. *Annu. Rev. Biochem.* 83, 409–439. doi: 10.1146/annurev-biochem-060713-035418

Casini, A., Olivieri, M., Petris, G., Montagna, C., Reginato, G., Maule, G., et al. (2018). A highly specific SpCas9 variant is identified by *in vivo* screening in yeast. *Nat. Biotechnol.* 36, 265–271. doi: 10.1038/nbt.4066

Cavazzana-Calvo, M., Hacein-Bey, S., De Saint Basile, G., Gross, F., Yvon, E., Nusbaum, P., et al. (2000). Gene therapy of human severe combined immunodeficiency (SCID)-X1 disease. *Science* 288, 669–672. doi: 10.1126/science.288.5466.669

Cavazzana-Calvo, M., Payen, E., Negre, O., Wang, G., Hehir, K., Fusil, F., et al. (2010). Transfusion independence and HMGA2 activation after gene therapy of human β-thalassaemia. *Nature* 467, 318–322. doi: 10.1038/nature09328

Ceccaldi, R., Briot, D., Larghero, J., Vasquez, N., D'Enghien, C. D., Chamousset, D., et al. (2011). Spontaneous abrogation of the G2 DNA damage checkpoint has clinical benefits but promotes leukemogenesis in Fanconi anemia patients. *J. Clin. Invest.* 121, 184–194. doi: 10.1172/JCI43836

Chapman, J. R., Taylor, M. R. G., and Boulton, S. J. (2012). Playing the end game: DNA double-strand break repair pathway choice. *Mol. Cell* 47, 497–510. doi: 10.1016/j.molcel.2012.07.029

Charlesworth, C. T., Camarena, J., Cromer, M. K., Vaidyanathan, S., Bak, R. O., Carte, J. M., et al. (2018). Priming human repopulating hematopoietic stem and progenitor cells for Cas9/sgRNA gene targeting. *Mol. Ther. Nucleic Acids* 12, 89–104. doi: 10.1016/j.omtn.2018.04.017

Charpentier, M., Khedher, A. H. Y., Menoret, S., Brion, A., Lamribet, K., Dardillac, E., et al. (2018). CtIP fusion to Cas9 enhances transgene integration by homology-dependent repair. *Nat. Commun.* 9:1133. doi: 10.1038/s41467-018-03475-7

Cho, S. W., Kim, S., Kim, Y., Kweon, J., Kim, H. S., Bae, S., et al. (2014). Analysis of off-target effects of CRISPR/Cas-derived RNA-guided endonucleases and nickases. *Genome Res.* 24, 132–141. doi: 10.1101/gr.162339.113

Chu, V. T., Weber, T., Wefers, B., Wurst, W., Sander, S., Rajewsky, K., et al. (2015). Increasing the efficiency of homology-directed repair for CRISPR-Cas9-induced precise gene editing in mammalian cells. *Nat. Biotechnol.* 33, 543–548. doi: 10.1038/nbt.3198

Cromer, M. K., Vaidyanathan, S., Ryan, D. E., Curry, B., Lucas, A. B., Camarena, J., et al. (2018). Global transcriptional response to CRISPR/Cas9-AAV6-based genome editing in CD34+ hematopoietic stem and progenitor cells. *Mol. Ther.* 26, 2431–2442. doi: 10.1016/j.ymthe.2018.06.002

Davis, K. M., Pattanayak, V., Thompson, D. B., Zuris, J. A., and Liu, D. R. (2015). Small molecule-triggered Cas9 protein with improved genome-editing specificity. *Nat. Chem. Biol.* 11, 316–318. doi: 10.1038/nchembio.1793

De Ravin, S. S., Brault, J., Meis, R. J., Liu, S., Li, L., Pavel-Dinu, M., et al. (2021). Enhanced homology-directed repair for highly efficient gene editing in hematopoietic stem/progenitor cells. *Blood*. doi: 10.1182/blood.2020008503

De Ravin, S. S., Li, L., Wu, X., Choi, U., Allen, C., Koontz, S., et al. (2017). CRISPR-Cas9 gene repair of hematopoietic stem cells from patients with X-linked chronic granulomatous disease. *Sci. Transl. Med.* 9:eaah3480. doi: 10.1126/scitranslmed.aah3480

De Ravin, S. S., Reik, A., Liu, P. Q., Li, L., Wu, X., Su, L., et al. (2016). Targeted gene addition in human CD34 + hematopoietic cells for correction of X-linked chronic granulomatous disease. *Nat. Biotechnol.* 34, 424–429. doi: 10.1038/nbt.3513

Demirci, S., Zeng, J., Wu, Y., Uchida, N., Shen, A. H., Pellin, D., et al. (2020). BCL11A enhancer–edited hematopoietic stem cells persist in rhesus monkeys without toxicity. *J. Clin. Invest.* 130, 6677–6687. doi: 10.1172/JCI140189

Dever, D. P., Bak, R. O., Reinisch, A., Camarena, J., Washington, G., Nicolas, C. E., et al. (2016). CRISPR/Cas9 β-globin gene targeting in human haematopoietic stem cells. *Nature* 539, 384–389. doi: 10.1038/nature20134

DeWitt, M. A., Magis, W., Bray, N. L., Wang, T., Berman, J. R., Urbinati, F., et al. (2016). Selection-free genome editing of the sickle mutation in human adult hematopoietic stem/progenitor cells. *Sci. Transl. Med.* 8:360ra134. doi: 10.1126/scitranslmed.aaf9336

Di Micco, R., Fumagalli, M., Cicalese, A., Piccinin, S., Gasparini, P., Luise, C., et al. (2006). Oncogene-induced senescence is a DNA damage response triggered by DNA hyper-replication. *Nature* 444, 638–642. doi: 10.1038/nature05327

Doudna, J. A. (2020). The promise and challenge of therapeutic genome editing. *Nature* 578, 229–236. doi: 10.1038/s41586-020-1978-5

Eichler, F., Duncan, C., Musolino, P. L., Orchard, P. J., De Oliveira, S., Thrasher, A. J., et al. (2017). Hematopoietic stem-cell gene therapy for cerebral adrenoleukodystrophy. *N. Engl. J. Med.* 377, 1630–1638. doi: 10.1056/NEJMoa1700554

Enache, O. M., Rendo, V., Abdusamad, M., Lam, D., Davison, D., Pal, S., et al. (2020). Cas9 activates the p53 pathway and selects for p53-inactivating mutations. *Nat. Genet.* 52, 662–668. doi: 10.1038/s41588-020-0623-4

Esrick, E. B., Lehmann, L. E., Biffi, A., Achebe, M., Brendel, C., Ciuculescu, M. F., et al. (2021). Post-Transcriptional genetic silencing of BCL11A to treat sickle cell disease. *N. Engl. J. Med.* 384, 205–215. doi: 10.1056/NEJMoa2029392

Essers, M. A. G., Offner, S., Blanco-Bose, W. E., Waibler, Z., Kalinke, U., Duchosal, M. A., et al. (2009). IFNα activates dormant haematopoietic stem cells *in vivo*. *Nature* 458, 904–908. doi: 10.1038/nature07815

Eyquem, J., Mansilla-Soto, J., Giavridis, T., Van Der Stegen, S. J. C., Hamieh, M., Cunanan, K. M., et al. (2017). Targeting a CAR to the TRAC locus with CRISPR/Cas9 enhances tumour rejection. *Nature* 543, 113–117. doi: 10.1038/nature21405

Fares, I., Chagraoui, J., Gareau, Y., Gingras, S., Ruel, R., Mayotte, N., et al. (2014). Pyrimidoindole derivatives are agonists of human hematopoietic stem cell self-renewal. *Science* 345, 1509–1512. doi: 10.1126/science.1256337

Fernandes, J. F., Nichele, S., Arcuri, L. J., Ribeiro, L., Zamperlini-Netto, G., Loth, G., et al. (2020). Outcomes after haploidentical stem cell transplantation with post-transplantation cyclophosphamide in patients with primary immunodeficiency diseases. *Biol. Blood Marrow Transplant.* 26, 1923–1929. doi: 10.1016/j.bbmt.2020.07.003

Ferrari, S., Jacob, A., Beretta, S., Unali, G., Albano, L., Vavassori, V., et al. (2020). Efficient gene editing of human long-term hematopoietic stem cells validated by clonal tracking. *Nat. Biotechnol.* 38, 1298–1308. doi: 10.1038/s41587-020-0551-y

Ferrua, F., Cicalese, M. P., Galimberti, S., Giannelli, S., Dionisio, F., Barzaghi, F., et al. (2019). Lentiviral haemopoietic stem/progenitor cell gene therapy for treatment of Wiskott-Aldrich syndrome: interim results of a non-randomised, open-label, phase 1/2 clinical study. *Lancet Haematol.* 6, e239–e253. doi: 10.1016/S2352-3026(19)30021-3

Fischer, A. (2019). Platelets are the achilles' heel of Wiskott-Aldrich syndrome. *J. Allergy Clin. Immunol.* 144, 668–670. doi: 10.1016/j.jaci.2019.06.039

Fraldi, A., Serafini, M., Sorrentino, N. C., Gentner, B., Aiuti, A., and Bernardo, M. E. (2018). Gene therapy for mucopolysaccharidoses: *in vivo* and *ex vivo* approaches. *Ital. J. Pediatr.* 44:130. doi: 10.1186/s13052-018-0565-y

Frangoul, H., Altshuler, D., Cappellini, M. D., Chen, Y.-S., Domm, J., Eustace, B. K., et al. (2021). CRISPR-Cas9 gene editing for sickle cell disease and β-thalassemia. *N. Engl. J. Med.* 384, 252–260. doi: 10.1056/NEJMoa2031054

Fu, Y., Sander, J. D., Reyon, D., Cascio, V. M., and Joung, J. K. (2014). Improving CRISPR-Cas nuclease specificity using truncated guide RNAs. *Nat. Biotechnol.* 32, 279–284. doi: 10.1038/nbt.2808

Gabriel, R., Lombardo, A., Arens, A., Miller, J. C., Genovese, P., Kaeppel, C., et al. (2011). An unbiased genome-wide analysis of zinc-finger nuclease specificity. *Nat. Biotechnol.* 29, 816–823. doi: 10.1038/nbt.1948

Gaj, T., Gersbach, C. A., and Barbas, C. F. (2013). ZFN, TALEN, and CRISPR/Cas-based methods for genome engineering. *Trends Biotechnol.* 31, 397–405. doi: 10.1016/j.tibtech.2013.04.004

Garaycoechea, J. I., Crossan, G. P., Langevin, F., Mulderrig, L., Louzada, S., Yang, F., et al. (2018). Alcohol and endogenous aldehydes damage chromosomes and mutate stem cells. *Nature* 553, 171–177. doi: 10.1038/nature25154

Garneau, J. E., Dupuis, M. È., Villion, M., Romero, D. A., Barrangou, R., Boyaval, P., et al. (2010). The CRISPR/cas bacterial immune system cleaves bacteriophage and plasmid DNA. *Nature* 468, 67–71. doi: 10.1038/nature09523

Gaspar, H. B., Cooray, S., Gilmour, K. C., Parsley, K. L., Zhang, F., Adams, S., et al. (2011). Immunodeficiency: Hematopoietic stem cell gene therapy for adenosine deaminase-deficient severe combined immunodeficiency leads to long-term immunological recovery and metabolic correction. *Sci. Transl. Med.* 3:97ra80. doi: 10.1126/scitranslmed.3002716

Genovese, P., Schiroli, G., Escobar, G., Di Tomaso, T., Firrito, C., Calabria, A., et al. (2014). Targeted genome editing in human repopulating haematopoietic stem cells. *Nature* 510, 235–240. doi: 10.1038/nature13420

Ghosh, S., Thrasher, A. J., and Gaspar, H. B. (2015). Gene therapy for monogenic disorders of the bone marrow. *Br. J. Haematol.* 171, 155–170. doi: 10.1111/bjh.13520

Greaves, M. (2018). A causal mechanism for childhood acute lymphoblastic leukaemia. *Nat. Rev. Cancer* 18, 471–484. doi: 10.1038/s41568-018-0015-6

Grieger, J. C., Soltys, S. M., and Samulski, R. J. (2016). Production of recombinant adeno-associated virus vectors using suspension HEK293 cells and continuous harvest of vector from the culture media for GMP FIX and FLT1 clinical vector. *Mol. Ther.* 24, 287–297. doi: 10.1038/mt.2015.187

Gutschner, T., Haemmerle, M., Genovese, G., Draetta, G. F., and Chin, L. (2016). Post-translational regulation of Cas9 during G1 enhances homology-directed repair. *Cell Rep.* 14, 1555–1566. doi: 10.1016/j.celrep.2016.01.019

Haapaniemi, E., Botla, S., Persson, J., Schmierer, B., and Taipale, J. (2018). CRISPR-Cas9 genome editing induces a p53-mediated DNA damage response. *Nat. Med.* 24, 927–930. doi: 10.1038/s41591-018-0049-z

Hacein-Bey-Abina, S., Garrigue, A., Wang, G. P., Soulier, J., Lim, A., Morillon, E., et al. (2008). Insertional oncogenesis in 4 patients after retrovirus-mediated gene therapy of SCID-X1. *J. Clin. Invest.* 118, 3132–3142. doi: 10.1172/JCI35700

Hacein-Bey-Abina, S., von Kalle, C., Schmidt, M., Le Deist, F., Wulffraat, N., McIntyre, E., et al. (2003a). A serious adverse event after successful gene therapy for X-linked severe combined immunodeficiency. *N. Engl. J. Med.* 348, 255–256. doi: 10.1056/NEJM200301163480314

Hacein-Bey-Abina, S., Von Kalle, C., Schmidt, M., McCormack, M. P., Wulffraat, N., Lebouch, P., et al. (2003b). LMO2-associated clonal T cell proliferation in two patients after gene therapy for SCID-X1. *Science* 302, 415–419. doi: 10.1126/science.1088547

Haeussler, M., Schönig, K., Eckert, H., Eschstruth, A., Mianné, J., Renaud, J. B., et al. (2016). Evaluation of off-target and on-target scoring algorithms and integration into the guide RNA selection tool CRISPOR. *Genome Biol.* 17:148. doi: 10.1186/s13059-016-1012-2

Handel, E.-M., and Cathomen, T. (2011). Zinc-finger nuclease based genome surgery: its all about specificity. *Curr. Gene Ther.* 11, 28–37. doi: 10.2174/156652311794520120

Hanlon, K. S., Kleinstiver, B. P., Garcia, S. P., Zaborowski, M. P., Volak, A., Spirig, S. E., et al. (2019). High levels of AAV vector integration into CRISPR-induced DNA breaks. *Nat. Commun.* 10:4439. doi: 10.1038/s41467-019-12449-2

Hendel, A., Bak, R. O., Clark, J. T., Kennedy, A. B., Ryan, D. E., Roy, S., et al. (2015). Chemically modified guide RNAs enhance CRISPR-Cas genome editing in human primary cells. *Nat. Biotechnol.* 33, 985–989. doi: 10.1038/nbt.3290

Heyer, W. D., Ehmsen, K. T., and Liu, J. (2010). Regulation of homologous recombination in eukaryotes. *Annu. Rev. Genet.* 44, 113–139. doi: 10.1146/annurev-genet-051710-150955

Hirsch, M. L. (2015). Adeno-associated virus inverted terminal repeats stimulate gene editing. *Gene Ther.* 22, 190–195. doi: 10.1038/gt.2014.109

Hoggatt, J., Singh, P., Sampath, J., and Pelus, L. M. (2009). Prostaglandin E2 enhances hematopoietic stem cell homing, survival, and proliferation. *Blood* 113, 5444–5455. doi: 10.1182/blood-2009-01-201335

Howe, S. J., Mansour, M. R., Schwarzwaelder, K., Bartholomae, C., Hubank, M., Kempski, H., et al. (2008). Insertional mutagenesis combined with acquired somatic mutations causes leukemogenesis following gene therapy of SCID-X1 patients. *J. Clin. Invest.* 118, 3143–3150. doi: 10.1172/JCI35798

Hsu, P. D., Scott, D. A., Weinstein, J. A., Ran, F. A., Konermann, S., Agarwala, V., et al. (2013). DNA targeting specificity of RNA-guided Cas9 nucleases. *Nat. Biotechnol.* 31, 827–832. doi: 10.1038/nbt.2647

Hu, J. H., Miller, S. M., Geurts, M. H., Tang, W., Chen, L., Sun, N., et al. (2018). Evolved Cas9 variants with broad PAM compatibility and high DNA specificity. *Nature* 556, 57–63. doi: 10.1038/nature26155

Hubbard, B. P., Badran, A. H., Zuris, J. A., Guilinger, J. P., Davis, K. M., Chen, L., et al. (2015). Continuous directed evolution of DNA-binding proteins to improve TALEN specificity. *Nat. Methods* 12, 939–942. doi: 10.1038/nmeth.3515

Hubbard, N., Hagin, D., Sommer, K., Song, Y., Khan, I., Clough, C., et al. (2016). Targeted gene editing restores regulated CD40L function in X-linked hyper-IgM syndrome. *Blood* 127, 2513–2522. doi: 10.1182/blood-2015-11-683235

Humbert, O., Radtke, S., Samuelson, C., Carrillo, R. R., Perez, A. M., Reddy, S. S., et al. (2019). Therapeutically relevant engraftment of a CRISPR-Cas9-edited HSC-enriched population with HbF reactivation in nonhuman primates. *Sci. Transl. Med.* 11:eaaw3768. doi: 10.1126/scitranslmed.aaw3768

Ihry, R. J., Worringer, K. A., Salick, M. R., Frias, E., Ho, D., Theriault, K., et al. (2018). p53 inhibits CRISPR-Cas9 engineering in human pluripotent stem cells. *Nat. Med.* 24, 939–946. doi: 10.1038/s41591-018-0050-6

Isalan, M. (2012). Zinc-finger nucleases: how to play two good hands. *Nat. Methods* 9, 32–34. doi: 10.1038/nmeth.1805

Jayavaradhan, R., Pillis, D. M., Goodman, M., Zhang, F., Zhang, Y., Andreassen, P. R., et al. (2019). CRISPR-Cas9 fusion to dominant-negative 53BP1 enhances HDR and inhibits NHEJ specifically at Cas9 target sites. *Nat. Commun.* 10:2866. doi: 10.1038/s41467-019-10735-7

Jinek, M., Chylinski, K., Fonfara, I., Hauer, M., Doudna, J. A., and Charpentier, E. (2012). A programmable dual-RNA-guided DNA endonuclease in adaptive bacterial immunity. *Science* 337, 816–821. doi: 10.1126/science.1225829

Kalhor, R., Kalhor, K., Mejia, L., Leeper, K., Graveline, A., Mali, P., et al. (2018). Developmental barcoding of whole mouse via homing CRISPR. *Science* 361:eaat9804. doi: 10.1126/science.aat9804

Kim, D., Bae, S., Park, J., Kim, E., Kim, S., Yu, H. R., et al. (2015). Digenome-seq: genome-wide profiling of CRISPR-Cas9 off-target effects in human cells. *Nat. Methods* 12, 237–243. doi: 10.1038/nmeth.3284

Kim, M. Y., Yu, K. R., Kenderian, S. S., Ruella, M., Chen, S., Shin, T. H., et al. (2018). Genetic Inactivation of CD33 in hematopoietic stem cells to enable CAR T cell immunotherapy for acute myeloid leukemia. *Cell* 173, 1439–1453.e19. doi: 10.1016/j.cell.2018.05.013

Kim, S., Kim, D., Cho, S. W., Kim, J., and Kim, J. S. (2014). Highly efficient RNA-guided genome editing in human cells via delivery of purified Cas9 ribonucleoproteins. *Genome Res.* 24, 1012–1019. doi: 10.1101/gr.171322.113

Kleinstiver, B. P., Pattanayak, V., Prew, M. S., Tsai, S. Q., Nguyen, N. T., Zheng, Z., et al. (2016). High-fidelity CRISPR-Cas9 nucleases with no detectable genome-wide off-target effects. *Nature* 529, 490–495. doi: 10.1038/nature16526

Kleinstiver, B. P., Prew, M. S., Tsai, S. Q., Topkar, V. V., Nguyen, N. T., Zheng, Z., et al. (2015). Engineered CRISPR-Cas9 nucleases with altered PAM specificities. *Nature* 523, 481–485. doi: 10.1038/nature14592

Kohn, D. B., Booth, C., Kang, E. M., Pai, S. Y., Shaw, K. L., Santilli, G., et al. (2020). Lentiviral gene therapy for X-linked chronic granulomatous disease. *Nat. Med.* 26, 200–206. doi: 10.1038/s41591-019-0735-5

Kosicki, M., Tomberg, K., and Bradley, A. (2018). Repair of double-strand breaks induced by CRISPR-Cas9 leads to large deletions and complex rearrangements. *Nat. Biotechnol.* 36, 765–771. doi: 10.1038/nbt.4192

Kotin, R. M., and Snyder, R. O. (2017). Manufacturing clinical grade recombinant adeno-associated virus using invertebrate cell lines. *Hum. Gene Ther.* 28, 350–360. doi: 10.1089/hum.2017.042

Kuo, C. Y., Long, J. D., Campo-Fernandez, B., de Oliveira, S., Cooper, A. R., Romero, Z., et al. (2018). Site-Specific gene editing of human hematopoietic stem cells for X-linked hyper-IgM syndrome. *Cell Rep.* 23, 2606–2616. doi: 10.1016/j.celrep.2018.04.103

Labun, K., Guo, X., Chavez, A., Church, G., Gagnon, J. A., and Valen, E. (2019). Accurate analysis of genuine CRISPR editing events with ampliCan. *Genome Res.* 29, 843–847. doi: 10.1101/gr.244293.118

Lee, C. M., Cradick, T. J., and Bao, G. (2016). The Neisseria meningitidis CRISPR-Cas9 system enables specific genome editing in mammalian cells. *Mol. Ther.* 24, 645–654. doi: 10.1038/mt.2016.8

Lee, H. J., Kim, E., and Kim, J. S. (2010). Targeted chromosomal deletions in human cells using zinc finger nucleases. *Genome Res.* 20, 81–89. doi: 10.1101/gr.099747.109

Lee, J. K., Jeong, E., Lee, J., Jung, M., Shin, E., Kim, Y., et al. (2018). Directed evolution of CRISPR-Cas9 to increase its specificity. *Nat. Commun.* 9:3048. doi: 10.1038/s41467-018-05477-x

Lim, Y., Bak, S. Y., Sung, K., Jeong, E., Lee, S. H., Kim, J. S., et al. (2016). Structural roles of guide RNAs in the nuclease activity of Cas9 endonuclease. *Nat. Commun.* 7:13350. doi: 10.1038/ncomms13350

Lipton, J. M., and Ellis, S. R. (2009). Diamond-Blackfan anemia: diagnosis, treatment, and molecular pathogenesis. *Hematol. Oncol. Clin. North Am.* 23, 261–282. doi: 10.1016/j.hoc.2009.01.004

Liu, J., Guo, Y. M., Hirokawa, M., Iwamoto, K., Ubukawa, K., Michishita, Y., et al. (2012). A synthetic double-stranded RNA, poly I: C, induces a rapid apoptosis of human CD34+ cells. *Exp. Hematol.* 40, 330–341. doi: 10.1016/j.exphem.2011.12.002

Lombardo, A., Genovese, P., Beausejour, C. M., Colleoni, S., Lee, Y. L., Kim, K. A., et al. (2007). Gene editing in human stem cells using zinc finger nucleases and integrase-defective lentiviral vector delivery. *Nat. Biotechnol.* 25, 1298–1306. doi: 10.1038/nbt1353

Mamcarz, E., Zhou, S., Lockey, T., Abdelsamed, H., Cross, S. J., Kang, G., et al. (2019). Lentiviral gene therapy combined with low-dose busulfan in infants with SCID-X1. *N. Engl. J. Med.* 380, 1525–1534. doi: 10.1056/NEJMoa1815408

Marktel, S., Scaramuzza, S., Cicalese, M. P., Giglio, F., Galimberti, S., Lidonnici, M. R., et al. (2019). Intrabone hematopoietic stem cell gene therapy for adult and pediatric patients affected by transfusion-dependent ß-thalassemia. *Nat. Med.* 25, 234–241. doi: 10.1038/s41591-018-0301-6

Maruyama, T., Dougan, S. K., Truttmann, M. C., Bilate, A. M., Ingram, J. R., and Ploegh, H. L. (2015). Increasing the efficiency of precise genome editing with CRISPR-Cas9 by inhibition of nonhomologous end joining. *Nat. Biotechnol.* 33, 538–542. doi: 10.1038/nbt.3190

McKenna, A., Findlay, G. M., Gagnon, J. A., Horwitz, M. S., Schier, A. F., and Shendure, J. (2016). Whole-organism lineage tracing by combinatorial and cumulative genome editing. *Science* 353:aaf7907. doi: 10.1126/science.aaf7907

Miller, J. C., Holmes, M. C., Wang, J., Guschin, D. Y., Lee, Y. L., Rupniewski, I., et al. (2007). An improved zinc-finger nuclease architecture for highly specific genome editing. *Nat. Biotechnol.* 25, 778–785. doi: 10.1038/nbt1319

Moehle, E. A., Rock, J. M., Lee, Y. L., Jouvenot, Y., DeKelver, R. C., Gregory, P. D., et al. (2007). Targeted gene addition into a specified location in the human genome using designed zinc finger nucleases. *Proc. Natl. Acad. Sci. U.S.A.* 104, 3055–3060. doi: 10.1073/pnas.0611478104

Montini, E., Cesana, D., Schmidt, M., Sanvito, F., Ponzoni, M., Bartholomae, C., et al. (2006). Hematopoietic stem cell gene transfer in a tumor-prone mouse model uncovers low genotoxicity of lentiviral vector integration. *Nat. Biotechnol.* 24, 687–696. doi: 10.1038/nbt1216

Mu, W., Tang, N., Cheng, C., Sun, W., Wei, X., and Wang, H. (2019). *In vitro* transcribed sgRNA causes cell death by inducing interferon release. *Protein Cell* 10, 461–465. doi: 10.1007/s13238-018-0605-9

Müller, M., Lee, C. M., Gasiunas, G., Davis, T. H., Cradick, T. J., Siksnys, V., et al. (2016). Streptococcus thermophilus CRISPR-Cas9 systems enable specific editing of the human genome. *Mol. Ther.* 24, 636–644. doi: 10.1038/mt.2015.218

Naldini, L. (2019). Genetic engineering of hematopoiesis: current stage of clinical translation and future perspectives. *EMBO Mol. Med.* 11:e9958. doi: 10.15252/emmm.201809958

Nasri, M., Ritter, M., Mir, P., Dannenmann, B., Aghaallaei, N., Amend, D., et al. (2020). CRISPR/Cas9-mediated ELANE knockout enables neutrophilic maturation of primary hematopoietic stem and progenitor cells and induced pluripotent stem cells of severe congenital neutropenia patients. *Haematologica* 105, 598–609. doi: 10.3324/haematol.2019.221804

Nelson, C. E., Wu, Y., Gemberling, M. P., Oliver, M. L., Waller, M. A., Bohning, J. D., et al. (2019). Long-term evaluation of AAV-CRISPR genome editing for duchenne muscular dystrophy. *Nat. Med.* 25, 427–432. doi: 10.1038/s41591-019-0344-3

Nihongaki, Y., Kawano, F., Nakajima, T., and Sato, M. (2015). Photoactivatable CRISPR-Cas9 for optogenetic genome editing. *Nat. Biotechnol.* 33, 755–760. doi: 10.1038/nbt.3245

Nishimasu, H., Shi, X., Ishiguro, S., Gao, L., Hirano, S., Okazaki, S., et al. (2018). Engineered CRISPR-Cas9 nuclease with expanded targeting space. *Science* 361, 1259–1262. doi: 10.1126/science.aas9129

Nozawa, T., Furukawa, N., Aikawa, C., Watanabe, T., Haobam, B., Kurokawa, K., et al. (2011). CRISPR inhibition of prophage acquisition in Streptococcus pyogenes. *PLoS ONE* 6:e19543. doi: 10.1371/journal.pone.0019543

Park, S. H., Lee, C. M., Dever, D. P., Davis, T. H., Camarena, J., Srifa, W., et al. (2019). Highly efficient editing of the β-globin gene in patient-derived hematopoietic stem and progenitor cells to treat sickle cell disease. *Nucleic Acids Res.* 47, 7955–7972. doi: 10.1093/nar/gkz475

Pattabhi, S., Lotti, S. N., Berger, M. P., Singh, S., Lux, C. T., Jacoby, K., et al. (2019). In Vivo Outcome of homology-directed repair at the HBB Gene in HSC using alternative donor template delivery methods. *Mol. Ther. Nucleic Acids* 17, 277–288. doi: 10.1016/j.omtn.2019.05.025

Pattanayak, V., Lin, S., Guilinger, J. P., Ma, E., Doudna, J. A., and Liu, D. R. (2013). High-throughput profiling of off-target DNA cleavage reveals RNA-programmed Cas9 nuclease specificity. *Nat. Biotechnol.* 31, 839–843. doi: 10.1038/nbt.2673

Pavani, G., Laurent, M., Fabiano, A., Cantelli, E., Sakkal, A., Corre, G., et al. (2020). *Ex vivo* editing of human hematopoietic stem cells for erythroid expression of therapeutic proteins. *Nat. Commun.* 11:3778. doi: 10.1038/s41467-020-17552-3

Pavel-Dinu, M., Wiebking, V., Dejene, B. T., Srifa, W., Mantri, S., Nicolas, C. E., et al. (2019). Gene correction for SCID-X1 in long-term hematopoietic stem cells. *Nat. Commun.* 10, 1634. doi: 10.1038/s41467-019-09614-y

Petrillo, C., Thorne, L. G., Unali, G., Schiroli, G., Giordano, A. M. S., Piras, F., et al. (2018). Cyclosporine H overcomes innate immune restrictions to improve lentiviral transduction and gene editing in human hematopoietic stem cells. *Cell Stem Cell* 23, 820–832.e9. doi: 10.1016/j.stem.2018.10.008

Piras, F., and Kajaste-Rudnitski, A. (2020). Antiviral immunity and nucleic acid sensing in haematopoietic stem cell gene engineering. *Gene Ther.* 28, 16–28. doi: 10.1038/s41434-020-0175-3

Piras, F., Riba, M., Petrillo, C., Lazarevic, D., Cuccovillo, I., Bartolaccini, S., et al. (2017). Lentiviral vectors escape innate sensing but trigger p53 in human hematopoietic stem and progenitor cells. *EMBO Mol. Med.* 9, 1198–1211. doi: 10.15252/emmm.201707922

Rai, R., Romito, M., Rivers, E., Turchiano, G., Blattner, G., Vetharoy, W., et al. (2020). Targeted gene correction of human hematopoietic stem cells for the treatment of Wiskott - Aldrich Syndrome. *Nat. Commun.* 11:4034. doi: 10.1038/s41467-020-17626-2

Ran, F. A., Cong, L., Yan, W. X., Scott, D. A., Gootenberg, J. S., Kriz, A. J., et al. (2015). *In vivo* genome editing using *Staphylococcus aureus* Cas9. *Nature* 520, 186–191. doi: 10.1038/nature14299

Richardson, C. D., Kazane, K. R., Feng, S. J., Zelin, E., Bray, N. L., Schäfer, A. J., et al. (2018). CRISPR–Cas9 genome editing in human cells occurs via the Fanconi anemia pathway. *Nat. Genet.* 50, 1132–1139. doi: 10.1038/s41588-018-0174-0

Román-Rodríguez, F. J., Ugalde, L., Álvarez, L., Díez, B., and Ramírez, M. J., Risueño, C., et al. (2019). NHEJ-Mediated repair of CRISPR-Cas9-induced DNA breaks efficiently corrects mutations in HSPCs from patients with fanconi anemia. *Cell Stem Cell* 25, 607–621.e7. doi: 10.1016/j.stem.2019.08.016

Romero, Z., Lomova, A., Said, S., Miggelbrink, A., Kuo, C. Y., Campo-Fernandez, B., et al. (2019). Editing the sickle cell disease mutation in human hematopoietic stem cells: comparison of endonucleases and homologous donor templates. *Mol. Ther.* 27, 1389–1406. doi: 10.1016/j.ymthe.2019.05.014

Roth, T. L., Puig-Saus, C., Yu, R., Shifrut, E., Carnevale, J., Li, P. J., et al. (2018). Reprogramming human T cell function and specificity with non-viral genome targeting. *Nature* 559, 405–409. doi: 10.1038/s41586-018-0326-5

Sacco, M. G., Ungari, M., Catò, E. M., Villa, A., Strina, D., Notarangelo, L. D., et al. (2000). Lymphoid abnormalities in CD40 ligand transgenic mice suggest the need for tight regulation in gene therapy approaches to hyper immunoglobulin M (IgM) syndrome. *Cancer Gene Ther.* 7, 1299–1306. doi: 10.1038/sj.cgt.7700232

Sadelain, M., Papapetrou, E. P., and Bushman, F. D. (2012). Safe harbours for the integration of new DNA in the human genome. *Nat. Rev. Cancer* 12, 51–58. doi: 10.1038/nrc3179

Sankaran, V. G., Menne, T. F., Xu, J., Akie, T. E., Lettre, G., Van Handel, B., et al. (2008). Human fetal hemoglobin expression is regulated by the developmental stage-specific repressor BCL11A. *Science* 322, 1839–1842. doi: 10.1126/science.1165409

Sato, T., Onai, N., Yoshihara, H., Arai, F., Suda, T., and Ohteki, T. (2009). Interferon regulatory factor-2 protects quiescent hematopoietic stem cells from type I interferon-dependent exhaustion. *Nat. Med.* 15, 696–700. doi: 10.1038/nm.1973

Schiroli, G., Conti, A., Ferrari, S., della Volpe, L., Jacob, A., Albano, L., et al. (2019). Precise gene editing preserves hematopoietic stem cell function following transient p53-mediated DNA damage response. *Cell Stem Cell* 24, 551–565.e8. doi: 10.1016/j.stem.2019.02.019

Schiroli, G., Ferrari, S., Conway, A., Jacob, A., Capo, V., Albano, L., et al. (2017). Preclinical modeling highlights the therapeutic potential of hematopoietic stem cell gene editing for correction of SCID-X1. *Sci. Transl. Med.* 9:eaan0820. doi: 10.1126/scitranslmed.aan0820

Sessa, M., Lorioli, L., Fumagalli, F., Acquati, S., Redaelli, D., Baldoli, C., et al. (2016). Lentiviral haemopoietic stem-cell gene therapy in early-onset metachromatic leukodystrophy: an ad-hoc analysis of a non-randomised, open-label, phase 1/2 trial. *Lancet* 388, 476–487. doi: 10.1016/S0140-6736(16)30374-9

Shapiro, J., Iancu, O., Jacobi, A. M., McNeill, M. S., Turk, R., Rettig, G. R., et al. (2020). Increasing CRISPR efficiency and measuring its specificity in HSPCs using a clinically relevant system. *Mol. Ther. Methods Clin. Dev.* 17, 1097–1107. doi: 10.1016/j.omtm.2020.04.027

Sharma, R., Dever, D. P., Lee, C. M., Azizi, A., Pan, Y., Camarena, J., et al. (2021). The TRACE-Seq method tracks recombination alleles and identifies clonal reconstitution dynamics of gene targeted human hematopoietic stem cells. *Nat. Commun.* 12:472. doi: 10.1038/s41467-020-20792-y

Shin, J. J., Schröder, M. S., Caiado, F., Wyman, S. K., Bray, N. L., Bordi, M., et al. (2020). Controlled cycling and quiescence enables efficient HDR in engraftment-enriched adult hematopoietic stem and progenitor cells. *Cell Rep.* 32:108093. doi: 10.1016/j.celrep.2020.108093

Slaymaker, I. M., Gao, L., Zetsche, B., Scott, D. A., Yan, W. X., and Zhang, F. (2016). Rationally engineered Cas9 nucleases with improved specificity. *Science* 351, 84–88. doi: 10.1126/science.aad5227

Soldi, M., Sergi Sergi, L., Unali, G., Kerzel, T., Cuccovillo, I., Capasso, P., et al. (2020). Laboratory-Scale lentiviral vector production and purification for enhanced *ex vivo* and *in vivo* genetic engineering. *Mol. Ther. Methods Clin. Dev.* 19, 411–425. doi: 10.1016/j.omtm.2020.10.009

Stein, S., Ott, M. G., Schultze-Strasser, S., Jauch, A., Burwinkel, B., Kinner, A., et al. (2010). Genomic instability and myelodysplasia with monosomy 7 consequent to EVI1 activation after gene therapy for chronic granulomatous disease. *Nat. Med.* 16, 198–204. doi: 10.1038/nm.2088

Sternberg, S. H., Redding, S., Jinek, M., Greene, E. C., and Doudna, J. A. (2014). DNA interrogation by the CRISPR RNA-guided endonuclease Cas9. *Nature* 507, 62–67. doi: 10.1038/nature13011

Sweeney, C. L., Zou, J., Choi, U., Merling, R. K., Liu, A., Bodansky, A., et al. (2017). Targeted Repair of CYBB in X-CGD iPSCs requires retention of intronic sequences for expression and functional correction. *Mol. Ther.* 25, 321–330. doi: 10.1016/j.ymthe.2016.11.012

Takahashi, K., Wang, F., Kantarjian, H., Doss, D., Khanna, K., Thompson, E., et al. (2017). Preleukaemic clonal haemopoiesis and risk of therapy-related myeloid neoplasms: a case-control study. *Lancet Oncol.* 18, 100–111. doi: 10.1016/S1470-2045(16)30626-X

Thompson, A. A., Walters, M. C., Kwiatkowski, J., Rasko, J. E. J., Ribeil, J.-A., Hongeng, S., et al. (2018). Gene therapy in patients with transfusion-dependent β-thalassemia. *N. Engl. J. Med.* 378, 1479–1493. doi: 10.1056/NEJMoa1705342

Touchot, N., and Flume, M. (2017). Early insights from commercialization of gene therapies in Europe. *Genes* 8:78. doi: 10.3390/genes8020078

Tsai, S. Q., Nguyen, N. T., Malagon-Lopez, J., Topkar, V. V., Aryee, M. J., and Joung, J. K. (2017). CIRCLE-seq: a highly sensitive *in vitro* screen for genome-wide CRISPR-Cas9 nuclease off-targets. *Nat. Methods* 14, 607–614. doi: 10.1038/nmeth.4278

Tsai, S. Q., Zheng, Z., Nguyen, N. T., Liebers, M., Topkar, V. V., Thapar, V., et al. (2015). GUIDE-seq enables genome-wide profiling of off-target cleavage by CRISPR-Cas nucleases. *Nat. Biotechnol.* 33, 187–198. doi: 10.1038/nbt.3117

Urnov, F. D., Miller, J. C., Lee, Y. L., Beausejour, C. M., Rock, J. M., Augustus, S., et al. (2005). Highly efficient endogenous human gene correction using designed zinc-finger nucleases. *Nature* 435, 646–651. doi: 10.1038/nature03556

Urnov, F. D., Rebar, E. J., Holmes, M. C., Zhang, H. S., and Gregory, P. D. (2010). Genome editing with engineered zinc finger nucleases. *Nat. Rev. Genet.* 11, 636–646. doi: 10.1038/nrg2842

Vakulskas, C. A., Dever, D. P., Rettig, G. R., Turk, R., Jacobi, A. M., Collingwood, M. A., et al. (2018). A high-fidelity Cas9 mutant delivered as a ribonucleoprotein complex enables efficient gene editing in human hematopoietic stem and progenitor cells. *Nat. Med.* 24, 1216–1224. doi: 10.1038/s41591-018-0137-0

van de Vrugt, H. J., Harmsen, T., Riepsaame, J., Alexantya, G., van Mil, S. E., de Vries, Y., et al. (2019). Effective CRISPR/Cas9-mediated correction of a Fanconi anemia defect by error-prone end joining or templated repair. *Sci. Rep.* 9:768. doi: 10.1038/s41598-018-36506-w

van Overbeek, M., Capurso, D., Carter, M. M., Thompson, M. S., Frias, E., Russ, C., et al. (2016). DNA repair profiling reveals nonrandom outcomes at Cas9-mediated breaks. *Mol. Cell* 63, 633–646. doi: 10.1016/j.molcel.2016.06.037

Vavassori, V., Mercuri, E., Marcovecchio, G. E., Castiello, M. C., Schiroli, G., Albano, L., et al. (2021). Modeling, optimization, and comparable efficacy of T cell and hematopoietic stem cell gene editing for treating hyper-IgM syndrome. *EMBO Mol. Med.* 13:e13545. doi: 10.15252/emmm.202013545

Villa, A., Capo, V., and Castiello, M. C. (2020). Innovative cell-based therapies and conditioning to cure RAG deficiency. *Front. Immunol.* 11:607926. doi: 10.3389/fimmu.2020.607926

Voit, R. A., Hendel, A., Pruett-Miller, S. M., and Porteus, M. H. (2014). Nuclease-mediated gene editing by homologous recombination of the human globin locus. *Nucleic Acids Res.* 42, 1365–1378. doi: 10.1093/nar/gkt947

Walasek, M. A., van Os, R., and de Haan, G. (2012). Hematopoietic stem cell expansion: challenges and opportunities. *Ann. N. Y. Acad. Sci.* 1266, 138–150. doi: 10.1111/j.1749-6632.2012.06549.x

Walton, R. T., Christie, K. A., Whittaker, M. N., and Kleinstiver, B. P. (2020). Unconstrained genome targeting with near-PAMless engineered CRISPR-Cas9 variants. *Science* 368, 290–296. doi: 10.1126/science.aba8853

Wang, C. X., and Cannon, P. M. (2016). The clinical applications of genome editing in HIV. *Blood* 127, 2546–2552. doi: 10.1182/blood-2016-01-678144

Wang, J., Exline, C. M., Declercq, J. J., Llewellyn, G. N., Hayward, S. B., Li, P. W. L., et al. (2015). Homology-driven genome editing in hematopoietic stem and progenitor cells using ZFN mRNA and AAV6 donors. *Nat. Biotechnol.* 33, 1256–1263. doi: 10.1038/nbt.3408

Wang, Q., Chen, S., Xiao, Q., Liu, Z., Liu, S., Hou, P., et al. (2017). Genome modification of CXCR4 by Staphylococcus aureus Cas9 renders cells resistance to HIV-1 infection. *Retrovirology* 14:51. doi: 10.1186/s12977-017-0375-0

Wilkinson, A. C., Dever, D. P., Baik, R., Camarena, J., Hsu, I., Charlesworth, C. T., et al. (2021). Cas9-AAV6 gene correction of beta-globin in autologous HSCs improves sickle cell disease erythropoiesis in mice. *Nat. Commun.* 12:686. doi: 10.1038/s41467-021-20909-x

Wilson, R. C., and Carroll, D. (2019). The daunting economics of therapeutic genome editing. *Cris. J.* 2, 280–284. doi: 10.1089/crispr.2019.0052

Xiao, Q., Chen, S., Wang, Q., Liu, Z., Liu, S., Deng, H., et al. (2019). CCR5 editing by Staphylococcus aureus Cas9 in human primary CD4+ T cells and hematopoietic stem/progenitor cells promotes HIV-1 resistance and CD4+ T cell enrichment in humanized mice. *Retrovirology* 16:15. doi: 10.1186/s12977-019-0477-y

Xu, K., Ren, C., Liu, Z., Zhang, T., Zhang, T., Li, D., et al. (2015). Efficient genome engineering in eukaryotes using Cas9 from Streptococcus thermophilus. *Cell. Mol. Life Sci.* 72, 383–399. doi: 10.1007/s00018-014-1679-z

Xu, L., Wang, J., Liu, Y., Xie, L., Su, B., Mou, D., et al. (2019). CRISPR-edited stem cells in a patient with HIV and acute lymphocytic leukemia. *N. Engl. J. Med.* 381, 1240–1247. doi: 10.1056/NEJMoa1817426

Xu, L., Yang, H., Gao, Y., Chen, Z., Xie, L., Liu, Y., et al. (2017). CRISPR/Cas9-MEDIATED ccr5 ablation in human hematopoietic stem/progenitor cells confers HIV-1 resistance *in vivo*. *Mol. Ther.* 25, 1782–1789. doi: 10.1016/j.ymthe.2017.04.027

Yeh, C. D., Richardson, C. D., and Corn, J. E. (2019). Advances in genome editing through control of DNA repair pathways. *Nat. Cell Biol.* 21, 1468–1478. doi: 10.1038/s41556-019-0425-z

Zetsche, B., Gootenberg, J. S., Abudayyeh, O. O., Slaymaker, I. M., Makarova, K. S., Essletzbichler, P., et al. (2015a). Cpf1 is a single RNA-guided endonuclease of a class 2 CRISPR-Cas system. *Cell* 163, 759–771. doi: 10.1016/j.cell.2015.09.038

Zetsche, B., Volz, S. E., and Zhang, F. (2015b). A split-Cas9 architecture for inducible genome editing and transcription modulation. *Nat. Biotechnol.* 33, 139–142. doi: 10.1038/nbt.3149

Zink, F., Stacey, S. N., Norddahl, G. L., Frigge, M. L., Magnusson, O. T., Jonsdottir, I., et al. (2017). Clonal hematopoiesis, with and without candidate driver mutations, is common in the elderly. *Blood* 130, 742–752. doi: 10.1182/blood-2017-02-769869

Zonari, E., Desantis, G., Petrillo, C., Boccalatte, F. E., Lidonnici, M. R., Kajaste-Rudnitski, A., et al. (2017). Efficient *ex vivo* engineering and expansion of highly purified human hematopoietic stem and progenitor cell populations for gene therapy. *Stem Cell Rep.* 8, 977–990. doi: 10.1016/j.stemcr.2017.02.010

9

Global and Local Manipulation of DNA Repair Mechanisms to Alter Site-Specific Gene Editing Outcomes in Hematopoietic Stem Cells

Elizabeth K. Benitez[1†], Anastasia Lomova Kaufman[1†], Lilibeth Cervantes[1],
Danielle N. Clark[1], Paul G. Ayoub[1], Shantha Senadheera[1], Kyle Osborne[1],
Julie M. Sanchez[1], Ralph Valentine Crisostomo[1], Xiaoyan Wang[2], Nina Reuven[3],
Yosef Shaul[3], Roger P. Hollis[1], Zulema Romero[1] and Donald B. Kohn[1*]

[1] Department of Microbiology, Immunology & Molecular Genetics, David Geffen School of Medicine, University of California, Los Angeles, Los Angeles, CA, United States, [2] Department of General Internal Medicine and Health Services Research, University of California, Los Angeles, Los Angeles, CA, United States, [3] Department of Molecular Genetics, Weizmann Institute of Science, Rehovot, Israel

*Correspondence:
Donald B. Kohn
dkohn1@mednet.ucla.edu

† These authors have contributed
equally to this work

Monogenic disorders of the blood system have the potential to be treated by autologous stem cell transplantation of *ex vivo* genetically modified hematopoietic stem and progenitor cells (HSPCs). The sgRNA/Cas9 system allows for precise modification of the genome at single nucleotide resolution. However, the system is reliant on endogenous cellular DNA repair mechanisms to mend a Cas9-induced double stranded break (DSB), either by the non-homologous end joining (NHEJ) pathway or by the cell-cycle regulated homology-directed repair (HDR) pathway. Here, we describe a panel of ectopically expressed DNA repair factors and Cas9 variants assessed for their ability to promote gene correction by HDR or inhibit gene disruption by NHEJ at the *HBB* locus. Although transient global overexpression of DNA repair factors did not improve the frequency of gene correction in primary HSPCs, localization of factors to the DSB by fusion to the Cas9 protein did alter repair outcomes toward microhomology-mediated end joining (MMEJ) repair, an HDR event. This strategy may be useful when predictable gene editing outcomes are imperative for therapeutic success.

Keywords: gene editing, hematopoietic stem cells, DNA repair, Cas9, HDR, sickle cell disease

INTRODUCTION

Inherited disorders of the hematopoietic system, such as primary immune deficiencies and hemoglobinopathies, have been historically treated by allogeneic hematopoietic stem cell transplantation (HSCT) of healthy HLA-matched donor cells (Griffith et al., 2008). The self-renewing hematopoietic stem and progenitor cells (HSPCs) engraft and repopulate the bone-marrow niche of a conditioned recipient, providing a steady supply of healthy blood cells. However, allogeneic HSCT does not come without risks; recipients may suffer graft rejection, graft-vs.-host disease, or complications due to immunosuppression (Dvorak and Cowan, 2008; Pai et al., 2014). Gene modification of autologous HSPCs for transplantation can circumvent these risks. Current approaches utilize site-specific endonucleases to facilitate precise gene editing, with the Cas family of RNA-guided nucleases emerging as the most promising for therapeutic gene editing. Of these, the *Streptococcus pyogenes* Cas9 (SpCas9) enzyme is recognized for its ease of use and production, and remarkable ability to hone in on a 20 base pair sequence among the ~3 billion base pairs in the human genome to create a directed double-stranded break (DSB; Doudna and Charpentier, 2014). Once the DSB is introduced, endogenous cell repair mechanisms are employed to mend the lesion.

Two main pathways compete to repair the break: non-homologous end joining (NHEJ), an imprecise repair pathway that can result in insertions and deletions (indels), or accurate homology-directed repair (HDR), which uses a donor template to seamlessly repair the break in S/G2 phases of cell cycle (Sartori et al., 2007; Branzei and Foiani, 2008; Heyer et al., 2010; Pietras et al., 2011; Symington and Gautier, 2011; Fradet-Turcotte et al., 2013; Jasin and Rothstein, 2013; Panier and Boulton, 2014; Polato et al., 2014; Anand et al., 2016; Cuella-Martin et al., 2016; Jasin and Haber, 2016; Symington, 2016; Lomova, 2019; Romero et al., 2019; Ceppi et al., 2020). Additionally, recent work suggests that microhomology-mediated end joining (MMEJ), an HDR event that results in deletions, is also a notable repair pathway in many cell types (McVey and Lee, 2008; Huertas, 2010; Iyer et al., 2019; Wu et al., 2019; Yeh et al., 2019). To accurately repair the DSB and introduce specific sequence changes to the gene, a DNA donor template designed with single nucleotide polymorphisms (SNPs) and flanked by homology arms can be incorporated into the genome via HDR. The activity of the repair pathways is not equivalent; NHEJ is more prevalent than HDR in mammalian cells (Chiruvella et al., 2013, Yeh et al., 2019). For certain diseases, where a knockout of a gene can result in therapeutic benefit, repair by the NHEJ pathway is favorable (Holt et al., 2010; Bauer et al., 2013; Bjurström et al., 2016; Chang et al., 2017). However, for site-specific gene correction of sickle cell disease (SCD), where disruption of the target *HBB* gene can result in a different or more severe disease phenotype, correction via HDR pathway is critical.

In the last several years, there have been many efforts to control DNA repair outcomes for genome editing by either globally inhibiting or activating DNA repair factors (DNA RFs; Yeh et al., 2019). Numerous studies have shown improvements in HDR or inhibition of NHEJ repair through overexpression of factors that promote or restrict these pathways, respectively (Orthwein et al., 2015; Canny et al., 2018; **Supplementary Figures 1A–C**). However, the effects of these manipulations on primary human HSPCs have not been previously reported. Local manipulation of DNA repair factors to control editing outcomes may prove to be a superior strategy over global manipulation of DNA repair. Cell cycle control of HDR to specific HDR-permissive states protects against loss of heterozygosity, while the NHEJ pathway is primarily in place as a protective mechanism against the estimated 10–50 DNA lesions that occur in a cell per day through natural causes (Ellis et al., 1995; Vilenchik and Knudson, 2003; Yeh et al., 2019). Localization of DNA RFs to a Cas9-induced DSB may reduce the risks associated with global manipulation of DNA repair (Jayavaradhan et al., 2019). Furthermore, tethering DNA RFs to Cas9 may ensure that the factors are present and active as soon as a Cas9-induced DSB occurs, thus controlling the fate of repair outcomes. Recent efforts of local manipulation of DNA repair

factors have reported successes in cell lines. Fusion of the "HDR enhancer element of CtIP" to Cas9 or Cas9-hGeminin (Cas9-hCtIP and Cas9-hGem-hCtIP, respectively) effectively increased HDR (Charpentier et al., 2018). Tethering of a dominant negative form of 53BP1 (DN1S) to Cas9 was able to inhibit NHEJ while maintaining levels of HDR (Jayavaradhan et al., 2019). To date, the only Cas9 fusion variant shown to improve the HDR/NHEJ ratio in primary HSPCs is Cas9-hGem (Gutschner et al., 2016; Lomova et al., 2019).

In this study, we investigated the cellular elements that govern the DNA repair pathway choice and how they can be exploited to shift the balance from NHEJ toward HDR while targeting the SCD causative mutation in *HBB*. We evaluated whether global overexpression of a series of DNA RFs can improve gene editing levels in a K562 cell line and primary CD34$^+$ human HSPCs. Interestingly, we observed no consistent improvement in HDR by over-expression of any of the DNA RF we examined, although there was non-specific improvement in HDR in K562 cells by the addition of plasmid DNA. In a parallel approach, we tested a panel of Cas9 variants fused to DNA RFs for their ability to promote HDR or inhibit NHEJ specifically at the DSB. Variants containing a fragment of the human Geminin (hGem) protein consistently reduced the frequency of NHEJ alleles compared to Cas9, while the levels of HDR remained similar. We observed an increase in MMEJ signature when HSPCs were edited with Cas9-hCtIP variants, suggesting that the CtIP fusion is biologically active but does not promote gene correction by canonical HDR.

RESULTS

Evaluating the Effects of DNA RF Overexpression on Gene Editing Levels in K562 Cells

In human cell lines, it has been shown that constitutively active phosphomimetic forms of CtIP (CtIP T847E, denoted as CtIP^E; CtIP S249D T847E, denoted as CtIP^{DE}), can promote end resection in G1 phase of the cell cycle and recruit BRCA1 irrespective of cell cycle stage (Huertas and Jackason, 2009; Orthwein et al., 2015). Furthermore, modifying PALB2 with mutations in the BRCA1 binding pocket (PALB2^{KR}) results in cell cycle-independent interaction with BRCA1; when coupled with activation of DSB end resection, HDR can occur in G1 (Orthwein et al., 2015). Inhibition of NHEJ factors can be beneficial by either limiting undesired indels or skewing repair toward HDR. Inhibitor of 53BP1 (i53) targets the ubiquitin-dependent recruitment (UDR) domain of 53BP1, preventing its recruitment to DSB and stimulating HDR (Canny et al., 2018; **Supplementary Figure 1B**). A truncated fragment of 53BP1 containing an identical tandem Tudor domain competitively antagonize the protein in a dominant negative fashion (dn53BP1). Coupled with ectopic expression of RAD52, dn53BP1 has been shown to improve HDR through the single strand template repair (SSTR) pathway (Paulsen et al., 2017).

To evaluate the effects of DNA RFs on HDR and NHEJ levels, factors were overexpressed from MND-LTR-U3-driven expression plasmids by co-electroporation with gene editing

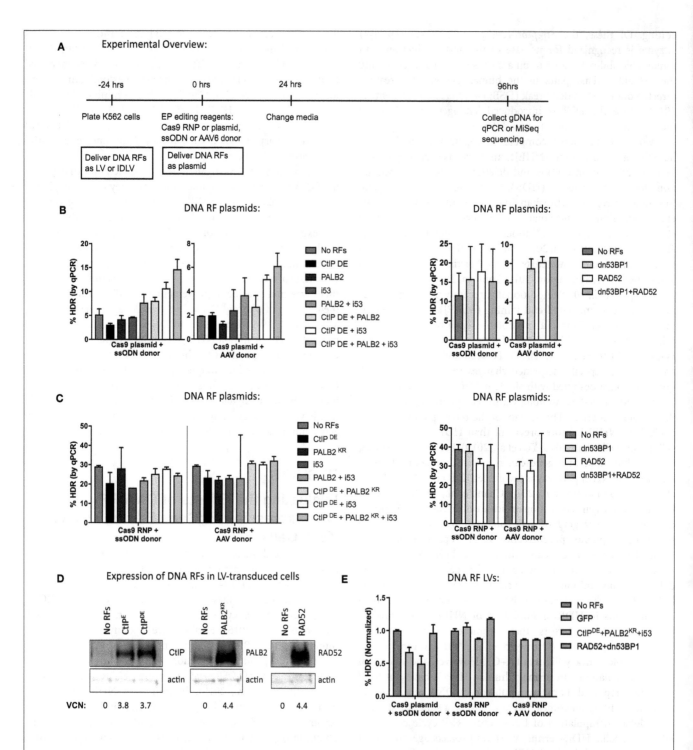

FIGURE 1 | The method for delivery of DNA repair factors (RFs) for global overexpression in K562 differentially affects gene editing outcomes. **(A)** Experimental overview of K562 cell transduction and electroporation for delivery of DNA RFs and editing reagents. DNA RFs delivered as plasmid were co-electroporated with editing reagents, while delivery of DNA RFs as LVs occurred 24 h prior to electroporation. **(B,C)** Cas9 nuclease was delivered either as plasmid (1 μg) or RNP (100 pmol Cas9 protein + 4.5 μg of IVT sgRNA); donor template was delivered either as ssODN (3 μM) or AAV6 (MOI 2e4). DNA RFs were delivered as a plasmid. HDR levels were measured by qPCR. $n = 2$ biological replicates for CtIP^{DE} + PALB2^{KR} + i53 experiments, $n = 6$ biological replicates for RAD52 + dn53BP1 experiments. Error bars, mean ± SD. **(D)** K562 cells were transduced with LVs expressing the indicated DNA RFs. Western Blot was performed on day 10 post-transduction. Vector copy number (VCN) was determined by droplet digital PCR (ddPCR). **(E)** K562 cells were transduced with DNA RF LVs and electroporated with editing reagents. $n = 2$ biological replicates. Data are normalized to "No RFs" conditions for each set of experiments. Error bars, mean ± SD.

TABLE 1 | Panel of DNA repair factors assessed in this study.

DNA RFs	Description
CtIP^E/CtIP^{DE}	T847E mutant acts as a CDK- mediated phosphomimetic.; S249D mutant increases BRCA2 recruitment to DSB (Orthwein et al., 2015)
PALB2^{KR}	KR mutation in the BRCA1 binding pocket allows for PALB2/BRCA1 binding irrespective of cell cycle (Orthwein et al., 2015)
i53	"Inhibitor of 53BP1" is an ubiquitin variant that binds to 53BP1 and prevents its accumulation at a DSB (Canny et al., 2018)
RAD52	Improves SSTR (Paulsen et al., 2017)
dn53BP1	Dominant negative form of 53BP1; inhibits NHEJ (Paulsen et al., 2017)

reagents into K562 cells, erythroleukemia cell line that is commonly used as a proxy for HSPCs (**Figure 1A**; see **Table 1** for a list of DNA RFs tested). Cas9 and the single guide RNA (sgRNA) to *HBB* were delivered either as expression plasmids or ribonucleoprotein (RNP), and donor template was delivered either as a single-stranded oligodeoxynucleotide (ssODN), or an adeno-associated virus 6 (AAV6; DeWitt et al., 2016; Lomova et al., 2019; Romero et al., 2019). The percentage of gene correction was measured by qPCR (Hoban et al., 2015).

When Cas9 was delivered as a plasmid, a combination of CtIP^{DE}, PALB2^{KR}, and i53 improved HDR levels almost 3-fold, compared to "No RFs" control with both ssODN and AAV donors. However, overexpression of the factors individually did not have any significant effects on HDR levels. Similar improvements in HDR levels were observed when RAD52 and dn53BP1 plasmids were co-electroporated with Cas9 plasmid (**Figure 1B**).

In contrast, when the same DNA RFs were co-delivered as plasmids with Cas9 RNP (**Figure 1C**), there were no improvements in HDR levels when CtIP^{DE}, PALB2^{KR}, and i53 were expressed in combination, irrespective of donor template used for repair. No improvements in HDR levels were detected in the context of ssODN donor when RAD52 and dn53BP1 were used in combination. A slight improvement (1.5-fold) in HDR levels in the context of AAV6 donor was observed with RAD52 and dn53BP1. We hypothesized that the reason for not achieving improvements in HDR levels when delivering Cas9 as RNP and DNA RFs as plasmids was due to delayed kinetics of DNA RF transcription and translation from the plasmid, relative to Cas9 RNP, which is already in its active protein form at the time of electroporation into the cells.

To synchronize expression of the DNA RFs during Cas9 RNP editing, cells were transduced with lentiviruses (LVs) expressing DNA RFs, 24 h prior to electroporation of gene editing reagents. To confirm overexpression, K562 cells were transduced with LVs at multiplicity of infection (MOI) of 1, and DNA RF protein expression was assessed by western blot analysis (**Figure 1D**). The results showed basal expression of CtIP^E, CtIP^{DE}, PALB2, and RAD52 proteins in "No RFs" condition (untransduced samples) and confirmed protein overexpression in LV-transduced samples.

Western blots for i53 and dn53BP1 were not performed due to unavailability of selective antibodies for these inhibitors. Analysis of editing outcomes revealed that expression of the DNA RFs from LVs did not have an effect on HDR levels, compared to "No RF" or GFP controls, independently of the way that Cas9 was delivered (plasmid vs. RNP) and the DNA donor template used (ssODN vs. AAV6; **Figure 1E**).

To test whether the improvements in HDR levels observed in **Figure 1B** were a true effect of the DNA RFs or merely a result of plasmid co-electroporation, we tested a GFP control plasmid co-electroporated at varying amounts (0.3–10 µg) with Cas9 and sgRNA plasmid delivery. The levels of gene editing were measured by high throughput sequencing (HTS) of the *HBB* target site. Increases in both HDR and NHEJ were detected with the addition of increasing amounts of GFP control plasmid (**Supplementary Figure 2A**). These data suggest that the increases in HDR levels observed earlier might be an artifact of plasmid co-electroporation and not the biological effect of DNA RFs.

Next, we went on to compare delivery of DNA RFs and GFP control as LV, integrase-defective lentiviral vector (IDLV) or plasmid. K562 cells were transduced with LV and IDLV 24 h prior to electroporation of gene editing reagents at a MOI that resulted in similar GFP expression to GFP plasmid electroporation at 24 h (refer to **Figure 1A** for timeline). Although not statistically significant, all plasmids (CtIP^{DE} + PALB2^{KR} + i53, RAD52 + dn53BP1, and GFP control) increased both HDR and NHEJ levels ∼2-fold, while none of the LVs or IDLVs had an effect on either HDR or NHEJ (**Supplementary Figure 2B**). Of note, additional transduction timepoints and varying MOIs were tested, but still did not improve HDR levels (data not shown). Together, these data suggest that plasmid co-electroporation induced a response in K562 cells that increased DNA repair levels via both HDR and NHEJ pathways. However, it does not appear that the overexpression of ectopic DNA RFs directly improved HDR levels.

Evaluating the Effects of DNA RF Overexpression on Gene Editing Levels in Primary Human HSPCs

To evaluate the effects of DNA RF overexpression on gene editing levels in primary human CD34$^+$ HSPCs, DNA RFs were delivered by either LVs or as *in vitro* transcribed (IVT) mRNAs due to the toxicity associated with plasmid electroporation in HSPCs (Hollis et al., 2006). Cas9 endonuclease was delivered as RNP (Cas9 protein + IVT sgRNA) or as mRNA (IVT Cas9 mRNA + IVT sgRNA), and donor template was delivered either as ssODN or AAV6. DNA RF were delivered as LVs to the HSPCs 24 h prior to electroporation, and IVT DNA RF mRNAs were co-electroporated with the gene editing reagents (**Figure 2A**).

No benefit in HDR or NHEJ levels were observed with the addition of DNA RFs compared to controls irrespective of delivery method (**Figures 2B,C**). Interestingly, while the levels of HDR achieved with Cas9 RNP and Cas9 mRNA ranged between 5 and 15%, the levels of NHEJ were higher with Cas9 RNP (35–60%) compared to Cas9 mRNA (12–15%). The HDR/NHEJ ratio

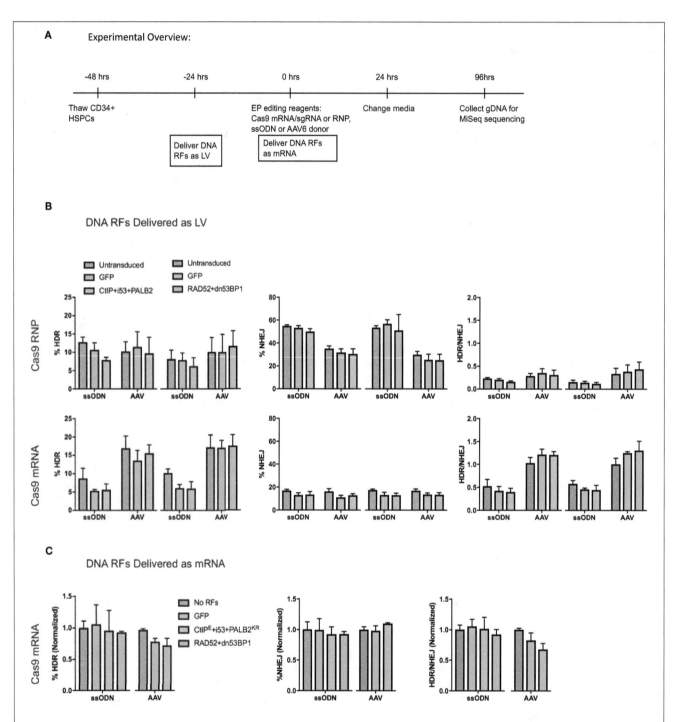

FIGURE 2 | (A) Experimental overview of CD34+ HSPC transduction and electroporation of DNA RFs and editing reagents. DNA RFs were co-expressed with the gene editing reagents. Cas9 nuclease was delivered either as RNP (100 pmol Cas9 protein + 4.5 μg of IVT sgRNA) or IVT Cas9 mRNA (5 μg) + IVT sgRNA (5 μg); donor template was delivered either as AAV6 (MOI 2e4) or ssODN (3 μg). HDR and NHEJ levels were measured by HTS four days post-electroporation. HDR/NHEJ ratio was calculated. **(B)** DNA repair factors delivered as LV 24 h prior to electroporation of editing reagents. n = 4 biological replicates for all CtIPDE+PALB2KR+i53 LV experiments (Cas9 RNP or Cas9mRNA); n = 8–12 for RAD52+dn53BP1 LV experiments using Cas9 RNP, or n = 4 for RAD52+dn53BP1 LV experiments using Cas9 mRNA. Error bars, mean ± SD. Differences are not significant if not specified, based on Wilcoxon rank sum test. **(C)** DNA RFs were co-delivered as IVT mRNA with editing reagents. n = 2–6 biological replicates for all conditions. Data are normalized to "no RFs" conditions for each set of experiments. Error bars, mean ± SD. Differences are not significant if not specified, based on Wilcoxon rank sum test.

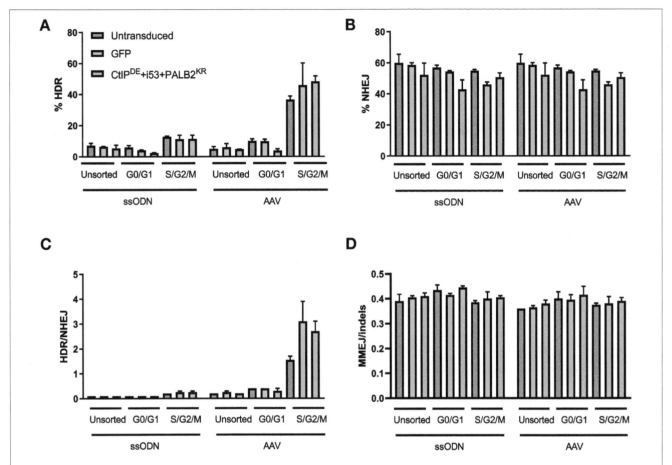

FIGURE 3 | CtIP^{DE}+PALB2^{KR} + i53 overexpression in G1 phase of the cell cycle does not activate HDR. **(A–D)** Gene editing levels in sorted populations. Hoescht stain was used to discriminate G0/G1 and S/G2/M phases. Cells were pre-transduced with the indicated DNA RFs or GFP LVs, sorted into cell cycle phases and then electroporated with Cas9 RNP and ssODN or transduced with an AAV6 donor template immediately after electroporation. HDR and NHEJ levels were measured by HTS. **(A)** HDR, **(B)** NHEJ, **(C)** HDR/NHEJ, **(D)** MMEJ/indels, in unsorted, G0/G1-sorted, or S/G2/M-sorted populations. $n = 2$ biological replicates. Error bars, mean ± SD.

was lower for all conditions edited with a ssODN compared to an AAV6 donor (**Figures 2B,C**). These differences in Cas9 nuclease delivery and donor template utilization, although beyond the scope of this study, suggest interesting distinctions in DNA damage repair pathways.

Because prior experiments were performed on unsorted CD34$^+$ HSPCs, the effects on gene editing outcomes from overexpression of the DNA RFs CtIP^{DE}, PALB2^{KR}, and i53, which we hypothesized would initiate HDR in G1 phase of the cell cycle, may have been overlooked (Orthwein et al., 2015). To evaluate whether these DNA RFs improved gene editing outcomes specifically in G0/G1 phases, HSPCs were transduced with the indicated DNA RFs or GFP LVs 24 h prior to fluorescence-activated cell sorting (FACS) into G0/G1 or S/G2/M populations, and the populations in the different cell cycle stages were immediately electroporated with editing reagents.

As expected, the levels of HDR were higher in the S/G2/M population compared to G0/G1-sorted and unsorted control for all conditions, while the levels of NHEJ were similar across all conditions and cell cycle stages (**Figures 3A,B**). Of note, while

the levels of HDR in unsorted and G0/G1-sorted cells were comparable for both donor templates (5–7%), the levels of HDR in the S/G2/M-sorted cells edited with an AAV6 donor were higher (36–50%) than in cells edited with a ssODN donor (11–13%), resulting in an increased HDR/NHEJ ratio with the AAV6 donor. However, there were no statistically significant differences in the levels of HDR, NHEJ, or MMEJ between cells transduced with the DNA RFs, GFP, or untransduced cells within a cell cycle stage population (**Figures 3A–D**). There was a slight increase in the HDR/NHEJ ratio in cells transduced with the DNA RFs (1.7-fold) or GFP (2-fold) relative to untransduced cells within the S/G2/M population edited with an AAV6 donor (**Figure 3C**). These data suggest that overexpression of CtIP^{DE}, PALB2^{KR} and i53 did not result in improved gene editing outcomes in G0/G1 cell cycle phase.

Evaluating a Panel of Cas9 Fusion Variants to Promote HDR or Decrease NHEJ

As previously stated, global, albeit transient, manipulation of DNA RFs may pose a threat to genome integrity (Jayavaradhan

TABLE 2 | Panel of Cas9-fusion variants assessed in this study.

Cas9 variant		Description
Cas9	Cas9	Wild-type Cas9
Cas9-hGem	Cas9-hGem	hGeminin is degraded by the APC/Cdh1 complex during G1 phase when the NHEJ pathway is selectively active over HDR (Gutschner et al., 2016)
Cas9-hCtIP	Cas9-hCtIP Cas9-GSG-CtIP* Cas9-TGS-CtIP**	hCtIP "HDR enhancer element" is involved in the DNA end resection. Involved in recruiting other factors to initiate repair (Charpentier et al., 2018).
	Cas9-hGem-hCtIP	
Cas9-UL12	Cas9-UL12	UL12 increases recombination by the single-strand annealing (SSA) pathway and inhibits NHEJ (Balasubramanian et al., 2010).
	Cas9-hGem-UL12	
Cas9-dn53BP1	Cas9-dn53BP1	A mouse dominant negative 53BP1 is expected to reduce accumulation of 53BP1 at the DSB site, thus suppressing NHEJ (Paulsen et al., 2017)
	Cas9-DN1S Cas9-GSG-DN1S*	Amino acids 1,231–1,644 of human 53BP1; (Jayavaradhan et al., 2019)

*GSG—signifies a 12 amino acid linker made up of repeating Gly-Ser-Gly residues (GGGS)×3.
**TGS—signifies a 12 amino acid linker made up of repeating Tyr-Gly-Ser residues (TGS)×4.

et al., 2019). Although extensive toxicity due to global overexpression of DNA RFs was not seen in this work (data not shown), no improvement in gene editing was observed either when these RFs were over-expressed, either stably (LV) or transiently (IVT mRNA). As an alternative approach to deliver these DNA RFs to the site of the Cas9-induced DSB, we have produced a series of novel Cas9 fusion proteins by adding sequences encoding proteins that may modulate DNA repair pathways by promoting HDR or inhibiting NHEJ (**Table 2**). One set of fusions contained the HDR enhancer element of hCtIP (Cas9-hCtIP; Charpentier et al., 2018). CtIP is necessary for DSB resection to generate single stranded-DNA (ssDNA), required for homology searching and strand invasion, and therefore is required for homologous recombination (HR). We have made modifications to this Cas9 variant by adding a flexible linker between the C-terminus of Cas9 and the N-terminus of the hCtIP fragment (**Supplementary Figure 3A**). The Cas9-GSG-CtIP variant contains a 12 amino acid linker made up of repeating Gly-Ser-Gly residues (GGGS)×3. Cas9-TGS-CtIP contains a 12 amino acid linker made up of repeating Tyr-Gly-Ser residues (TGS)×4. Moreover, we have constructed a double fusion variant containing a fragment of the hGem protein fused between Cas9 and the hCtIP fragment (Cas9-hGem-hCtIP).

We have also constructed a Cas9 variant which contains a 126 amino acid N-terminal fragment from the Herpes Simplex Virus protein UL12, fused to the C-terminus of Cas9 (Reuven et al., 2019). UL12 may recruit subsets of the critical HDR complex proteins to the nuclease-mediated cleavage site, increasing the yield of HDR–mediated editing outcomes. We have made

subsequent modifications to the Cas9-UL12 variant by adding the hGem fragment (Cas9-hGem-UL12).

The Cas9-dn53BP1 variant contains a fragment of the mouse 53BP1, a DNA repair protein involved in the recruitment of NHEJ factors to a DSB, fused to Cas9. Previous reports have shown that global transient expression of dn53BP1 in cell lines can decrease NHEJ. We have fused this fragment to the C-terminus of Cas9 to assess its ability to block the recruitment of 53BP1 specifically at a Cas9-induced break site. We have tested other dominant negative 53BP1 Cas9 fusion variants, namely Cas9-DN1S (Jayavaradhan et al., 2019; **Supplementary Figure 3B**). To date, this Cas9-variant has only been assessed in cell lines.

Editing in a K562 BFP Reporter Cell Line for Preliminary Assessment of Cas9 Variants

To initially screen a panel of these novel Cas9 fusion variants, as well as the fusion of Cas9 to a fragment from hGem to destabilize Cas9 in the G1 phase as we previously described (Lomova et al., 2019), for their ability to promote HDR or limit NHEJ, the sequences encoding these Cas9 fusion proteins were cloned into MND-LTR-U3-expression plasmids. These were co-electroporated with a plasmid encoding a sgRNA targeting a stably integrated monoallelic BFP reporter gene in a K562 cell line (Richardson et al., 2018; **Figure 4A**). Cas9 editing at the BFP locus results in either disruption of the BFP gene by NHEJ or modification to the eGFP gene by HDR, depending on the activated DNA repair pathway and presence of a donor template. Formation of either in-frame or frameshift indels by the NHEJ pathway at the target site will result in disruption of the BFP gene, resulting in non-fluorescent cells [BFP−/GFP−; non-fluorescent {NF}; Glaser et al., 2016]. The addition of a ssODN donor template containing a single point mutation that alters the 66th amino acid of the BFP gene from a histidine to a tyrosine results in conversion of the BFP gene to eGFP upon HDR (BFP−/GFP+; "GFP"). The donor also contains an additional single nucleotide polymorphism (SNP) at the PAM recognition site to prevent re-cleavage by the Cas9 nuclease of the HDR-edited sequence. Unedited cells will remain BFP+/GFP− ("BFP").

Preliminary comparison of the Cas9 fusion variants by phenotypic assessment of edited cells using flow cytometry resulted in baseline wild-type Cas9 editing of 68.2–79% NF cells (NHEJ) and 13.5–18.4% GFP+ (HDR) cells. Editing with the Cas9-hGem fusion resulted in slightly reduced gene disruption (61.5–69.5%), and similar levels of GFP+ cells as with wild-type Cas9 (16.3–19.1%; **Figures 4B,D,F**). We have previously reported that the Cas9-hGem fusion reduces NHEJ by 50% in primary human HSPCs at the *HBB* locus (Lomova et al., 2019). We believe that the limited decrease in NHEJ with Cas9-hGem seen using this K562 BFP reporter assay is due to the differences in cell cycle distribution of K562 cells relative to HSPCs (**Supplementary Figure 4**).

Among the Cas9-hCtIP variants tested, editing with the Cas9-hCtIP and the Cas9-GSG-hCtIP fusion proteins resulted in a ~15% reduction of NF cells (NHEJ), with a slight reduction in GFP+ cells compared to Cas9 editing. Cas9-TGS-hCtIP had a

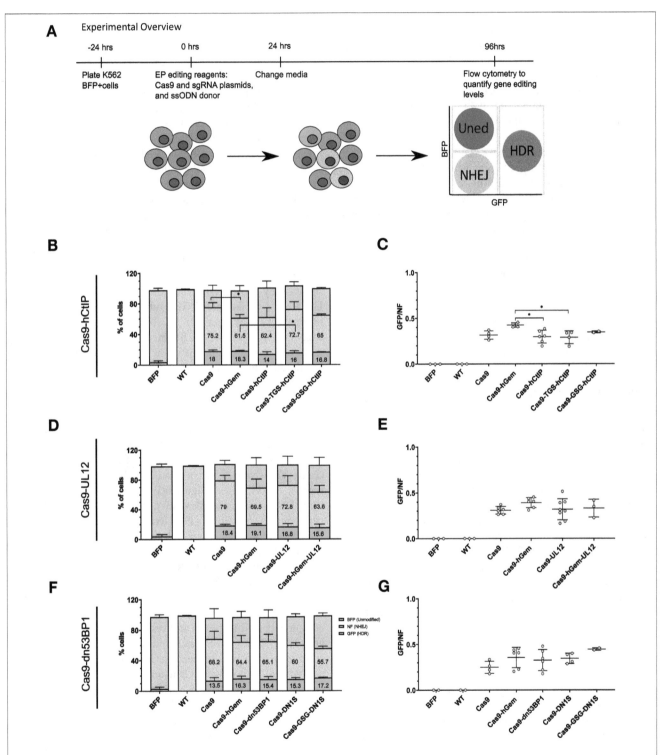

FIGURE 4 | Preliminary assessment of Cas9 variants to modulate local gene editing outcomes in a K562 BFP reporter cell line. **(A)** Experimental overview of electroporation of Cas9 variants as plasmid into a K562 BFP reporter cell line. K562 BFP cells were electroporated with 1 μg Cas9 variant plasmid, 1 μg of sgRNA plasmid targeting the BFP gene, and a ssODN donor (3 μM). Cells were cultured for 4 days post-electroporation prior to analysis by flow cytometry. **(B–G)** Proportion of GFP+, BFP+, or NF cells and GFP/NF ratio of cells edited with Cas9-hCtIP variants, $n = 2$–6 biological replicates **(B,C)**, and Cas9-UL12 variants, $n = 3$–8 biological replicates **(D,E)**, and Cas9-dn53BP1, $n = 2$–6 biological replicates **(F,G)**. Error bars, mean ± SD. Differences are not significant if not specified, $^*p < 0.05$, based on Wilcoxon rank sum test.

similar editing profile to Cas9 alone (**Figure 4B**). In this reporter system, the GFP/NF ratio is used to estimate the HDR/NHEJ ratio. Cas9-hCtIP and Cas9-TGS-CtIP has significantly reduced GFP/NF ratios compared to Cas9-hGem (**Figure 4C**).

Among the Cas9-UL12 variants tested, the Cas9-UL12 fusion did not alter repair pathway choice compared to Cas9 or Cas9-hGem. Interestingly, editing with the Cas9-hGem-UL12 fusion led to a 20% decrease in BFP disruption (63.6% compared to 79%), with a modest decline in HDR levels compared to Cas9 (15.6% compared to 18.4%; **Figure 4D**). However, the GFP/NF ratio was not significantly different among these Cas9-UL12 variants compared to Cas9 or Cas9-hGem (**Figure 4E**).

Among the Cas9-dn53BP1 variants tested, all variants reduced the percentage of resulting NF cells compared to Cas9. Cas9-dn53BP1 editing resulted in a 4.5% relative decrease in NF cells (65.1% compared to 68.2%), while maintaining the level of GFP$^+$ cells. Cas9-DN1S and Cas9-GSG-DN1S editing resulted in a 12 and 18.3% reduction of NF cells, respectively, compared to Cas9 alone. Cas9-GSG-DN1S had similar levels of GFP$^+$ cells to Cas9-hGem, with a 13.5% reduction in NF cells (55.7% compared to 69.2%). These findings suggest that Cas9-DN1S and Cas9-GSG-DN1S are the most effective variants at reducing NHEJ compared to Cas9 and Cas9-hGem when editing cell lines. (**Figures 4F,G**).

Assessing Cas9 Variant Editing in Primary Human CD34$^+$ HSPCs

Following preliminary assessment of the Cas9 variants in a K562 BFP reporter cell line, a subset of Cas9 variants [Cas9-hGem, Cas9-hCtIP, Cas9-hGem-hCtIP, Cas9-UL12, Cas9-hGem-UL12, Cas9-dn53BP1, Cas9-DN1S] were tested in primary human CD34$^+$ HSPCs by targeted editing of the SCD causative mutation at the *HBB* locus. HSPCs were edited with IVT Cas9 mRNA and IVT sgRNA targeting exon 1 of the *HBB* locus, along with a ssODN or AAV6 donor conferring modifications at the site of the sickle mutation and the PAM site (**Figure 5A**). Since the Cas9 variant transcripts vary in length (4–6 kb), going forward, we modified the protocol to test these variants at equimolar amounts rather than equal weight (**Supplementary Figures 5A,B**). Editing outcomes were assessed by HTS of the *HBB* target site. Viability of HSPCs at 24 h post-electroporation was unaffected by the Cas9 variants compared to Cas9 or Cas9-hGem (**Figure 5B**).

Gene editing with Cas9 mRNA and an AAV6 donor led to ~14% HDR and 15% NHEJ in HSPCs edited with Cas9 on average across all experiments (**Figures 6A,D,G**). Cas9-hGem editing with the AAV6 donor maintained levels of HDR and decreased the frequency of NHEJ by one third compared to Cas9 (10 vs. 15%, respectively), as previously reported (Lomova et al., 2019).

Editing by the Cas9-hCtIP was consistently low, presumably due to reduced nuclease activity compared to Cas9; this was partially rescued by the addition of the hGem fragment between Cas9 and hCtIP (Cas9-hGem-hCtIP). Interestingly, while the hGem-hCtIP double fusion did not result in an increase in HDR relative to Cas9 or Cas9-hGem, similar levels of NHEJ were achieved between the Cas9-hGem-hCtIP and Cas9-hGem variants (**Figure 6A**). There was consistently significantly improved HDR/NHEJ ratio for variants containing

hGem compared to Cas9 alone (Cas9-hGem, Cas9-hGem-hCtIP; **Figure 6B**).

CtIP has been implicated in stimulating significant MMEJ, an HDR-mediated event that leads to specific sized indels, in the presence of homologous sequences flanking a DSB. We have noted a frequent 9 base pair deletion in *HBB* among the indels around the Cas9-induced DSB that is presumed to be an MMEJ event. When assessing MMEJ out of total indel-forming events (MMEJ/indels), we noted that Cas9 variants containing the hCtIP fragment had higher levels of MMEJ, suggesting that the hCtIP fragment is biologically active but is not inducing HR or SSTR (**Figure 6C, Supplementary Figure 6**). This finding may be valuable for targeted gene editing in which the end goal is to induce a specific MMEJ-mediated deletion (Métais et al., 2019).

When comparing Cas9 variants containing a UL12 fusion in the context of an AAV6 donor, there were no remarkable differences in HDR or NHEJ by either Cas9-UL12 or Cas9-hGem-UL12 relative to Cas9, while Cas9-UL12 lead to significantly higher NHEJ than Cas9-hGem (**Figure 6D**). Cas9-UL12 had a similar HDR/NHEJ ratio to Cas9 alone, while Cas9-hGem-UL12 had a similar HDR/NHEJ ratio to Cas9-hGem, suggesting that the hGem fragment, and not UL12, is driving these differences (**Figure 6E**). The ratios of MMEJ/indels were not different between Cas9 and Cas9-UL12, or Cas9-hGem and Cas9-hGem-UL12 (**Figure 6F**).

Among the dn53BP1 variants tested, Cas9-dn53BP1 resulted in significantly reduced NHEJ levels, compared to Cas9, but still higher than Cas9-hGem (**Figure 6G**). Editing with Cas9-DN1S using an AAV6 donor resulted in decreased levels of HDR (10% from 14%) while similar levels of NHEJ relative to Cas9, contrary to what was seen previously in this work and in previous reports in cell lines (**Figure 6G**; Jayavaradhan et al., 2019). Cas9-DN1S editing resulted in a decreased HDR/NHEJ ratio compared to Cas9 and Cas9-hGem (**Figure 6H**). No differences in MMEJ/indels ratios were observed with the Cas9-dn53BP1 variants (**Figure 6I**).

Gene editing with Cas9 mRNA and a ssODN donor resulted in ~7% HDR and 13% NHEJ in human HSPCs, while Cas9-hGem editing lead to a slight increase in HDR (10%) with no reduction in NHEJ (11%; **Figure 7A**). As previously reported, Cas9-hCtIP editing appeared impaired and resulted in lower levels of HDR and NHEJ relative to Cas9 and Cas9-hGem. However, the addition of the hGem fragment to Cas9-hCtIP improved nuclease activity similar to Cas9-hGem levels. Levels of HDR did not change for the Cas9-UL12 variants when compared to Cas9-hGem in these experiments; however, Cas9-UL12 editing did result in an increase in NHEJ (from ~12.5 to ~17%), suggesting that the addition of UL12 may be promoting exonuclease activity (as described in Schumacher et al., 2012), but expression of UL12 alone may not be sufficient to promote HDR with a ssODN donor. Among the Cas9-dn53BP1 variants tested, there was a slight decrease in HDR with Cas9-dn53BP1 compared to Cas9-hGem, falling to similar levels as Cas9 alone. Interestingly, editing with Cas9-DN1S did not reduce NHEJ in the context of editing primary HSPCs with a ssODN donor (**Figure 7A**).

Overall, the HDR/NHEJ ratio increased relative to Cas9 for all variants containing the hGem fragment; there was no further improvement to the HDR/NHEJ ratio by the additional fusion

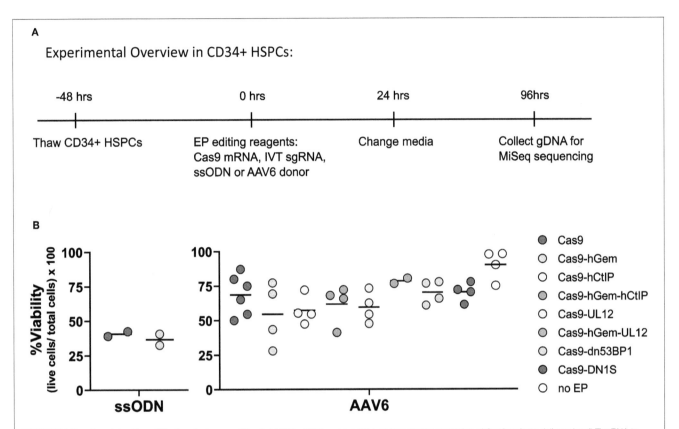

FIGURE 5 | Experimental outline of Cas9 variant gene editing in HSPCs. **(A)** Experimental overview of electroporation of Cas9 variants delivered as IVT mRNA to CD34$^+$ HSPCs. Cas9 variants were electroporated at equimolar amounts (3 pmol) with 120 pmol of IVT sgRNA targeting the SCD mutation at the *HBB* locus, and either a ssODN (3 μM) or AAV6 donor (MOI 2e4). Editing outcomes were measured by MiSeq HTS 4 days post-electroporation. **(B)** Viability of CD34$^+$ HSPCs edited with Cas9 variants, and an ssODN or AAV6 donor 24 h post-electroporation. $n = 2$–6 biological replicates. Center line represents mean. Differences are not significant if not specified, based on Wilcoxon rank sum test.

proteins (**Figure 7B**). All variants containing the CtIP fragment had increased MMEJ/indel ratios relative to Cas9 and Cas9-hGem (**Figure 7C**). In summary, the Cas9 variants containing hGem had the most favorable HDR/NHEJ ratios irrespective of donor template type (AAV6 or ssODN; **Figures 8A,B**).

DISCUSSION

In this study, we investigated whether gene editing outcomes can be modified by manipulating DNA repair pathways. Specifically, we aimed to increase the frequency of HDR and/or reduce NHEJ-mediated repair by global and local manipulation of endogenous DNA repair pathways in human hematopoietic stem and progenitor cells. A panel of DNA RFs that have been shown to promote HDR or inhibit NHEJ in various cell lines were assessed for their ability to manipulate gene editing outcomes in K562 cells and in primary human CD34$^+$ HSPCs, when co-expressed with editing. To synchronize DNA RF expression to the time of Cas9-induced DSB and DNA repair, K562s were pre-transduced with LVs expressing DNA RFs. Constitutive overexpression of the DNA RFs was demonstrated by western blots. However, the expressed DNA RFs had no effect on HDR or NHEJ levels when cells were edited with Cas9 plasmid or Cas9

RNP targeting the site of the SCD mutation at the *HBB* locus relative to cells that were untransduced or transduced with a GFP control LV.

Similar gene editing trends were seen when DNA RFs were globally overexpressed in CD34$^+$ HSPCs edited with Cas9 mRNA or Cas9 RNP targeting the *HBB* locus. Delivery of the DNA RFs as either constitutively expressed LVs or transiently expressed mRNA did not alter HDR or NHEJ relative to "no RFs" or GFP control conditions. This signified that the combination of DNA RFs used in this study was unable to manipulate endogenous DNA repair to favor HDR over NHEJ.

We hypothesized that the combination of CtIP^{DE} + PALB2^{KR} + i53 DNA, would specifically promote HDR in the G1 phase of the cell cycle. Sequencing of editing outcomes in bulk (unsynchronized) HSPCs may mask this phenomenon. To overcome this, we sorted pre-transduced HSPCs that expressed the various factors of interest immediately prior to gene editing into different cell cycle populations, and assessed editing outcomes in the G0/G1 and S/G2/M sorted populations. As expected, levels of HDR were higher in the S/G2/M sorted population relative to G0/G1 or unsorted populations, as HDR is selectively active in S/G2 phases of the cell cycle. However, no further improvement in HDR was seen with the expression

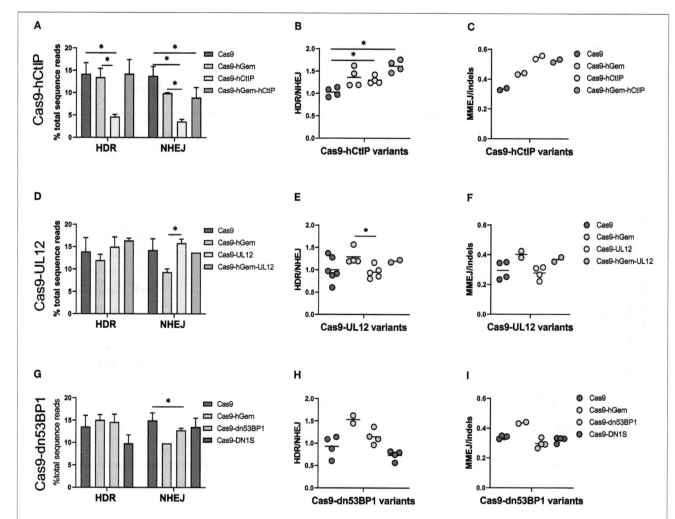

FIGURE 6 | Cas9 variant gene editing of the β-globin locus with an AAV6 donor reveals distinctive DNA repair outcomes in HSPCs. CD34+ HSPCs edited with Cas9 variants (3 pmol Cas9 mRNA + 120 pmol IVT sgRNA) and an AAV6 donor (MOI 2e4). Editing outcomes were measured by MiSeq HTS 4 days post-electroporation. Cas9 and Cas9-hGem were used as controls. **(A–C)** Gene editing outcomes with Cas9-hCtIP variants. **(A)** HDR and NHEJ. $n = 4$ biological replicates). Error bars, mean ± SD. **(B)** HDR/NHEJ. $n = 4$ biological replicates Center line represents mean **(C)** MMEJ/indels. $n = 2$ biological replicates. Center line represents mean. **(D–F)** Gene editing outcomes with Cas9-UL12 variants. **(D)** HDR and NHEJ. $n = 2–6$ biological replicates. Error bars, mean ± SD. **(E)** HDR/NHEJ. $n = 2–6$ biological replicates Center line represents mean **(F)** MMEJ/indels. $n = 2–4$ biological replicates. Center line represents mean. **(G–I)** Gene editing outcomes with Cas9-dn53BP1 variants. **(G)** HDR and NHEJ. $n = 2–4$ biological replicates. Error bars, mean ± SD. **(H)** HDR/NHEJ, $n = 2–4$ biological replicates. Center line represents mean **(I)** MMEJ/indels. $n = 2–4$ biological replicates. Center line represents mean. Differences are not significant if not specified, *$p < 0.05$, based on Wilcoxon rank sum test.

of combined CtIP^{DE} + PALB2^{KR} + i53, suggesting that the expression of these combination of factors alone is not enough to manipulate DNA repair pathways in primary HSPCs.

In a parallel approach, we assessed how localization of DNA RFs to the Cas9-induced DSB site by fusing DNA RFs directly to the C- terminus of Cas9 would affect gene editing outcomes. We tested a panel of Cas9 fusion protein variants for their ability to promote HDR or to inhibit NHEJ initially in a K562 BFP reporter cell line, then in primary human HSPCs. As previously reported, editing HSPCs with Cas9-hGem and an AAV6 consistently improved the HDR/NHEJ ratio compared to Cas9 editing, predominantly by a decrease in NHEJ alleles (Lomova et al., 2019). A similar increase in the HDR/NHEJ ratio was seen with Cas9-hGem editing and

a ssODN donor; however, these results seem to be driven by an increase in HDR, rather than a decrease in NHEJ. An increase in the MMEJ/indels ratio was also seen in Cas9-hGem edited cells.

Cas9-hCtIP editing in K562 BFP cells was comparable to Cas9 editing; however, Cas9-hCtIP nuclease activity was severely impaired in the context of HSPCs gene editing. This may suggest differential DNA repair states between K562 cells and primary HSPCs, where CtIP expression during an HDR non-permissive state may impair canonical HDR and NHEJ repair systems. Gene editing by Cas9-hGem-hCtIP had a similar profile to Cas9-hGem when assessing HDR, NHEJ, and the HDR/NHEJ ratio. However, both CtIP-containing Cas9 fusions promoted an increase in MMEJ-mediated repair outcomes, confirming

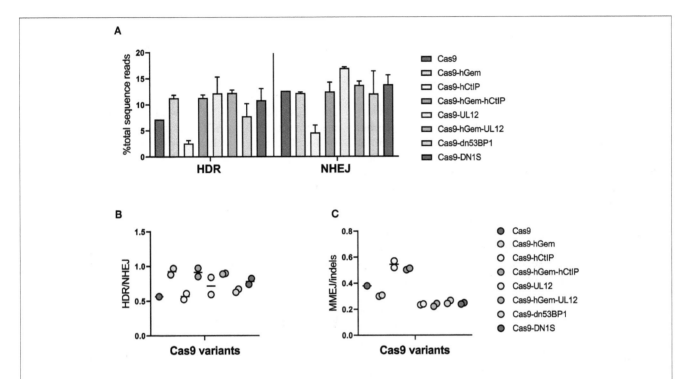

FIGURE 7 | Cas9 variant gene editing of the *HBB* locus with a ssODN donor. CD34+ HSPCs edited with Cas9 variants (3 pmol Cas9 mRNA + 120 pmol IVT sgRNA) and ssODN donor (3 μM). Editing outcomes were measured by MiSeq HTS 4 days post-electroporation. Cas9 and Cas9-hGem were used as controls. **(A)** HDR and NHEJ. **(B)** HDR/NHEJ n = 2 biological replicates. Error bars, mean ± SD. **(C)** MMEJ/indels. n = 2 biological replicates. Center line represents mean.

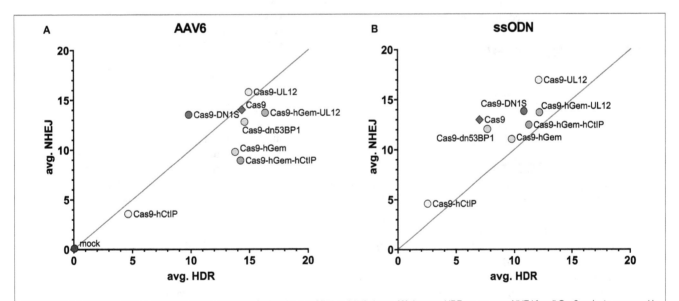

FIGURE 8 | Comparison of averageCas9 variant editing in HSPCs with a ssODN or AAV6 donor. **(A)** Average HDR vs. average NHEJ for all Cas9 variants assessed in this study. The *y* axis reflects average NHEJ editing, and the *x* axis reflects the average HDR editing of each variant at the *HBB* locus. Average editing of Cas9 variants targeting the SCD mutation in CD34+ HSPCs with an AAV6 donor **(A)** or an ssODN donor **(B)**.

that the CtIP element is biologically active and is able to shift repair toward an error-prone HDR pathway. Cas9-UL12 editing resulted in higher NHEJ relative to Cas9 and Cas9-hGem when a ssODN donor was used. The N-terminal domain of UL12 used in this study is sufficient to recruit the MRN complex, a vital step toward HDR (Reuven et al., 2019). However, it does not possess

exonuclease activity which may further stimulate the production of 3′ overhangs and have a stronger influence on shifting repair outcomes toward HDR. Cas9-DN1S, expressing dominant negative 53BP1 fragment, effectively decreased the frequency of NHEJ in K562 cells, but did not have a similar effect in primary HSPCs.

Interestingly, we noted that HDR levels increased in K562 cells that were edited using a Cas9/sgRNA plasmid and DNA RFs or GFP expressed as plasmid, suggesting that the increase in editing is not directly related to the DNA RFs but to plasmid co-delivery. No increase in HDR was seen when K562 cells were edited with Cas9 RNP and plasmid DNA RFs. A recent report suggests that co-transfection of large plasmid cassettes with small plasmid vectors (3 kb) can improve transfection efficiency and viability of cell lines and primary cell types (Søndergaard et al., 2020). These findings could explain our observation of increased editing in K562 cells only when Cas9 plasmid was used in combination with DNA RF or GFP plasmids. However, other potential hypotheses remain and need to be tested; plasmid electroporation may increase transcription and/or translation of Cas9 plasmid, thus increasing total Cas9 activity and thereby increasing HDR, or plasmid electroporation may enhance the DNA damage response in K562 cells, enhancing DNA repair pathways and increasing HDR and NHEJ levels in the cells.

Overall, this work underlines the complexity of DNA repair regulation and the challenges to harnessing it to achieve curative gene editing levels in therapeutically relevant cell types. The consistent performance of the Cas9 fusions with the fragment of human Geminin domain to improve the ratio of HDR to NHEJ events strongly supports further evaluation of this variant for potential clinical applications. The ability of the CtIP fusions to promote MMEJ may also have specific indications. Continued efforts to successfully manipulate DNA repair pathways may lead to improved methods of gene editing for gene therapy.

MATERIALS AND METHODS

K562 Cells

K562 cells were modified to contain sickle cell disease-causing mutation, as described previously (Hoban et al., 2016). K562 BFP cells were modified to contain monoallelic copy of the BFP gene, as described in Richardson et al. (2016).

Primary Human CD34+ Cells

Leukopaks from healthy donors were purchased from HemaCare (HemaCare BioResearch Products; Van Nuys, CA). Mobilized peripheral blood (mPB) was collected from normal, healthy donors on days 5 and 6 after 5 days of stimulation with granulocyte-colony stimulating factor (G-CSF). Briefly, leukapheresis bags were washed three times with PBS/EDTA at room temperature (RT) and spun down at 150×g. Platelet depletion was performed from the centrifuged bags at each wash step using a plasma expressor extractor (Fenwal). The subsequent enrichment of CD34+ cells was done by using the CliniMACS Plus (Miltenyi; Bergish Gladbach, Germany). Cells were cryopreserved in CryoStor CS5 (Stemcell Technologies; Vancouver, Canada) using a CryoMed controlled-rate freezer (Thermo Fisher Scientific; Waltham, MA).

Cell Culture

K562 cells were cultured in RPMI medium + 10% heat-inactivated fetal bovine serum [HI FBS (Gibco/ThermoFisher; Waltham, MA)] + 1% penicillin, streptomycin, glutamine [PSQ (Gemini Bio-Products; Sacramento, CA)], and were kept at a density between 1×10^5 and 1×10^6 cells per ml. Healthy human CD34+ cells from mPB (peripheral blood stem cells, PBSCs) were thawed in pre-warmed X-Vivo 15 medium (Lonza; Basel, Switzerland) with 1% PSQ, pelleted at 500×g for 5 min, and resuspended at 5×10^5 cells/mL in pre-warmed X-Vivo 15 medium with PSQ and SFT cytokines [50 ng/mL stem cell factor (SCF), 50 ng/mL fms-related tyrosine kinase 3 ligand (Flt3-L), and 50 ng/mL thrombopoietin (TPO)] (Peprotech; Rocky Hill, NJ). Cells were pre-stimulated at 37°C and 5% CO_2 incubator for 48 h.

LV/IDLV Transduction

To deliver LV/IDLV DNA RFs, cells were transduced with the MOIs indicated in figure legends for 24 h (additional time points were tested, but data not shown). Transduction enhancers (PGE2 and Poloxamer Synperonic F108) were added during transduction, as described elsewhere (Masiuk et al., 2019).

K562 Cell Electroporation With DNA RFs

K562 cells were split 1:5 1 day before the electroporation. Where indicated, the cells were transduced with LV or IDLV 24 h prior to electroporation. On the day of electroporation, the cells were counted on ViCell (Beckman Coulter; Brea, CA), 2×10^5 cells per condition were centrifuged at 90×g for 15 min at RT, resuspended in 20 µl of SF electroporation buffer (Lonza; Basel, Switzerland), combined with Cas9 plasmid or RNP, 3 µM ssODN (where applicable), and DNA RF or GFP plasmids (where applicable). The cells were electroporated on Amaxa 4D Nucleofector X Unit (Lonza; Basel, Switzerland) using FF-120 setting. After electroporation, the cells were rested in electroporation strips for 10 min at RT, and then recovered with 500 µl of RPMI medium + 10% HI FBS (Gibco/ThermoFisher; Waltham, MA) + 1% PSQ (Gemini BioProducts; Sacramento, CA). AAV6 donor template was added to recovery medium where applicable. Twenty-four hours post electroporation, the cells were re-plated into fresh medium. The cells were harvested 4 days post electroporation for gDNA extraction to evaluate gene editing levels. gDNA was extracted using PureLink Genomic DNA Mini Kit (Invitrogen/ThermoFisher Scientific; Carlsbad, CA).

CD34+ HSPC Cell Electroporation With DNA RFs

For electroporation, 2×10^5 (or 1×10^6 for FACS experiment) cells per condition were pelleted at 90×g for 15 min at RT, resuspended in 100 µl of BTXpress Electroporation buffer (Harvard Bioscience, Inc; Holliston, MA), combined with pre-aliquoted ssODN (where applicable), RNP (100 pmol Cas9 protein + 4.5 µg of IVT sgRNA) or 5 µg Cas9 mRNA + 5 µg of IVT sgRNA, kept on ice, and pulsed once at 250 V for 5 ms in the BTX ECM 830 Square Wave Electroporator (Harvard Apparatus; Holliston, MA). After electroporation, cells were rested in cuvettes for 10 min at RT, and then recovered with 400 µl (or 2.4 mL, for 1×10^6 cells) of X-Vivo 15 medium (with PSQ and SFT cytokines). Where applicable, recovery media contained AAV6 (multiplicity of infection, MOI = 2e4) to introduce 4 SNPs (Virovek; Hayward, CA). The cells were cultured in a 24-well (or 6-well, for 1×10^6 cells) plate at 37°C, 5% CO_2 incubator. Twenty-four hours post electroporation, the cells were diluted 1:2 with trypan blue and counted manually using a hemocytometer to determine viability (number of live cells/number of total cells $\times$ 100) and fold expansion (number of cells 24 h after electroporation/number of cells before electroporation). Cells were re-plated into 1 mL (or 5 mL, for 1×10^6 cells) of myeloid expansion medium [Iscove's Modified Dulbecco's Medium (IMDM, Thermo Fisher Scientific; Waltham, MA) + 20% FBS (HI FBS, Gibco/ThermoFisher; Waltham, MA) + 5 ng/mL Interleukin 3 (IL3), 10 ng/mL Interleukin 6 (IL6), 25 ng/mL SCF (Peprotech; Rocky Hill, NJ)], and cultured for 4 days prior to harvesting for genomic DNA (gDNA). gDNA was extracted using PureLink Genomic DNA Mini Kit (Invitrogen/ThermoFisher Scientific; Carlsbad, CA).

Determination of Vector Copy Number (VCN)

VCN was evaluating using Psi and SDC4 primers as described previously (Masiuk et al., 2019).

mRNA/sgRNA Production

To make mRNA template, maxi-prepped expression plasmids were linearized with SpeI (NEB; Ipswitch, MA), and purified using PCR purification kit according to manufacturer's protocol. In vitro transcription was carried out using mMessage Machine T7 Ultra Transcription Kit (ThermoFisher Scientific; Waltham, MA). mRNA product was purified using the RNeasy MinElute Cleanup Kit (Qiagen; Valencia, CA) following the manufacturer's protocol.

sgRNA template was prepared as previously described (dx.doi.org/10.17504/protocols.io.hdrb256). RNA was purified using the RNeasy MinElute Cleanup Kit (Qiagen; Valencia, CA) following manufacturer's protocol.

DNA RF and Cas9 Variant Production

DNA RF sequences were cloned into pCCL-MNDU3 (Logan et al., 2004) or pT7 plasmids using Gibson Assembly Cloning Kit (NEB; Ipswich, MA). Gene blocks were ordered from IDT to include homology arms for NEBuilder cloning.

Flow Cytometry/Fluorescence-Activated Cell Sorting (FACS)

All flow cytometry analysis and FACS were performed on the following instruments: BD LSRII, BD LSRFortessa, BD FACS Aria II, all with the similar 5-laser configurations: UV 355 nm, Violet 405 nm, Blue 488 nm, Yel-Grn 561 nm, Red 633 nm.

Cell Cycle

Cell cycle FACS was performed as described previously (Lomova et al., 2019). Briefly, CD34$^+$ cells were cultured at 5×10^5-1×10^6 cells/mL and stained with 5 µg/mL Hoechst 33342 for 45–60 min at 37°C. Cells were washed with PBS + 2% HI FBS and resuspended at 5×10^6 cells/mL in X-Vivo 15 + 5 µg/mL Hoechst 33342. Cells were sorted into G0/G1 or S/G2/M populations and recovered in X-Vivo15 medium.

Immediately after sort, cells were counted, centrifuged at 90×g and electroporated.

K562 BFP Cell Electroporation and Gene Editing Assessment With Cas9 variants

K562 BFP cells were split 1:5 1 day before the electroporation. On the day of electroporation, the cells were counted on ViCell (Beckman Coulter; Brea, CA), 2×10^5 cells per condition were centrifuged at 90×g for 15 min at RT, resuspended in 20 µl of SF electroporation buffer (Lonza; Basel, Switzerland), combined with 1 µg Cas9 plasmid and 3 µM ssODN ultramer donor (GCCACCTACGGCAAGC TGACCCTGAAGTTCATCTGCACCACC GGCAAGCTGCCC GTGCCCTGGCCCACCCTCGTGACCACCCTGACGTAC GGCGTGCAGTGCTTCAGCCGCTACCCCGACCACATGA; Integrated DNA Technologies). The cells were electroporated on Amaxa 4D Nucleofector X Unit (Lonza; Basel, Switzerland) using FF-120 setting. After electroporation, the cells were rested in electroporation strips for 10 min at RT, and then recovered with 500 µl of RPMI medium + 10% HI FBS (Gibco/ThermoFisher; Waltham, MA) + 1% PSQ (Gemini BioProducts; Sacramento, CA).Editing outcomes were measured 4 days post-electroporation by flow cytometry. Cells were sorted into BFP$^+$GFP$^-$ (unedited), BFP$^-$GFP$^-$ (non-fluorescent, NHEJ) and BFP$^-$GFP$^+$ (HDR) populations for gene editing outcomes analysis.

CD34$^+$ HSPC Electroporation With Cas9 Variants

For electroporation, 2×10^5 cells per condition were pelleted at 90×g for 15 min at RT, resuspended in 100 µl of BTXpress Electroporation buffer (Harvard Bioscience, Inc; Holliston, MA), combined with pre-aliquoted ssODN (where applicable), Cas9 mRNA (3 pmol) and IVT sgRNA (120 pmol), and pulsed once at 250 V for 5 ms in the BTX ECM 830 Square Wave Electroporator (Harvard Apparatus; Holliston, MA). After electroporation, cells were rested in cuvettes for 10 min at RT, and then recovered with 400 µl of X-Vivo 15 medium (with PSQ and SFT cytokines). If applicable, cells were recovered with media containing AAV6 (multiplicity of infection, MOI = 2e4) to introduce 4 SNPs (Virovek; Hayward, CA). The cells were cultured in a 24-well plate at 37°C, 5% CO_2 incubator. Twenty-four hours post electroporation, the cells were diluted 1:2 with trypan blue and counted manually using a hemocytometer to determine viability (number of live cells/number of total cells $\times$ 100) and fold expansion (number of cells 24 h after electroporation/number of cells before electroporation). Cells were re-plated into 1 mL (or 5 mL, for 1×10^6 cells) of myeloid expansion medium (Iscove's Modified Dulbecco's Medium (IMDM, Thermo Fisher Scientific; Waltham, MA) + 20% FBS [HI FBS, Gibco/ThermoFisher; Waltham, MA] + 5 ng/mL Interleukin 3 (IL3), 10 ng/mL Interleukin 6 (IL6), 25 ng/mL SCF (Peprotech; Rocky Hill, NJ)], and cultured for 4 days prior to harvesting for genomic DNA (gDNA). gDNA was extracted using PureLink Genomic DNA Mini Kit (Invitrogen/ThermoFisher Scientific; Carlsbad, CA).

Illumina MiSeq Library Preparation

DNA library for HTS was prepared as described previously (Hoban et al., 2015; Lomova et al., 2019). Briefly, an outer PCR was performed on genomic DNA to amplify a 1.1 kb region of interest (using Outer PCR Forward (Fwd) and Reverse (Rev) primers). A second PCR was performed to add a unique index to the PCR product of each sample to be sequenced (read1/read2 and P5/P7 primers). The PCR products with the indexes were mixed at equal concentrations, which was determined by densitometry of the PCR products and analyzed by gel electrophoresis, to create a pooled library. The pooled library was purified twice using AMPure XP beads (Beckman Coulter Inc.; Brea, CA) and then quantified using ddPCR (QX 200; Bio-Rad Laboratories Inc.; Hercules, CA). HTS was performed at UCLA Technology Center for Genomics & Bioinformatics (TCGB) using MiSeq 2 × 150 paired-end reads (Illumina Inc; San Diego, CA). The sequences for all HSPC editing experiments were deposited to NCBI Sequence Read Archive (SRA): **PRJNA672655**.

Sequencing Analysis and Calculations

Analysis of sequencing data was performed as described elsewhere (Hoban et al., 2015, 2016; Lomova et al., 2019). Percentage of HDR was calculated as the (number of sequence reads containing a sickle change)/(total reads for that sample)*100. Percentage of NHEJ was calculated as the frequency of sequence reads containing an insertion or deletion −50/+36 bases around the nuclease cut site. CRISPResso2 was used for visualization of select experimental samples (Clement et al., 2019).

Statistical Analysis

Summary statistics including mean and standard deviation were calculated and presented in figures for quantitative measures. For experiments with small n, interpretations of the result were mostly descriptive. Statistical tests between experimental group and control group were carried out via Wilcoxon rank sum test to properly account for non-normality of the data. An alpha of 0.05 was chosen as the significance cut-off for two-tailed statistical testing. All statistical analyses were performed using statistical software R Version 4.0.0 (http://www.R-project.org/).

AUTHOR CONTRIBUTIONS

EB, AL, ZR, RH, and DK conceived these studies. EB and AL performed the laboratory studies with assistance from LC, DC, PA, SS, KO, JS, RC, NR, and YS. Biostatistical analyses by XW. EB and AL primarily wrote the paper, with assistance from ZR and DK. All authors contributed to the article and approved the submitted version.

ACKNOWLEDGMENTS

The contents of this manuscript have been published in part as part of the thesis of Lomova (2019).

REFERENCES

Anand, R., Ranjha, L., Cannavo, E., and Cejka, P. (2016). Phosphorylated CtIP functions as a co-factor of the MRE11-RAD50-NBS1 endonuclease in DNA end resection. *Mol. Cell* 64, 940–950. doi: 10.1016/j.molcel.2016.10.017

Balasubramanian, N., Bai, P., Buchek, G., Korza, G., and Weller, S. K. (2010). Physical Interaction between the Herpes Simplex Virus Type 1 Exonuclease, UL12, and the DNA Double-Strand Break-Sensing MRN Complex. *J. Virol.* 84, 12504–12514. doi: 10.1128/jvi.01506-10

Bauer, D. E., Kamran, S. C., Lessard, S., Xu, J., Fujiwara, Y., Lin, C., et al. (2013). An erythroid enhancer of BCL11A subject to genetic variation determines fetal hemoglobin level. *Science* 342, 253–257. doi: 10.1126/science.1242088

Bjurström, C. F., Mojadidi, M., Phillips, J., Kuo, C., Lai, S., Lill, G. R., et al. (2016). Reactivating fetal hemoglobin expression in human adult erythroblasts through BCL11A knockdown using targeted endonucleases. *Mol. Ther. Nucl. Acids* 5:e351. doi: 10.1038/mtna.2016.52

Branzei, D., and Foiani, M. (2008). Regulation of DNA repair throughout the cell cycle. *Nat. Rev. Mol. Cell Biol.* 9, 297–308. doi: 10.1038/nrm2351

Canny, M. D., Moatti, N., Wan, L. C. K., Fradet-Turcotte, A., Krasner, D., Mateos-Gomez, P. A., et al. (2018). Inhibition of 53BP1 favors homology-dependent DNA repair and increases CRISPR-Cas9 genome-editing efficiency. *Nat. Biotechnol.* 36, 95–102. doi: 10.1038/nbt.4021

Ceppi, I., Howard, S. M., Kasaciunaite, K., Pinto, C., Anand, R., Seidel, R., et al. (2020). CtIP promotes the motor activity of DNA2 to accelerate long-range DNA end resection. *Proc. Natl. Acad. Sci. U.S.A.* 117, 8859–8869. doi: 10.1073/pnas.2001165117

Chang, K. H., Smith, S. E., Sullivan, T., Chen, K., Zhou, Q., West, J. A., et al. (2017). Long-term engraftment and fetal globin induction upon BCL11A gene editing in bone-marrow-derived CD34+ hematopoietic stem and progenitor cells. *Mol. Ther. Methods Clin. Dev.* 4, 137–148. doi: 10.1016/j.omtm.2016.12.009

Charpentier, M., Khedher, A. H. Y., Menoret, S., Brion, A., Lamribet, K., Dardillac, E., et al. (2018). CtIP fusion to Cas9 enhances transgene integration by homology-dependent repair. *Nat. Commun.* 9:113. doi: 10.1038/s41467-018-03475-7

Chiruvella, K. K., Liang, Z., Birkeland, S. R., Basrur, V., and Wilson, T. E. (2013). Saccharomyces cerevisiae DNA ligase IV supports imprecise end joining independently of its catalytic activity. *PLoS Genet.* 9:e1003599. doi: 10.1371/journal.pgen.1003599

Clement, K., Rees, H., Canver, M. C., Gehrke, J. M., Farouni, R., Hsu, J. Y., et al. (2019). CRISPResso2 provides accurate and rapid genome editing sequence analysis. *Nat. Biotechnol.* 37, 224–226. doi: 10.1038/s41587-019-0032-3

Cuella-Martin, R., Oliveira, C., Lockstone, H. E., Snellenberg, S., Grolmusova, N., and Chapman, J. R. (2016). 53BP1 Integrates DNA repair and p53-dependent cell fate decisions via distinct mechanisms. *Mol. Cell* 64, 51–64. doi: 10.1016/j.molcel.2016.08.002

DeWitt, M. A., Magis, W., Bray, N. L., Wang, T., Berman, J. R., Urbinati, F., et al. (2016). Selection-free genome editing of the sickle mutation in human adult hematopoietic stem/progenitor cells. *Sci. Transl. Med.* 8:360ra134. doi: 10.1126/scitranslmed.aaf9336

Doudna, J. A., and Charpentier, E. (2014). The new frontier of genome engineering with CRISPR-Cas9. *Science* 346:1258096. doi: 10.1126/science.1258096

Dvorak, C. C., and Cowan, M. J. (2008). Hematopoietic stem cell transplantation for primary immunodeficiency disease. *Bone Marrow Transplant.* 41, 119–126. doi: 10.1038/sj.bmt.1705890

Ellis, N. A., Groden, J., Ye, T.-Z., Straughen, J., Lennon, D. J., Ciocci, S., et al. (1995). The bloom's syndrome gene product is homologous to RecQ helicases. *Cell* 83, 655–666. doi: 10.1016/0092-8674(95)90105-1

Fradet-Turcotte, A., Canny, M. D., Escribano-Díaz, C., Orthwein, A., Leung, C. C. Y., Huang, H., et al. (2013). 53BP1 is a reader of the DNA-damage-induced H2A Lys 15 ubiquitin mark. *Nature* 499, 50–54. doi: 10.1038/nature12318

Glaser, A., McColl, B., and Vadolas, J. (2016). GFP to BFP conversion: a versatile assay for the quantification of CRISPR/Cas9-mediated genome editing. *Mol. Ther. Nucl. Acids* 5:e334. doi: 10.1038/mtna.2016.48

Griffith, L. M., Cowan, M. J., Kohn, D. B., Notarangelo, L. D., Puck, J. M., Schultz, K. R., et al. (2008). Allogeneic hematopoietic cell transplantation for primary immune deficiency diseases: current status and critical needs. *J. Allergy Clin. Immunol.* 122, 1087–1096. doi: 10.1016/j.jaci.2008.09.045

Gutschner, T., Haemmerle, M., Genovese, G., Draetta, G. F., and Chin, L. (2016). Post-translational regulation of Cas9 during G1 enhances homology-directed repair. *Cell Rep.* 14, 1555–1566. doi: 10.1016/j.celrep.2016.01.019

Heyer, W. D., Ehmsen, K. T., and Liu, J. (2010). Regulation of homologous recombination in eukaryotes. *Annu. Rev. Genet.* 44, 113–139. doi: 10.1146/annurev-genet-051710-150955

Hoban, M. D., Cost, G. J., Mendel, M. C., Romero, Z., Kaufman, M. L., Joglekar, A. V., et al. (2015). Correction of the sickle cell disease mutation in human hematopoietic stem/progenitor cells. *Blood* 125, 2597–2604. doi: 10.1182/blood-2014-12-615948

Hoban, M. D., Lumaquin, D., Kuo, C. Y., Romero, Z., Long, J., Ho, M., et al. (2016). CRISPR/Cas9-mediated correction of the sickle mutation in human CD34+ cells. *Mol. Ther.* 24, 1561–1569. doi: 10.1038/mt.2016.148

Hollis, R. P., Nightingale, S. J., Wang, X., Pepper, K. A., Yu, X. J., Barsky, L., et al. (2006). Stable gene transfer to human CD34+ hematopoietic cells using the Sleeping beauty transposon. *Exp. Hematol.* 34, 1333–1343. doi: 10.1016/j.exphem.2006.05.023

Holt, N., Wang, J., Kim, K., Friedman, G., Wang, X., Taupin, V., et al. (2010). Human hematopoietic stem/progenitor cells modified by zinc-finger nucleases targeted to CCR5 control HIV-1 *in vivo*. *Nat. Biotechnol.* 28, 839–847. doi: 10.1038/nbt.1663

Huertas, P. (2010). DNA resection in eukaryotes: deciding how to fix the break. *Nat. Struct. Mol. Biol.* 17, 11–16. doi: 10.1038/nsmb.1710

Huertas, P., and Jackason, S. P. (2009). Human CtIP mediates cell cycle control of DNA end resection and double strand break repair. *J. Biol. Chem.* 284, 9558–9565. doi: 10.1074/jbc.M808906200

Iyer, S., Suresh, S., Guo, D., Daman, K., Chen, J. C. J., Liu, P., et al. (2019). Precise therapeutic gene correction by a simple nuclease-induced double-stranded break. *Nature* 568, 561–565. doi: 10.1038/s41586-019-1076-8

Jasin, M., and Haber, J. E. (2016). The democratization of gene editing: Insights from site-specific cleavage and double-strand break repair. *DNA Repair* 44, 6–16. doi: 10.1016/j.dnarep.2016.05.001

Jasin, M., and Rothstein, R. (2013). Repair of strand breaks by homologous recombination. *Cold Spring Harb. Perspect. Biol.* 5:a012740. doi: 10.1101/cshperspect.a012740

Jayavaradhan, R., Pillis, D. M., Goodman, M., Zhang, F., Zhang, Y., Andreassen, P. R., et al. (2019). CRISPR-Cas9 fusion to dominant-negative 53BP1 enhances HDR and inhibits NHEJ specifically at Cas9 target sites. *Nat. Commun.* 10:2866. doi: 10.1038/s41467-019-10735-7

Logan, A. C., Nightingale, S. J., Haas, D. L., Cho, G. J., Pepper, K. A., and Kohn, D. B. (2004). Factors influencing the titer and infectivity of lentiviral vectors. *Hum. Gene Ther.* 15, 976–988. doi: 10.1089/hum.2004.15.976

Lomova, A. (2019). *UCLA UCLA Electronic Theses and Dissertations Title Improving Nuclease-Mediated Gene Editing Outcomes in Human Hematopoietic Stem Cells*. Available online at: https://escholarship.org/uc/item/1tm222z0 (accessed September 15, 2020).

Lomova, A., Clark, D. N., Campo-Fernandez, B., Flores-Bjurström, C., Kaufman, M. L., Fitz-Gibbon, S., et al. (2019). Improving gene editing outcomes in human hematopoietic stem and progenitor cells by temporal control of DNA repair. *Stem Cells* 37, 284–294. doi: 10.1002/stem.2935

Masiuk, K. E., Zhang, R., Osborne, K., Hollis, R. P., Campo-Fernandez, B., and Kohn, D. B. (2019). PGE2 and poloxamer synperonic F108 enhance transduction of human HSPCs with a β-globin lentiviral vector. *Mol. Ther. Methods Clin. Dev.* 13, 390–398. doi: 10.1016/j.omtm.2019.03.005

McVey, M., and Lee, S. E. (2008). MMEJ repair of double-strand breaks (director's cut): deleted sequences and alternative endings. *Trends Genet.* 24, 529–538. doi: 10.1016/j.tig.2008.08.007

Métais, J. Y., Doerfler, P. A., Mayuranathan, T., Bauer, D. E., Fowler, S. C., Hsieh, M. M., et al. (2019). Genome editing of HBG1 and HBG2 to induce fetal hemoglobin. *Blood Adv.* 3, 3379–3392. doi: 10.1182/bloodadvances.2019000820

Orthwein, A., Noordermeer, S. M., Wilson, M. D., Landry, S., Enchev, R. I., Sherker, A., et al. (2015). A mechanism for the suppression of homologous recombination in G1 cells. *Nature* 528, 422–426. doi: 10.1038/nature16142

Pai, S. Y., Logan, B. R., Griffith, L. M., Buckley, R. H., Parrott, R. E., Dvorak, C. C., et al. (2014). Transplantation outcomes for severe combined immunodeficiency, 2000-2009. *N. Engl. J. Med.* 371, 434–446. doi: 10.1056/NEJMoa1401177

Panier, S., and Boulton, S. J. (2014). Double-strand break repair: 53BP1 comes into focus. *Nat. Rev. Mol. Cell Biol.* 15, 7–18. doi: 10.1038/nrm3719

Paulsen, B. S., Mandal, P. K., Frock, R. L., Boyraz, B., Yadav, R., Upadhyayula, S., et al. (2017). Ectopic expression of RAD52 and dn53BP1 improves homology-directed repair during CRISPR/Cas9 genome editing. *Nat. Biomed. Eng.* 1, 878–888. doi: 10.1038/s41551-017-0145-2

Pietras, E. M., Warr, M. R., and Passegué, E. (2011). Cell cycle regulation in hematopoietic stem cells. *J. Cell Biol.* 195, 709–720. doi: 10.1083/jcb.201102131

Polato, F., Callen, E., Wong, N., Faryabi, R., Bunting, S., Chen, H. T., et al. (2014). CtIP-mediated resection is essential for viability and can operate independently of BRCA1. *J. Exp. Med.* 211, 1027–1036. doi: 10.1084/jem.20131939

Reuven, N., Adler, J., Broennimann, K., Myers, N., and Shaul, Y. (2019). Recruitment of DNA repair MRN complex by intrinsically disordered protein domain fused to Cas9 improves efficiency of CRISPR-mediated genome editing. *Biomolecules* 9:584. doi: 10.3390/biom9100584

Richardson, C. D., Kazane, K. R., Feng, S. J., Zelin, E., Bray, N. L., Schäfer, A. J., et al. (2018). CRISPR–Cas9 genome editing in human cells occurs via the Fanconi anemia pathway. *Nat. Genet.* 50, 1132–1139. doi: 10.1038/s41588-018-0174-0

Richardson, C. D., Ray, G. J., DeWitt, M. A., Curie, G. L., and Corn, J. E. (2016). Enhancing homology-directed genome editing by catalytically active and inactive CRISPR-Cas9 using asymmetric donor DNA. *Nat. Biotechnol.* 34, 339–344. doi: 10.1038/nbt.3481

Romero, Z., Lomova, A., Said, S., Miggelbrink, A., Kuo, C. Y., Campo-Fernandez, B., et al. (2019). Editing the sickle cell disease mutation in human hematopoietic stem cells: comparison of endonucleases and homologous donor templates. *Mol. Ther.* 27, 1389–1406. doi: 10.1016/j.ymthe.2019.05.014

Sartori, A. A., Lukas, C., Coates, J., Mistrik, M., Fu, S., Bartek, J., et al. (2007). Human CtIP promotes DNA end resection. *Nature* 450, 509–514. doi: 10.1038/nature06337

Schumacher, A. J., Mohni, K. N., Kan, Y., Hendrickson, E. A., Stark, J. M., and Weller, S. K. (2012). The HSV-1 exonuclease, UL12, stimulates recombination by a single strand annealing mechanism. *PLoS Pathog.* 8:e1002862. doi: 10.1371/journal.ppat.1002862

Søndergaard, J. N., Geng, K., Sommerauer, C., Atanasoai, I., Yin, X., and Kutter, C. (2020). Successful delivery of large-size CRISPR/Cas9 vectors in hard-to-transfect human cells using small plasmids. *Commun. Biol.* 3:319. doi: 10.1038/s42003-020-1045-7

Symington, L. S. (2016). Mechanism and regulation of DNA end resection in eukaryotes. *Crit. Rev. Biochem. Mol. Biol.* 51, 195–212. doi: 10.3109/10409238.2016.1172552

Symington, L. S., and Gautier, J. (2011). Double-strand break end resection and repair pathway choice. *Annu. Rev. Genet.* 45, 247–271. doi: 10.1146/annurev-genet-110410-132435

Vilenchik, M. M., and Knudson, A. G. (2003). Endogenous DNA double-strand breaks: production, fidelity of repair, and induction of cancer. *Proc. Natl. Acad. Sci. U.S.A.* 100, 12871–12876. doi: 10.1073/pnas.2135498100

Wu, Y., Zeng, J., Roscoe, B. P., Liu, P., Yao, Q., Lazzarotto, C. R., et al. (2019). Highly efficient therapeutic gene editing of human hematopoietic stem cells. *Nat. Med.* 25, 776–783. doi: 10.1038/s41591-019-0401-y

Yeh, C. D., Richardson, C. D., and Corn, J. E. (2019). Advances in genome editing through control of DNA repair pathways. *Nat. Cell Biol.* 21, 1468–1478. doi: 10.1038/s41556-019-0425-z

10

From Basic Biology to Patient Mutational Spectra of *GATA2* Haploinsufficiencies: What are the Mechanisms, Hurdles and Prospects of Genome Editing for Treatment

Cansu Koyunlar and Emma de Pater*

Department of Hematology, Erasmus MC, Rotterdam, Netherlands

*Correspondence:
Emma de Pater
e.depater@erasmusmc.nl

Inherited bone marrow failure syndromes (IBMFS) are monogenetic disorders that result in a reduction of mature blood cell formation and predisposition to leukemia. In children with myeloid leukemia the gene most often mutated is *Gata binding protein 2* (*GATA2*) and 80% of patients with *GATA2* mutations develop myeloid malignancy before the age of forty. Although *GATA2* is established as one of the key regulators of embryonic and adult hematopoiesis, the mechanisms behind the leukemia predisposition in *GATA2* haploinsufficiencies is ambiguous. The only curative treatment option currently available is allogeneic hematopoietic stem cell transplantation (allo-SCT). However, allo-SCT can only be applied at a relatively late stage of the disease as its applicability is compromised by treatment related morbidity and mortality (TRM). Alternatively, autologous hematopoietic stem cell transplantation (auto-SCT), which is associated with significantly less TRM, might become a treatment option if repaired hematopoietic stem cells would be available. Here we discuss the recent literature on leukemia predisposition syndromes caused by *GATA2* mutations, current knowledge on the function of *GATA2* in the hematopoietic system and advantages and pitfalls of potential treatment options provided by genome editing.

Keywords: *GATA2*, Inherited bone marrow failure syndrome, MDS, AML, *GATA2* haploinsufficiency syndrome, genome editing, HSCs, autologous HSC transplantation

INTRODUCTION

IBMFS are a heterogeneous cluster of disorders manifested by an ineffective blood production and concurrent cytopenias that eventually result in a hypoplastic bone marrow (BM). These syndromes constitute an increased propensity to develop hematological malignancies such as myelodysplastic syndrome (MDS) and acute myeloid leukemia (AML) (Dokal and Vulliamy, 2010; Wilson et al., 2014; Cook, 2018). Mutations in *GATA2* are the most common genetic defects in pediatric MDS (Spinner et al., 2014). *GATA2* is one of the master regulators of blood production and patients that carry a mutation in one of the two alleles of *GATA2* often manifest with immunodeficiency syndromes and increased lifetime risk for MDS/AML (Wlodarski et al., 2016; Donadieu et al., 2018; McReynolds et al., 2018). Once malignant transformation becomes overt, survival rates are below 50% (Spinner et al., 2014). Due to the inherited mutation, allo-SCT is the only curative treatment option for these patients (Simonis et al., 2018; van Lier et al., 2020).

Unfortunately, the use of allo-SCT is compromised by TRM and not applicable for patients who have not progressed to leukemia yet. Uncovering the *modus operandi* of *GATA2* and other (epi)genetic factors in the complex network of blood regulation is essential to design non-invasive and preventive treatment options for IBMFS patients.

Genome editing strategies, especially the implementation of clustered regularly interspaced short palindromic repeat/associated protein 9 (CRISPR/Cas9) nuclease platforms, improve rapidly and progress toward efficient therapies for several genetic diseases (Cong et al., 2013; Mali et al., 2013; Anzalone et al., 2019). In this review, we will summarize clinical symptoms of *GATA2* haploinsufficiency patients and results from *Gata2* experimental models to inspect the function of *GATA2* in leukemogenesis. Our aim is to explore the potential and pitfalls of genome editing methods to treat *GATA2* deficiency syndromes in the light of current technologies.

THE TRANSCRIPTION FACTOR *GATA2*

GATA2 is a zinc finger transcription factor that contains 2 first exons; a hematopoietic and neuronal cell specific distal first exon and a proximal first exon that is utilized ubiquitously. These two transcript variants encode the same protein (Minegishi et al., 1998; Pan et al., 2000). *GATA2* binds a highly conserved (A/T)GATA(A/G) DNA sequence and other protein partners through two multifunctional zinc finger (ZF) domains; ZF1 and ZF2 that are encoded by exon 4 and exon 5, respectively (Evans and Felsenfeld, 1989; Alfayez et al., 2019). Two *GATA2* protein isoforms can be formed, one lacking exon 5 and consequently

lacking the ZF2 domain (Vicente et al., 2012) (**Figure 1**). To date, the functional consequence of this remains unclear.

GERMLINE *GATA2* MUTATIONS

In 2011, four different studies described germline heterozygous *GATA2* mutations in a total of 44 patients with various syndromes; monocytopenia and mycobacterial infection (MonoMAC) syndrome (Hsu et al., 2011), monocyte, B cell, NK cell and dendritic cell deficiencies (DCML) (Dickinson et al., 2011), Emberger Syndrome, which is characterized by primary lymphedema with a predisposition to AML (Ostergaard et al., 2011) and familial MDS/AML predisposition (Hahn et al., 2011). Distinct clinical perspectives discerned in these studies coalesce under the theme of the loss of one allele of *GATA2* resulting in the *GATA2* haploinsufficiency syndrome, which can present with immunodeficiency, lymphedema and 80% predisposition to develop MDS/AML.

Taken together, 60% of patients present with a truncating mutation in *GATA2* before the ZF2 domain and 30% of patients present with a non-synonymous mutation in ZF2. However, some patients develop MonoMAC syndrome without mutations in the coding region of *GATA2* but have reduced *GATA2* expression levels (Hsu et al., 2013). These patients harbor mutations in the intronic region, specifically in intron 4. Mutations in this region abrogate the function of a conserved +9.5 cis-element, that regulates *GATA2* transcription levels resulting in *GATA2* haploinsufficiency (Hsu et al., 2013) and intron 4 mutations represent 10% of all *GATA2* haploinsufficiency cases (Wlodarski et al., 2017) (**Figure 1**).

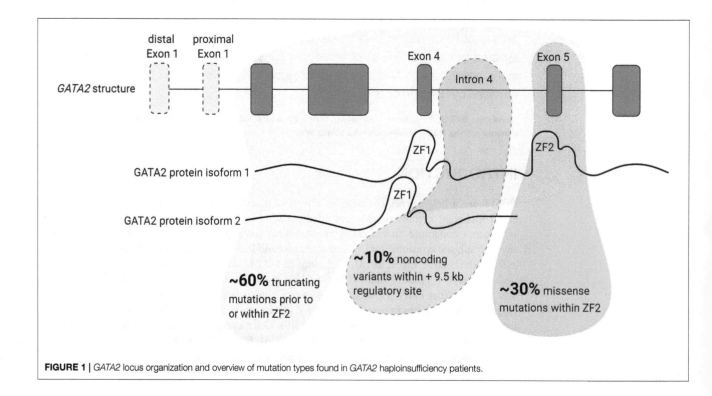

FIGURE 1 | *GATA2* locus organization and overview of mutation types found in *GATA2* haploinsufficiency patients.

GATA2 mutations are also present in a subset of patients with chronic neutropenia and aplastic anemia (AA) (Townsley et al., 2012; Pasquet et al., 2013). However, BM of AA patients with *GATA2* mutations encompasses noticeably different types of altered hematopoietic populations than idiopathic AA patients, such as the complete loss of lymphoid progenitors and atypical megakaryocytes (Ganapathi et al., 2015).

Both familial and sporadic mutations in the coding and cis-regulatory regions of *GATA2* are found and are the underlying cause in 15% of advanced and 7% of all pediatric MDS cases (Wlodarski et al., 2016). Most of these mutations can be found in the ClinVar database (https://www.ncbi.nlm.nih.gov/clinvar). Currently, despite the improving definition of the phenotypic characteristics of *GATA2* deficiency syndromes and high penetrance of myeloid malignancy, the mutational background and phenotypic outcome observed in these patients do not correlate, suggesting that additional events are important for disease progression (Collin et al., 2015; Wlodarski et al., 2016). Evidence for this is found in a cohort of pediatric MDS-*GATA2* patients that acquired additional somatic mutations in *ASXL1*, *RUNX1*, *SETBP1*, *IKZF1*, and *CRLF2* genes, which resulted in an increased progression to AML. Furthermore, 72% of adolescents with MDS and monosomy 7 had an underlying *GATA2* mutation (Wlodarski et al., 2016; Fisher et al., 2017; Yoshida et al., 2020).

SOMATIC *GATA2* MUTATIONS

Although truncating germline *GATA2* mutations occur most often, a few somatic mutations are reported that phenocopy germline loss-of-function mutations (Sekhar et al., 2018; Alfayez et al., 2019). These cause a relatively milder form of the immunodeficiency phenotype observed in germline mutant *GATA2* patients, along with a common presentation of AML, atypical chronic myeloid leukemia and in some cases acute erythroid leukemia (Ping et al., 2017; Sekhar et al., 2018; Alfayez et al., 2019).

Somatic *GATA2* mutations are found both in ZF1 and ZF2 and all patients with somatic *GATA2* mutations harbor mutations in other genes, predominantly *CEBPA* with an incidence of 18–21% (Fasan et al., 2013; Hou et al., 2015; Theis et al., 2016). In one cohort of AML patients, ZF1 but not ZF2 mutations in *GATA2* closely associate with biallelic *CEBPA* mutations (Tien et al., 2018). This implies that ZF1 is crucial for *GATA2* function in disease progression in combination with *CEBPA* mutations.

THE FUNCTION OF THE TRANSCRIPTION FACTOR *GATA2* IN MAMMALIAN HEMATOPOIESIS

The Function of *GATA2* in Embryonic Hematopoiesis

In mouse, homozygous deletion of *Gata2* results in 67% lethality at embryonic day (E) 10.5 and none survive beyond E11.5, due to severe anemia. Chimeras of WT and *Gata2*$^{-/-}$ embryonic stem (ES) cells show that *Gata2*-null cells cannot contribute to hematopoiesis in adult blood, fetal liver, BM and thymus revealing a requirement for *Gata2* in embryonic hematopoiesis (Tsai et al., 1994). Besides the embryonic lethality of *Gata2*-null embryos, the number and function of hematopoietic stem and progenitor cells from germline heterozygous *Gata2* mutant mice at E10.5–E12 is impaired (Ling et al., 2004).

Both in human and mouse embryos, *Gata2* is expressed in a specialized endothelial cell population called hemogenic endothelium (HE) and in the first transplantable hematopoietic stem cells (HSCs) that differentiate from HE (Marshall et al., 1999; Yokomizo and Dzierzak, 2010; Eich et al., 2018; Vink et al., 2020). Conditional deletion of *Gata2* in HE cells resulted in reduced hematopoietic cluster formation in the embryo and long-term repopulating HSCs were not formed. Conditional deletion of *Gata2* in HSCs induced apoptosis indicating that *GATA2* is required both for HSC generation and maintenance (de Pater et al., 2013).

Gata2 expression is regulated by the enhancer activity of multiple conserved cis-regulatory elements. The disruption of the +9.5 element of *Gata2* impaired vascular integrity and formation of HSCs from HE in the mouse embryo (Lim et al., 2012; Gao et al., 2013).

Although both number and functionality of HSCs were reduced in embryonic *Gata2* haploinsufficiency, it is yet to be discovered whether and how the propensity for MDS/AML observed in *GATA2* haploinsufficiency patients is influenced by these early embryonic functions.

The Function of *GATA2* in Adult Bone Marrow Hematopoiesis

The function of *GATA2* in adult hematopoiesis is still abstruse. In BM, *Gata2* is highly expressed in HSCs and downregulated during lineage commitment (Akashi et al., 2000; Miyamoto et al., 2002; Guo et al., 2013). HSCs in the BM of *Gata2*$^{+/-}$ mice are impaired in number and functionality as shown by serial transplantation assays (Rodrigues et al., 2005; Guo et al., 2013). In addition, *Gata2*-heterozygosity in BM HSCs is associated with a decreased proliferation ability together with increased quiescence and apoptosis (Ling et al., 2004; Rodrigues et al., 2005). Moreover, *Gata2* haploinsufficiency reduces the function of granulocyte-macrophage progenitors but not of other myeloid committed progenitors (Rodrigues et al., 2008). However, *Gata2*$^{+/-}$ mice do not develop MDS/AML. This makes it difficult to study the contribution of *GATA2* haploinsufficiency to leukemic progression in these models.

On the other hand, *Gata2* overexpression results in the self-renewal of myeloid progenitors and blocks lymphoid differentiation in mouse BM (Nandakumar et al., 2015). In addition, overexpression of *GATA2* in human ES cells (hESC) promotes proliferation in hESCs, but quiescence in hESC-derived HSCs (Zhou et al., 2019). Furthermore, increased *GATA2* expression is also observed in adult and pediatric AML patients with poor prognosis (Ayala et al., 2009; Luesink et al., 2012; Vicente et al., 2012; Menendez-Gonzalez et al., 2019). These findings indicate that, next to its tumor suppressor role, *GATA2* might act as an oncogene when overexpressed.

GENOME EDITING: A CURE FOR *GATA2* HAPLOINSUFFICIENCIES?

GATA2 Repair Strategies

Allo-SCT is a powerful approach to treat malignancies in *GATA2* haploinsufficiency patients (Simonis et al., 2018; van Lier et al., 2020). However, finding a matched donor and TRM compromises the use of allo-SCT and is therefore not suitable before the onset of malignancy (Bogaert et al., 2020). Regulation of *GATA2* expression is crucial in HSCs and in leukemia predisposition. This makes overexpression of WT *GATA2* using lenti-viral transgenic approaches not suitable as gene therapy method. An auto-SCT approach, after *ex vivo* correction of the underlying patient specific *GATA2* mutation by genome editing tools is possibly a more effective treatment option for these patients (**Figure 2**).

Genome editing, since it was pioneered in the previous century, is developing meteorically as a revolutionary therapeutic tool for genetic defects, including hematological disorders

(Xie et al., 2014; Hoban et al., 2016; De Ravin et al., 2017; Orkin and Bauer, 2019) CRISPR/Cas9, a part of the bacterial acquired immune system, was adapted as a breakthrough genome engineering technology and has since been extensively used to engineer eukaryotic cells in basic research and holds great potential for gene therapy (Gasiunas et al., 2012; Jinek et al., 2012; Cong et al., 2013; Barrangou and Doudna, 2016). CRISPR/Cas9 mediated genome editing relies on sequence specific guide RNAs that assemble with Cas9 protein to create double strand breaks (DSBs) in the targeted sequence. DSBs activates cell intrinsic repair mechanisms if the cell is to undergo proliferation and repaired by one of two mechanisms: non-homologous end joining (NHEJ) in which random insertions/deletions (InDels) are introduced or homology-directed repair (HDR) which uses the other DNA strand as template to restore its original sequence. This system can be hijacked by providing an exogenous repair template containing any desired sequence. Because HDR is rare, a selection cassette can be inserted for positive selection of the desired repair (Doudna and Charpentier, 2014).

Because heterogeneity of mutations in *GATA2* haploinsufficieny patients (https://www.ncbi.nlm.nih.gov/clinvar), these mutations would need to be restored at the

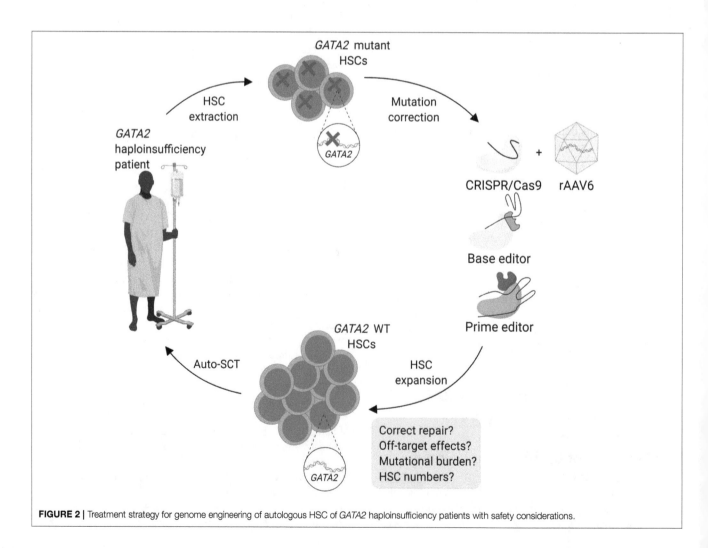

FIGURE 2 | Treatment strategy for genome engineering of autologous HSC of *GATA2* haploinsufficiency patients with safety considerations.

endogenous locus, requiring HDR as repair mechanism. Therefore, optimizing an editing strategy by using large HDR donor templates that cover various *GATA2* mutation regions found in patients or the whole gene, containing homologous regions covering several exons, could provide treatment for a substantial group of *GATA2* patients. An efficient method for gene correction in HSCs with CRISPR/Cas9 and large HDR donor delivered by rAAV6 (adeno-associated viral vectors of serotype 6) was used to correct a *HBB* gene mutation causing sickle cell disease and has potential to correct *GATA2* mutations in HSCs using the same strategy (Dever et al., 2016; DeWitt et al., 2016; Bak et al., 2018) (**Figure 2**).

Hurdles

GATA2 haploinsufficiencies result in a diminished number of HSCs in both embryonic and adult stages. Additionally, HDR mediated repair works with low efficiencies and studies showed that it is more efficient in hematopoietic progenitor cells rather than long-term repopulating HSCs (Genovese et al., 2014; Hoban et al., 2015). Together this implicates the biggest hurdle to treat *GATA2* haploinsufficiency patients would be to obtain sufficient number of corrected HSCs for auto-SCT. An enrichment method, possibly a reporter-based selection followed by an *ex vivo* expansion of *GATA2*-corrected HSCs, could potentially solve this problem. For this purpose, small molecule drugs promoting *ex vivo* expansion of HSCs, like SR1 or UM171, could be used to obtain higher number of corrected HSCs prior to auto-SCT (Boitano et al., 2010; Fares et al., 2014).

Furthermore, in *GATA2* haploinsufficiency patients, additional mutations in other genes could be the driver of leukemia which brings challenges to treat these patients by only correcting the mutant *GATA2* allele. Therefore, a preliminary genetic screening for additional mutations should be compulsory in *GATA2* haploinsufficiency patients to elucidate if correcting only the mutant *GATA2* allele would eliminate the disease phenotype of the patient.

Another hurdle when using genome editing tools for clinical applications is the off-target effects (OTEs) that might occur in undesired parts of the DNA. Detection of OTEs with whole genome sequencing are often challenging due to high background of random reads in combination with low sequence depth (<10-fold) (Kim et al., 2015). More screening strategies for OTEs, like GUIDE-seq (Genome wide, Unbiased Identification of DSB Enabled by sequencing), CIRCLE-seq (Circularization for *in vitro* Reporting of Cleavage Effects) and DISCOVER-seq (Discovery of *in situ* Cas Off-targets and VERification by Sequencing), are shown to overcome these obstacles and could be used to efficiently identify OTEs that might result from *GATA2*-editing strategy before its clinical translation (Tsai et al., 2015, 2017; Wienert et al., 2019).

Prospects

Fortunately, recent improvements of CRISPR/Cas9 genome editing may overcome some of these hurdles for patient applications. Base editing methods are developed by the addition of enzymes to Cas9 to provide single base pair changes without making DSBs (Komor et al., 2016; Gaudelli et al., 2017). Although base editing can correct point mutations that are also found in *GATA2* patients, the off-target effects caused by the broad activity of cytidine deaminases used in this method should be considered carefully (Zuo et al., 2019; Yu et al., 2020). More recently Anzalone et al. (2019) described prime editing that introduces specific insertions, deletions and point mutations to a variety of genomic regions with high efficiency without DSBs. Prime editing was successfully used in human cells to correct mutations that cause sickle cell disease and Tay-Sachs disease and only 1–10% of prime-edited cells are found to have unwanted off-target InDels throughout the genome (Anzalone et al., 2019). These recent advances in genome editing techniques anticipate the improvement of a safer and more efficient correction of the patient mutations in HSCs prior to auto-SCT, and should be considered for the treatment of *GATA2* haploinsufficiencies (**Figure 2**).

Currently, the minimum level of donor chimerism necessary to reverse the disease phenotype in *GATA2* haploinsufficiency patients remains unclear (Hickstein, 2018). For sickle cell disease however, it was shown that clinical benefits might be observed when as few as 2–5 HSCs are engrafted (Walters et al., 2001; DeWitt et al., 2016). Interestingly, an asymptomatic germline *GATA2* mutant individual acquired a somatic mutation reversing the harmful *GATA2* mutation. This resulted in a selective advantage of the corrected HSCs and prevented from developing malignancy (Catto et al., 2020). Together this implicates having a few mutation-corrected HSCs might already have clinical significance for *GATA2* haploinsufficiency patients.

CRISPR/Cas9 technology has been approved in patient treatment for various types of malignancies including hematological diseases (https://clinicaltrials.gov). Currently, clinical trials are performed where CRISPR/Cas9 is used to remove erythroid expression of the fetal hemoglobin repressor *BCL11A* in the treatment of hemaglobinopathies, implicating a highly promising potential for genome editing to treat various hematological disorders (Orkin and Bauer, 2019; The Lancet Haematology, 2019).

Careful consideration of possible challenges discussed for *GATA2* haploinsufficiency patients could lead to a beneficial clinical translation of genome editing to treat these patients in the near future.

DISCUSSION

Although *GATA2* haploinsufficiency depletes the HSC compartment in humans and mice, the function of *GATA2* haploinsufficiency in MDS/AML progression is poorly understood. A possibility could be that *GATA2* haploinsufficiency provides a fertile ground for the emergence of additional mutations in HSCs and these acquired mutations promote leukemogenesis. Evidence that support this hypothesis is the inconsistent penetrance of leukemia in *GATA2* haploinsufficiency patients that cannot be explained solely by the mutations in the *GATA2* locus and MDS/AML patients with germline *GATA2* mutation presented with additional mutations which are linked to hematological malignancies (Wlodarski et al., 2016; Fisher et al., 2017; Yoshida et al., 2020). In order to understand the concept of fertile ground as a driver of MDS/AML in *GATA2* deficiency syndromes, more fundamental research is needed to reveal the clonal origin (embryonic and/or adult) of leukemogenic driver mutations to help us choose an appropriate time frame and strategy to treat these patients using genome editing. If leukemic driver mutations arise early during hematopoietic development, targeting leukemic clones will be challenging.

in vivo Gata2$^{+/-}$ models have not developed an MDS/AML phenotype (Ling et al., 2004; Rodrigues et al., 2005). This could be due to differences governing HSC mechanisms in these models or due to differences in lifespan, infection status, genetic background or a combination of these factors. Perhaps aged *Gata2$^{+/-}$* models could provide more insight, since this would challenge the HSC compartment and increase the chances of additional events that would promote leukemogenesis to occur.

Base editing and prime editing are the recent promising and rigorous refinements of genome editing technologies which could provide and improve a patient specific mutation correction for *GATA2* mutations or any other gene mutations that predispose to hematological malignancies when potentials and risks of these tools are tested sufficiently prior to the actual patient treatments. In addition to their potential for gene therapy discussed in this review, CRISPR base and prime editing technologies are also fantastic tools for basic research to introduce additional predicted leukemia driver mutations to HSCs in *GATA2* haploinsufficiency models in order to identify their potential role in malignant transformation.

AUTHOR CONTRIBUTIONS

CK and EP wrote the manuscript.

ACKNOWLEDGMENTS

We thank Dr. IP Touw and Dr. T Cupedo for careful reading of the manuscript. Figures are created with BioRender.com.

REFERENCES

Akashi, K., Reya, T., Dalma-Weiszhausz, D., and Weissman, I. L. (2000). Lymphoid precursors. *Curr. Opin. Immunol.* 12, 144–150. doi: 10.1016/S0952-7915(99)00064-3

Alfayez, M., Wang, S. A., Bannon, S. A., Kontoyiannis, D. P., Kornblau, S. M., Orange, J. S., et al. (2019). Myeloid malignancies with somatic *GATA2* mutations can be associated with an immunodeficiency phenotype. *Leuk. Lymphoma* 60, 2025–2033. doi: 10.1080/10428194.2018.1551535

Anzalone, A. V., Randolph, P. B., Davis, J. R., Sousa, A. A., Koblan, L. W., Levy, J. M., et al. (2019). Search-and-replace genome editing without double-strand breaks or donor DNA. *Nature* 576, 149–157. doi: 10.1038/s41586-019-1711-4

Ayala, R. M., Martínez-López, J., Albízua, E., Diez, A., and Gilsanz, F. (2009). Clinical significance of Gata-1, Gata-2, EKLF, and c-MPL expression in acute myeloid leukemia. *Am. J. Hematol.* 84, 79–86. doi: 10.1002/ajh.21332

Bak, R. O., Dever, D. P., and Porteus, M., H. (2018). CRISPR/Cas9 genome editing in human hematopoietic stem cells. *Nat. Protoc.* 13, 358–376. doi: 10.1038/nprot.2017.143

Barrangou, R., and Doudna, J. A. (2016). Applications of CRISPR technologies in research and beyond. *Nat. Biotechnol.* 34, 933–941. doi: 10.1038/nbt.3659

Bogaert, D. J., Laureys, G., Naesens, L., Mazure, D., De Bruyne, M., Hsu, A. P., et al. (2020). *GATA2* deficiency and haematopoietic stem cell transplantation: challenges for the clinical practitioner. *Br. J. Haematol.* 188, 768–773. doi: 10.1111/bjh.16247

Boitano, A. E., Wang, J., Romeo, R., Bouchez, L. C., Parker, A. E., Sutton, S. E., et al. (2010). Aryl hydrocarbon receptor antagonists promote the expansion of human hematopoietic stem cells. *Science* 329, 1345–1348. doi: 10.1126/science.1191536

Catto, L. F. B., Borges, G., Pinto, A. L., Clé, D., V., Chahud, F., et al. (2020). Somatic genetic rescue in hematopoietic cells in *GATA2* deficiency. *Blood* 136, 1002–1005. doi: 10.1182/blood.2020005538

Collin, M., Dickinson, R., and Bigley, V. (2015). Haematopoietic and immune defects associated with *GATA2* mutation. *Br. J. Haematol.* 169, 173–187. doi: 10.1111/bjh.13317

Cong, L., Ran, F. A., Cox, D., Lin, S., Barretto, R., Habib, N., et al. (2013). Multiplex genome engineering using CRISPR/Cas systems. *Science* 339, 819–823. doi: 10.1126/science.1231143

Cook, J. R. (2018). "5 - bone marrow failure syndromes," in *Hematopathology, 3rd Edn.* ed. E. D. Hsi (Philadelphia, PA: Elsevier), 167–183.e161. doi: 10.1016/B978-0-323-47913-4.00005-7

de Pater, E., Kaimakis, P., Vink, C. S., Yokomizo, T., Yamada-Inagawa, T., R., et al. (2013). Gata2 is required for HSC generation and survival. *J. Exp. Med.* 210, 2843–2850. doi: 10.1084/jem.20130751

De Ravin, S. S., Li, L., Wu, X., Choi, U., Allen, C., Koontz, S., et al. (2017). CRISPR-Cas9 gene repair of hematopoietic stem cells from patients with X-linked chronic granulomatous disease. *Sci. Transl. Med.* 9:aah3480. doi: 10.1126/scitranslmed.aah3480

Dever, D. P., Bak, R. O., Reinisch, A., Camarena, J., Washington, G., Nicolas, C. E., et al. (2016). CRISPR/Cas9 β-globin gene targeting in human haematopoietic stem cells. *Nature* 539, 384–389. doi: 10.1038/nature20134

DeWitt, M. A., Magis, W., Bray, N. L., Wang, T., Berman, J. R., Urbinati, F., et al. (2016). Selection-free genome editing of the sickle mutation in human adult hematopoietic stem/progenitor cells. *Sci. Transl. Med.* 8:360ra134. doi: 10.1126/scitranslmed.aaf9336

Dickinson, R. E., Griffin, H., Bigley, V., Reynard, L. N., Hussain, R., Haniffa, M., et al. (2011). Exome sequencing identifies GATA-2 mutation as the cause of dendritic cell, monocyte, B and NK lymphoid deficiency. *Blood* 118, 2656–2658. doi: 10.1182/blood-2011-06-360313

Dokal, I., and Vulliamy, T. (2010). Inherited bone marrow failure syndromes. *Haematologica* 95, 1236–1240. doi: 10.3324/haematol.2010.025619

Donadieu, J., Lamant, M., Fieschi, C., de Fontbrune, F. S., Caye, A., Ouachee, M., et al. (2018). Natural history of *GATA2* deficiency in a survey of 79 French and Belgian patients. *Haematologica* 103, 1278–1287. doi: 10.3324/haematol.2017.181909

Doudna, J. A., and Charpentier, E. (2014). The new frontier of genome engineering with CRISPR-Cas9. *Science* 346:1258096. doi: 10.1126/science.1258096

Eich, C., Arlt, J., Vink, C. S., Solaimani Kartalaei, P., Kaimakis, P., Mariani, S. A., et al. (2018). *In vivo* single cell analysis reveals Gata2 dynamics in cells transitioning to hematopoietic fate. *J. Exp. Med.* 215, 233–248. doi: 10.1084/jem.20170807

Evans, T., and Felsenfeld, G. (1989). The erythroid-specific transcription factor Eryf1: a new finger protein. *Cell* 58, 877–885. doi: 10.1016/0092-8674(89)90940-9

Fares, I., Chagraoui, J., Gareau, Y., Gingras, S., Ruel, R., Mayotte, N., et al. (2014). Cord blood expansion. Pyrimidoindole derivatives are agonists of human hematopoietic stem cell self-renewal. *Science* 345, 1509–1512. doi: 10.1126/science.1256337

Fasan, A., Eder, C., Haferlach, C., Grossmann, V., Kohlmann, A., Dicker, F., et al. (2013). *GATA2* mutations are frequent in intermediate-risk karyotype AML with biallelic CEBPA mutations and are associated with favorable prognosis. *Leukemia* 27, 482–485. doi: 10.1038/leu.2012.174

Fisher, K. E., Hsu, A. P., Williams, C. L., Sayeed, H., Merritt, B. Y., Elghetany, M. T., et al. (2017). Somatic mutations in children with *GATA2*-associated myelodysplastic syndrome who lack other features of *GATA2* deficiency. *Blood Adv.* 1, 443–448. doi: 10.1182/bloodadvances.2016002311

Ganapathi, K. A., Townsley, D. M., Hsu, A. P., Arthur, D. C., Zerbe, C. S., Cuellar-Rodriguez, J., et al. (2015). *GATA2* deficiency-associated bone marrow disorder differs from idiopathic aplastic anemia. *Blood* 125, 56–70. doi: 10.1182/blood-2014-06-580340

Gao, X., Johnson, K. D., Chang, Y. I., Boyer, M. E., Dewey, C. N., Zhang, J., et al. (2013). *Gata2* cis-element is required for hematopoietic stem cell generation in the mammalian embryo. *J. Exp. Med.* 210, 2833–2842. doi: 10.1084/jem.20130733

Gasiunas, G., Barrangou, R., Horvath, P., and Siksnys, V. (2012). Cas9-crRNA ribonucleoprotein complex mediates specific DNA cleavage for adaptive immunity in bacteria. *Proc. Natl. Acad. Sci. U.S.A.* 109, E2579–2586. doi: 10.1073/pnas.1208507109

Gaudelli, N. M., Komor, A. C., Rees, H. A., Packer, M. S., Badran, A. H., Bryson, D. I., et al. (2017). Programmable base editing of A•T to G•C in genomic DNA without DNA cleavage. *Nature* 551, 464–471. doi: 10.1038/nature24644

Genovese, P., Schiroli, G., Escobar, G., Tomaso, T. D., Firrito, C., Calabria, A., et al. (2014). Targeted genome editing in human repopulating haematopoietic stem cells. *Nature* 510, 235–240. doi: 10.1038/nature13420

Guo, G., Luc, S., Marco, E., Lin, T. W., Peng, C., Kerenyi, M. A., et al. (2013). Mapping cellular hierarchy by single-cell analysis of the cell surface repertoire. *Cell Stem Cell* 13, 492–505. doi: 10.1016/j.stem.2013.07.017

Hahn, C. N., Chong, C. E., Carmichael, C. L., Wilkins, E. J., Brautigan, P. J., Li, X. C., et al. (2011). Heritable *GATA2* mutations associated with familial myelodysplastic syndrome and acute myeloid leukemia. *Nat. Genet.* 43, 1012–1017. doi: 10.1038/ng.913

Hickstein, D. (2018). HSCT for *GATA2* deficiency across the pond. *Blood* 131, 1272–1274. doi: 10.1182/blood-2018-02-826461

Hoban, M. D., Cost, G. J., Mendel, M. C., Romero, Z., Kaufman, M. L., Joglekar, A. V., et al. (2015). Correction of the sickle cell disease mutation in human hematopoietic stem/progenitor cells. *Blood* 125, 2597–2604. doi: 10.1182/blood-2014-12-615948

Hoban, M. D., Lumaquin, D., Kuo, C. Y., Romero, Z., Long, J., Ho, M., et al. (2016). CRISPR/Cas9-mediated correction of the sickle mutation in human CD34+ cells. *Mol. Ther.* 24, 1561–1569. doi: 10.1038/mt.2016.148

Hou, H. A., Lin, Y. C., Kuo, Y. Y., Chou, W. C., Lin, C. C., Liu, C. Y., et al. (2015). *GATA2* mutations in patients with acute myeloid leukemia-paired samples analyses show that the mutation is unstable during disease evolution. *Ann. Hematol.* 94, 211–221. doi: 10.1007/s00277-014-2208-8

Hsu, A. P., Johnson, K. D., Falcone, E. L., Sanalkumar, R., Sanchez, L., Hickstein, D. D., et al. (2013). *GATA2* haploinsufficiency caused by mutations in a conserved intronic element leads to MonoMAC syndrome. *Blood* 121, 3830–3837. doi: 10.1182/blood-2012-08-452763

Hsu, A. P., Sampaio, E. P., Khan, J., Calvo, K. R., Lemieux, J. E., Patel, S. Y., et al. (2011). Mutations in *GATA2* are associated with the autosomal dominant and sporadic monocytopenia and mycobacterial infection (MonoMAC) syndrome. *Blood* 118, 2653–2655. doi: 10.1182/blood-2011-05-356352

Jinek, M., Chylinski, K., Fonfara, I., Hauer, M., Doudna, J. A., and Charpentier, E. (2012). A programmable dual-RNA-guided DNA endonuclease in adaptive bacterial immunity. *Science* 337, 816–821. doi: 10.1126/science.1225829

Kim, D., Bae, S., Park, J., Kim, E., Kim, S., Yu, H. R., et al. (2015). Digenome-seq: genome-wide profiling of CRISPR-Cas9 off-target effects in human cells. *Nat. Methods* 12, 237–243. doi: 10.1038/nmeth.3284

Komor, A. C., Kim, Y. B., Packer, M. S., Zuris, J. A., and Liu, D., R. (2016). Programmable editing of a target base in genomic DNA without double-stranded DNA cleavage. *Nature* 533, 420–424. doi: 10.1038/nature17946

Lim, K. C., Hosoya, T., Brandt, W., Ku, C. J., Hosoya-Ohmura, S., Camper, S. A., et al. (2012). Conditional *Gata2* inactivation results in HSC loss and lymphatic mispatterning. *J. Clin. Invest.* 122, 3705–3717. doi: 10.1172/JCI61619

Ling, K. W., Ottersbach, K., van Hamburg, J. P., Oziemlak, A., Tsai, F. Y., Orkin, S. H., et al. (2004). GATA-2 plays two functionally distinct roles during the ontogeny of hematopoietic stem cells. *J. Exp. Med.* 200, 871–882. doi: 10.1084/jem.20031556

Luesink, M., Hollink, I. H., V. H., van der Velden, Knops, R. H., Boezeman, J. B., de Haas, V., et al. (2012). High *GATA2* expression is a poor prognostic marker in pediatric acute myeloid leukemia. *Blood* 120, 2064–2075. doi: 10.1182/blood-2011-12-397083

Mali, P., Yang, L., Esvelt, K. M., Aach, J., Guell, M., DiCarlo, J. E., et al. (2013). RNA-guided human genome engineering via Cas9. *Science* 339, 823–826. doi: 10.1126/science.1232033

Marshall, C. J., Moore, R. L., Thorogood, P., Brickell, P. M., Kinnon, C., Thrasher, A., et al. (1999). Detailed characterization of the human aorta-gonad-mesonephros region reveals morphological polarity resembling a hematopoietic stromal layer. *Dev. Dyn.* 215, 139–147. doi: 10.1002/(SICI)1097-0177(199906)215:2<139::AID-DVDY6>3.0.CO;2-#

McReynolds, L. J., Calvo, K. R., and Holland, S., M. (2018). Germline *GATA2* mutation and bone marrow failure. *Hematol. Oncol. Clin. North Am.* 32, 713–728. doi: 10.1016/j.hoc.2018.04.004

Menendez-Gonzalez, J. B., Vukovic, M., Abdelfattah, A., Saleh, L., Almotiri, A., Thomas, L. A., et al. (2019). *Gata2* as a crucial regulator of stem cells in adult hematopoiesis and acute myeloid leukemia. *Stem Cell Rep.* 13, 291–306. doi: 10.1016/j.stemcr.2019.07.005

Minegishi, N., Ohta, J., Suwabe, N., Nakauchi, H., Ishihara, H., Hayashi, N., et al. (1998). Alternative promoters regulate transcription of the mouse GATA-2 gene. *J. Biol. Chem.* 273, 3625–3634. doi: 10.1074/jbc.273.6.3625

Miyamoto, T., Iwasaki, H., Reizis, B., Ye, M., Graf, T., Weissman, I. L., et al. (2002). Myeloid or lymphoid promiscuity as a critical step in hematopoietic lineage commitment. *Dev. Cell* 3, 137–147. doi: 10.1016/S1534-5807(02)00201-0

Nandakumar, S. K., Johnson, K., Throm, S. L., Pestina, T. I., Neale, G., Persons, D., et al. (2015). Low-level *GATA2* overexpression promotes myeloid progenitor self-renewal and blocks lymphoid differentiation in mice. *Exp. Hematol.* 43, 565–577.e561–e510. doi: 10.1016/j.exphem.2015.04.002

Orkin, S. H., and Bauer, D. E. (2019). Emerging genetic therapy for sickle cell disease. *Annu. Rev. Med.* 70, 257–271. doi: 10.1146/annurev-med-041817-125507

Ostergaard, P., Simpson, M. A., Connell, F. C., Steward, C. G., Brice, G., Woollard, W. J., et al. (2011). Mutations in *GATA2* cause primary lymphedema associated with a predisposition to acute myeloid leukemia (Emberger syndrome). *Nat. Genet.* 43, 929–931. doi: 10.1038/ng.923

Pan, X., Minegishi, N., Harigae, H., Yamagiwa, H., Minegishi, M., Akine, Y., et al. (2000). Identification of human GATA-2 gene distal IS exon and its expression in hematopoietic stem cell fractions. *J. Biochem.* 127, 105–112. doi: 10.1093/oxfordjournals.jbchem.a022570

Pasquet, M., Bellanné-Chantelot, C., Tavitian, S., Prade, N., Beaupain, B., Larochelle, O., et al. (2013). High frequency of *GATA2* mutations in patients with mild chronic neutropenia evolving to MonoMac syndrome, myelodysplasia, and acute myeloid leukemia. *Blood* 121, 822–829. doi: 10.1182/blood-2012-08-447367

Ping, N., Sun, A., Song, Y., Wang, Q., Yin, J., Cheng, W., et al. (2017). Exome sequencing identifies highly recurrent somatic *GATA2* and CEBPA mutations in acute erythroid leukemia. *Leukemia* 31, 195–202. doi: 10.1038/leu.2016.162

Rodrigues, N. P., Boyd, A. S., Fugazza, C., May, G. E., Guo, Y., Tipping, A. J., et al. (2008). GATA-2 regulates granulocyte-macrophage progenitor cell function. *Blood* 112, 4862–4873. doi: 10.1182/blood-2008-01-136564

Rodrigues, N. P., Janzen, V., Forkert, R., Dombkowski, D. M., Boyd, A. S., Orkin, S. H., et al. (2005). Haploinsufficiency of GATA-2 perturbs adult hematopoietic stem-cell homeostasis. *Blood* 106, 477–484. doi: 10.1182/blood-2004-08-2989

Sekhar, M., Pocock, R., Lowe, D., Mitchell, C., Marafioti, T., Dickinson, R., et al. (2018). Can somatic *GATA2* mutation mimic germ line *GATA2* mutation? *Blood Adv.* 2, 904–908. doi: 10.1182/bloodadvances.2017012617

Simonis, A., Fux, M., Nair, G., Mueller, N. J., Haralambieva, E., Pabst, T., et al. (2018). Allogeneic hematopoietic cell transplantation in patients with *GATA2* deficiency-a case report and comprehensive review of the literature. *Ann. Hematol.* 97, 1961–1973. doi: 10.1007/s00277-018-3388-4

Spinner, M. A., Sanchez, L. A., Hsu, A. P., Shaw, P. A., Zerbe, C. S., Calvo, K. R., et al. (2014). *GATA2* deficiency: a protean disorder of hematopoiesis, lymphatics, and immunity. *Blood* 123, 809–821. doi: 10.1182/blood-2013-07-515528

The Lancet Haematology (2019). CRISPR-Cas9 gene editing for patients with haemoglobinopathies. *Lancet Haematol.* 6:e438. doi: 10.1016/S2352-3026(19)30169-3

Theis, F., Corbacioglu, A., Gaidzik, V. I., Paschka, P., Weber, D., Bullinger, L., et al. (2016). Clinical impact of *GATA2* mutations in acute myeloid leukemia patients harboring CEBPA mutations: a study of the AML study group. *Leukemia* 30, 2248–2250. doi: 10.1038/leu.2016.185

Tien, F. M., Hou, H. A., Tsai, C. H., Tang, J. L., Chiu, Y. C., Chen, C. Y., et al. (2018). *GATA2* zinc finger 1 mutations are associated with distinct clinico-biological features and outcomes different from *GATA2* zinc finger 2 mutations in adult acute myeloid leukemia. *Blood Cancer J.* 8:87. doi: 10.1038/s41408-018-0123-2

Townsley, D. M., Hsu, A., Dumitriu, B., Holland, S. M., and Young, N., S. (2012). Regulatory mutations in *GATA2* associated with aplastic anemia. *Blood* 120, 3488–3488. doi: 10.1182/blood.V120.21.3488.3488

Tsai, F. Y., Keller, G., Kuo, F. C., Weiss, M., Chen, J., Rosenblatt, M., et al. (1994). An early haematopoietic defect in mice lacking the transcription factor GATA-2. *Nature* 371, 221–226. doi: 10.1038/371221a0

Tsai, S. Q., Nguyen, N. T., Malagon-Lopez, J., Topkar, V. V., Aryee, M. J., Joung, J., et al. (2017). CIRCLE-seq: a highly sensitive in vitro screen for genome-wide CRISPR-Cas9 nuclease off-targets. *Nat. Methods* 14, 607–614. doi: 10.1038/nmeth.4278

Tsai, S. Q., Zheng, Z., Nguyen, N. T., Liebers, M., Topkar, V. V., Thapar, V., et al. (2015). GUIDE-seq enables genome-wide profiling of off-target cleavage by CRISPR-Cas nucleases. *Nat. Biotechnol.* 33, 187–197. doi: 10.1038/nbt.3117

van Lier, Y. F., de Bree, G. J., Jonkers, R. E., Roelofs, J., Ten Berge, I. J., M., et al. (2020). Allogeneic hematopoietic cell transplantation in the management of *GATA2* deficiency and pulmonary alveolar proteinosis. *Clin. Immunol.* 218:108522. doi: 10.1016/j.clim.2020.108522

Vicente, C., Conchillo, A., García-Sánchez, M. A., and Odero, M., D. (2012). The role of the *GATA2* transcription factor in normal and malignant hematopoiesis. *Crit. Rev. Oncol. Hematol.* 82, 1–17. doi: 10.1016/j.critrevonc.2011.04.007

Vink, C. S., Calero-Nieto, F. J., Wang, X., Maglitto, A., Mariani, S. A., Jawaid, W., et al. (2020). Iterative single-cell analyses define the transcriptome of the first functional hematopoietic stem cells. *Cell Rep.* 31:107627. doi: 10.1016/j.celrep.2020.107627

Walters, M. C., Patience, M., Leisenring, W., Rogers, Z. R., Aquino, V. M., Buchanan, G. R., et al. (2001). Stable mixed hematopoietic chimerism after bone marrow transplantation for sickle cell anemia. *Biol. Blood Marrow Transplant* 7, 665–673. doi: 10.1053/bbmt.2001.v7.pm11787529

Wienert, B., Wyman, S. K., Richardson, C. D., Yeh, C. D., Akcakaya, P., Porritt, M. J., et al. (2019). Unbiased detection of CRISPR off-targets in vivo using DISCOVER-Seq. *Science* 364, 286–289. doi: 10.1101/469635

Wilson, D. B., Link, D. C., Mason, P. J., and Bessler, M. (2014). Inherited bone marrow failure syndromes in adolescents and young adults. *Ann. Med.* 46, 353–363. doi: 10.3109/07853890.2014.915579

Wlodarski, M. W., Collin, M., and Horwitz, M., S. (2017). *GATA2* deficiency and related myeloid neoplasms. *Semin. Hematol.* 54, 81–86. doi: 10.1053/j.seminhematol.2017.05.002

Wlodarski, M. W., Hirabayashi, S., Pastor, V., Star,ý, J., Hasle, H., Masetti, R., et al. (2016). Prevalence, clinical characteristics, and prognosis of *GATA2*-related myelodysplastic syndromes in children and adolescents. *Blood* 127, 1387–1397; quiz 1518. doi: 10.1182/blood-2015-09-669937

Xie, F., Ye, L., Chang, J. C., Beyer, A. I., Wang, J., Muench, M. O., et al. (2014). Seamless gene correction of β-thalassemia mutations in patient-specific iPSCs using CRISPR/Cas9 and piggyBac. *Genome Res.* 24, 1526–1533. doi: 10.1101/gr.173427.114

Yokomizo, T., and Dzierzak, E. (2010). Three-dimensional cartography of hematopoietic clusters in the vasculature of whole mouse embryos. *Development* 137, 3651–3661. doi: 10.1242/dev.051094

Yoshida, M., Tanase-Nakao, K., Shima, H., Shirai, R., Yoshida, K., Osumi, T., et al. (2020). Prevalence of germline *GATA2* and SAMD9/9L variants in paediatric haematological disorders with monosomy 7. *Br. J. Haematol.* doi: 10.1111/bjh.17006. [Epub ahead of print].

Yu, Y., Leete, T. C., Born, D. A., Young, L., Barrera, L. A., Lee, S. J., et al. (2020). Cytosine base editors with minimized unguided DNA and RNA off-target events and high on-target activity. *Nat. Commun.* 11:2052. doi: 10.1038/s41467-020-15887-5

Zhou, Y., Zhang, Y., Chen, B., Dong, Y., Zhang, Y., Mao, B., et al. (2019). Overexpression of *GATA2* enhances development and maintenance of human embryonic stem cell-derived hematopoietic stem cell-like progenitors. *Stem Cell Rep.* 13, 31–47. doi: 10.1016/j.stemcr.2019.05.007

Zuo, E., Sun, Y., Wei, W., Yuan, T., Ying, W., Sun, H., et al. (2019). Cytosine base editor generates substantial off-target single-nucleotide variants in mouse embryos. *Science* 364, 289–292. doi: 10.1126/science.aav9973

11

Targeted Gene Delivery: Where to Land

Giulia Pavani[†] and Mario Amendola[*]

INTEGRARE, UMR_S951, Genethon, Inserm, Univ Evry, Univ Paris-Saclay, Evry, France

*Correspondence:
Mario Amendola
mamendola@genethon.fr

†Present address:
Giulia Pavani,
The Children's Hospital of
Philadelphia, Raymond G. Perelman
Center for Cellular and Molecular
Therapeutics, Philadelphia, PA,
United States

Genome-editing technologies have the potential to correct most genetic defects involved in blood disorders. In contrast to mutation-specific editing, targeted gene insertion can correct most of the mutations affecting the same gene with a single therapeutic strategy (gene replacement) or provide novel functions to edited cells (gene addition). Targeting a selected genomic harbor can reduce insertional mutagenesis risk, while enabling the exploitation of endogenous promoters, or selected chromatin contexts, to achieve specific transgene expression levels/patterns and the modulation of disease-modifier genes. In this review, we will discuss targeted gene insertion and the advantages and limitations of different genomic harbors currently under investigation for various gene therapy applications.

Keywords: genome editing, gene therapy, nuclease, CRISPR, targeted integration (TI), knock-in, safe harbor, homologous recombination (HR)

INTRODUCTION

Blood genetic disorders are caused by mutations in genes or in their regulatory elements that result in a dysfunctional, dysregulated, or absent protein. Conventional gene therapy approach consists of the addition of a functional copy of a mutated gene to patients' cells using viral vectors, such as adeno-associated virus (AAV) (Mingozzi and High, 2011) and lentivirus (LV)-derived vectors (Naldini, 2011). These modified viruses can deliver the transgene expression cassettes encoded in their genome to the cell nucleus, where the genetic information is used. This gene replacement strategy is mutation-independent and thus can benefit patients with the same condition regardless of their genotype.

Despite its remarkable success for *ex vivo* and *in vivo* treatment of several monogenic disorders (Dunbar et al., 2018), there are still major hurdles to overcome to improve therapeutic outcomes and treat challenging monogenic (e.g., hemoglobinopathies, immunodeficiencies, and congenital anemias) as well as multifactorial blood diseases (e.g., cancer, autoimmune, and infectious disorders). Apart from vector-specific issues such as immunogenicity and tropism (Masat et al., 2013; Colella et al., 2018), which are beyond the scope of this review, classic gene replacement has a major limitation: it is hard to faithfully re-create characteristics of endogenous promoters and gene-specific regulation within the context of a viral vector. Tissue-, developmental-, and stimulus-specific gene expression requires the complex interaction of different genomic elements (promoters, enhancers, and silencers) that can be located in distant regions of the genome and span several kilobases (Schoenfelder and Fraser, 2019).

AAV vectors are small viruses (~4.7 kb), limiting the choice of regulatory elements to include in the expression cassette, especially when delivering large transgenes (Li and Samulski, 2020). Moreover, they persist mainly as episomes in non-dividing cells and are progressively lost through cell division (Nakai et al., 2001; Ehrhardt et al., 2003; Bortolussi et al., 2014)—a major obstacle for treating infantile disorders and tissues undergoing rapid proliferation (e.g., hematopoietic and epithelial cells). On the other hand, LV have larger cargo capacity (~8 kb), stably integrate in the genome, and persist through cell replication (Naldini et al., 1996), but they carry the intrinsic risk of insertional mutagenesis and oncogene transactivation (mainly when strong promoters/enhancers are present (Cavazzana et al., 2019; Bushman, 2020)). In addition, their semi-random integration (Schroder et al., 2002) results in transduction mosaicism and heterogeneous transgene expression due to chromatin position effects (Chen et al., 2017; Vansant et al., 2020), making therapeutic levels harder to reach.

When combining AAV and nucleases, both transgene expression cassettes and genomic integration sites contribute to the corrective strategy, dramatically expanding therapeutic possibilities. Primarily, targeting a functional copy of a gene to its endogenous locus, under the control of its own promoter and in the right chromatin context, can result in physiological expression and minimize genotoxic integrations. Alternatively, transgenes can be targeted to safe integration sites or specific genomic elements of interest to engineer cells with novel functions, further improving safety and increasing potential applications of gene replacement/addition therapy (Cox et al., 2015).

Sequence-specific endonucleases (such as ZNF, TALEN, or CRISPR/Cas9) (Gaj et al., 2016) can induce genomic DNA double-strand breaks (DSB) in proximity to pathological mutations and activate cellular DNA repair pathways to correct them. The inclusion of short single-stranded oligodeoxynucleotide (ssODN) donors is a simple and effective approach for precise correction of single-nucleotide mutations (DeWitt et al., 2016; De Ravin et al., 2017; Romero et al., 2019). Although their short size currently limits their application for diseases caused by multiple pathological variants (e.g., β-thalassemia, ~300 different mutations across the β-globin locus), technological advances in long ssODN synthesis would most likely expand their therapeutic potential (Praetorius et al., 2017; Roth et al., 2018).

DSB generated by endonucleases can also facilitate integration of therapeutic transgenes to selected genomic locations (targeted gene replacement). AAV has a tendency to integrate at pre-existing chromosomal breaks that provide free DNA ends for non-homologous end joining (NHEJ) (Miller et al., 2004). To increase efficiency, specificity, and precision of integration, homology arms derived from genomic regions flanking the target site are introduced on each side of the AAV cassette with the aim of leveraging the homologous DNA repair pathway (Hirata et al., 2002). Although effective in proliferating cells, homologous recombination is quite inefficient in quiescent hematopoietic stem cells (HSC) and postmitotic cells or tissues (Nishiyama, 2019; Shin et al., 2020). Therefore, alternative DNA repair mechanisms based on NHEJ or microhomology-mediated end joining (MMEJ) are now being investigated (Suzuki et al., 2016; Banan, 2020). In both cases, AAV are the gold-standard DNA delivery system for gene-targeted integration *in vivo* (Li et al., 2011) and *ex vivo* (Wang et al., 2015), though the exact molecular mechanism underpinning this process remains unknown (Deyle and Russell, 2009).

INTEGRATION STRATEGIES

Selecting a suitable genomic site for transgene integration depends on many factors, such as the expression level required, the target cells/tissue, and the disease to be treated.

We have subdivided integration sites in four groups according to functional characteristics: (i) endogenous promoters, when promoterless transgenes are inserted under the control of endogenous enhancers/promoters; (ii) safe genomic harbors, when transgenes and their promoters are integrated into genomic regions that allow robust expression without affecting cell physiology; (iii) disease modifier genes, when transgenes integrate into coding sequence of endogenous genes, whose inactivation benefits disease-affected cells; and (iv) specificity exchange, when transgenes are integrated into coding sequence of endogenous genes to change their function.

It is worth noting that this subdivision is only a working framework, as the same integration site can fall into two or more categories, and it is not exhaustive, as new integration strategies are described every day.

ENDOGENOUS PROMOTERS
Correction of Dysfunctional Genes

A straightforward approach for targeted gene replacement consists in inserting a functional copy of a gene downstream of its endogenous promoter. This strategy can correct most pathological mutations that are scattered along the gene body (such as substitutions and frameshift mutations), while maintaining physiological gene expression (**Table 1A**), which can be hard to achieve with artificial promoters used in classical gene therapy vectors (Toscano et al., 2011).

The first proof of concept was obtained using ZFN on primary T cells *ex vivo* to replace interleukin-2 receptor subunit gamma (*IL2RG*), whose mutational inactivation causes X-linked severe combined immunodeficiency (X-SCID) (Urnov et al., 2005; Lombardo et al., 2007). X-SCID represents an ideal model for testing this approach, as correction of only a small fraction of treated cells, given their strong growth advantage, should allow expansion and restoration of T cell function *in vivo*.

However, for effective clinical translation, targeted gene replacement should be performed in hematopoietic stem cells (HSC), the life-long source of all the different blood progenitors. Genovese via ZFN (Genovese et al., 2014) and Schiroli via CRISPR/Cas9 (Schiroli et al., 2017) were the first to report successful integration of a functional copy of *IL2RG* gene downstream its endogenous promoter in HSC, with the idea of restoring the endogenous lineage specificity and expression level of *IL2RG* without the risk of insertional mutagenesis (Hacein-Bey-Abina et al., 2003, 2008). Following this example, additional strategies have been developed for many blood diseases, including thalassemia (Voit et al., 2014; Dever et al., 2016), chronic granulomatous disease (De Ravin et al., 2017; Sweeney et al., 2017), hyper-immunoglobulin (Ig) M syndrome

TABLE 1 | (A–F) The advantages and disadvantages of different integration strategies.

	Integration strategies		Advantages	Disadvantages	References
A	Endogenous locus		Physiological transgene expression Corrects multiple mutations	Gene-specific strategy Limited to gene body mutations	Urnov et al., 2005; Lombardo et al., 2007; Li et al., 2011; Genovese et al., 2014; Voit et al., 2014; Dever et al., 2016; Hubbard et al., 2016; Schiroli et al., 2017; Sweeney et al., 2017; Kuo et al., 2018; Wang et al., 2019; Rai et al., 2020; Wang L. et al., 2020
B	Superactive promoters (ALB, HBA)		Accommodates different transgenes Supraphysiological expression Few integrations required	Partial gene disruption Limited to non-cell autonomous disorders Extensive validation required	Barzel et al., 2015; Sharma et al., 2015; Davidoff and Nathwani, 2016; Laoharawee et al., 2018; Chen et al., 2019; Conway et al., 2019; De Caneva et al., 2019; Ou et al., 2019, 2020; Zhang et al., 2019; Wang Q. et al., 2020
C	Tolerant to integration (AAVS1, CCR5, Rosa26)		Accommodates different transgenes	Artificial promoters required Variable expression	De Ravin et al., 2016; Diez et al., 2017; Stephens et al., 2018, 2019; Gomez-Ospina et al., 2019; Scharenberg et al., 2020
D	Chromatin domains (NAD)		Fine gene regulation Far from oncogenic genes	No proof-of-principle in clinically relevant models	Schenkwein et al., 2020
E	Disease-modifier genes (CCR5, HBA)		Improve therapeutic effect Lower therapeutic threshold	Extensive validation required Limited to well-known diseases	Voit et al., 2013; Wiebking et al., 2018
F	Specificity Exchange (TCR, BCR)		Improved CAR expression and potency	Off-targets Translocations risk (for multiple edits)	Eyquem et al., 2017; MacLeod et al., 2017; Greiner et al., 2019; Hartweger et al., 2019; Moffett et al., 2019; Voss et al., 2019

Scissors: nuclease; Solid arrows: promoters; Enh, enhancers; TAD, topologically associating; d, domain; Solid ovals: histone modifications; Solid squares: DNA modifications.

(Hubbard et al., 2016; Kuo et al., 2018), and Wiskott–Aldrich Syndrome (Rai et al., 2020).

Beside HSC and terminally differentiated blood cells, like B and T cells (Wang et al., 2016; Hung et al., 2018), AAV and nucleases have been the preferred method to achieve targeted transgene integration in many tissues *in vivo* (Suzuki et al., 2019; Kohama et al., 2020; Nishiguchi et al., 2020), especially the liver.

Li et al. were the first to demonstrate targeted gene correction *in vivo* by delivering ZFN and a partial *F9* (coagulation factor IX, FIX) cDNA cassette with AAV8 to the liver of a humanized mouse model of hemophilia B (Li et al., 2011). While correction was performed in newborn mice, FIX expression was maintained in adults and even persisted after partial hepatectomy, demonstrating stable genomic integration. This approach was later replicated using CRISPR/Cas9 to integrate a hyperactive FIX variant in the mouse *F9* locus (Wang et al., 2019).

Targeted gene replacement can also be combined with classical gene therapy to improve therapeutic outcome. In a neonatal mouse model of ornithine transcarbamylase (OTC) deficiency, an AAV carrying a liver-specific promoter and a human OTC transgene was integrated via CRISPR/Cas9 in the murine OTC locus (Wang L. et al., 2020). Prompt, short-term expression from episomal AAV protected newborn mice from fatal hyperammonemia crisis, whereas its genomic integration allowed long-term disease correction.

Although targeting transgenes to their genomic loci is an effective therapeutic approach, it requires the development of countless gene-tailored editing strategies. Moreover, it can be difficult to reach and correct a number of cells that is sufficient to achieve a therapeutic benefit. Finally, its efficacy is limited in the presence of deletions/inversions that affect large portions of the locus or when regulatory elements controlling gene expression are mutated.

Over/Expression by Superactive Promoters

Although gene-editing technologies are evolving at a fast pace, it can be challenging to correct enough cells to reach a clinical benefit even using high doses of nuclease and donor DNA, which increase chances of off-target genomic cleavage, immune responses, and donor random integration. An alternative strategy consists in "hijacking" strong endogenous promoters to overexpress therapeutic cassettes from few modified cells (**Table 1B**). An elegant example of this approach is the targeted integration of AAV-delivered transgenes under the control of the endogenous albumin promoter in the liver (Barzel et al., 2015; Sharma et al., 2015; Davidoff and Nathwani, 2016). Even with <1% of targeted integration events, the terrific transcriptional activity of this superactive promoter was sufficient to achieve 5–20% of FIX levels and correct bleeding in hemophilia B mice (Barzel et al., 2015). Until today, this strategy has been successfully applied in different preclinical models of hemophilia A and B (Barzel et al., 2015; Sharma et al., 2015; Chen et al., 2019; Conway et al., 2019; Zhang et al., 2019; Wang Q. et al., 2020) and metabolic disorders (Laoharawee et al., 2018; Conway et al., 2019; De Caneva et al., 2019; Ou et al., 2019). Importantly, this is also the first genome-editing strategy undergoing *in vivo* testing in humans to treat mucopolysaccharidosis I and II (NTC02702115, NTC03041324).

Although promising, this approach still presents some concerns. First, targeted integration can lower serum albumin levels (Zhang et al., 2019; Ou et al., 2020) and albumin mutations have been observed in human hepatocellular carcinoma (Cancer Genome Atlas Research Network, 2017; Rao et al., 2017). Second, long-term AAV-mediated expression of endonucleases can result in off-target editing and unwanted AAV insertions (Li et al., 2019; Breton et al., 2020; Wang H. et al., 2020). Finally, pre-existing liver conditions and immune responses against AAV vectors used to deliver transgenes or nucleases severely limit the number of eligible patients (Boutin et al., 2010; Simhadri et al., 2018).

To avoid these issues, we have recently proposed to integrate therapeutic transgenes in the α-globin locus of HSC

(Pavani et al., 2020). Similar to albumin targeting, the idea is to combine the strong transcriptional output of the α-globin promoter with the abundance of transgene-expressing erythroblasts to maximize protein production, reducing the number of integration events required to reach therapeutic levels. Moreover, differently from the liver, autologous HSC can be recovered from patients and edited *ex vivo* before re-administration, thus circumventing immunological issues. Additional experiments in preclinical disease models will elucidate the therapeutic potential of this novel HSC platform for treating genetic diseases.

Following these examples, additional endogenous promoters with specific expression levels/patterns can be exploited for transgene expression. Although promoter hijacking has many advantages over other approaches, it is important to functionally validate the dispensability of the disrupted gene, as nuclease-mediated targeting can result in bi-allelic gene knock out, or to consider safer editing alternatives (e.g., nicking endonucleases Ran et al., 2013).

SAFE GENOMIC HARBORS

Tolerant to the Integration of an Expression Cassette

Genomic safe harbors are intragenic or intergenic regions of the human genome that enable stable expression of integrated transgenes without negatively affecting the host cell (Sadelain et al., 2011). Targeting expression cassettes to these loci is an efficient way to develop a "one-fits-all" platform to express different therapeutic transgenes using the same nuclease(s), therefore optimizing efficiency and improving safety.

By far, the most widely targeted genomic loci are AAVS1, CCR5, and Rosa26 (**Table 1C**).

The *AAVS1 locus* (chromosome 19 q13.42) was historically identified as the preferential integration site of wild-type AAV in human cell lines (Kotin et al., 1992). It encodes the PPP1R12C gene, a subunit of myosin phosphatase whose functions are not fully elucidated (Surks et al., 2003), but probably redundant (Smith et al., 2008). Stable and corrective editing of patients' HSC at this locus has been obtained by integrating a transgene cassette with (Fanconi anemia (Diez et al., 2017)) or without an exogenous promoter (X-CGD (De Ravin et al., 2016)). It is worth noting that the AAVS1 locus is an extremely gene-rich region and, although the presence of an insulator in the promoter of PPP1R12C could shield the genome from the action of the inserted promoter/enhancer (Ogata et al., 2003; Li et al., 2009), it requires a carefully designed transgene expression cassette to avoid transcriptional perturbation of neighboring genes (Lombardo et al., 2011). Moreover, several studies showed that variable expression and promoter silencing can occur at this site in different cell types (Lamartina et al., 2000; Smith et al., 2008; Ordovas et al., 2018; Bhagwan et al., 2019; Klatt et al., 2020), thus potentially limiting transgene expression.

The *CCR5* gene (chromosome 3 p21.31) encodes for the main HIV co-receptor. Since a bi-allelic null mutation of this receptor (CCR5Δ32) confers HIV-1 resistance and is not associated with any major pathology (Hutter et al., 2009), this locus was first targeted/disrupted with nucleases in T cells and HSC to provide protection against AIDS ((Perez et al., 2008; Yu et al., 2020), NCT00842634, NCT02500849, and NCT03164135) and later exploited for targeted gene addition. Therapeutic transgenes involved in lysosomal storage disorders were inserted in the *CCR5* gene of human HSC, under the control of exogenous ubiquitous or tissue-specific promoters. Upon transplantation, edited HSC engrafted, differentiated, and corrected the pathological phenotype in mouse models of MPS I (Gomez-Ospina et al., 2019) and Gaucher (Scharenberg et al., 2020). Although promising, the safety of this approach needs to be further validated, as CCR5 deficiency can result in increased susceptibility to West Nile (Lim et al., 2006; Cahill et al., 2018), influenza (Falcon et al., 2015), and Japanese encephalitis viruses (Larena et al., 2012).

The *Rosa26 locus* (chromosome 3 p25.31) was serendipitously discovered in mice as a reliable site to integrate DNA cassettes for transgenesis (Zambrowicz et al., 1997). This locus was then successfully targeted *in vivo* with CRISPR/Cas9 to knock-in human alpha-1-antitrypsin or FIX in mouse liver (Stephens et al., 2018, 2019). The human homolog was identified on chromosome 3 (position 3p25.3) (Irion et al., 2007); however, the efficacy and safety of this site for targeted integration is still undetermined.

While genomic safe harbors could represent a universal platform for gene targeting and thus expedite clinical development, so far no site of the human genome has been fully validated. The described loci may be acceptable for research applications, but clinical translation will require extensive validation as they localize in gene-dense areas and in proximity of cancer-related genes.

Chromatin Domains With Specific Expression Patterns

The genomic location of transgene integration can change its transcription up to 1,000-fold, according to some well-studied aspects of large-scale domain organization of chromatin (Akhtar et al., 2013; Brueckner et al., 2016; Corrales et al., 2017). Recent evidence for targeting 3D chromatin domains comes from the work of Schenkwein et al. showing that in primary human T cells genomic regions distant from one another linearly, but near in the three-dimensional genome, became jointly affected when site-specific transgene integration was performed (Schenkwein et al., 2020). In this work, transgenes were targeted to nucleolar-associated domains (NAD), which are distant from protein-encoding genes with oncogenic potential and thus represent safe genomic loci for inserting therapeutic transgenes.

The increasing knowledge of chromatin functions and dynamics (Moore et al., 2020) might soon allow us to select integration sites to obtain a certain transcriptional activity and cell/tissue/developmental specificity, as predicted by the presence/absence of certain histone marks (Talbert et al., 2019), DNA methylation, transcriptional factor binding sites, nuclear lamina interaction (Amendola and van Steensel, 2014), chromatin accessibility, and topology (Zheng and Xie, 2019; Zhang et al., 2020) (**Table 1D**). We can easily envision that the combination of selected chromatin locations and expression cassettes will allow fine-tuning of therapeutic transgene expression to unprecedented levels.

DISEASE-MODIFIER GENES

Inactivation of Pathogen Receptors

A disease-modifier gene alters the expression of another gene involved in a genetic/infectious disorder, therefore changing the penetrance, dominance, and severity of the disease itself (Genin et al., 2008). Novel genome-editing strategies can combine transgene expression with modulation of disease-modifier genes to improve therapeutic outcomes and provide cells with novel functions (**Table 1E**). Voit et al. were the first to describe the use of ZFN to integrate transgenes encoding for HIV restriction factors into the HIV co-receptor gene CCR5 (Voit et al., 2013). With this strategy, treated T cells were resistant to HIV infection thanks to the concomitant expression of protective transgenes and knockout of CCR5 (disease-modifier).

Restoring Balance in Disease Pathways

A second example of this approach involves β-thalassemias, a group of blood disorders caused by mutations in the β-globin gene. β-globin associates with α-globin to form adult hemoglobin (HbA, α2β2) and, when β-globin chains are absent or limiting, free α-globin precipitates causing hemolysis and ineffective erythropoiesis. Reduction of α-globin has been shown to ameliorate the β-thalassemia phenotype (Mettananda et al., 2015); hence, we and others have proposed to target the integration of a β-globin transgene into the α-globin site (disease-modifier) of HSC to simultaneously express the therapeutic gene while reducing α-globin production in differentiated erythroblasts (**Table 1E**) (Pavani et al.; Cromer et al.; Molecular Therapy Vol 27 No 4S1, April 2019). The full potential of this combination therapy for these and other genetic diseases will be more clear in the future (Hightower and Alexander, 2018; Rahit and Tarailo-Graovac, 2020).

While the possibility of combining gene replacement and endogenous gene regulation could attain unparalleled additive or synergic therapeutic effects, it is limited to the treatment of diseases for which a deep knowledge of the underlying molecular mechanism is available, and it requires careful examination.

Providing Novel Functions

Targeted integration can also provide cells with novel functions, such as a "safety-switch" for cell therapy applications. Transgene integration can be directed to inactivate an essential metabolic enzyme, the uridine monophosphate synthetase, which makes T cells dependent on supplemented uridine for their growth and survival (Wiebking et al., 2018). This approach could help therapies based on chimeric antigen receptor T cells by introducing a metabolic control of their proliferation and persistence. Further experiments are required to evaluate the clinical readiness of the approach.

SPECIFICITY EXCHANGE

A special case of gene targeting is represented by the "specificity exchange" (**Table 1F**). Chimeric antigen receptors (CARs) are synthetic receptors that redirect and reprogram T cells to recognize specific antigens for tumor rejection (June and Sadelain, 2018). Initially, CARs were introduced in T cells using retroviral and lentiviral vectors (gene addition), with the risk of insertional mutagenesis. In addition, these CAR-T cells had two antigen specificities, the engineered one and the physiological one encoded by the endogenous $\alpha\beta$ T cell receptor (TCR) chains, which may induce graft-vs-host disease when allogenic T cells are used (Torikai et al., 2012).

New CAR-T cells are generated by targeting the integration of the CAR transgene under the transcriptional control of TCR α-chain gene promoter to simultaneously achieve physiological expression of CAR and disruption of the endogenous TCR, thus maintaining only CAR antigen specificity (specificity exchange) (Eyquem et al., 2017; MacLeod et al., 2017). Overall, this strategy allows uniform CAR expression in human T cells and enhances T cell potency, outperforming conventional CAR-T cells.

A similar strategy has also been described to integrate and express a sequence encoding for a defined monoclonal antibody (Ab) of interest under the control of the heavy or light immunoglobulin chain promoter to reprogram B cells to secrete broadly neutralizing Ab against pathogens, for which no protective Ab has been isolated (Greiner et al., 2019; Hartweger et al., 2019; Moffett et al., 2019; Voss et al., 2019).

CONCLUSIONS

Over the past decades, gene therapy for blood disorders has mainly focused on the optimization of transgenes and synthetic promoters to improve expression and achieve therapeutic effects using gene replacement. However, this strategy is associated with the risk of insertional mutagenesis (LV) and episomal vector loss (AAV). The advent of the first generation of DNA endonucleases allowed the integration of transgenes in few selected genomic loci, mainly to achieve stable expression while minimizing insertional mutagenesis risk. Now, thanks to

easily programmable nucleases such as CRISPR/Cas9, we have dramatically expanded our integration options and can creatively exploit different genomic locations to finely tune transgene expression or modulate disease-modifier genes to improve gene therapy outcomes.

A common strategy to target transgene integration combines nucleases with a donor DNA template (generally AAV) and leverages the homologous recombination pathway. However, before clinical translation, strict functional validation will be necessary to reduce potential adverse events associated with each individual component of this system. In particular, nucleases can induce potential off-targets (Kleinstiver et al., 2016; Carroll, 2019) and chromosomal alterations induced by on-target cleavage (Adikusuma et al., 2018; Kosicki et al., 2018; Cullot et al., 2019; Ledford, 2020); nucleases and AAV activate p53 response and trigger cell cycle arrest (Schwartz et al., 2007; Haapaniemi et al., 2018; Ihry et al., 2018); donor DNA integration can occur by different DNA repair mechanisms with outcomes sometimes difficult to predict (Canaj et al., 2019; Hanlon et al., 2019; Nelson et al., 2019); the target site needs to be functionally validated for safety and disposability (Papapetrou and Schambach, 2016).

Additional studies and further optimization of existing editing technologies will remove these hurdles and allow a broad clinical application of the described strategies to treat both monogenic and multifactorial blood diseases.

AUTHOR CONTRIBUTIONS

GP and MA wrote the manuscript. All authors contributed to the article and approved the submitted version.

ACKNOWLEDGMENTS

MA thanks the members of his laboratory at the Genethon Institute.

REFERENCES

Adikusuma, F., Piltz, S., Corbett, M. A., Turvey, M., McColl, S. R., Helbig, K. J., et al. (2018). Large deletions induced by Cas9 cleavage. *Nature* 560, E8–E9. doi: 10.1038/s41586-018-0380-z

Akhtar, W., de Jong, J., Pindyurin, A. V., Pagie, L., Meuleman, W., de Ridder, J., et al. (2013). Chromatin position effects assayed by thousands of reporters integrated in parallel. *Cell* 154, 914–927. doi: 10.1016/j.cell.2013.07.018

Amendola, M., and van Steensel, B. (2014). Mechanisms and dynamics of nuclear lamina-genome interactions. *Curr. Opin. Cell Biol.* 28, 61–68. doi: 10.1016/j.ceb.2014.03.003

Banan, M. (2020). Recent advances in CRISPR/Cas9-mediated knock-ins in mammalian cells. *J. Biotechnol.* 308, 1–9. doi: 10.1016/j.jbiotec.2019.11.010

Barzel, A., Paulk, N. K., Shi, Y., Huang, Y., Chu, K., Zhang, F., et al. (2015). Promoterless gene targeting without nucleases ameliorates haemophilia B in mice. *Nature* 517, 360–364. doi: 10.1038/nature13864

Bhagwan, J. R., Collins, E., Mosqueira, D., Bakar, M., Johnson, B. B., Thompson, A., et al. (2019). Variable expression and silencing of CRISPR-Cas9 targeted transgenes identifies the AAVS1 locus as not an entirely safe harbour. *F1000Res* 8:1911. doi: 10.12688/f1000research.19894.1

Bortolussi, G., Zentillin, L., Vanikova, J., Bockor, L., Bellarosa, C., Mancarella, A., et al. (2014). Life-long correction of hyperbilirubinemia with a neonatal liver-specific AAV-mediated gene transfer in a lethal mouse model of Crigler-Najjar Syndrome. *Hum. Gene Ther.* 25, 844–855. doi: 10.1089/hum.2013.233

Boutin, S., Monteilhet, V., Veron, P., Leborgne, C., Benveniste, O., Montus, M. F., et al. (2010). Prevalence of serum IgG and neutralizing factors against adeno-associated virus (AAV) types 1, 2, 5, 6, 8, and 9 in the healthy population:

implications for gene therapy using AAV vectors. *Hum. Gene Ther.* 21, 704–712. doi: 10.1089/hum.2009.182

Breton, C., Clark, P. M., Wang, L., Greig, J. A., and Wilson, J. M. (2020). ITR-Seq, a next-generation sequencing assay, identifies genome-wide DNA editing sites *in vivo* following adeno-associated viral vector-mediated genome editing. *BMC Genom.* 21:239. doi: 10.1186/s12864-020-6655-4

Brueckner, L., van Arensbergen, J., Akhtar, W., Pagie, L., and van Steensel, B. (2016). High-throughput assessment of context-dependent effects of chromatin proteins. *Epigenet. Chromatin* 9:43. doi: 10.1186/s13072-016-0096-y

Bushman, F. D. (2020). Retroviral insertional mutagenesis in humans: evidence for four genetic mechanisms promoting expansion of cell clones. *Mol. Ther.* 28, 352–356. doi: 10.1016/j.ymthe.2019.12.009

Cahill, M. E., Conley, S., DeWan, A. T., and Montgomery, R. R. (2018). Identification of genetic variants associated with dengue or West Nile virus disease: a systematic review and meta-analysis. *BMC Infect. Dis.* 18:282. doi: 10.1186/s12879-018-3186-6

Canaj, H., Hussmann, J. A., Li, H., Beckman, K. A., Goodrich, L., Cho, N. H., et al. (2019). Deep profiling reveals substantial heterogeneity of integration outcomes in CRISPR knock-in. *bioRxiv [Preprint]. bioRxiv:* 841098. doi: 10.1101/841098

Cancer Genome Atlas Research Network (2017). Comprehensive and integrative genomic characterization of hepatocellular carcinoma. *Cell* 169, 1327–1341 e23. doi: 10.1016/j.cell.2017.05.046

Carroll, D. (2019). Collateral damage: benchmarking off-target effects in genome editing. *Genome Biol.* 20:114. doi: 10.1186/s13059-019-1725-0

Cavazzana, M., Bushman, F. D., Miccio, A., Andre-Schmutz, I., and Six, E. (2019). Gene therapy targeting haematopoietic stem cells for inherited diseases: progress and challenges. *Nat. Rev. Drug Discov.* 18, 447–462. doi: 10.1038/s41573-019-0020-9

Chen, H., Shi, M., Gilam, A., Zheng, Q., Zhang, Y., Afrikanova, I., et al. (2019). Hemophilia A ameliorated in mice by CRISPR-based *in vivo* genome editing of human factor. *Sci. Rep.* 9:16838. doi: 10.1038/s41598-019-53198-y

Chen, H. C., Martinez, J. P., Zorita, E., Meyerhans, A., and Filion, G. J. (2017). Position effects influence HIV latency reversal. *Nat. Struct. Mol. Biol.* 24, 47–54. doi: 10.1038/nsmb.3328

Colella, P., Ronzitti, G., and Mingozzi, F. (2018). Emerging issues in AAV-mediated *in vivo* gene therapy. *Mol. Ther. Methods Clin. Dev.* 8, 87–104. doi: 10.1016/j.omtm.2017.11.007

Conway, A., Mendel, M., Kim, K., McGovern, K., Boyko, A., Zhang, L., et al. (2019). Non-viral delivery of zinc finger nuclease mRNA enables highly efficient *in vivo* genome editing of multiple therapeutic gene targets. *Mol. Ther.* 27, 866–877. doi: 10.1016/j.ymthe.2019.03.003

Corrales, M., Rosado, A., Cortini, R., van Arensbergen, J., van Steensel, B., and Filion, G. J. (2017). Clustering of Drosophila housekeeping promoters facilitates their expression. *Genome Res.* 27, 1153–1161. doi: 10.1101/gr.211433.116

Cox, D. B., Platt, R. J., and Zhang, F. (2015). Therapeutic genome editing: prospects and challenges. *Nat. Med.* 21, 121–131. doi: 10.1038/nm.3793

Cullot, G., Boutin, J., Toutain, J., Prat, F., Pennamen, P., Rooryck, C., et al. (2019). CRISPR-Cas9 genome editing induces megabase-scale chromosomal truncations. *Nat. Commun.* 10:1136. doi: 10.1038/s41467-019-09006-2

Davidoff, A. M., and Nathwani, A. C. (2016). Genetic targeting of the albumin locus to treat Hemophilia. *N. Engl. J. Med.* 374, 1288–1290. doi: 10.1056/NEJMcibr1600347

De Caneva, A., Porro, F., Bortolussi, G., Sola, R., Lisjak, M., Barzel, A., et al. (2019). Coupling AAV-mediated promoterless gene targeting to SaCas9 nuclease to efficiently correct liver metabolic diseases. *JCI Insight.* 5:128863. doi: 10.1172/jci.insight.128863

De Ravin, S. S., Li, L., Wu, X., Choi, U., Allen, C., Koontz, S., et al. (2017). CRISPR-Cas9 gene repair of hematopoietic stem cells from patients with X-linked chronic granulomatous disease. *Sci. Transl. Med.* 9:aah3480. doi: 10.1126/scitranslmed.aah3480

De Ravin, S. S., Reik, A., Liu, P. Q., Li, L., Wu, X., Su, L., et al. (2016). Targeted gene addition in human CD34(+) hematopoietic cells for correction of X-linked chronic granulomatous disease. *Nat. Biotechnol.* 34, 424–429. doi: 10.1038/nbt.3513

Dever, D. P., Bak, R. O., Reinisch, A., Camarena, J., Washington, G., Nicolas, C. E., et al. (2016). CRISPR/Cas9 beta-globin gene targeting in human haematopoietic stem cells. *Nature* 539, 384–389. doi: 10.1038/nature20134

DeWitt, M. A., Magis, W., Bray, N. L., Wang, T., Berman, J. R., Urbinati, F., et al. (2016). Selection-free genome editing of the sickle mutation in human adult hematopoietic stem/progenitor cells. *Sci. Transl. Med.* 8:360ra134. doi: 10.1126/scitranslmed.aaf9336

Deyle, D. R., and Russell, D. W. (2009). Adeno-associated virus vector integration. *Curr Opin Mol Ther.* 11, 442–447.

Diez, B., Genovese, P., Roman-Rodriguez, F. J., Alvarez, L., Schiroli, G., Ugalde, L., et al. (2017). Therapeutic gene editing in CD34(+) hematopoietic progenitors from Fanconi anemia patients. *EMBO Mol. Med.* 9, 1574–1588. doi: 10.15252/emmm.201707540

Dunbar, C. E., High, K. A., Joung, J. K., Kohn, D. B., Ozawa, K., and Sadelain, M. (2018). Gene therapy comes of age. *Science* 359:aan4672. doi: 10.1126/science.aan4672

Ehrhardt, A., Xu, H., and Kay, M. A. (2003). Episomal persistence of recombinant adenoviral vector genomes during the cell cycle *in vivo. J. Virol.* 77, 7689–7695. doi: 10.1128/JVI.77.13.7689-7695.2003

Eyquem, J., Mansilla-Soto, J., Giavridis, T., van der Stegen, S. J., Hamieh, M., Cunanan, K. M., et al. (2017). Targeting a CAR to the TRAC locus with CRISPR/Cas9 enhances tumour rejection. *Nature* 543, 113–117. doi: 10.1038/nature21405

Falcon, A., Cuevas, M. T., Rodriguez-Frandsen, A., Reyes, N., Pozo, F., Moreno, S., et al. (2015). CCR5 deficiency predisposes to fatal outcome in influenza virus infection. *J. Gen. Virol.* 96, 2074–2078. doi: 10.1099/vir.0.000165

Gaj, T., Sirk, S. J., Shui, S. L., and Liu, J. (2016). Genome-editing technologies: principles and applications. *Cold Spring Harb. Perspect. Biol.* 8:a023754. doi: 10.1101/cshperspect.a023754

Genin, E., Feingold, J., and Clerget-Darpoux, F. (2008). Identifying modifier genes of monogenic disease: strategies and difficulties. *Hum. Genet.* 124, 357–368. doi: 10.1007/s00439-008-0560-2

Genovese, P., Schiroli, G., Escobar, G., Tomaso, T. D., Firrito, C., Calabria, A., et al. (2014). Targeted genome editing in human repopulating haematopoietic stem cells. *Nature* 510, 235–240. doi: 10.1038/nature13420

Gomez-Ospina, N., Scharenberg, S. G., Mostrel, N., Bak, R. O., Mantri, S., Quadros, R. M., et al. (2019). Human genome-edited hematopoietic stem cells phenotypically correct Mucopolysaccharidosis type. *Nat. Commun.* 10:4045. doi: 10.1038/s41467-019-11962-8

Greiner, V., Bou Puerto, R., Liu, S., Herbel, C., Carmona, E. M., and Goldberg, M. S. (2019). CRISPR-mediated editing of the B cell receptor in primary human B cells. *iScience* 12, 369–378. doi: 10.1016/j.isci.2019.01.032

Haapaniemi, E., Botla, S., Persson, J., Schmierer, B., and Taipale, J. (2018). CRISPR-Cas9 genome editing induces a p53-mediated DNA damage response. *Nat. Med.* 24, 927–930. doi: 10.1038/s41591-018-0049-z

Hacein-Bey-Abina, S., Garrigue, A., Wang, G. P., Soulier, J., Lim, A., Morillon, E., et al. (2008). Insertional oncogenesis in 4 patients after retrovirus-mediated gene therapy of SCID-X1. *J. Clin. Invest.* 118, 3132–3142. doi: 10.1172/JCI35700

Hacein-Bey-Abina, S., Von Kalle, C., Schmidt, M., McCormack, M. P., Wulffraat, N., Leboulch, P., et al. (2003). LMO2-associated clonal T cell proliferation in two patients after gene therapy for SCID-X1. *Science* 302, 415–419. doi: 10.1126/science.1088547

Hanlon, K. S., Kleinstiver, B. P., Garcia, S. P., Zaborowski, M. P., Volak, A., Spirig, S. E., et al. (2019). High levels of AAV vector integration into CRISPR-induced DNA breaks. *Nat. Commun.* 10:4439. doi: 10.1038/s41467-019-12449-2

Hartweger, H., McGuire, A. T., Horning, M., Taylor, J. J., Dosenovic, P., Yost, D., et al. (2019). HIV-specific humoral immune responses by CRISPR/Cas9-edited B cells. *J. Exp. Med.* 216, 1301–1310. doi: 10.1084/jem.20190287

Hightower, R. M., and Alexander, M. S. (2018). Genetic modifiers of Duchenne and facioscapulohumeral muscular dystrophies. *Muscle Nerve.* 57, 6–15. doi: 10.1002/mus.25953

Hirata, R., Chamberlain, J., Dong, R., and Russell, D. W. (2002). Targeted transgene insertion into human chromosomes by adeno-associated virus vectors. *Nat. Biotechnol.* 20, 735–738. doi: 10.1038/nbt0702-735

Hubbard, N., Hagin, D., Sommer, K., Song, Y., Khan, I., Clough, C., et al. (2016). Targeted gene editing restores regulated CD40L function in X-linked hyper-IgM syndrome. *Blood* 127, 2513–2522. doi: 10.1182/blood-2015-11-683235

Hung, K. L., Meitlis, I., Hale, M., Chen, C. Y., Singh, S., Jackson, S. W., et al. (2018). Engineering protein-secreting plasma cells by homology-directed repair in primary human B cells. *Mol. Ther.* 26, 456–467. doi: 10.1016/j.ymthe.2017.11.012

Hutter, G., Nowak, D., Mossner, M., Ganepola, S., Mussig, A., Allers, K., et al. (2009). Long-term control of HIV by CCR5 Delta32/Delta32 stem-cell transplantation. *N. Engl. J. Med.* 360, 692–698. doi: 10.1056/NEJMoa0802905

Ihry, R. J., Worringer, K. A., Salick, M. R., Frias, E., Ho, D., Theriault, K., et al. (2018). p53 inhibits CRISPR-Cas9 engineering in human pluripotent stem cells. *Nat. Med.* 24, 939–946. doi: 10.1038/s41591-018-0050-6

Irion, S., Luche, H., Gadue, P., Fehling, H. J., Kennedy, M., and Keller, G. (2007). Identification and targeting of the ROSA26 locus in human embryonic stem cells. *Nat. Biotechnol.* 25, 1477–1482. doi: 10.1038/nbt1362

June, C. H., and Sadelain, M. (2018). Chimeric antigen receptor therapy. *N. Engl. J. Med.* 379, 64–73. doi: 10.1056/NEJMra1706169

Klatt, D., Cheng, E., Hoffmann, D., Santilli, G., Thrasher, A. J., Brendel, C., et al. (2020). Differential transgene silencing of myeloid-specific promoters in the AAVS1 safe harbor locus of induced pluripotent stem cell-derived myeloid cells. *Hum. Gene Ther.* 31, 199–210. doi: 10.1089/hum.2019.194

Kleinstiver, B. P., Pattanayak, V., Prew, M. S., Tsai, S. Q., Nguyen, N. T., Zheng, Z., et al. (2016). High-fidelity CRISPR-Cas9 nucleases with no detectable genome-wide off-target effects. *Nature* 529, 490–495. doi: 10.1038/nature16526

Kohama, Y., Higo, S., Masumura, Y., Shiba, M., Kondo, T., Ishizu, T., et al. (2020). Adeno-associated virus-mediated gene delivery promotes S-phase entry-independent precise targeted integration in cardiomyocytes. *Sci. Rep.* 10:15348. doi: 10.1038/s41598-020-72216-y

Kosicki, M., Tomberg, K., and Bradley, A. (2018). Repair of double-strand breaks induced by CRISPR-Cas9 leads to large deletions and complex rearrangements. *Nat. Biotechnol.* 36, 765–771. doi: 10.1038/nbt.4192

Kotin, R. M., Linden, R. M., and Berns, K. I. (1992). Characterization of a preferred site on human chromosome 19q for integration of adeno-associated virus DNA by non-homologous recombination. *EMBO J.* 11, 5071–5078. doi: 10.1002/j.1460-2075.1992.tb05614.x

Kuo, C. Y., Long, J. D., Campo-Fernandez, B., de Oliveira, S., Cooper, A. R., Romero, Z., et al. (2018). Site-specific gene editing of human hematopoietic stem cells for X-linked hyper-IgM syndrome. *Cell Rep.* 23, 2606–2616. doi: 10.1016/j.celrep.2018.04.103

Lamartina, S., Sporeno, E., Fattori, E., and Toniatti, C. (2000). Characteristics of the adeno-associated virus preintegration site in human chromosome 19: open chromatin conformation and transcription-competent environment. *J. Virol.* 74, 7671–7677. doi: 10.1128/JVI.74.16.7671-7677.2000

Laoharawee, K., DeKelver, R. C., Podetz-Pedersen, K. M., Rohde, M., Sproul, S., Nguyen, H. O., et al. (2018). Dose-dependent prevention of metabolic and neurologic disease in murine MPS II by ZFN-mediated *in vivo* genome editing. *Mol. Ther.* 26, 1127–1136. doi: 10.1016/j.ymthe.2018.03.002

Larena, M., Regner, M., and Lobigs, M. (2012). The chemokine receptor CCR5, a therapeutic target for HIV/AIDS antagonists, is critical for recovery in a mouse model of Japanese encephalitis. *PLoS ONE* 7:e44834. doi: 10.1371/journal.pone.0044834

Ledford, H. (2020). CRISPR gene editing in human embryos wreaks chromosomal mayhem. *Nature* 583, 17–18. doi: 10.1038/d41586-020-01906-4

Li, A., Lee, C. M., Hurley, A. E., Jarrett, K. E., De Giorgi, M., Lu, W., et al. (2019). A self-deleting AAV-CRISPR system for *in vivo* genome editing. *Mol. Ther. Methods Clin. Dev.* 12, 111–122. doi: 10.1016/j.omtm.2018.11.009

Li, C., Hirsch, M., Carter, P., Asokan, A., Zhou, X., Wu, Z., et al. (2009). A small regulatory element from chromosome 19 enhances liver-specific gene expression. *Gene Ther.* 16, 43–51. doi: 10.1038/gt.2008.134

Li, C., and Samulski, R. J. (2020). Engineering adeno-associated virus vectors for gene therapy. *Nat. Rev. Genet.* 21, 255–272. doi: 10.1038/s41576-019-0205-4

Li, H., Haurigot, V., Doyon, Y., Li, T., Wong, S. Y., Bhagwat, A. S., et al. (2011). *In vivo* genome editing restores haemostasis in a mouse model of haemophilia. *Nature* 475, 217–221. doi: 10.1038/nature10177

Lim, J. K., Glass, W. G., McDermott, D. H., and Murphy, P. M. (2006). CCR5: no longer a "good for nothing" gene–chemokine control of West Nile virus infection. *Trends Immunol.* 27, 308–312. doi: 10.1016/j.it.2006.05.007

Lombardo, A., Cesana, D., Genovese, P., Di Stefano, B., Provasi, E., Colombo, D. F., et al. (2011). Site-specific integration and tailoring of cassette design for sustainable gene transfer. *Nat. Methods* 8, 861–869. doi: 10.1038/nmeth.1674

Lombardo, A., Genovese, P., Beausejour, C. M., Colleoni, S., Lee, Y. L., Kim, K. A., et al. (2007). Gene editing in human stem cells using zinc finger nucleases and integrase-defective lentiviral vector delivery. *Nat. Biotechnol.* 25, 1298–1306. doi: 10.1038/nbt1353

MacLeod, D. T., Antony, J., Martin, A. J., Moser, R. J., Hekele, A., Wetzel, K. J., et al. (2017). Integration of a CD19 CAR into the TCR alpha chain locus streamlines production of allogeneic gene-edited CAR T cells. *Mol. Ther.* 25, 949–961. doi: 10.1016/j.ymthe.2017.02.005

Masat, E., Pavani, G., and Mingozzi, F. (2013). Humoral immunity to AAV vectors in gene therapy: challenges and potential solutions. *Discov. Med.* 15, 379–389.

Mettananda, S., Gibbons, R. J., and Higgs, D. R. (2015). alpha-Globin as a molecular target in the treatment of beta-thalassemia. *Blood* 125, 3694–3701. doi: 10.1182/blood-2015-03-633594

Miller, D. G., Petek, L. M., and Russell, D. W. (2004). Adeno-associated virus vectors integrate at chromosome breakage sites. *Nat. Genet.* 36, 767–773. doi: 10.1038/ng1380

Mingozzi, F., and High, K. A. (2011). Therapeutic *in vivo* gene transfer for genetic disease using AAV: progress and challenges. *Nat. Rev. Genet.* 12, 341–355. doi: 10.1038/nrg2988

Moffett, H. F., Harms, C. K., Fitzpatrick, K. S., Tooley, M. R., Boonyaratanakornkit, J., and Taylor, J. J. (2019). B cells engineered to express pathogen-specific antibodies protect against infection. *Sci. Immunol.* 4:aax0644. doi: 10.1126/sciimmunol.aax0644

Moore, J. E., Purcaro, M. J., Pratt, H. E., Epstein, C. B., Shoresh, N., Adrian, J., et al. (2020). Expanded encyclopaedias of DNA elements in the human and mouse genomes. *Nature* 583, 699–710. doi: 10.1038/s41586-020-2493-4

Nakai, H., Yant, S. R., Storm, T. A., Fuess, S., Meuse, L., and Kay, M. A. (2001). Extrachromosomal recombinant adeno-associated virus vector genomes are primarily responsible for stable liver transduction *in vivo*. *J. Virol.* 75, 6969–6976. doi: 10.1128/JVI.75.15.6969-6976.2001

Naldini, L. (2011). *Ex vivo* gene transfer and correction for cell-based therapies. *Nat. Rev. Genet.* 12, 301–315. doi: 10.1038/nrg2985

Naldini, L., Blomer, U., Gallay, P., Ory, D., Mulligan, R., Gage, F. H., et al. (1996). *In vivo* gene delivery and stable transduction of non-dividing cells by a lentiviral vector. *Science* 272, 263–267. doi: 10.1126/science.272.5259.263

Nelson, C. E., Wu, Y., Gemberling, M. P., Oliver, M. L., Waller, M. A., Bohning, J. D., et al. (2019). Long-term evaluation of AAV-CRISPR genome editing for Duchenne muscular dystrophy. *Nat. Med.* 25, 427–432. doi: 10.1038/s41591-019-0344-3

Nishiguchi, K. M., Fujita, K., Miya, F., Katayama, S., and Nakazawa, T. (2020). Single AAV-mediated mutation replacement genome editing in limited number of photoreceptors restores vision in mice. *Nat. Commun.* 11:482. doi: 10.1038/s41467-019-14181-3

Nishiyama, J. (2019). Genome editing in the mammalian brain using the CRISPR-Cas system. *Neurosci. Res.* 141, 4–12. doi: 10.1016/j.neures.2018.07.003

Ogata, T., Kozuka, T., and Kanda, T. (2003). Identification of an insulator in AAVS1, a preferred region for integration of adeno-associated virus DNA. *J. Virol.* 77, 9000–9007. doi: 10.1128/JVI.77.16.9000-9007.2003

Ordovas, L., Boon, R., Pistoni, M., Chen, Y., Wolfs, E., Guo, W., et al. (2018). Efficient recombinase-mediated cassette exchange in hPSCs to study the hepatocyte lineage reveals AAVS1 locus-mediated transgene inhibition. *Stem Cell Rep.* 10:673. doi: 10.1016/j.stemcr.2018.01.034

Ou, L., DeKelver, R. C., Rohde, M., Tom, S., Radeke, R., St Martin, S. J., et al. (2019). ZFN-mediated *in vivo* genome editing corrects murine hurler syndrome. *Mol. Ther.* 27, 178–187. doi: 10.1016/j.ymthe.2018.10.018

Ou, L., Przybilla, M. J., Ahlat, O., Kim, S., Overn, P., Jarnes, J., et al. (2020). A highly efficacious PS gene editing system corrects metabolic and neurological complications of Mucopolysaccharidosis type I. *Mol. Ther.* 28, 1442–1454. doi: 10.1016/j.ymthe.2020.03.018

Papapetrou, E. P., and Schambach, A. (2016). Gene insertion into genomic safe harbors for human gene therapy. *Mol. Ther.* 24, 678–684. doi: 10.1038/mt.2016.38

Pavani, G., Laurent, M., Fabiano, A., Cantelli, E., Sakkal, A., Corre, G., et al. (2020). *Ex vivo* editing of human hematopoietic stem cells for erythroid expression of therapeutic proteins. *Nat. Commun.* 11:3778. doi: 10.1038/s41467-020-17552-3

Perez, E. E., Wang, J., Miller, J. C., Jouvenot, Y., Kim, K. A., Liu, O., et al. (2008). Establishment of HIV-1 resistance in CD4+ T cells by genome editing using zinc-finger nucleases. *Nat. Biotechnol.* 26, 808–816. doi: 10.1038/nbt1410

Praetorius, F., Kick, B., Behler, K. L., Honemann, M. N., Weuster-Botz, D., and Dietz, H. (2017). Biotechnological mass production of DNA origami. *Nature* 552, 84–87. doi: 10.1038/nature24650

Rahit, K., and Tarailo-Graovac, M. (2020). Genetic modifiers and rare mendelian disease. *Genes.* 11:30239. doi: 10.3390/genes11030239

Rai, R., Romito, M., Rivers, E., Turchiano, G., Blattner, G., Vetharoy, W., et al. (2020). Targeted gene correction of human hematopoietic stem cells for the treatment of Wiskott - Aldrich Syndrome. *Nat. Commun.* 11:4034. doi: 10.1038/s41467-020-17626-2

Ran, F. A., Hsu, P. D., Lin, C. Y., Gootenberg, J. S., Konermann, S., Trevino, A. E., et al. (2013). Double nicking by RNA-guided CRISPR Cas9 for enhanced genome editing specificity. *Cell* 154, 1380–1389. doi: 10.1016/j.cell.2013.08.021

Rao, C. V., Asch, A. S., and Yamada, H. Y. (2017). Frequently mutated genes/pathways and genomic instability as prevention targets in liver cancer. *Carcinogenesis* 38, 2–11. doi: 10.1093/carcin/bgw118

Romero, Z., Lomova, A., Said, S., Miggelbrink, A., Kuo, C. Y., Campo-Fernandez, B., et al. (2019). Editing the sickle cell disease mutation in human hematopoietic stem cells: comparison of endonucleases and homologous donor templates. *Mol. Ther.* 27, 1389–1406. doi: 10.1016/j.ymthe.2019.05.014

Roth, T. L., Puig-Saus, C., Yu, R., Shifrut, E., Carnevale, J., Li, P. J., et al. (2018). Reprogramming human T cell function and specificity with non-viral genome targeting. *Nature* 559, 405–409. doi: 10.1038/s41586-018-0326-5

Sadelain, M., Papapetrou, E. P., and Bushman, F. D. (2011). Safe harbours for the integration of new DNA in the human genome. *Nat. Rev. Cancer.* 12, 51–58. doi: 10.1038/nrc3179

Scharenberg, S. G., Poletto, E., Lucot, K. L., Colella, P., Sheikali, A., Montine, T. J., et al. (2020). Engineering monocyte/macrophage-specific glucocerebrosidase expression in human hematopoietic stem cells using genome editing. *Nat. Commun.* 11:3327. doi: 10.1038/s41467-020-17148-x

Schenkwein, D., Afzal, S., Nousiainen, A., Schmidt, M., and Yla-Herttuala, S. (2020). Efficient nuclease-directed integration of lentivirus vectors into the human ribosomal DNA locus. *Mol. Ther.* 28, 1858–1875. doi: 10.1016/j.ymthe.2020.05.019

Schiroli, G., Ferrari, S., Conway, A., Jacob, A., Capo, V., Albano, L., et al. (2017). Preclinical modeling highlights the therapeutic potential of hematopoietic stem cell gene editing for correction of SCID-X1. *Sci. Transl. Med.* 9:aan0820. doi: 10.1126/scitranslmed.aan0820

Schoenfelder, S., and Fraser, P. (2019). Long-range enhancer-promoter contacts in gene expression control. *Nat. Rev. Genet.* 20, 437–455. doi: 10.1038/s41576-019-0128-0

Schroder, A. R., Shinn, P., Chen, H., Berry, C., Ecker, J. R., and Bushman, F. (2002). HIV-1 integration in the human genome favors active genes and local hotspots. *Cell* 110, 521–529. doi: 10.1016/S0092-8674(02)00864-4

Schwartz, R. A., Palacios, J. A., Cassell, G. D., Adam, S., Giacca, M., and Weitzman, M. D. (2007). The Mre11/Rad50/Nbs1 complex limits adeno-associated virus transduction and replication. *J. Virol.* 81, 12936–12945. doi: 10.1128/JVI.01523-07

Sharma, R., Anguela, X. M., Doyon, Y., Wechsler, T., DeKelver, R. C., Sproul, S., et al. (2015). *In vivo* genome editing of the albumin locus as a platform for protein replacement therapy. *Blood* 126, 1777–1784. doi: 10.1182/blood-2014-12-615492

Shin, J. J., Schroder, M. S., Caiado, F., Wyman, S. K., Bray, N. L., Bordi, M., et al. (2020). Controlled cycling and quiescence enables efficient HDR in engraftment-enriched adult hematopoietic stem and progenitor cells. *Cell Rep.* 32:108093. doi: 10.1016/j.celrep.2020.108093

Simhadri, V. L., McGill, J., McMahon, S., Wang, J., Jiang, H., and Sauna, Z. E. (2018). Prevalence of pre-existing antibodies to CRISPR-associated nuclease Cas9 in the USA population. *Mol. Ther. Methods Clin. Dev.* 10, 105–112. doi: 10.1016/j.omtm.2018.06.006

Smith, J. R., Maguire, S., Davis, L. A., Alexander, M., Yang, F., Chandran, S., et al. (2008). Robust, persistent transgene expression in human embryonic stem cells is achieved with AAVS1-targeted integration. *Stem Cells* 26, 496–504. doi: 10.1634/stemcells.2007-0039

Stephens, C. J., Kashentseva, E., Everett, W., Kaliberova, L., and Curiel, D. T. (2018). Targeted *in vivo* knock-in of human alpha-1-antitrypsin cDNA using adenoviral delivery of CRISPR/Cas9. *Gene Ther.* 25, 139–156. doi: 10.1038/s41434-018-0003-1

Stephens, C. J., Lauron, E. J., Kashentseva, E., Lu, Z. H., Yokoyama, W. M., and Curiel, D. T. (2019). Long-term correction of hemophilia B using adenoviral delivery of CRISPR/Cas9. *J. Contr. Release.* 298, 128–141. doi: 10.1016/j.jconrel.2019.02.009

Surks, H. K., Richards, C. T., and Mendelsohn, M. E. (2003). Myosin phosphatase-Rho interacting protein. A new member of the myosin phosphatase complex that directly binds RhoA. *J. Biol. Chem.* 278, 51484–51493. doi: 10.1074/jbc.M305622200

Suzuki, K., Tsunekawa, Y., Hernandez-Benitez, R., Wu, J., Zhu, J., Kim, E. J., et al. (2016). *In vivo* genome editing *via* CRISPR/Cas9 mediated homology-independent targeted integration. *Nature* 540, 144–149. doi: 10.1038/nature20565

Suzuki, K., Yamamoto, M., Hernandez-Benitez, R., Li, Z., Wei, C., Soligalla, R. D., et al. (2019). Precise *in vivo* genome editing *via* single homology arm donor mediated intron-targeting gene integration for genetic disease correction. *Cell Res.* 29, 804–819. doi: 10.1038/s41422-019-0213-0

Sweeney, C. L., Zou, J., Choi, U., Merling, R. K., Liu, A., Bodansky, A., et al. (2017). Targeted repair of CYBB in X-CGD iPSCs requires retention of intronic sequences for expression and functional correction. *Mol. Ther.* 25, 321–330. doi: 10.1016/j.ymthe.2016.11.012

Talbert, P. B., Meers, M. P., and Henikoff, S. (2019). Old cogs, new tricks: the evolution of gene expression in a chromatin context. *Nat. Rev. Genet.* 20, 283–297. doi: 10.1038/s41576-019-0105-7

Torikai, H., Reik, A., Liu, P. Q., Zhou, Y., Zhang, L., Maiti, S., et al. (2012). A foundation for universal T-cell based immunotherapy: T cells engineered to express a CD19-specific chimeric-antigen-receptor and eliminate expression of endogenous TCR. *Blood* 119, 5697–5705. doi: 10.1182/blood-2012-01-405365

Toscano, M. G., Romero, Z., Munoz, P., Cobo, M., Benabdellah, K., and Martin, F. (2011). Physiological and tissue-specific vectors for treatment of inherited diseases. *Gene Ther.* 18, 117–127. doi: 10.1038/gt.2010.138

Urnov, F. D., Miller, J. C., Lee, Y. L., Beausejour, C. M., Rock, J. M., Augustus, S., et al. (2005). Highly efficient endogenous human gene correction using designed zinc-finger nucleases. *Nature* 435, 646–651. doi: 10.1038/nature03556

Vansant, G., Chen, H. C., Zorita, E., Trejbalova, K., Miklik, D., Filion, G., et al. (2020). The chromatin landscape at the HIV-1 provirus integration site determines viral expression. *Nucl. Acids Res.* 48, 7801–7817. doi: 10.1093/nar/gkaa536

Voit, R. A., Hendel, A., Pruett-Miller, S. M., and Porteus, M. H. (2014). Nuclease-mediated gene editing by homologous recombination of the human globin locus. *Nucl. Acids Res.* 42, 1365–1378. doi: 10.1093/nar/gkt947

Voit, R. A., McMahon, M. A., Sawyer, S. L., and Porteus, M. H. (2013). Generation of an HIV resistant T-cell line by targeted "stacking" of restriction factors. *Mol. Ther.* 21, 786–795. doi: 10.1038/mt.2012.284

Voss, J. E., Gonzalez-Martin, A., Andrabi, R., Fuller, R. P., Murrell, B., McCoy, L. E., et al. (2019). Reprogramming the antigen specificity of B cells using genome-editing technologies. *Elife* 8:42995. doi: 10.7554/eLife.42995

Wang, H., Lu, H., Lei, Y. S., Gong, C. Y., Chen, Z., Luan, Y. Q., et al. (2020). Development of a self-restricting CRISPR-Cas9 system to reduce off-target effects. *Mol. Ther. Methods Clin. Dev.* 18, 390–401. doi: 10.1016/j.omtm.2020.06.012

Wang, J., DeClercq, J. J., Hayward, S. B., Li, P. W., Shivak, D. A., Gregory, P. D., et al. (2016). Highly efficient homology-driven genome editing in human T cells by combining zinc-finger nuclease mRNA and AAV6 donor delivery. *Nucl. Acids Res.* 44:e30. doi: 10.1093/nar/gkv1121

Wang, J., Exline, C. M., DeClercq, J. J., Llewellyn, G. N., Hayward, S. B., Li, P. W., et al. (2015). Homology-driven genome editing in hematopoietic stem and progenitor cells using ZFN mRNA and AAV6 donors. *Nat. Biotechnol.* 33, 1256–1263. doi: 10.1038/nbt.3408

Wang, L., Yang, Y., Breton, C., Bell, P., Li, M., Zhang, J., et al. (2020). A mutation-independent CRISPR-Cas9-mediated gene targeting approach to treat a murine model of ornithine transcarbamylase deficiency. *Sci. Adv.* 6:eaax5701. doi: 10.1126/sciadv.aax5701

Wang, L., Yang, Y., Breton, C. A., White, J., Zhang, J., Che, Y., et al. (2019). CRISPR/Cas9-mediated *in vivo* gene targeting corrects hemostasis in newborn and adult factor IX-knockout mice. *Blood* 133, 2745–2752. doi: 10.1182/blood.2019000790

Wang, Q., Zhong, X., Li, Q., Su, J., Liu, Y., Mo, L., et al. (2020). CRISPR-Cas9-mediated *in vivo* gene integration at the albumin locus recovers hemostasis in neonatal and adult hemophilia B mice. *Mol. Ther. Methods Clin. Dev.* 18, 520–531. doi: 10.1016/j.omtm.2020.06.025

Wiebking, V., Patterson, J. O., Martin, R., Chanda, M. K., Lee, C. M., Srifa, W., et al. (2018). Metabolic engineering generates a transgene-free safety switch for cell therapy. *Nat. Biotechnol* 2020:6. doi: 10.1038/s41587-020-0580-6

Yu, S., Ou, Y., Xiao, H., Li, J., Adah, D., Liu, S., et al. (2020). Experimental treatment of SIV-infected macaques *via* autograft of CCR5-disrupted hematopoietic stem and progenitor cells. *Mol. Ther. Methods Clin. Dev.* 17, 520–531. doi: 10.1016/j.omtm.2020.03.004

Zambrowicz, B. P., Imamoto, A., Fiering, S., Herzenberg, L. A., Kerr, W. G., and Soriano, P. (1997). Disruption of overlapping transcripts in the ROSA beta geo 26 gene trap strain leads to widespread expression of beta-galactosidase in mouse embryos and hematopoietic cells. *Proc. Natl. Acad. Sci. U. S. A.* 94, 3789–3794. doi: 10.1073/pnas.94.8.3789

Zhang, D., Huang, P., Sharma, M., Keller, C. A., Giardine, B., Zhang, H. (2020). Alteration of genome folding *via* contact domain boundary insertion. *Nat. Genet.* 52, 1076–1087. doi: 10.1038/s41588-020-0680-8

Zhang, J. P., Cheng, X. X., Zhao, M., Li, G. H., Xu, J., Zhang, F., et al. (2019). Curing hemophilia A by NHEJ-mediated ectopic F8 insertion in the mouse. *Genome Biol.* 20:276. doi: 10.1186/s13059-019-1907-9

Zheng, H., and Xie, W. (2019). The role of 3D genome organization in development and cell differentiation. *Nat. Rev. Mol. Cell Biol.* 20, 535–550. doi: 10.1038/s41580-019-0132-4

12

The Promise and the Hope of Gene Therapy

Eleni Papanikolaou [1,2]* and Andreas Bosio [1]

[1] Department of Molecular Technologies and Stem Cell Therapy, Miltenyi Biotec, Bergisch Gladbach, Germany, [2] Laboratory of Biology, School of Medicine, National and Kapodistrian University of Athens, Athens, Greece

*Correspondence:
Eleni Papanikolaou
elinapapanikolaou@gmail.com

It has been over 30 years since visionary scientists came up with the term "Gene Therapy," suggesting that for certain indications, mostly monogenic diseases, substitution of the missing or mutated gene with the normal allele via gene addition could provide long-lasting therapeutic effect to the affected patients and consequently improve their quality of life. This notion has recently become a reality for certain diseases such as hemoglobinopathies and immunodeficiencies and other monogenic diseases. However, the therapeutic wave of gene therapies was not only applied in this context but was more broadly employed to treat cancer with the advent of CAR-T cell therapies. This review will summarize the gradual advent of gene therapies from bench to bedside with a main focus on hemopoietic stem cell gene therapy and genome editing and will provide some useful insights into the future of genetic therapies and their gradual integration in the everyday clinical practice.

Keywords: genome editing, hemopoietic stem cell, retroviral vectors, designer nucleases, CRISPR

INTRODUCTION

The idea that a gene can be delivered into specific cell types and its expression can lead to therapeutic efficacy, dramatically improving the patients' quality of life, was originally introduced by Theodore Friedmann 45 years ago and was later strongly encouraged and realized by George Stamatoyannopoulos, one of the founding members of the American Society of Gene and Cell Therapy (ASGCT). In this setting, the drug, which in the case of gene therapy is a gene, is packaged within a vector used to facilitate its entrance into the patients' cells. Of course, the notion of gene therapy has evolved, and in general, we refer to gene therapy when a therapeutic process involves genetic manipulation of the patients' cells with the use of a nucleic acid. This is actually the most important difference between cell and gene therapy: in cell therapy, the cells are not genetically modified but instead are subjected to a certain manipulation involving cell culture and exposure to specific types of media whereas gene therapy is mediated by the addition of any nucleic acid. For obvious reasons, the idea of gene addition was particularly applicable in monogenic diseases based on the simplified notion of "adding the missing gene or the normal allele to compensate for the expression of the mutated allele." However, under the view of the latest advancements, gene therapy does not correspond to an addition of a gene, otherwise missing in the patient's cells, but with a gene that could offer therapeutic benefit to the affected individual.

There are basically three types of gene therapy: *ex vivo*, *in vivo*, and *in situ*. In *ex vivo* gene therapy, the target cells are removed from the patient's body, engineered either by the addition of the therapeutic gene or by other genetic manipulations that allow correction of the phenotype of the disease. The "corrected" cells are subsequently re-infused to the patient. This type of intervention is also termed *in vitro* gene therapy and is particularly applicable to blood diseases: in the case of blood cancer, the target cell may be T and, most recently, NK cells, and the therapeutic gene is the chimeric antigen receptor (CAR). In the case of monogenic diseases, the target cell is the hemopoietic stem cell (HSC) and the transgene varies analogous to the disease. The viral vectors utilized in both cases are mostly retroviral vectors, belonging either in the lentiviral or the oncoretroviral families of *Retroviridae*. However, depending on the affected tissue, *ex vivo* gene therapy is not always the intended type of corrective approach. For example, if the target organ is the brain, the spinal canal, or the liver, another type of therapy is employed, termed *in vivo* gene therapy. In this setting, the therapeutic vector is administered systemically in the blood circulation or the cerebrospinal fluid of the patient, and depending on the disease, different types of viral vectors are utilized, such as adenoviral vectors (AVs) or adeno-associated viral vectors (AAVs). Finally, there is a last scheme of gene therapy, in which the viral vector is administered *in situ*, i.e., to a specific organ or area in the body of the patient either through direct injection, e.g., into the tumor (in the case of melanoma) or into suitable brain areas (in the case of neuropathies) or by an insertion of a catheter in the case that the organ to be treated is the heart. The selection of the procedure depends entirely on the type of indication, the affected tissue, and the cell type that requires correction. In contrast to HSCs, namely, CD34$^+$ cells, that can be easily isolated from the patients, nerve stem cells are difficult to obtain for *ex vivo* manipulation. In addition, stem cells are only partially characterized in the liver. Hence, gene therapy for specific organs or indications is dependent on systemic or *in situ* administration of the therapeutic vector.

Although the idea of genome correction was quite innovative in its nature, especially during the 90s, clinical translation involving genome correction is still rare and adoption of the application of gene therapy at a wider scale and in the context of a medical routine has been only partial. To date, there are more than 2,600 clinical trials concerning gene therapy and/or genome editing, but very few therapeutic drugs have acquired marketing authorization for different indications (summarized in **Table 1**).

Innovation

During the early times of its development, the gene therapy field has faced a lot of skepticism specifically after the unfortunate death of Jesse Gelsinger (Teichler Zallen, 2000) but also later on during the leukemic events recorded on the X-SCID clinical trial (Papanikolaou and Anagnou, 2010) in the early 2000s. The death of Jesse Gelsinger not only had a profound impact on the gene therapy field, it also underlined the general lack of knowledge about the vector–host interactions and ultimately pointed out the weak spots within the collaboration between the researchers and the regulatory agencies. Eventually, the case of Gelsinger has been quoted relatively recently for a number of times[1] (Baker and Herzog, 2020) specifically in view of the coronavirus pandemic and the

generation of a new and effective vaccine. Of note, one of these reports[1] correlates the safety issues raised around the time of Gelsinger's death with the genome editing approaches currently employed, rather successfully, by a number of companies and academic institutions.

The scientific community is characterized by a heterogeneity in terms of taking risks, since there are scientists who intensely question the safety of any novel therapeutic approach and scientists who pave the way toward innovative and frequently risky treatments. A striking example of such risks and their potential to shape the policies around genetic therapies has recently happened in China, where the regulatory norms originally comprised mostly technical management methods or ethical guidelines under a broad legal framework issued by Commissions of the State Council in combination with departmental regulations and regulatory documents issued by individual ministries (Wang et al., 2020). It was only after the incidence with the CRISPR (Clustered Regularly Interspaced Short Palindromic Repeats) babies in November of 2018 (Lander et al., 2019) that urged China to advance legislation in areas of biosecurity, genetic technology, and biomedicine. To this end, the "Biosafety Law" was approved in 2019 by the Standing Committee of the National People's Congress. The aim of this law is to become a basic, systematic, comprehensive, and dominant legal framework on biosafety. Therefore, the regulatory landscape in genetic therapies is currently being shaped in China.

On the other hand, in Europe and in the USA, any new drug, regardless if it is gene therapy related, is not judged by the number or even the quality of publications, but eventually by the regulatory authorities who have the legal capacity to determine the marketing authorization of the formulation. However, the regulatory authorities have different views from the researchers in terms of innovation and safety. It is also important to keep in mind that regulators are basing their decisions on data and always compare those to the pre-existing state of the art of a specific indication in terms of equivalency. Hence, any new therapy, from a regulatory aspect will be thoroughly investigated and examined on the safety profile it presents and eventually on the extent of comparability between the currently authorized therapeutic treatments. This approach is employed both by the European Medicines Agency (EMA) in Europe and the Food and Drug Administration (FDA) in the United States (Iglesias-Lopez et al., 2020).

One strategy that can be utilized by regulators, including governments, health technology assessment (HTA) bodies, and health care decision makers, in order to advance and promote the development of novel medicinal treatments, is to recognize and award innovation. In the review of De Solà-Morales et al. (2018), the authors try to investigate how innovation is defined with respect to new medicines. Their conclusion is that innovation is differentially defined through countries, depending on independent political and societal factors. Hence, it is challenging to achieve common alignment, although coordination between countries and among regulators should be strongly encouraged as it would eventually help researchers

---

[1] https://www.sciencehistory.org/distillations/the-death-of-jesse-gelsinger-20-years-later

TABLE 1 | Gene therapy products that have acquired marketing authorization.

Name (Brand name)	Vendor	Indication	Type of indication	Approval region	Price (kE§)
Onasemnogene abeparvovec (ZOLGENSMA®)	Novartis	Spinal muscular atrophy	Rare disease	2019 (USA)	2.125
Betibeglogene autotemcel (ZYNTEGLO®)	bluebird bio	Transfusion dependent β-thalassemia	Rare disease	2019 (EU)	1.575
Voretigene neparvovec (LUXTURNA®)	Spark Therapeutics	Leber's congenital amaurosis	Rare disease	2017 (USA)	850
Alipogene tiparvovec (GLYBERA®)	UniQure	Lipoprotein lipase deficiency	Rare disease	2012 (EU*)	1.000
STRIMVELIS®	Orchard Therapeutics	Severe combined immunodeficiency due to adenosine deaminase deficiency (ADA-SCID)	Rare disease	2016 (EU)	594
Tisagenlecleucel (KYMRIAH®)	Novartis	B acute lymphoblastic leukemia	Cancer	2017 (USA)	475
Axicabtagene ciloleucel (YESCARTA®)	Kite Pharma	Type of non-Hodgkin lymphoma	Cancer	2017 (USA)	373
Talimogene laherparepvec (IMLYGIC®)	Amgen Inc	Melanoma	Cancer	2015 (USA and EU)	65

*Withdrawn in 2017, kE§ thousands of euros.

and/or manufacturers toward determining mutually applicable research policies that can drive innovation. In their review (De Solà-Morales et al., 2018), components and dimensions of innovation are mentioned and include notions such as unmet need, health outcomes, novelty, step change, availability of existing treatments, efficacy, new molecular entity, molecular novelty, therapeutic value, market share, cost-saving, disease severity, clinical benefit, safety, pharmacological/technological differences from current treatments, etc.

Innovation in other industrial sectors is defined usually as any improvement of the end product either in terms of manufacturing or in terms of cost reduction in the long term. However, this usually does not apply in the health care sector: a new product is often substantially different from existing therapies and improvements in patients' quality of life; i.e., the therapeutic benefit, as a result of the application of the innovative approach, is of the greatest importance. Another major aspect is the overall expenditure associated with development of the novel approach by the health industry, which is usually high and is currently the focus of specific discussions in Europe and in the United States and ultimately points toward the affordability within the public health budgets (McCabe et al., 2009). However, as considerations about the costs are not usually included during the original design of the novel approach as a key component of innovation, there is the probability that innovation in pharmaceuticals and cell/gene therapy may not be aligned with the requirements of public or insurance health budgets and by extrapolation of society as a whole. Specifically for gene therapy approaches, the term "financial toxicity" is already circulating among the policy makers, the industry, and, consequently, the researchers.

Paradigms of definitions of innovations in different European countries are listed below: In France, the HAS (Haute Autorité de Santé) defines innovative products as those for which the producers assert a medium to major improvement of the clinical benefit compared to the currently available treatments [i.e., Amélioration du Service Médical Rendu (ASMR) of level I, II, or III] (O'Connor et al., 2016). Other agencies such as the Swedish Tandvårds–och läkemedelsförmånsverket (TLV), the Scottish Medicines Consortium (SMC), and the National Health Service in England (NHS) take into consideration the novelty of the approach but in combination with the improvement of patients' quality of life and any potential reformation of the health care system; i.e., the new therapeutic approach should present palpable added value (De Solà-Morales et al., 2018). Surprisingly, in the Netherlands, the Zorginstituut Nederland (ZINL) characterizes a product as innovative when it seems to be promising from a scientific point of view, but for which even insufficient data can overall provide a reasonably positive outlook and consequently effect a constructive response by the agency (De Solà-Morales et al., 2018). Finally in Germany, innovation is not referenced within the legal framework and in general the focus lies on the additional therapeutic benefits provided by the novel approach (De Solà-Morales et al., 2018).

To summarize, the definition of a novel medical approach as innovative in essence lies in its truly innovative nature. However, ideally, it should combine additional features such as (a) be at least as safe as the current treatments, (b) dramatically improve the patients' quality of life, and (c) be affordable by reimbursement bodies (payers). Finally, another important aspect would be to distinguish between price and the true value of the novel approach.

Early Insights From Commercialization of Gene Therapies in Europe

Toward a better understanding of the impact that gene therapy presents at a societal level, one should keep in mind that in terms of innovation, any gene therapy approach is considered highly innovative. Consequently, in the context of genome editing, identification of the nucleases that generate targeted double strand DNA breaks that can, in a subsequent process, be repaired by indels or via homologous recombination and correct any genetic mutation was not only innovative but also considered a scientific breakthrough.

However, any marketing authorization of these products is expected to be scrutinized by the regulatory agencies as it was previously the case for other gene therapy products. Under the existing regulatory framework, cellular products that have been subjected to more-than-minimal manipulation are broadly classified as either medicinal products (EU) or biologics (USA). In Europe, cell-based medicinal products are regulated under the Advanced Therapy Medicinal Product (ATMP) Regulation, which mandates that all ATMPs are subject to a centralized marketing authorization procedure (Coopman, 2008). All marketing authorization applications are subject to a 210-day assessment procedure by the EMA, supported by the Committee for Advanced Therapies (CAT), before a license can be granted. Member states retain responsibility for authorization of clinical trials occurring within their borders and have the option to exempt certain products used on a non-routine basis for unmet clinical need, referred to as the "Hospital Exemption" based on Article 28 of Regulation (EC) 1394/2007. As with all medicines, the EMA continues to monitor the safety and efficacy of ATMPs after they are approved and marketed and provides scientific support to developers for designing pharmacovigilance and risk management strategies used to monitor the safety of these medicines.

Regulatory approval, however, does not guarantee availability to patients or reimbursement by European health systems, because novel therapies, regardless of their mechanism of action, have to undergo formal Health Technology Assessment (Touchot and Flume, 2017). From a time perspective, the first marketing authorization for gene therapy products for rare diseases occurred in 2012 with Glybera® (EU), followed by Imlygic® (EU and USA) in 2015 and Strimvelis® (EU) in 2016. Therefore, these products have not only undergone meticulous evaluation from regulatory agencies, they have been also subjected to Health Technology Assessment by the reimbursement bodies and have received positive opinions from regulators and payers, and thus, a comprehensive analysis of their life cycle can now be conducted.

Glybera (alipogene tiparvovec) was the very first gene therapy agent to officially receive marketing authorization in Europe for treatment of lipoprotein lipase deficiency, a deadly disease causing severe pancreatitis to the affected patients. LPL deficiency (LPLD) is classified as a rare disease, estimated to occur in ~1 in 250,000 people in the general population and has been described in all races. Glybera was an adeno-associated serotype 1 vector (AAV-1), designed to deliver *in vivo* to the patients several copies of the normal allele (gene addition) by injection to several parts of the muscle areas of the body. Each vial of the vector had an estimated cost of ~100,000 euros, and to achieve a therapeutic quantity in the body of the patient, it was necessary to inject at least 10 vials. This fact raised the price of the therapy to 1 million euros. The drug was originally marketed by uniQure and, after going through formal evaluation through Health Technology Assessment in Germany and in France, failed

to achieve a recognition of benefit in either country (Touchot and Flume, 2017). In France, the HAS Transparency Commission stated that (Touchot and Flume, 2017):

➤ "A moderate effect on triglycerides and on episodes of pancreatitis has been observed but this effect was not sustained in the medium–and long-term" (in line with submitted efficacy data showing only transient efficacy);
➤ "The clinical relevance of the chosen primary efficacy endpoint (reduction in the triglyceride level) is debatable;"
➤ "Uncertainties about the short–and medium-term safety of this gene therapy, which cannot be re-administered because of its action mechanism, remain."

As a result, the HAS concluded that the actual benefit of Glybera is insufficient to justify reimbursement by the French national health insurance and thus the product was not commercialized in France.

In Germany, it was initially assessed as a community product but was evaluated by AMNOG (the German Health Technology Assessment process) to confer "unquantifiable additional benefit" because of lack of proper clinical data that would adequately justify the actual therapeutic potency of the product (Touchot and Flume, 2017). This led to a repositioning of the drug to a hospital-only product and allowed price negotiations directly between hospitals and payers. In the case of Germany, these discussions were fruitful only for a single patient that was treated at Charité in Berlin in September 2015 with an estimated price of 900,000 euros after an agreement with DAK (Deutschen Angestellten-Krankenkasse), a large German health insurance provider. This patient, was a woman with LPLD who suffered consecutive debilitating pancreatitis and was hospitalized in intensive care more than 40 times, and thus, she qualified for gene therapy because of the severity of her overall clinical status. The woman was fully cured and never suffered from pancreatitis again (Crowe, 2018). Despite these hopeful events and taking into account the very low number of patients, uniQure decided in 2015 not to apply for approval in the USA and exclusively licensed rights in Europe to Chiesi Farmaceuticals for €31 million (Regalado, 2016). A total of three remaining doses left on the shelf were basically given away in one patient from Italy and two German patients who received doses for 1 euro each. Since October 2017, the utilization of Glybera was discontinued in EU because marketing authorization to Chiesi Farmaceuticals was not renewed, for financial reasons.

Imlygic (Talimogene laherparepvec), which has been authorized for treatment of melanoma, is a vector based on a strain of Herpes Simplex Virus 1 (HSV-1) that possesses oncolytic properties in combination with the expression of granulocyte-macrophage colony-stimulating factor (GM-CSF) to attract antigen-presenting cells (APCs) in the affected area. Upon administration *in situ*, Imlygic lyses tumor cells, enhances antigen loading of MHC class I molecules, and express GM-CSF to increase tumor antigen presentation by dendritic cells (Conry et al., 2018). Therefore, although it is administered *in situ*, it provokes a systemic anti-tumor immunity. It was approved by the EMA and FDA in October and December of 2018, respectively (Touchot and Flume, 2017). Upon approval of the regulatory agencies, evaluation of Imlygic has been completed so far in the UK (Touchot and Flume, 2017). Initially, the NICE (National Institute of Clinical Excellence) concluded that Imlygic, despite its truly innovative mechanism of action, was not cost-effective and did not confer significant advantage in terms of the overall survival of the patients compared to the existing therapies for melanoma. This evaluation prompted the company to discuss a respective discount with the Department of Health (Touchot and Flume, 2017), to agree to a patient access scheme, and to narrow the indication of coverage to patients who did not qualify for systemically administered immunotherapies. Imlygic is currently still being evaluated in Germany by IQWiG (the German health technology assessment body) and the Federal Joint Committee (G-BA), which requested additional data to complete the assessment including comparison with administration of GM-CSF alone. Of note, previously in clinical trials, the overall response rate (ORR) was increased in the Imlygic arm (26.4%) compared to the GM-CSF arm (5.7%). The mean overall survival (OS) was 23.3 months in the Imlygic arm, vs. 18.9 months on the GM-CSF arm ($p = 0.051$), showing a marginal statistical trend in favor of Imlygic (Andtbacka et al., 2015). However, administration of GM-CSF is also not an authorized treatment for melanoma. This poses a risk toward the final positive evaluation of Imlygic as it could be again classified as providing "no quantifiable additional benefit," suggesting that it is probable that it will face challenges in reaching a wider number of patients, unless newly generated data provide an undisputable therapeutic benefit compared to the standard treatment, as this is defined by each individual payer (Touchot and Flume, 2017).

The aforementioned products are employed in *in vivo* and *in situ* gene therapy, respectively. However, one of the greatest achievements in the history of the field was the case of Strimvelis®. Strimvelis®, is a product derived from genetic engineering of HSCs isolated from patients suffering from severe combined immunodeficiency due to adenosine deaminase deficiency (ADA-SCID). In this case, genetic correction of HSCs is mediated by gene addition of the normal allele packaged inside an oncoretroviral (also termed gamma retroviral) vector. In terms of safety, the gene therapy field has been severely hampered by the unfortunate leukemic events that occurred during the clinical trial for another form of SCID, namely, the X-SCID. In the early 2000s, four cases of leukemia in the French X-SCID clinical trial were recorded out of the initial seven infants that were recruited for the study. These events were attributed to the vector's integration into the proto-oncogene LMO2 (Hacein-Bey-Abina et al., 2003a; Kohn et al., 2003) and triggered a new field of research resulting in a comprehensive characterization of the preference to integrate of lentiviral vectors and oncoretroviral vectors (Montini et al., 2006; Biasco et al., 2017) within the human genome. Surprisingly, although lymphoproliferative aberrations were also observed in the trials of HSC gene therapy for Wiskott–Aldrich syndrome (Braun et al., 2014) and for chronic granulomatous disease (CGD, Stein et al., 2010), no case of leukemic events for ADA-SCID in the context of clinical trials has been recorded, despite the fact that all the aforementioned indications employed oncoretroviral vectors.

Unfortunately, 4 years after Strimvelis® received marketing authorization, lymphoid T cell leukemia has been reported in one patient in October of 2020, and its relationship to the gene therapy is currently under investigation (Ferrari G. et al., 2020). Strimvelis® was originally developed in Ospedale San Raffaele in Milan (Aiuti et al., 2002, 2009) in collaboration with Fondazione Telethon before it was acquired by GlaxoSmithKline and, in May 2016, received approval in Europe. GSK initially collaborated with MolMed a clinical biotech company, to develop a robust process for commercializing the product. Because Strimvelis® contains essentially HSCs that need to be engineered within a very short period of time (not more than 2 days), until today, it was authorized only in Italy (MolMed) and patients from other European countries are supposed to travel to Italy to receive the treatment (Touchot and Flume, 2017). The Italian medicines agency (AIFA) agreed to a reimbursement of 594,000 euros based on the substantial clinical benefit for the patients in combination with the overall amount spared from a lifetime treatment with enzyme replacement therapy, as Strimvelis was beneficial for the public health budget in the long run (Touchot and Flume, 2017). In 2018, GSK transferred all the assets associated with Strimvelis to Orchard Therapeutics (Paton, 2018). Although the product has to undergo evaluation also in other European countries, and despite the small number of patients treated so far, it should be mentioned that the short time period between the approval and the reimbursement decision by the Italian authorities indicates that good clinical practice, good manufacturing practice, and robust clinical data combined with reasonable pricing can pave the way toward integrating gene therapies in medical routine. Of course, the report of the leukemic event is expected to create delays toward authorization in other countries until the results of the investigations are announced.

Last but not least, another important achievement for HSC gene therapy is Zynteglo®, which received marketing authorization for treatment of transfusion dependent β-thalassemia (TDT), a disease that was the first candidate for HSC gene therapy. Significant research efforts toward the generation of erythroid-specific globin expressing lentiviral vectors were employed that were eventually successfully translated to clinical trials in 2006 (Ferrari G. et al., 2020). Zynteglo®, similar to Strimvelis®, is a product derived from genetic engineering of HSCs isolated from patients suffering from TDT, transduced with BB305 lentiviral vector, which encodes a β-globin transgene (βT87Q globin), which also has antisickling properties. The results of phase I and phase II trials were reported and showed that gene therapy was efficacious in 80% of patients with non-β^0/β^0 genotypes and 38% of patients with β^0/β^0 genotypes, measured by transfusion independence at the 2-year follow-up (Ferrari G. et al., 2020), while the rest of the participants reached various levels of transfusion reduction. On the basis of these results, Zynteglo® received conditional marketing authorization for use in patients with transfusion-dependent β-thalassemia with non-β^0/β^0 genotypes in 2019 in Europe, while the respective authorization by the FDA is still pending.

Undisputable success stories in the field of CAR-T gene therapy are also Kymriah and Yescarta. However, Zynteglo®,

Kymriah®, and Yescarta® have relatively recently received regulatory approval, and their assessment in terms of reimbursement is currently ongoing in EU and USA.

Excellent Science and Safety

Gene therapy based on viral vectors utilizes the natural ability of viruses to deliver genetic material to cells, and a large part of research has been devoted toward generating novel, more efficient, and safer delivery tools employing gammaretroviruses, lentiviruses, adenoviruses, and adeno-associated viruses. Retroviruses are particularly applicable in the case of HSC gene therapy because they have the unique capability to fully integrate their genome intact into the genome of the host cell. However, as with any new therapeutic approach, gene transfer using viral vectors also introduced new side effects. One of these side effects, known as insertional mutagenesis or genotoxicity, involves activation of proto-oncogenes or disruption of tumor suppressor genes due to retroviral vector integration. Of course, genotoxicity is a natural phenomenon that has been described since the discovery of retrotransposons, as transpositions of Long Interspersed Nuclear Elements (LINEs) were (i) detected as *de novo* insertions into the coding regions of factor VIII gene resulting in hemophilia A, (ii) integrated into the adenomatous polyposis coli tumor suppressor gene causing its disruption and generating colon cancer, (iii) detected into the myc locus in a breast cancer, and (iv) inserted into exon 48 of the dystrophin gene (Löwer et al., 1996). These transpositions were detected in extremely very low frequency within the overall population and even within the population suffering from these specific indications. Regarding the utilization of retroviral vectors into gene therapy protocols, although the possibility of insertional mutagenesis was originally discussed as theoretically possible, such risks had been estimated to be extremely low, based on (a) the fact that over 90% of human genome is non-coding and (b) the assumption that proviral integration into the human genome would be random (Papanikolaou et al., 2015). Unfortunately, these hypotheses were not verified after the reports of lymphoproliferation due to insertional activation of the LMO2 gene following gene therapy in the French X-SCID clinical trial (Hacein-Bey-Abina et al., 2003a,b), the leukemias developed in the Wiskott–Aldrich gene therapy trial (Braun et al., 2014), and myelodysplasia attributed to EVI1 activation after gene therapy for CGD (Stein et al., 2010). All these events highlighted the importance of understanding the underlying mechanisms that are responsible for integration into the preferred genomic loci but also the components that contribute toward the repair of the genome during the integration events. From a phenotypic standpoint, this lack of knowledge was translated as leukemic events only during clinical trials, as such events were not detectable during the pre-clinical development of gene therapies of the aforementioned indications. From a regulatory standpoint, the clonal dominance observed during the French β-thalassemia trial (Cavazzana-Calvo et al., 2010) led to a clinical hold of the specific trial as per FDA guidelines for 5 years, until it was clear that the respective clonal dominance did not evolve to any kind of dysplasia or leukemia and it was safe to proceed and recruit more patients to the study.

All the aforementioned cases underlined the non-random integration patterns of retroviral vectors and sparked the field's interest toward characterizing the potential mechanisms. Therefore, it was comprehensively shown that gammaretroviral vectors preferentially locate around transcription start sites while HIV-based vectors strongly favor integration in transcriptional units and gene-dense regions of the human genome (Papanikolaou et al., 2015). These properties rendered lentiviral vectors safer for gene therapy approaches compared to oncoretroviral vectors and paved the way toward substitution of oncoretroviral by lentiviral vectors. Indeed, lentiviral vector-based gene transfer into HSCs has subsequently been applied in the treatment of X-linked adrenoleukodystrophy (Cartier et al., 2009), metachromatic leukodystrophy (Biffi et al., 2013; Sessa et al., 2016), and Wiskott–Aldrich syndrome (Aiuti et al., 2013) without any vector-related adverse events. Therefore, the clonal dominance observed in the β-thalassemia trial is still an open question regarding whether this was purely coincidental or was truly attributable to a clonal proliferation as a result of the HMGA-2 dysregulation.

Aside from the comprehensive characterization of the integration preference of onco- and lentiviral vectors, the field furthermore strengthened the efforts toward making gene therapy safer by generation of self-inactivating (SIN) vectors. Because activation of the LMO2 oncogene was attributed to the strong enhancer elements within the U3 region of the retroviral Long Terminal Repeats (LTRs) (Hacein-Bey-Abina et al., 2003a), part of the U3 enhancer was removed in order to minimize the probability of activating neighboring oncogenes. In addition, alternative genetic elements, such as chromatin insulators, were gradually incorporated in the remaining U3 region of the LTR. Chromatin insulators are DNA sequences capable of maintaining the expression of a gene region independently of the expression of the neighboring gene region, by inhibiting their natural interactions (insulation). Insulator sequences have two main characteristics: (a) barrier activity, i.e., gene expression of a chromatin region is not affected by the adjacent heterochromatin region if an insulator is inserted between them, and (b) enhancer blocking activity, i.e., inhibition of the concerted action between a promoter and an adjacent enhancer (Heger and Wiehe, 2014). Therefore, the incorporation of a chromatin insulator into the U3 region of the LTR, on the one hand, offers additional protection against the activation of neighboring oncogenes and, on the other hand, ensures the expression of the therapeutic gene in case of integration in a heterochromatic region. For globin gene therapy, significant efforts have been employed to this end due to long-standing knowledge that the expression of globin genes was variable due to the integration of the vector into transcriptionally inactive regions of chromatin, i.e., dependent on "position effects" (Persons et al., 2003). Additional efforts deriving from the group of Dr. Stamatoyannopoulos have demonstrated the need to incorporate chromatin insulators into vectors intended for the gene therapy of hemoglobinopathies (Aker et al., 2007). However, later studies showed that incorporation of chromatin insulators leads to a significant loss of titer of the lentiviral vector (Urbinati et al., 2009), which typically translates to greater manufacturing costs as more vector is necessary to achieve the ideal transduction efficiency that would suffice to exhibit therapeutic efficacy. Currently, in the ongoing clinical trials of bluebird bio, the globin vector utilized is insulator-free (Negre et al., 2015), and as previously stated, it remains unclear whether the initial clonal dominance was because of the higher proliferation rate of a specific clone as a result of the vector integration into the HMGA gene or whether this observation merely reflects the effects of incorporating a limited number of genetically modified hematopoietic stem cells into the patient's marrow. Thus, bluebird's vector format is not considered dangerous from a regulatory standpoint.

Excluding genotoxicity, in clinical protocols that utilize lentiviral vectors, the regulatory agencies are also concerned about recombination events that might occur during the manufacturing process of the vectors and require extensive data demonstrating the lack of replication-competent retroviruses or lentiviruses (RCRs/RCLs) partly because the agencies assume higher probability for genotoxicity if RCRs or RCLs are present (Milone and O'Doherty, 2018). In addition, they request long-term follow-up monitoring of the patients participating in cell and gene therapy studies for the presence or RCRs/RCLs, new incidence or re-appearance of autoimmune, rheumatologic, and neurological disorders, or delayed malignancies, as a result of genotoxicity. Toward generating safer tools to reduce the risk of insertional mutagenesis, integration-deficient lentiviral vectors (IDLVs) or non-integrating lentiviral vectors (NILVs) have been generated (Wanisch and Yáñez-Muñoz, 2009; Milone and O'Doherty, 2018), which present lower probability of causing either genotoxicity or generating RCRs. Unfortunately, their use is rather limited because they provide merely transient transgene expression in proliferating cells, but they can still be employed to promote stable expression in non-dividing cells or to induce RNA interference and mediate homologous recombination (Wanisch and Yáñez-Muñoz, 2009).

To summarize, clinical trials in gene therapy via gene addition were initiated in the early 1990s, and until the late 2010s, a significant amount of effort combining excellent science and extensive assessment of potential risk factors have managed to make gene therapy more robust and simultaneously achieve great advancements toward clinical benefit.

THE ERA OF GENOME EDITING: CHALLENGES AND PROSPECTS

Prospects

Over the last decade, the discovery of important novel regulatory elements of the human genome, combined with the continuous developments of novel technologies in the field of molecular biology and biotechnology, has conferred important conceptual insights for the implementation of new molecular approaches for the treatment of monogenic disorders. The advent of induced pluripotent stem cells and the design of novel nucleases that target specific areas in the genome have rendered gene editing approaches pivotal players in the field of therapy of inherited diseases. Gene targeting that is currently mediated by genome editing, is anticipated to outperform the classical approach of

gene therapy via gene addition utilizing retroviral vectors, mainly due to the inability of the latter to establish targeted vector integration into the host genome.

Gene editing technology allows site-specific genome modifications, ranging from single-nucleotide edits to large deletions/inversions or targeted integration of entire genes, and is anticipated to outperform the classical approach of gene therapy via gene addition utilizing retroviral vectors, in part due to the inherent risk of insertional mutagenesis of gene addition by retroviral vectors and its limitations to treat gain-of-function mutations or defects in large genes. Moreover, in contrast to gene addition, most gene editing approaches maintain the natural genomic regulation of the gene of interest and thus physiological expression.

The original and still most prevalent application of gene editing for therapy relies on double strand breaks in DNA, which are introduced by engineered nucleases that act at predetermined and targeted genomic loci (Genovese et al., 2014). Such nucleases are:

- Zinc Finger Nucleases (ZFNs)
- Transcription Activator-Like Effector Nucleases (TALENs)
- Cas nuclease of the CRISPR/Cas9 system.

Their mode of action is to induce a double strand break (DSB) on the DNA molecule followed by respective repair either through the non-homologous end joining (NHEJ) or via homologous recombination (HR). Through NHEJ, repair of the DSBs leads to disruption of the target sequence by generation of small insertions or deletions, which collectively are called "indels." Repair through HR leads to full reconstitution of the target sequence if a template donating a homologous sequence, that serves as a matrix for the repair to take place, is provided.

It should be noted, however, that a DSB is actually the initiating step in natural genome editing and occurs in mammalian cells on several occasions, such as the V(D)J recombination through the RAG1/RAG2 enzymes (Jasin and Rothstein, 2013), during the meiotic recombination mediated by the Spo11 nuclease (Jasin and Rothstein, 2013) and finally during the natural gene drives, managed by homing endonucleases (Burt, 2003). Also, all mammalian cells possess robust DNA repair mechanisms; however, the frequency of repair either through NHEJ or HR increases at least by a 100-fold following a double strand break (Jasin and Rothstein, 2013). Therefore, the novel engineered nucleases are necessary to achieve adequate gene correction to reach the anticipated therapeutic levels required. This aspect is of particular interest for the clinical applications of engineered HSCs, because the number of $CD34^+$ cells that need to be infused to patients are in the range of 5×10^6-10^7 cells/kg and 80% of those should be genetically corrected. For example, for a thalassemic patient with an average weight of 70 kg, one would need to infuse $5 \times 10^6 \times 70$, i.e., a total of 3.5×10^8 viable $CD34^+$ cells, of which at least 80% should be genetically corrected. Thus, in order to have a final total cell count of ~ 4-5×10^8 cells in the final cell product, it is anticipated that optimization toward mobilization of HSCs to the periphery specifically from patients suffering from rare diseases, optimization of infusion protocols, as well as optimization of the editing process *per se* are absolutely necessary. These are current challenges that will increasingly appear as we pave the way toward clinical genome editing applications. For example, even optimized transfer of nucleases by electroporation leads to a significant loss of cell viability, which, in turn, necessitates efficient mobilization and collection of high numbers of HSCs as editing substrate. Unfortunately, because in certain cases, such as in the case of sickle cell disease, patients mobilize poorly or due to innate characteristics of the disease *per se* use of granulocyte colony stimulating factor (G-CSF) is not recommended, one of the first challenges toward clinical translation would be the existence of a validated freezing protocol followed by a validated thawing protocol as it is possible that certain patients would need to undergo multiple rounds of mobilization.

A second notable challenge is the process of genome editing in terms of culture conditions including media, cytokines, timelines, and inclusion of several means of molecules or strategies to enhance the efficiency of the editing. To this end, several amendments have been published. Dever et al. (2016) reported a CRISPR/Cas9-based gene editing approach that combines Cas9 ribonucleoproteins (RNPs) and delivery of a homologous template via an AAV to achieve homologous recombination at the β-globin gene in HSCs combined with a concomitant purification method that generates a population of hemopoietic stem and progenitor cells with more than 90% targeted integration. Respective results were also obtained for SCID-X1 (Pavel-Dinu et al., 2019) following the same approach, i.e., the CRISPR/Cas9-AAV6-based strategy to insert the cDNA of the normal gene into the endogenous start codon. This approach aims to functionally correct disease-causing mutations throughout the genomic locus. Unfortunately, a similar strategy could not be employed for hemoglobinopathies as the presence of genomic introns is mandatory to achieve tissue specificity as well as therapeutic expression levels (Uchida et al., 2019).

Another interesting approach to achieve higher editing efficiency is to modulate the cellular pathways responsible for DSB repair. More specifically, the efficiency of HR by genome editing is limited by DSB repair pathways that compete with homology-directed repair (HDR), such as non-homologous end joining (NHEJ) (Nambiar et al., 2019). The choice of the type of the DSB repair pathway is mostly determined by the DSB resection, a nucleolytic process that converts DSB ends into 3′-single-stranded DNA overhangs (Nambiar et al., 2019). Certain NHEJ factors, including 53BP1, promote the direct joining of DSBs by protecting DNA ends from resection. Limited resection of DSB ends can expose regions of sequence microhomology, which favor DSB repair through microhomology-mediated end joining (MMEJ), while more extensive DSB resection generates the long 3′-single-stranded DNA tails required for HDR (Nambiar et al., 2019). Thus, cellular factors that impede DSB resection represent major barriers to HDR-mediated precision genome editing. Toward this direction, the authors characterized RAD18 as a stimulator of CRISPR-mediated HDR and identified its mechanism of action that involved suppression of the localization of the NHEJ-promoting factor 53BP1 to DSBs (Nambiar et al., 2019).

An alternative strategy to enhance the efficiency of genome editing was to transiently silence p53 (Schiroli et al., 2019). More specifically, Schiroli et al. challenged the successful use of the combination of AAV and generation of DSBs by engineered nucleases such as ZFNs and CRISPR/Cas9 by claiming that they cause excessive DNA damage response (DDR) across all hemopoietic stem and progenitor cell subtypes analyzed (Schiroli et al., 2019). DDR consequently induced cumulative p53 pathway activation, constraining proliferation, yield, and engraftment of edited HSPCs, which could be overcome by transient inactivation of p53. Of note, DDR is reported to be activated also under conditions of viral infections or vector transduction as there are recent reports correlating immune responses within the cells that undergo DNA damage (Piras et al., 2017; Dunphy et al., 2018). Immune responses have also been detected in the context of gene therapy via gene addition (Papanikolaou et al., 2015) after transduction of CD34+ cells with a GFP encoding lentiviral vector. It is not unprecedent that such immune responses are linked to DNA damage repair mechanisms, since retroviral integration presupposes breaks on the DNA chain. However, it should be noted that DDR is not always activated: For example, in the study by Papanikolaou et al. (2015), transduction with the GFP lentiviral vector activated immune responses without significant DDR. On the contrary, in the study by Piras et al. (2017), there was significant upregulation of DDR. One important difference between the two studies was the multiplicity of infection (MOI); in the first study, an MOI = 10 was employed, while in the second study, the authors experimented with MOI = 100. These results immediately suggest that the MOI plays a crucial role during the manufacturing process since both studies employed a VSV-G pseudotyped GFP encoding lentiviral vector and used cord blood CD34+ cells. Obviously, a better understanding of the interplay between vectors or nucleic acid molecules with the host cell in terms of both quality and quantity would be necessary to advance the field of gene engineering. An important aspect that is linked to clinical translation is that activation of vector-mediated DDR can induce significant, albeit mild, increase in apoptosis of human HSCs in culture (Piras et al., 2017), which typically results in lower engraftment of engineered HSCs *in vivo*, particularly during the early phases of hemopoietic reconstitution (Piras et al., 2017; Piras and Kajaste-Rudnitski, 2020). Therefore, induction of DDR mechanisms in the context of genome editing should be taken into serious consideration, and strategies toward achieving robust and efficient editing without interfering with the stem cell-like character of CD34+ should be generated.

As reviewed by Piras and Kajaste-Rudnitski (2020), HSCs have devised several strategies of responding to RNA molecules as well as ssDNA and dsDNA molecules. Indeed, a plausible approach to increase the efficiency of retroviral transduction or gene editing would be to assess the mechanisms of innate immunity and nucleic acid sensing in HSCs and harness their potential. For example, transient silencing of cellular nucleic acid sensors could increase the level of transduction or the efficiency of the editing. To that end, many researchers have focused on several transduction enhancers such as 16,16-dimethyl prostaglandin E2 (PGE2) and LentiBOOST™, poloxamers, the polycationic protamine sulfate, cyclosporine A and cyclosporine H, and rapamycin (Piras and Kajaste-Rudnitski, 2020). PGE2 and LentiBOOST™ are already employed in the context of clinical trials (Tisdale John et al., 2018), but it should be emphasized that the exact mechanism of action of the majority of these transduction enhancers is not fully elucidated. Besides the employment of transduction enhancers, additional strategies exist in terms of culture conditions that urge HSCs to move toward the S phase of the cell cycle in order to increase the successful HR. One strategy employed by Ferrari S. et al. (2020) was to transiently downregulate p53 with GSE56 in addition to including the E4orf6/7 protein of adenovirus, a known interactor with cellular components involved in survival and cell cycle (Ferrari S. et al., 2020) to successfully enhance the efficiency of editing. From another perspective toward advancing safety, Wiebking et al. (2020) disrupted the uridine monophosphate synthetase (UMPS) involved in the pyrimidine *de novo* synthesis pathway rendering proliferation dependent on external uridine and providing thus the possibility to control cell growth by modulating the uridine supply. However, it should be noted that disruption of UMPS would be an additional genome editing process on top of any other correction, suggesting that to manufacture cell products that have been genetically engineered and present advanced safety features, one would have to edit at least two genomic loci. Although both strategies (Ferrari S. et al., 2020; Wiebking et al., 2020) certainly assume great potential, they involve genetic manipulation beyond the current state of the art, and the transition to the clinic will probably be challenging from a regulatory standpoint.

A final aspect of great importance is the type of mutations that are introduced in the human genome in the context of therapy. One idea would be to add the desired transgene into a safe harbor. Papapetrou et al. (2011) characterized as safe harbors specific genomic loci based on their position relative to contiguous coding genes, microRNAs, and ultraconserved regions. Genomic safe harbors should fulfill the following criteria: (i) distance of at least 50 kb from the 5' end of any mapped gene, (ii) distance of at least 300 kb from any cancer-related gene, (iii) distance of at least 300 kb from any microRNA (miRNA), (iv) location outside a transcription unit, and (v) location outside ultraconserved regions (UCRs) of the human genome (i.e., enhancers, exons, regulatory sequences, etc.). The idea is promising and has been widely employed in the context of induced pluripotent stem cells, and most lately, it was capitalized by Gomez-Ospina et al. (2019) toward showing therapeutic benefit for Mucopolysaccharidosis type I by generating a CRISPR/Cas9 approach that targets the lysosomal enzyme iduronidase to the CCR5 safe harbor locus in human CD34$^+$ hematopoietic stem and progenitor cells. The authors demonstrated adequate therapeutic efficacy in an immunocompromised mouse model of Mucopolysaccharidosis type I and showed that the modified cells could secrete supra-endogenous enzyme levels, maintain long-term repopulation and multi-lineage differentiation potential, and provide biochemical and phenotypic improvement *in vivo*.

Therefore, one approach is to introduce the therapeutic transgene into a safe harbor locus. Another approach is to introduce the therapeutic gene exactly in its natural position in the genome, thus ensuring lifelong regulation by the naturally occurring expression modulating elements affecting the respective region. This was already described to treat X-SCID 1 (Pavel-Dinu et al., 2019) but is a particularly plausible approach for hemoglobinopathies aiming to correct either mutations within the β-globin gene in the case of β-thalassemia, or the specific point mutation for sickle cell disease. To that end, at least two successful strategies have been developed aiming to correct the IVS I-110 (G>A) mutation in β-thalassemia (Patsali et al., 2019) via either CRISPR/Cas9 or TALENS or the sickle cell mutation (Park et al., 2019). However, the most widely employed approach applicable for both sickle cell disease and thalassemia is the induction of fetal hemoglobin via genome editing. In 2013, the group of Stewart Orkin mapped a regulator of expression of BCL11A specific for the erythroid lineage (Bauer et al., 2013), and a follow-up study employing genome editing proved that targeted disruption of the critical GATA1 binding motif within the +58 intronic BCL11A enhancer leads to indel generation and thereby to reduced BCL11A expression with associated induction of γ-globin expression in erythroid cells (Wu et al., 2019). This notion was moved to the clinic by two ongoing clinical trials, NCT03745287 by CRISPR Therapeutics and NCT03653247 by Bioverativ. The two trials differ in the designer nucleases used to target the enhancer in that CRISPR Therapeutics utilizes a CRISPR approach, while Bioverative utilizes a ZFN. Regarding the CRISPR trial, short-term results of 15–18 months of follow-up reported two patients, one with thalassemia and a second with sickle cell disease, who demonstrated significant increase in hemoglobin values (expressed in g/dl) after gene therapy, combined with the presence of over 95% F-cells in peripheral blood (Frangoul et al., 2020). This recapitulation of the HPFH (Hereditary Persistence of Fetal Hemoglobin) phenotype has become a common approach and was also employed as a therapeutic alternative by other researchers as well, first by disrupting the BCL11A binding motifs in the promoters of γ-globin genes by CRISPR (Métais et al., 2019) or TALENs (Lux et al., 2018), so as to inhibit the binding of BCL11A and hence prevent the silencing of γ-globin and also by comparing disruption of different HbF repressors, including KLF1 (Lamsfus-Calle et al., 2020) and LRF (Weber et al., 2020). Finally, efforts to reconstitute naturally occurring deletions that lead to loss of putative silencers located at the 3' end of the γ-globin genes have been employed, including the 7.2-kb "Corfu" deletion of the γ-δ intergenic region and the 13.6-kb deletion including the γ-δ intergenic region and extending to the first intron of the β-globin gene, similar to the "Sicilian" 12.9-kb HPFH-5 deletion (Lattanzi et al., 2019).

Last but not least, another promising option is base editing by nucleotide deaminases linked to programmable DNA-binding proteins. These proteins function by fusing inactive or nickase Cas9 to deaminases that catalyze the enzymatic conversion of C to T (G-to-A on the opposing strand) or A to G (T-to-C on the opposing strand) (Gaudelli et al., 2017). Because this approach does not involve generation of DNA double strand breaks, it is supposedly safer compared to "classical" genome editing; however, certain limitations exist, as the currently available range of base editors cannot enable conversion of the sickle cell mutation, i.e., direct T-to-A correction. Nevertheless, the strategy can be employed to disrupt alternative sequence elements, analogous to NHEJ-mediated methods, to correct specific mutations of β-thalassemia (Zeng et al., 2020). Subsequent work by Liu and co-workers led to the concept of prime editing, which improved upon the versatility of their base editing tools by inclusion in the RNP particle of a reverse transcriptase and a template for reverse transcription. The resulting tools can precisely introduce all conceivable 12 nucleotide changes as well as small indels (Anzalone et al., 2019). Of note, an extremely interesting study was published in 2016 by Bahal et al. (2016) introducing the use of triplex-forming peptide nucleic acids (PNAs). PNAs are designed in a way that permits their binding to specific genomic DNA sites via strand invasion and formation of PNA/DNA/PNA triplexes (via both Watson–Crick and Hoogsteen binding) with a displaced DNA strand. PNAs are essentially nanoparticles consisting of a charge-neutral peptide-like backbone and nucleobases, enabling hybridization with DNA with high affinity. These PNA/DNA/PNA triplexes are potent in recruiting the cell's endogenous DNA repair systems to initiate site-specific modification of the genome when single-stranded "donor DNAs" are co-delivered as templates containing the desired sequence modifications (Anzalone et al., 2019). The results of this study proved the efficacy of nanoparticles in terms of phenotype correction in the context of monogenic diseases.

Challenges

Undoubtedly, the research regarding all potential applications in the field of genome editing is very promising and perhaps has better long-term prospects compared to gene therapy by retroviral vectors. Gene addition by designer nucleases outperforms the classical gene addition by retroviral vectors because it provides targeted integration, which, so far, cannot be achieved with retroviral vectors. However, despite potentially higher safety, caveats still exist for genome editing.

The first very important challenge in terms of safety is the identification of the off-target effects. To that end, major efforts have been described including Digenome-seq (Kim et al., 2015) and CIRCLE-seq (Tsai et al., 2017; Lazzarotto et al., 2018). Both methods are based on adapter ligation to the CRISPR generated ends: Digenome-seq generates *in vitro* Cas9-digested whole-genome fragments and then proceeds to profile genome-wide Cas9 off-target effects in human cells. CIRCLE-seq generates a library of circularized genomic DNA with minimized numbers of free ends and subsequent treatment of purified circles with CRISPR/Cas9 RNP complexes followed by adapter ligation and high-throughput sequencing. Although both approaches are highly promising, there are limiting steps such as the length of reads during NGS. Additional efforts such as BLISS (Yan et al., 2017) involve fixation of cells and it is doubtful if there is high accuracy in introducing DSBs as part of the screening (and not the therapeutic) process at high accuracy. Finally the DISCOVER-SEQ (Wienert et al., 2019) approach is based on recruitment of specific DNA repair proteins; hence, it is questionable if all DSBs can be identified, given the fact that even the amount of the engineering agent can have a profound impact

on the same cell type: For example, there have been differences described between engineered cord blood CD34[+] by lentiviral vectors with low MOI (Papanikolaou et al., 2015) compared to high MOI (Piras et al., 2017). Excluding the actual limitations existing in the current approaches, another point of concern is the fact that some off-targets may be completely benign, whereas others could have serious consequences depending on the cell context or the indication. This is a well-recognized issue in the field and is currently being addressed by engineering the CRISPR payload at both the protein and gRNA level with simultaneous optimization of the ideal window of active exposure of the cells of interest to the functional RNP complex (Tay et al., 2020).

Therefore, the burden from a regulatory aspect is major for the following reasons: (a) Even a single genetic disease caused by knockout of a single gene or sequence may be associated with several mutations, even unrelated ones, in different patients. For example, nobody knows or can accurately predict what can be caused by disruption of the erythroid specific enhancer within the second intron of BCL11A at a population scale. (b) Depending on the indication, even the most well-characterized agents in the field of gene therapy still present surprises. The latest manifestation of tumor generation after lentiviral mediated gene addition in the context of CGD is alarming (Jofra Hernández et al., 2020), as the authors described the development of T cell lymphoblastic lymphoma and myeloid leukemia in 2.94% and 5.88% of the mice tested, respectively, and oligoclonal composition with rare dominant clones harboring vector insertions near oncogenes in these mice. (c) Genetic engineering of HSCs presents additional hurdles as CD34[+] cells are difficult to be tested for karyotypic analysis, as most of the cells reside in Go phase. This poses a certain challenge toward identification of large chromosomal rearrangements as a result of designer nuclease action in the patients' genome, suggesting the need for development of surrogate assays. For example, approaches introducing chromosomal deletions and not indels will most probably face several difficulties during the transition toward a clinical trial. (d) Last but not least, gene therapy products are often described as "living drugs" and possess totally different pharmacokinetics compared to classical small molecules, and therefore even the regulatory agencies are not streamlined for assessments of such products.

Hence, the transition from bench to the clinic and accordingly for industry toward acquiring marketing authorization will require collaboration between different disciplines including researchers, physicians, industrial stakeholders, regulatory agencies, and policy makers.

DISCUSSION—FUTURE PERSPECTIVES

The development of therapeutic approaches based on genome editing by designer nucleases is proceeding with great speed and utilizes as a foundation knowledge produced from decades of traditional gene therapy research. However, any new curative scheme faces new challenges many of which are not foreseen particularly by research labs developing the proof of principle for these important new modalities.

The first perspective under discussion for the entire progress of the field is the actual location at which the therapy will take place. Currently, there are two different models that serve this cause: The centralized model assumes collection of the initial cell product from the patient at a local hospital, shipment of this product to a centralized facility in which the genetic engineering takes place, followed by freezing of the cell therapy product and shipment back to the original location. Thereby, the administering physician thaws the cell engineered product and reinfuses it to the patient. There are several advantages as well as disadvantages with this approach. First, centralized manufacturing is much more familiar with the existing mentality of both regulatory agencies as well as policy makers and governmental or societal stakeholders. However, there are serious limitations: This manufacturing model is intended for products with long shelf life and low degree of personalization, which obviously are not applicable for cell and gene therapy products for which transport can have a profound effect on the underlying biology of the cells of interest. Moreover, there is a high risk of incurring issues related from the distance of the user both geographically and in terms of responsiveness to end user requirements and logistics might face the serious issue of biological waste generation. Generally, the centralized model creates opportunities for errors and mistiming of the cell product delivery.

On the other hand, decentralized manufacturing assumes cell collection and processing locally. Equivalent approaches are currently being employed by hospitals in the context of blood transfusion and transplantation of HSCs. This manufacturing model also has pros and cons: the main advantage of this approach is the general flexibility brought about by being closer to the end user, therefore providing responsiveness to evolving requirements and greater personalization according to patient needs. The area of HSC transplantation has contributed enormously to the progress of the gene therapy field, and from that aspect, the decentralized model is closer to the mentality of tissue transplants, a medical routine since 1975 (Dunbar et al., 2018) and shares a lot of common challenges. However, most of these products are under specific tissue or transplant regulations, and these regulations have debatable applicability on gene therapy products. A key limitation to the decentralized model is exactly one of its assets: the flexibility. For such a manufacturing process to be successful from every possible aspect, it is of critical importance to demonstrate robustness. Therefore, a key question is how it is possible to simultaneously be robust and flexible, specifically taking into account that decentralized manufacturing is based on the expertise and skills of each specialized personnel undertaking the manufacturing in different locations. Another most obvious consideration is the starting material and the variability associated with it. Moreover, the type of culture, the differences in the cultivation media and cytokines used, and the timing of the culture generate additional fluctuations. One plausible approach to decrease user variability or bias would be to apply automation during the manufacturing preferably by closed systems with minimal user interaction. This mentality, ideally could be adopted even from early developments in research labs, suggesting that it would be of great benefit to the field if the cell product was produced already under mock-GMP conditions utilizing automated closed systems and GMP-like grade of media and cytokines. A process of this kind would provide a higher degree of maturity of the cell product and the only open variable step would be the starting material. It should be emphasized that once researchers streamline their processes, they should take into consideration that transfer of a research grade manufacturing to a GMP-like manufacturing would include specific documentation from media and cytokine providers, from retroviral vector providers, and from manufacturers of plasmids or RNPs in the case of genome editing. Also, it is generally advisable to utilize one module in the automation step and not different modules, because the regulatory authorities will ask for specific documentation and accreditation from every single module. Therefore, semi-automation will only create delays during any upcoming evaluation from a regulatory agency compared to full automation. Finally, researchers should keep in mind early on that fetal bovine serum, a material widely used in cell and tissue culture, is not characterized as GMP and therefore it would be eliminated from any future step in the process, requiring optimization of the whole process from the beginning.

As a last remark, successful decentralization would most probably require a new set of highly skilled personnel, possibly creating "technology transfer champions" (Harrison et al., 2018) from the current pool of researchers or students and most importantly students of medical sciences who are young, motivated, and eager to undertake the transition between manufacturing and practice in translational medicine. Additionally, centralized managed control standards and certified operators who receive mandatory re-training and licensing of remote site operations should be seriously considered by the universities, the industry, the government, and the society in general.

CONCLUDING REMARKS

The medical field is surely evolving fast and toward the direction of treating diseases previously incurable by the use of genetic manipulations in the form of classical gene therapy by gene addition but also with the advent of designer nucleases by genome editing. Over the past 20 years, significant milestones have been reached in terms of marketing authorization of gene therapy products and real benefit for a large number of patients has been established. However, the field is still in an immature phase, indicating its huge potential for future growth. To that end, researchers should focus early on toward generating true innovative solutions for patients that have the potential to transfer under GMP conditions and are also comparable price wise to the current state of the art. Super expensive solutions, albeit truly innovative in nature, will most certainly face challenges toward achieving proper reimbursement, thereby jeopardizing their eventual availability to patients. It should be emphasized that adoption of poor organization strategies and lack of risk mitigation measures early in the development has the potential to undermine the future success of an otherwise promising strategy or product, specifically in the area of genome editing. If such strategies are adopted early on from researchers, it is possible that previously unforeseen or unanticipated obstacles on the path to approval, often taking decades to address, will be omitted, increasing the wider applicability of genetic therapies, and unlocking their true potential.

AUTHOR CONTRIBUTIONS

EP researched the literature and wrote the manuscript. AB read the manuscript, provided feedback and final approval. Both authors contributed to the article and approved the submitted version.

REFERENCES

Aiuti, A., Biasco, L., Scaramuzza, S., Ferrua, F., Cicalese, M. P., Baricordi, C., et al. (2013). Lentiviral hematopoietic stem cell gene therapy in patients with Wiskott-Aldrich syndrome. *Science* 341:1233151. doi: 10.1126/science.1233151

Aiuti, A., Cattaneo, F., Galimberti, S., Benninghoff, U., Cassani, B., Callegaro, L., et al. (2009). Gene therapy for immunodeficiency due to adenosine deaminase deficiency. *N. Engl. J. Med.* 360, 447–458. doi: 10.1056/NEJMoa0805817

Aiuti, A., Slavin, S., Aker, M., Ficara, F., Deola, S., Mortellaro, A., et al. (2002). Correction of ADA-SCID by stem cell gene therapy combined with nonmyeloablative conditioning. *Science* 296, 2410–2413. doi: 10.1126/science.1070104

Aker, M., Tubb, J., Groth, A. C., Bukovsky, A. A., Bell, A. C., Felsenfeld, G. et al. (2007). Extended core sequences from the cHS4 insulator are necessary for protecting retroviral vectors from silencing position effects. *Hum. Gene Ther.* 18, 333–343. doi: 10.1089/hum.2007.021

Andtbacka, R. H., Kaufman, H. L., Collichio, F., Amatruda, T., Senzer, N., Chesney, J., et al. (2015). Talimogene laherparepvec improves durable response rate in patients with advanced melanoma. *J. Clin. Oncol.* 33, 2780–2788. doi: 10.1200/JCO.2014.58.3377

Anzalone, A. V., Randolph, P. B., Davis, J. R., Sousa, A. A., Koblan, L. W., Levy, J. M., et al. (2019). Search-and-replace genome editing without double-strand breaks or donor DNA. *Nature* 576, 149–157. doi: 10.1038/s41586-019-1711-4

Bahal, R., Ali McNeer, N., Quijano, E., Liu, Y., Sulkowski, P., Turchick, A., et al. (2016). *In vivo* correction of anaemia in β-thalassemic mice by γPNA-mediated gene editing with nanoparticle delivery. *Nat Commun.* 7:13304. doi: 10.1038/ncomms13304

Baker, A. H., and Herzog, R. W. (2020). Did dendritic cell activation, induced by adenovirus-antibody complexes, play a role in the death of jesse gelsinger? *Mol. Ther.* 28, 704–706. doi: 10.1016/j.ymthe.2020.02.010

Bauer, D. E., Kamran, S. C., Lessard, S., Xu, J., Fujiwara, Y., Lin, C., et al. (2013). An erythroid enhancer of BCL11A subject to genetic variation determines fetal hemoglobin level. *Science* 342, 253–257. doi: 10.1126/science.1242088

Biasco, L., Rothe, M., Büning, H., and Schambach, A. (2017). Analyzing the genotoxicity of retroviral vectors in hematopoietic cell gene therapy. *Mol. Ther. Methods Clin. Dev.* 8, 21–30. doi: 10.1016/j.omtm.2017.10.002

Biffi, A., Montini, E., Lorioli, L., Cesani, M., Fumagalli, F., Plati, T., et al. (2013). Lentiviral hematopoietic stem cell gene therapy benefits metachromatic leukodystrophy. *Science* 341:1233158. doi: 10.1126/science.1233158

Braun, C. J., Boztug, K., Paruzynski, A., Witzel, M., Schwarzer, A., Rothe, M., et al. (2014). Gene therapy for Wiskott-Aldrich syndrome–long-term efficacy and genotoxicity. *Sci. Transl. Med.* 6:227ra33. doi: 10.1126/scitranslmed.3007280

Burt, A. (2003). Site-specific selfish genes as tools for the control and genetic engineering of natural populations. *Proc. Biol. Sci.* 1518, 921–928. doi: 10.1098/rspb.2002.2319

Cartier, N., Hacein-Bey-Abina, S., Bartholomae, C. C., Veres, G., Schmidt, M., Kutschera, I., et al. (2009). Hematopoietic stem cell gene therapy with a lentiviral vector in X-linked adrenoleukodystrophy. *Science* 326, 818–823. doi: 10.1126/science.1171242

Cavazzana-Calvo, M., Payen, E., Negre, O., Wang, G., Hehir, K., Fusil, F., et al. (2010). Transfusion independence and HMGA2 activation after gene therapy of human β-thalassaemia. *Nature* 467, 318–322. doi: 10.1038/nature09328

Conry, R. M., Westbrook, B., McKee, S., and Norwood, T. G. (2018). Talimogene laherparepvec: first in class oncolytic virotherapy. *Hum. Vaccin. Immunother.* 14, 839–846. doi: 10.1080/21645515.2017.1412896

Coopman, K, and Medcalf, N. (2008). *From Production to Patient: Challenges and Approaches for Delivering Cell Therapies*. Cambridge, MA: Harvard Stem Cell Institute. Available online at: https://www.ncbi.nlm.nih.gov/books/NBK208660/ (accessed February 12, 2021).

Crowe, K. (2018). The million-dollar drug. *CBC News*. Available online at: https://newsinteractives.cbc.ca/longform/glybera (accessed February 12, 2021).

De Solà-Morales, O., Cunningham, D., Flume, M., Overton, P., Shalet, N., and Capri, S. (2018). Defining innovation with respect to new medicines: a systematic review from a payer perspective. *Int. J. Technol. Assess. Health Care* 34, 224–240. doi: 10.1017/S0266462318000259

Dever, D. P., Bak, R. O., Reinisch, A., Camarena, J., Washington, G., Nicolas, C. E., et al. (2016). CRISPR/Cas9 β-globin gene targeting in human haematopoietic stem cells. *Nature* 539, 384–389. doi: 10.1038/nature20134

Dunbar, C. E., High, K. A., Joung, J. K., Kohn, D. B., Ozawa, K., and Sadelain, M. (2018). Gene therapy comes of age. *Science* 359:eaan4672. doi: 10.1126/science.aan4672

Dunphy, G., Flannery, S. M., Almine, J. F., Connolly, D. J., Paulus, C., Jonsson, K. L., et al. (2018). Non-canonical activation of the DNA sensing adaptor STING by ATM and IFI16 Mediates NF-kappaB signaling after nuclear DNA damage. *Mol. Cell.* 71, 745–760. doi: 10.1016/j.molcel.2018.07.034

Ferrari, G., Thrasher, A. J., and Aiuti, A. (2020). Gene therapy using haematopoietic stem and progenitor cells. *Nat. Rev. Genet.* doi: 10.1038/s41576-020-00298-5 [Epub ahead of print].

Ferrari, S., Jacob, A., Beretta, S., Unali, G., Albano, L., Vavassori, V. et al. (2020). Efficient gene editing of human long-term hematopoietic stem cells validated by clonal tracking. *Nat. Biotechnol.* 38, 1298–1308. doi: 10.1038/s41587-020-0551-y

Frangoul, H., Altshuler, D., Cappellini, M. D., Chen, Y. S., Domm, J., Eustace, B. K., et al. (2020). CRISPR-Cas9 Gene Editing for Sickle Cell Disease and β-Thalassemia. *N. Engl. J. Med.* 384, 252–260. doi: 10.1056/NEJMoa2031054

Gaudelli, N. M., Komor, A. C., Rees, H. A., Packer, M. S., Badran, A. H., Bryson, D. I., et al. (2017). Programmable base editing of A·T to G·C in genomic DNA without DNA cleavage. *Nature* 551, 464–471. doi: 10.1038/nature24644

Genovese, P., Schiroli, G., Escobar, G., Di Tomaso, T., Firrito, C., Calabria, A., et al. (2014). Targeted genome editing in human repopulating haematopoietic stem cells. *Nature* 510, 235–240. doi: 10.1038/nature13420

Gomez-Ospina, N., Scharenberg, S. G., Mostrel, N., Bak, R. O., Mantri, S., Quadros, R. M., et al. (2019). Human genome-edited hematopoietic stem cells phenotypically correct Mucopolysaccharidosis type I. *Nat. Commun.* 10:4045. doi: 10.1038/s41467-019-11962-8

Hacein-Bey-Abina, S., von Kalle, C., Schmidt, M., Le Deist, F., Wulffraat, N., McIntyre, E., et al. (2003b). A serious adverse event after successful gene therapy for X-linked severe combined immunodeficiency. *N. Engl. J. Med.* 348, 255–256. doi: 10.1056/NEJM200301163480314

Hacein-Bey-Abina, S., Von Kalle, C., Schmidt, M., McCormack, M. P., Wulffraat, N., Leboulch, P., et al. (2003a). LMO2-associated clonal T cell proliferation in two patients after gene therapy for SCID-X1. *Science* 302, 415–419. doi: 10.1126/science.1088547

Harrison, R. P., Ruck, S., Rafiq, Q. A., and Medcalf, N. (2018). Decentralised manufacturing of cell and gene therapy products: learning from other healthcare sectors. *Biotechnol. Adv.* 2, 345–357. doi: 10.1016/j.biotechadv.2017.12.013

Heger, P., and Wiehe, T. (2014). New tools in the box: an evolutionary synopsis of chromatin insulators. *Trends Genet.* 30, 161–171. doi: 10.1016/j.tig.2014.03.004

Iglesias-Lopez, C., Agustí A., Obach, M., and Vallano, A. (2020). Corrigendum: regulatory framework for advanced therapy medicinal products in Europe and United States. *Front. Pharmacol.* 11:766. doi: 10.3389/fphar.2020.00766

Jasin, M., and Rothstein, R. (2013). Repair of strand breaks by homologous recombination. *Cold Spring Harb. Perspect. Biol.* 11:a012740. doi: 10.1101/cshperspect.a012740

Jofra Hernández, R., Calabria, A., Sanvito, F., De Mattia, F., Farinelli, G., Scala, S., et al. (2020). Hematopoietic tumors in a mouse model of X-linked chronic granulomatous disease after lentiviral vector-mediated gene therapy. *Mol. Ther.* 29, 86–102. doi: 10.1016/j.ymthe.2020.09.030

Kim, D., Bae, S., Park, J., Kim, E., Kim, S., Yu, H. R., et al. (2015). Digenome-seq: genome-wide profiling of CRISPR-Cas9 off-target effects in human cells. *Nat. Methods* 3, 237–243. doi: 10.1038/nmeth.3284

Kohn, D. B., Sadelain, M., and Glorioso, J. C. (2003). Occurrence of leukaemia following gene therapy of X-linked SCID. *Nat. Rev. Cancer* 3, 477–488. doi: 10.1038/nrc1122

Lamsfus-Calle, A., Daniel-Moreno, A., Antony, J. S., Epting, T., Heumos, L., Baskaran, P., et al. (2020). Comparative targeting analysis of KLF1, BCL11A, and HBG1/2 in CD34+ HSPCs by CRISPR/Cas9 for the induction of fetal hemoglobin. *Sci. Rep.* 10:10133. doi: 10.1038/s41598-020-66309-x

Lander, E. S., Baylis, F., Zhang, F., Charpentier, E., Berg, P., Bourgain, C., et al. (2019). Adopt a moratorium on heritable genome editing. *Nature* 567, 165–168. doi: 10.1038/d41586-019-00726-5

Lattanzi, A., Meneghini, V., Pavani, G., Amor, F., Ramadier, S., Felix, T., et al. (2019). Optimization of CRISPR/cas9 delivery to human hematopoietic stem and progenitor cells for therapeutic genomic rearrangements. *Mol. Ther.* 27, 137–150. doi: 10.1016/j.ymthe.2018.10.008

Lazzarotto, C. R., Nguyen, N. T., Tang, X., Malagon-Lopez, J., Guo, J. A., Aryee, M. J., et al. (2018). Defining CRISPR-Cas9 genome-wide nuclease activities with CIRCLE-seq. *Nat. Protoc.* 11, 2615–2642. doi: 10.1038/s41596-018-0055-0

Löwer, R., Löwer, J., and Kurth, R. (1996). The viruses in all of us: characteristics and biological significance of human endogenous retrovirus sequences. *Proc. Natl. Acad. Sci. U.S.A.* 93, 5177–5184. doi: 10.1073/pnas.93.11.5177

Lux, C. T., Pattabhi, S., Berger, M., Nourigat, C., Flowers, D. A., Negre, O., et al. (2018). TALEN-Mediated Gene Editing of HBG in Human Hematopoietic Stem Cells Leads to Therapeutic Fetal Hemoglobin Induction. *Mol. Ther. Methods Clin. Dev.* 12, 175–183. doi: 10.1016/j.omtm.2018.12.008

McCabe, C., Bergmann, L., Bosanquet, N., Ellis, M., Enzmann, H., von Euler, M., et al. (2009). Market and patient access to new oncology products in Europe: a current, multidisciplinary perspective. *Ann. Oncol.* 20, 403–412. doi: 10.1093/annonc/mdn603

Métais, J. Y., Doerfler, P. A., Mayuranathan, T., Bauer, D. E., Fowler, S. C., Hsieh, M. M., et al. (2019). Genome editing of HBG1 and HBG2 to induce fetal hemoglobin. *Blood Adv.* 3, 3379–3392. doi: 10.1182/bloodadvances.2019000820

Milone, M. C., and O'Doherty, U. (2018). Clinical use of lentiviral vectors. *Leukemia* 32, 1529–1541. doi: 10.1038/s41375-018-0106-0

Montini, E., Cesana, D., Schmidt, M., Sanvito, F., Ponzoni, M., Bartholomae, C., et al. (2006). Hematopoietic stem cell gene transfer in a tumor-prone mouse model uncovers low genotoxicity of lentiviral vector integration. *Nat. Biotechnol.* 24, 687–696. doi: 10.1038/nbt1216

Nambiar, T. S., Billon, P., Diedenhofen, G., Hayward, S. B., Taglialatela, A., Cai, K., et al. (2019). Stimulation of CRISPR-mediated homology-directed repair by an engineered RAD18 variant. *Nat. Commun.* 10:3395. doi: 10.1038/s41467-019-11105-z

Negre, O., Bartholomae, C., Beuzard, Y., Cavazzana, M., Christiansen, L., Courne, C., et al. (2015). Preclinical evaluation of efficacy and safety of an improved lentiviral vector for the treatment of β-thalassemia and sickle cell disease. *Curr. Gene Ther.* 1, 64–81. doi: 10.2174/1566523214666141127095336

O'Connor, D. J., McDonald, K., and Lam, S. P. (2016). A regulator's guide to the UK early access to medicines scheme. *Regul. Rapp.* 13, 10–13. Available online at: https://www.topra.org/TOPRA/TOPRA_Member/regulatory_rapporteur.aspx

Papanikolaou, E., and Anagnou, N. P. (2010). Major challenges for gene therapy of thalassemia and sickle cell disease. *Curr. Gene Ther.* 10, 403–411. doi: 10.2174/156652310793180724

Papanikolaou, E., Paruzynski, A., Kasampalidis, I., Deichmann, A., Stamateris, E., Schmidt, M., et al. (2015). Cell cycle status of CD34(+) hemopoietic stem cells determines lentiviral integration in actively transcribed and development-related genes. *Mol. Ther.* 4, 683–696. doi: 10.1038/mt.2014.246

Papapetrou, E. P., Lee, G., Malani, N., Setty, M., Riviere, I., Tirunagari, L. M., et al. (2011). Genomic safe harbors permit high β-globin transgene expression in thalassemia induced pluripotent stem cells. *Nat. Biotechnol.* 1, 73–78. doi: 10.1038/nbt.1717

Park, S. H., Lee, C. M., Dever, D. P., Davis, T. H., Camarena, J., Srifa, W., et al. (2019). Highly efficient editing of the β-globin gene in patient-derived hematopoietic stem and progenitor cells to treat sickle cell disease. *Nucleic Acids Res.* 47, 7955–7972. doi: 10.1093/nar/gkz475

Paton, J (2018). *Tiny U.K. Biotech Takes On Glaxo's $730,000 Gene Therapy.* New York, NY: Bloomberg.

Patsali, P., Turchiano, G., Papasavva, P., Romito, M., Loucari, C. C., Stephanou, C., et al. (2019). Correction of IVS I-110(G>A) β-thalassemia by CRISPR/Cas- and TALEN-mediated disruption of aberrant regulatory elements in human hematopoietic stem and progenitor cells. *Haematologica* 104, e497–e501. doi: 10.3324/haematol.2018.215178

Pavel-Dinu, M., Wiebking, V., Dejene, B. T., Srifa, W., Mantri, S., Nicolas, C. E., et al. (2019). Gene correction for SCID-X1 in long-term hematopoietic stem cells. *Nat Commun.* 10:1634. doi: 10.1038/s41467-019-10080-9

Persons, D. A., Hargrove, P. W., Allay, E. R., Hanawa, H., Nienhuis, A. W. (2003). The degree of phenotypic correction of murine β-thalassemia intermedia following lentiviral-mediated transfer of a human γ-globin gene is influenced by chromosomal position effects and vector copy number. *Blood* 101, 2175–2183. doi: 10.1182/blood-2002-07-2211

Piras, F., and Kajaste-Rudnitski, A. (2020). Antiviral immunity and nucleic acid sensing in haematopoietic stem cell gene engineering. *Gene Ther.* 13, 1–13. doi: 10.1038/s41434-020-0175-3

Piras, F., Riba, M., Petrillo, C., Lazarevic, D., Cuccovillo, I., Bartolaccini, S., et al. (2017). Lentiviral vectors escape innate sensing but trigger p53 in human hematopoietic stem and progenitor cells. *EMBO Mol. Med.* 9, 1198–1211. doi: 10.15252/emmm.201707922

Regalado, A. (2016). *The World's Most Expensive Medicine Is a Bust. MIT Technology Review.* Available online at: https://www.technologyreview.com/2016/05/04/245988/the-worlds-most-expensive-medicine-is-a-bust/ (accessed February 12, 2021).

Schiroli, G., Conti, A., Ferrari, S., Della Volpe, L., Jacob, A., Albano, L., et al. (2019). Precise gene editing preserves hematopoietic stem cell function following transient p53-mediated DNA damage response. *Cell Stem Cell* 24, 551–565. doi: 10.1016/j.stem.2019.02.019

Sessa, M., Lorioli, L., Fumagalli, F., Acquati, S., Redaelli, D., Baldoli, C., et al. (2016). Lentiviral haemopoietic stem-cell gene therapy in earlyonset metachromatic leukodystrophy: an ad-hoc analysis of a non-randomised, open-label, phase 1/2 trial. *Lancet* 388, 476–487. doi: 10.1016/S0140-6736(16)30374-9

Stein, S., Ott, M. G., Schultze-Strasser, S., Jauch, A., Burwinkel, B., Kinner, A., et al. (2010). Genomic instability and myelodysplasia with monosomy 7 consequent to EVI1 activation after gene therapy for chronic granulomatous disease. *Nat. Med.* 16, 198–204. doi: 10.1038/nm.2088

Tay, L. S., Palmer, N., Panwala, R., Chew, W. L., and Mali, P. (2020). Translating CRISPR-Cas therapeutics: approaches and challenges. *CRISPR J.* 4, 253–275. doi: 10.1089/crispr.2020.0025

Teichler Zallen, D. (2000). US gene therapy in crisis. *Trends Genet.* 6, 272–275. doi: 10.1016/S0168-9525(00)02025-4

Tisdale John, K. J., Markus, M., Janet, K., Lakshmanan, K., Manfred, S., Alexandra, M., et al. (2018). Current results of lentiglobin gene therapy in patients with severe sickle cell disease treated under a refined protocol in the Phase 1 Hgb-206 study. *Blood* 132(Suppl. 1):1026. doi: 10.1182/blood-2018-99-113480

Touchot N., and Flume, M. (2017). Early Insights from Commercialization of Gene Therapies in Europe. *Genes* 8:78. doi: 10.3390/genes8020078

Tsai, S. Q., Nguyen, N. T., Malagon-Lopez, J., Topkar, V. V., Aryee, M. J., and Joung, J. K. (2017). CIRCLE-seq: a highly sensitive *in vitro* screen for genome-wide CRISPR-Cas9 nuclease off-targets. *Nat. Methods* 6, 607–614. doi: 10.1038/nmeth.4278

Uchida, N., Hsieh, M. M., Raines, L., Haro-Mora, J. J., Demirci, S., Bonifacino, A. C., et al. (2019). Development of a forward-oriented therapeutic lentiviral vector for hemoglobin disorders. *Nat. Commun.* 10:4479. doi: 10.1038/s41467-019-12456-3

Urbinati, F., Arumugam, P., Higashimoto, T., Perumbeti, A., Mitts, K., Xia, P., et al. (2009). Mechanism of reduction in titers from lentivirus vectors carrying large inserts in the 3' LTR. *Mol. Ther.* 9, 1527–1536. doi: 10.1038/mt.2009.89

Wang, D., Wang, K., and Cai, Y. (2020). An overview of development in gene therapeutics in China. *Gene Ther.* 7-8, 338–348. doi: 10.1038/s41434-020-0163-7

Wanisch, K., and Yáñez-Muñoz, R. J. (2009). Integration-deficient lentiviral vectors: a slow coming of age. *Mol. Ther.* 17, 1316–1332. doi: 10.1038/mt.2009.122

Weber, L., Frati, G., Felix, T., Hardouin, G., Casini, A., Wollenschlaeger, C., et al. (2020). Editing a γ-globin repressor binding site restores fetal hemoglobin synthesis and corrects the sickle cell disease phenotype. *Sci. Adv.* 6:eaay9392. doi: 10.1126/sciadv.aay9392

Wiebking, V., Patterson, J. O., Martin, R., Chanda, M. K., Lee, C. M., Srifa, W., et al. (2020). Metabolic engineering generates a transgene-free safety switch for cell therapy. *Nat. Biotechnol.* 38, 1441–1450. doi: 10.1038/s41587-020-0580-6

Wienert, B., Wyman, S. K., Richardson, C. D., Yeh, C. D., Akcakaya, P., Porritt, M. J., et al. (2019). Unbiased detection of CRISPR off-targets *in vivo* using DISCOVER-Seq. *Science* 364, 286–289. doi: 10.1101/469635

Wu, Y., Zeng, J., Roscoe, B. P., Liu, P., Yao, Q., Lazzarotto, C. R., et al. (2019). Highly efficient therapeutic gene editing of human hematopoietic stem cells. *Nat. Med.* 5, 776–783. doi: 10.1038/s41591-019-0401-y

Yan, W. X., Mirzazadeh, R., Garnerone, S., Scott, D, Schneider, M. W., Kallas, T., et al. (2017). BLISS is a versatile and quantitative method for genome-wide profiling of DNA double-strand breaks. *Nat. Commun.* 8:15058. doi: 10.1038/ncomms15058

Zeng, J., Wu, Y., Ren, C., Bonanno, J., Shen, A. H., Shea, D., et al. (2020). Therapeutic base editing of human hematopoietic stem cells. *Nat. Med.* 4, 535–541. doi: 10.1038/s41591-020-0790-y

13

Base and Prime Editing Technologies for Blood Disorders

Panagiotis Antoniou, Annarita Miccio* and Mégane Brusson*

Université de Paris, Imagine Institute, Laboratory of Chromatin and Gene Regulation During Development, INSERM UMR 1163, Paris, France

*Correspondence:
Annarita Miccio
annarita.miccio@institutimagine.org
Mégane Brusson
megane.brusson@institutimagine.org

Nuclease-based genome editing strategies hold great promise for the treatment of blood disorders. However, a major drawback of these approaches is the generation of potentially harmful double strand breaks (DSBs). Base editing is a CRISPR-Cas9-based genome editing technology that allows the introduction of point mutations in the DNA without generating DSBs. Two major classes of base editors have been developed: cytidine base editors or CBEs allowing C>T conversions and adenine base editors or ABEs allowing A>G conversions. The scope of base editing tools has been extensively broadened, allowing higher efficiency, specificity, accessibility to previously inaccessible genetic loci and multiplexing, while maintaining a low rate of Insertions and Deletions (InDels). Base editing is a promising therapeutic strategy for genetic diseases caused by point mutations, such as many blood disorders and might be more effective than approaches based on homology-directed repair, which is moderately efficient in hematopoietic stem cells, the target cell population of many gene therapy approaches. In this review, we describe the development and evolution of the base editing system and its potential to correct blood disorders. We also discuss challenges of base editing approaches–including the delivery of base editors and the off-target events–and the advantages and disadvantages of base editing compared to classical genome editing strategies. Finally, we summarize the recent technologies that have further expanded the potential to correct genetic mutations, such as the novel base editing system allowing base transversions and the more versatile prime editing strategy.

Keywords: genome editing, base editing, CRISPR/Cas9, genetic disorders, blood diseases

INTRODUCTION

The vast majority of human genetic diseases are due to point mutations. In fact, amongst the 54,444 human disease-causing variants described in ClinVar, 33,739 are point mutations (Rees and Liu, 2018).

Human blood genetic disorders are due to mutations affecting hematopoietic stem cells (HSCs) or their committed progeny leading to general hematopoiesis defects or lineage-specific damages (e.g., in leukocytes or erythrocytes). For example, β-hemoglobinopathies are due to >300 mutations affecting the β-globin gene (*HBB*), resulting in red blood cell (RBC) defects and anemia (Cavazzana et al., 2017; Amaya-Uribe et al., 2019). Allogeneic HSC transplantation is the only curative treatment for many blood genetic disorders. However, it is limited by the availability of sibling donors and is associated with risks of graft rejection and graft vs. host disease (Cavazzana et al., 2017; Castagnoli et al., 2019). Therefore, *ex vivo* gene therapy approaches based on autologous transplantation of genetically corrected HSCs have been developed to offer a permanent and safer therapeutic solution. Many clinical studies using lentiviral-based gene addition approaches have proven to be beneficial for patients with genetic blood disorders. Nevertheless, some limitations still exist; for example, the expression of the transgene might be insufficient to cure the disease. The CRISPR/Cas9 nuclease allows the correction of genetic mutations, therefore achieving a physiological expression of the target endogenous gene; however, it introduces double-strand breaks (DSBs) that can be deleterious for the target cells (Cromer et al., 2018; Kosicki et al., 2018).

Hematological malignancies have been successfully treated using chimeric antigen receptor (CAR) T-cell therapies. This approach is based on the engineering of autologous or allogenic T-cells that express a CAR recognizing antigens on tumor cells (e.g., CD19 in B-cell malignancies). In allogenic CAR T-cell therapies, several genes involved in alloreactivity can be inactivated using nuclease-based approaches. Nonetheless, DSBs can lead to genomic translocations, when simultaneous edits of different loci occur (Stadtmauer et al., 2020).

Base editing is a newly developed tool able to precisely edit DNA sequences in a specific locus without inducing DSBs. Interestingly, around 60% of the pathogenic point mutations can be potentially corrected by base editors (BEs) (Rees and Liu, 2018). Notably, base editing is a new therapeutic tool able to precisely and safely correct genetic mutations and to target disease modifiers and inactivate genes or cis-regulatory regions in hematopoietic cells. Therefore, base editing can potentially provide a cure for many blood diseases.

Different BEs have been created allowing base conversions in a variety of target regions. The cytosine BEs (CBEs) allow the conversion of a C:G to a T:A base pair (bp), while adenine BEs (ABEs) convert an A:T into a G:C bp. BEs are composed by a catalytically dead Cas9 (dCas9) or a nickase Cas9 (nCas9) fused to a deaminase and guided by a single guide RNA (sgRNA) to the locus of interest (**Figure 1**). The d/nCas9 recognizes a specific sequence named protospacer adjacent motif (PAM) and the DNA unwinds thanks to the complementarity between the sgRNA and the DNA sequence usually located upstream of the PAM ("protospacer"). Then, the opposite DNA strand is accessible to the deaminase that converts the bases located in a specific DNA stretch of the protospacer ("editing window," **Figure 1**).

One of the major advantages of BEs compared to the CRISPR/Cas9 nuclease system is their ability to introduce precise point mutations without generating DSBs. In fact, despite the high efficiency, CRISPR/Cas9 treatment of human hematopoietic stem/progenitor cells (HSPCs) induces a DNA damage response (Cromer et al., 2018) that can lead to apoptosis. CRISPR/Cas9 can cause P53-dependent cell toxicity (Haapaniemi et al., 2018; Ihry et al., 2018; Schiroli et al., 2019) and cell cycle arrest, resulting in negative selection of cells with a functional P53 pathway. Furthermore, the generation of several on-target DSBs, simultaneous on-target and off-target DSBs, or even a single on-target DSB is associated with a risk of deletion, inversion, and translocation (Kosicki et al., 2018; Cullot et al., 2019; Blattner et al., 2020; Leibowitz et al., 2020). These events impair gene correction and might result in the complete inactivation of the target gene or even have long-range transcriptional consequences

that could constitute a first carcinogenic hit. Therefore, the absence or the very low frequency of DSBs, confer to BEs the potential to perform safer genome edits. Moreover, BEs accurately convert specific bases in a wide range of cell types and at different stages along the cell cycle. On the contrary, nuclease-based correction of genetic mutations via homology-directed repair (HDR) is limited mainly to dividing cells (Zhang et al., 2017). Compared to HDR-based strategies, base editing is a promising therapeutic tool to precisely correct genetic mutations as it avoids gene disruption by non-homologous end-joining (NHEJ) associated with failed HDR-mediated gene correction (Yeh et al., 2018). Finally, this DSB-free strategy can potentially allow simultaneous targeting of multiple regions in the genome without generating chromosomal rearrangements such as large deletions and translocations (Stadtmauer et al., 2020).

DEVELOPMENT OF CYTOSINE AND ADENINE BASE EDITORS

Different versions of CBEs have been created with the goal of improving their efficiency and safety. The original BE1 is composed of a catalytically dCas9 from *Streptococcus pyogenes* (*Sp*) fused with the rat deaminase (rAPOBEC1). This enzyme was selected amongst several deaminases for its high deaminase activity (Komor et al., 2016). The dCas9 contains amino acid substitutions (D10A and H840A) that abolish the nuclease activity avoiding DSB generation without interfering with its DNA binding capacity. BE1 recognizes the cytosine at the target locus and converts it into a uracil. The U:G bp is recognized as a mismatch by the cellular repair machinery that usually removes the U. To protect this newly formed U from excision, BE2 was developed by fusing a uracil glycosylase inhibitor (UGI) to the dCas9 C-terminus (Komor et al., 2016). In BE3, the dCas9 was modified to generate a Cas9 nickase (Cas9n containing the D10A amino acid substitution) that nicks the non-edited G-containing DNA strand without generating DSBs (Komor et al., 2016). The nicking step favors the replacement of the G in the nicked strand by an A by the DNA repair machinery. Then, the uracil from the U:A bp is converted to T by the host repair machinery allowing the formation of the desired T:A bp. These modifications improved the efficiency of CBEs in mammalian cells (Komor et al., 2016). Finally, the fourth-generation BE4 differs from BE3 as it carries a second UGI conferring a higher editing efficiency and improved product purity (percentage of C converted to T over the total base conversion events (C>T, C>G, and C>A) (Komor et al., 2017). The editing window of these CBEs is located at positions 4–8 of the protospacer (with the PAM's first nucleotide located at position 21). The use of alternative cytosine deaminases was also explored, such as the *P.marinus* activation-induced cytidine deaminase (AID or PmCDA1; editing window at positions 2–8) and the human APOBEC3A (hA3A; editing window at positions 2–13) (Gehrke et al., 2018; Nishimasu et al., 2018; Wang et al., 2018).

The absence of a DNA adenine deaminase to target and convert an A:T bp to a G:C bp prompted Liu and coworkers to create an engineered enzyme (Gaudelli et al., 2017). A dimeric

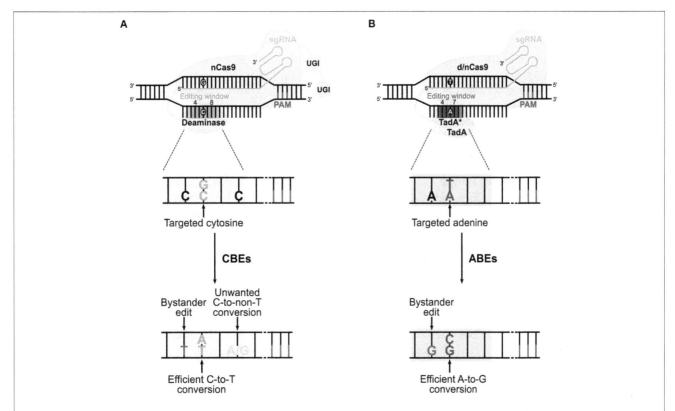

FIGURE 1 | Cytosine and adenine base editors. **(A)** Cytosine base editors (CBEs), composed of a nickase Cas9 (nCas9) fused to a deaminase and one (in BE3s) or two (in BE4s) UGI (uracil glycosylase inhibitor), convert C:G into T:A base pairs in the editing window (nucleotide 4 to 8 in the protospacer, in green). **(B)** Adenine base editors (ABEs) are composed of a dead (d) or nickase (n) Cas9 (d/nCas9) fused to two TadA, one evolved to edit adenine in DNA (TadA*) and one wild type (TadA). ABEs convert A:T into G:C base pairs in the editing window (nucleotide 4 to 7 in the protospacer, in purple). Cas9 is guided by the sgRNA to the protospacer [which is followed by the PAM (protospacer adjacent motif)], unwinds the DNA and the deaminase converts the target base. Undesired events (bystander edits, in blue, and unwanted base conversion, in yellow) of CBEs and ABEs are shown in **(A,B)**, respectively. The addition of the second UGI in CBEs (in BE4) and the removal of TadA in ABEs (ABE8) are highlighted with a gray dotted line. The gradient color of the editing window in the upper panels of **(A,B)** represents the enlarged editing window observed with novel BEs.

tRNA adenine deaminase from *E. coli* (TadA) was modified to generate TadA* that efficiently deaminates adenine in the DNA. TadA∗ was then fused to the SpCas9n (D10A) to create ABEs. As TadA works natively as a homodimer, an enzyme composed of wild-type TadA and TadA* was fused to SpCas9n and various mutations were introduced in the TadA* domain. This resulted in the development of four ABEs (ABE6.3, ABE7.8, ABE7.9, and ABE7.10) with increased editing efficiency. The editing window is located at positions 8-10 of the protospacer for ABE6.3, ABE7.8, and ABE7.9 and at position 4–7 for ABE7.10. Therefore, for the same sgRNA, the choice of the ABE can be dictated by the position of the target bases (Gaudelli et al., 2017). Interestingly, at the same loci, ABEs were able to introduce point mutations with a higher efficiency and reduced InDel formation compared to Cas9 nuclease-mediated HDR approaches (Gaudelli et al., 2017).

BE3, BE4, and ABE7.10 are the most commonly used base editors nowadays and have been extensively improved in the last years (Gaudelli et al., 2020; Miller et al., 2020; Richter et al., 2020). These base editors have been optimized by modifying the codon usage and the nuclear localization sequences to enhance base editing in mammalian cells [e.g., BE4max, AncBE4max, and

ABEmax (Koblan et al., 2018)]. For instance, BE4 was improved by the addition of a bipartite NLS at both N- and C-termini and by codon optimization to generate BE4max. Replacement of rAPOBEC1 with an optimized ancestor rAPOBEC1 homolog— Anc689 that contains 36 amino acid substitutions compared to rAPOBEC1–resulted in the generation of AncBE4max. Both BE4max and AncBE4max exhibit a higher editing efficiency compared to BE4 (Koblan et al., 2018). Furthermore, the use of alternative Cas variants or the engineering of Cas enzymes allowed the development of BEs recognizing a greater variety of PAMs, thus expanding the targeting scope of BEs. Finally, modifications of the deaminase domain led to the generation of more precise BEs with increased product purity and a narrower activity window.

Improving the Targeting Scope of Base Editors

One of the limitations to the use of BEs is the requirement of a suitable PAM adjacent to the target sequence and in a position that places the target bases in the optimal editing window. The first CBEs and ABEs were designed using the SpCas9n (that is the most commonly used Cas for genome editing) limiting the editing to genomic loci containing NGG PAMs. To increase the number of potential targets, BEs harboring orthologous Cas9n or engineered Cas9n variants have been developed. These enzymes recognize non-NGG PAMs and for some of them, the editing window is shifted or enlarged to target bases that otherwise would be inaccessible due to the lack of an optimal PAM. Finally, the use of alternative or engineered deaminase variants was also explored to enlarge the editing window.

CBEs With Expanded Targeting Range

To broaden the targeting scope of CBEs, new Cas9n variants have been introduced in CBEs allowing the editing of non-NGG PAM sites.

BE3s harboring the engineered SpCas9n variants SpCas9n-VQR (NGA PAM), SpCas9n-VRQR (NGA PAM), SpCas9n-EQR (NGAG PAM), and SpCas9n-VRER (NGCG PAM) allowed the targeting of genomic regions containing non-NGG PAMs (Kim et al., 2017b).

Furthermore, Kim et al. created SaBE3 harboring the nickase version of the *Staphylococcus aureus* Cas9 (SaCas9n, containing the D10A amino acid substitution), which edits sites containing NNGRRT PAMs (Ran et al., 2015). SaBE3 effectively converts C to T in human cells with a high conversion efficiency at NNGRRT PAM compared to BE3 (Kim et al., 2017b). The SaCas9n was also introduced in BE4 to create SaBE4, resulting in higher editing efficiency and product purity compared to SaBE3 (Komor et al., 2017). A SaCas9n mutant harboring three mutations (SaCas9n-KKH, SaKKHn) was used to develop CBEs that can target loci containing NNNRRT PAMs (Kim et al., 2017b). Importantly, Sa BEs have an expanded editing window compared to Sp BEs (positions 3–12) allowing the editing of bases located closer to the PAM.

Interestingly, a small Cas9 nickase from *Staphylococcus auricularis* (SauriCas9n containing the D15A amino acid substitution) was inserted in the BE4max (SauriBE4max). Its reduced size allowed the packaging in adeno-associated virus (AAV) vectors. In addition, this novel CBE allows the targeting of loci containing NNGG PAMs (Hu et al., 2020).

To enlarge the number of editable loci that lack G/C-rich PAM sequences, Li et al. fused the dead Cas12a from *Lachnospiraceae bacterium* (dLbCas12a or dLbCpf1) to rAPOBEC1 to generate dCas12a-BE3. This CBE can edit loci containing T-rich PAMs (TTTV) and efficiently convert cytosines located downstream of the PAM (from position 8–13, counting the base next to the PAM as position 1) with minimal InDels and undesired base conversions (Li et al., 2018b). Another engineered Cas12a variant from *Acidaminococcus sp.* (enAsCas12a) was used to generate CBEs that recognize TTTV as well as additional PAMs (e.g., TTYN, VTTV TRTV). These BEs show improved C>T conversion compared to the original AsCas12a (Kleinstiver et al., 2019). Finally, the insertion of an engineered SpCas9n containing the PAM-interacting region of *Streptococcus macacae* Cas9 (Spy-macCas9n) in BE4max led to the development of Spy-mac-BE4max, which is capable of targeting sites containing TAAA PAMs (Liu et al., 2019).

To further increase the number of genomic regions accessible to CBEs, Hu et al. developed new SpCas9 variants harboring mutations that expand the PAM compatibility. In particular, the use of the xCas9 variant recognizing a large range of PAMs (including NG, GAA, and GAT) in the BE3 enzyme (xCas9-BE3) greatly increased cytosine base editing scope. However, this BE was proved efficient in a limited number of genomic sites (Hu et al., 2018). Another engineered Cas9 variant recognizing NG PAMs [SpCas9n-NG (Nishimasu et al., 2018)] was incorporated in CBEs harboring rAPOBEC1, APOBEC3A or PmCDA1 (Nishimasu et al., 2018; Thuronyi et al., 2019). In particular, Nishimasu et al. showed that a fusion of PmAID and SpCas9n-NG (Target-AID-NG) is more active than the xCas9-BEs in human cells (Nishimasu et al., 2018). Recently, novel CBEs compatible with NRCH, NRTH or NRRH PAMs (including non-G PAMs) allowed the targeting of previously inaccessible genomic loci (Miller et al., 2020).

Besides expanding the PAM compatibility of CBEs, several studies aimed at targeting cytosines outside the classical editing window. A larger editing window can allow the installation of point mutations in previously inaccessible regions to disrupt genes or regulatory regions; however, if the goal is to generate a precise mutation (e.g., in the coding region of a gene), only silent mutations of non-target bases should be permitted. Huang et al. generated novel circularly permutated (CP)-SpCas9n BE variants with a broadened or shifted editing window. These variants were used to generate CP-BE4max enzymes that can efficiently edit bases that otherwise would be inaccessible (Huang et al., 2019). Interestingly, the introduction of the RAD51 single-stranded DNA binding domain (ssDBD) in BE4max, dramatically increased the editing frequency and extended the editing window to cytosines in positions 9–15 (hyBE4max) (Zhang et al., 2020a). Similar results were obtained by inserting the RAD51 ssDBD in BE4max harboring APOBEC3A (hyA3A-BE4max) (Zhang et al., 2020a).

Different deaminase variants can also be employed to target previously inaccessible sites. The introduction of human APOBEC3A (hA3A) deaminase in BE3 (hA3A-BE3) improved C-to-T base conversion in highly methylated genomic regions and enlarged the editing window to 12 nucleotides (position 2–13 in the protospacer) (Wang et al., 2018). Thuronyi et al. generated several rAPOBEC1 and PmCDA1 variants with improved context compatibility (i.e., allowing editing of GC motifs) and enlarged editing window. EvoFERNY (an ancestor of rAPOBEC1), evoAPOBEC1 (a rAPOBEC1 variant) and evoCDA1 (a PmCDA1 deaminase variant) deaminases were introduced in BE4max to test their activity in GC motifs, which were usually poorly edited by the previously developed CBEs. EvoCDA1-BE4max and evoFERNY-BE4max outperformed evoAPOBEC1-BE4max at GC target sites, while offering similar or even higher efficiency in non-GC targets. An advantage of evoFERNY-BE4max is the smaller size of its deaminase allowing its delivery by viral particles. While evoFERNY-BE4max and evoAPOBEC1-BE4max present an editing window comparable to BE4max, evoCDA1-BE4max offers an enlarged editing window (position 1–13 of the protospacer) and enables the conversion of cytosines located in

GC or TC motifs far from the classical editing window (Thuronyi et al., 2019).

ABEs With Expanded Targeting Range

The use of orthologous or engineered Cas9n in ABEs increased the number of PAMs compatible with these enzymes, thus broadening the range of adenine base editing targets.

Several Cas9n variants were introduced in ABEs to generate A>G conversions at genomic sites containing non-NGG PAMs (Chatterjee et al., 2018; Hu et al., 2018; Yang et al., 2018; Jeong et al., 2019). SpCas9n was replaced by SaKKHn or SpCas9n-VQR in ABE7.10 to generate SaKKH-ABE and VQR-ABE that target sites harboring the NNNRRT and the NGA PAM, respectively (Yang et al., 2018). Similarly, Hu et al. introduced xCas9 in ABE7.10 and created xCas9-ABE offering improved editing efficiency at NGG PAM-containing sites as well as at loci harboring NGC, NGA, and GAT PAMs (Hu et al., 2018). ABEmax versions containing Cas9 variants recognizing NG (xCas9 in xABEmax or SpCas9n-NG in NG-ABE max) or NR PAMs (SpCas9n-NRCH, SpCas9n-NRTH, and SpCas9n-NRRH) have also been generated (Huang et al., 2019; Miller et al., 2020). ABEmax was further improved by replacing SpCas9n with SaCas9n or with the engineered SaKKHn, SpCas9n-VRER and SpCas9n-VRQR allowing the targeting of loci containing non-NGG PAMs. SpCas9n-VRER and SpCas9n-VRQR induce A-to-G conversions in many target sites containing PAMs other than NGG. Sa-ABEmax and SaKKH-ABEmax present a large editing window (position 4–14 of the protospacer) although the editing efficiency is modest (Huang et al., 2019). To target bases located outside the canonical editing window, Huang et al. generated CP-ABEmax enzymes with a broadened or shifted activity window (Huang et al., 2019).

Recently, Richter et al. developed a novel ABE (ABE8e) with enhanced activity and compatibility with different Cas homologs, which was limited with the previously described ABEs (Richter et al., 2020). ABE8e contains eight additional mutations in the TadA* deaminase domain that confer a higher processing activity (Lapinaite et al., 2020). ABE8e showed greatly increased editing efficiency when combined with SpCas9n and different Cas9 variants (e.g., SaCas9n, SaKKHn, SpCas9n-NG, and LbCas12a) compared to the corresponding ABEmax-based enzymes (Richter et al., 2020). Furthermore, removal of the wild type TadA did not affect ABE8e editing activity, indicating that the optimized TadA* can efficiently work as a monomer (Richter et al., 2020). Interestingly, Gaudelli et al. also generated ABE8 variants offering improved editing efficiency and extended editing window (position 3–10) compared to ABEmax (Gaudelli et al., 2020). The SpCas9n of ABE8s was replaced by the engineered SpCas9n-NG or SaCas9n, broadening the editing scope of ABE8s, while maintaining their preference for adenine editing in a wide editing window (position 5–14) (Gaudelli et al., 2020). Of note, ABE8 enzymes showed increased DNA and RNA off-target activity. However, this was reduced by delivering the BE as mRNA or ribonucleoprotein (RNP) (compared to plasmid delivery) or by inserting amino acid substitutions that enhance the genome-wide specificity (see paragraph "BE off-target activity") (Gaudelli et al., 2020; Richter et al., 2020).

Virtually PAMless CBEs and ABEs

In a recent study, Walton et al. used structure-guided engineering to relax the PAM requirement of SpCas9, resulting in a near-PAMless variant (SpRY). SpRY is compatible with both CBEs and ABEs and with nearly all the possible PAMs (NRN and NYN, with low but substantial activity with NYN) (Walton et al., 2020). As expected, the PAM relaxation reduced specificity and increased the number of DNA off-targets (Walton et al., 2020). However, insertion of amino acid substitutions conferring a reduced or absent off-target activity can be envisioned to improve the precision of SpRY-based BEs (see paragraph "BE off-target activity").

Improving Product Purity of BEs

Base editing is a powerful tool to efficiently correct point mutations at a specific locus. However, at certain genomic targets, CBEs and, to a lesser extent, ABEs generate unwanted base conversions, thus reducing the product purity. In fact, the initial study describing CBEs reports that BE3 generates unwanted C>non-T edits inside the activity window (Komor et al., 2016). In a second study, Komor et al. improved BE3 by inserting a second UGI and by increasing the length of the linkers between rAPOBEC1 and Cas9n (32 amino acids), between Cas9n and UGI (9 amino acids), and between the 2 UGI (9 amino acids) (Komor et al., 2017). The new BE4 enzyme showed improved C-to-T editing efficiency and product purity and decreased InDel formation compared to BE3. Moreover, the introduction of CP-SpCas9 in BE4max to generate CP-BE4max improved product purity compared to BE4max (Huang et al., 2019). Finally, the Gam protein of the Mu bacteriophage, known to protect DSB ends from degradation, was fused to the N-terminal part of BE3, SaBE3, BE4, and SaBE4 via a linker of 16 amino acids. These four novel enzymes displayed lower InDel frequency and increased product purity without affecting C>T editing efficiency compared to their unmodified versions (Komor et al., 2017). Interestingly, the product purity was particularly high in human *bona fide* HSCs–the target cell population in gene therapy approaches for hematological genetic disorders (Zeng et al., 2020).

Contrary to CBEs, ABEs have a high product purity. Only one study describes ABEs as a generator of aberrant edits. Surprisingly, ABEs was not responsible for A>non-G edits but for C>G or C>T conversions (Kim et al., 2019).

Reducing Bystander Edits and Narrowing the Activity Window of BEs

The vast majority of BEs convert cytosines or adenines located in a precise editing window of 4 to 6 nucleotides. The original BEs (BE3, BE4, and ABE7.10) display an editing window ranging from position 4–8 for CBEs and 4–7 for ABEs (**Figure 1**). However, if multiple C or A are present in the editing window, their conversion by BEs can potentially introduce undesired mutations (Komor et al., 2016). These bystander edits should be taken into consideration when base editing is used as a therapeutic strategy because they could create aberrant gene variants. Deaminase engineering was mainly used to narrow or shift the editing window and reduce bystander edits.

In the case of rAPOBEC1-based CBEs, mutations have been inserted in rAPOBEC1 to develop new BEs that precisely edit specific cytosines in the protospacer without modifying adjacent cytosines. Among all the mutants tested, the triple mutant YEE-BE3 (W90Y, R126E, and R132E) exhibits a restricted editing window of 1 to 2 nucleotides mainly editing cytosine at position 6 in the protospacer. If two C are present in the editing window, YEE-BE3 favors the conversion of only one of them (Kim et al., 2017b). However, this engineered BE displays reduced editing efficiency. Similarly, the introduction of the YEE mutations in the deaminase of BE4-Gam (YEE-BE4-Gam) and BE4max (YEE-BE4max) narrows the editing window to position 5 or 6 but lowers the editing efficiency (Liu et al., 2020). By removing the R132E mutation (known to reduce the editing efficiency) and introducing the Y120F mutation (known to narrow the editing window), Liu et al. created YFE-BE4max that presents a restricted editing window (position 4–6) and a high editing efficiency (Liu et al., 2020). The YE mutations were also introduced in the dCas12a-BE (dCas12a-BE-YE) to narrow the width of the editing window from 6 to 3 nucleotides (position 10-12 of the protospacer counting the base next to the PAM as position 1) (Li et al., 2018b).

Interestingly, the substitution of the original flexible linker between rAPOBEC1 and Cas9n by a rigid linker of 5–7 amino acids in BE3 greatly shortens the editing window and favors editing at positions 5 and 7 (Tan et al., 2019). Furthermore, truncation of PmCDA1 in the BE3-based enzyme restricted the editing window to position 2 (Tan et al., 2019).

Finally, to restrict the editing window and reduce the high InDel frequency associated with hA3A-BE3, Y130F, or Y132D mutations (known to partially reduce hA3A activity) and 3 UGI were inserted in hA3A-BE3 to generate BEs with a narrowed editing window (position 3–8) and lower InDel frequency (Wang et al., 2018). Gehrke et al. also introduced in BE3 an engineered hA3A (eA3A) containing the N57G amino acid substitution that improved the editing precision. This engineered eA3A-BE3 favors conversion of the C located in a TCR motif and reduces bystander mutations compared to BE3 and YE-BE3 variants (Gehrke et al., 2018).

Concerning the ABEs, no variant with a narrower editing window has been described up to date.

BASE EDITING FOR THE TREATMENT OF BLOOD DISORDERS

Base Editing Strategies for β-Hemoglobinopathies

β-hemoglobinopathies, β-thalassemia, and sickle cell disease (SCD), are monogenic diseases caused by mutations in the β-globin locus and affect the synthesis, the structure or the properties of the adult hemoglobin (HbA). β-thalassemia is caused by mutations in the β-globin locus that reduce (β^+) or abolish (β^0) the production of adult β-globin chains composing the HbA tetramer. This leads to the precipitation of uncoupled α-globin chains, ineffective erythropoiesis, erythroid cell death, and anemia (Weatherall, 2001; Cappellini et al., 2018; Taher et al.,

2018). In SCD, an A>T mutation in the *HBB* gene causes the substitution of valine for glutamic acid at position 6 of the β-globin chain (β^S) that is responsible for deoxygenation-induced polymerization of the sickle hemoglobin (HbS). This primary event drives RBC sickling, hemolysis, vaso-occlusive crises, multi-organ damage, often associated with severely reduced life expectancy (Piel et al., 2017; Kato et al., 2018).

Allogenic HSC transplantation is the only curative therapy for β-hemoglobinopathies; however, the absence of sibling donors and the risk of immunological complications prevent its use in a large fraction of patients (Locatelli et al., 2013, 2016; Leonard and Tisdale, 2018). Because of their high prevalence, β-hemoglobinopathies are a common study model for developing genetic treatments. Transplantation of lentiviral-corrected HSCs containing a functional β-globin gene is a promising therapeutic solution for patients lacking sibling donors. However, the low expression level of the therapeutic transgene per viral copy is associated with a variable clinical outcome (Miccio et al., 2008; Thompson et al., 2018; Weber et al., 2018; Cavazzana et al., 2019; Magrin et al., 2019; Marktel et al., 2019). Promising genome editing-based therapies were developed to directly modify endogenous genes and induce therapeutic β-like globin expression. Current nuclease-based strategies can reactivate the expression of fetal γ-globin genes or correct the defective β-globin gene. CRISPR/Cas9-mediated editing strategies raising γ-globin levels take advantage of the NHEJ pathway to disrupt genes or *cis*-regulatory regions involved in γ-globin silencing. As NHEJ is an active DNA repair pathway in HSCs, NHEJ-based strategies are highly efficient (Wu et al., 2019; Weber et al., 2020). On the contrary, HDR-based approaches are modestly efficient in quiescent HSCs. For instance, the SCD-causing mutation was efficiently corrected by CRISPR/Cas9 combined with a donor template in HSPCs. However, the efficiency of gene correction was drastically reduced after xenotransplantation in immunodeficient mice, confirming the low HDR rate in long-term repopulating HSCs (Dever et al., 2016; Antony et al., 2018; Pattabhi et al., 2019; Romero et al., 2019). Finally, one of the major limitations of nuclease-based approaches is the potential DSB-induced toxicity (see introduction). Therefore, BEs could provide safer therapeutic strategies (**Figure 2, Table 1**). Notably, these approaches could be more efficacious than HDR-based strategies in correcting β-hemoglobinopathy-causing mutations, as base editing is efficient in quiescent cells, as are HSCs (Zeng et al., 2020).

Correcting β-Hemoglobinopathy-Causing Mutations With Base Editing
Correcting a β-Thalassemia-Causing HBB −28 Mutation Using CBEs

The *HBB* −28 (A>G) mutation is highly prevalent in β-thalassemia patients from China and East Asia. This mutation maps to the ATAA box of the *HBB* promoter and prevents β-globin expression. An HDR-based CRISPR/Cas9 approach was developed to revert this mutation in iPSCs, and restored *HBB* expression in their erythroid progeny (Xie et al., 2014). However, this strategy was not tested in clinically-relevant HSPCs.

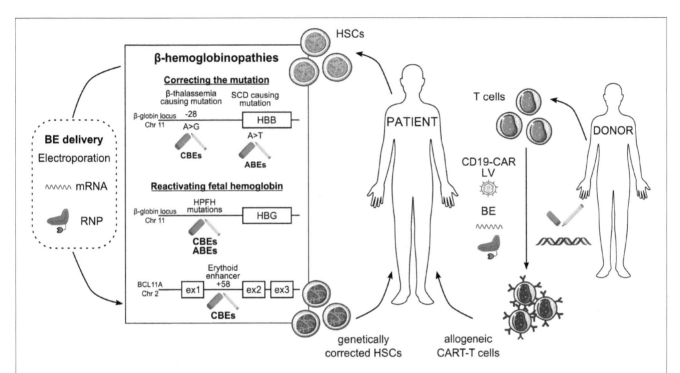

FIGURE 2 | Potential *ex vivo* base editing approaches for genetic blood disorders. Schematic representation of base editing approaches to genetically correct HSCs from SCD and β-thalassemia patients (left) or to generate allogeneic CAR-T cells (right). (Left) Correction of the A>G β-thalassemic mutation (in position-28) and reversion of the SCD A>T mutation can be performed using CBEs and ABEs, respectively. HbF reactivation can be achieved (i) upon generation of HPFH mutations in *HBG1/2* promoters by ABEs or CBEs or (ii) upon disruption of the *BCL11A* erythroid enhancer (located at position +58 kb from *BCL11A* transcription start site) by CBEs. BEs are delivered to HSCs as mRNA or RNP complexes. In *ex vivo* gene therapy approaches, HSCs genetically modified by BEs will be transplanted to the patient as a definitive therapy. (Right) Multiplex base editing of loci involved in alloreactivity (e.g., *TRAC, B2M, PDC1D, CD7*) and lentiviral vectors (LV)-mediated CAR expression to safely generate allogeneic CAR-T cells, which will be infused into patients to kill cancer cells.

Liang et al. used BE3 to correct this mutation in patients' fibroblasts (Liang et al., 2017). However, bystander editing was observed at the −25 position leading to the generation of a mutation causing β-thalassemia in humans. These results highlighted the need to use BEs with a narrower activity window to improve edit precision. Mutation correction was observed also in 23% of human embryos generated by nuclear transfer using a BE with a narrower editing window (YEE-BE3). No bystander edits were observed, suggesting that this BE allows a more precise editing of the *HBB* promoter.

Gehrke et al. compared the efficacy and the precision of BE3, different YE-BE3 variants and eA3A-BE3 in HEK293T cells harboring the *HBB*−28 (A>G) mutation (Gehrke et al., 2018). eA3A-BE3 (containing the N57G amino acid substitution) showed the highest efficacy, followed by BE3 and YE-BE3s. eA3A-BE3 also appeared to be more precise than BE3 and YE-BE3s because of the N57G mutation in A3A that minimizes bystander editing activity. The efficacy and precision of different BEs were also compared in erythroid precursors from a compound heterozygous β-thalassemia patient harboring a deletion in exon 1 in one *HBB* allele and the *HBB* −28 (A>G) mutation in the other allele. eA3A-BE3 and eA3A(N57Q)-BE3 (another BE3 variant with a N57Q mutation in hA3A) preferentially edited the−28 position compared to the −25 position (around 20% of alleles carried only the −28 mutation

for both enzymes) and eA3A-BE3 showing the lowest bystander activity. However, eA3A(N57Q)-BE3 was more efficient than eA3A-BE3 at the on-target position. In differentiated erythroid precursors, correction of this mutation by eA3A-BE3 and eA3A(N57Q)-BE3 increased *HBB* expression by 2.6- and 4.0-fold, respectively. Finally, eA3A-BE3 caused off-target edits at one out of six analyzed sites, while eA3A(N57Q)-BE3 caused off-target edits at four of the six sites and with higher frequency than eA3A-BE3. Altogether, these results show that CBEs can be used to correct the *HBB* −28 (A>G) mutation and increase β-globin production in β-thalassemia erythroid cells. However, further studies should be conducted to minimize the off-target effects, while maintaining a high base editing efficiency (see paragraph "BE off-target activity").

The *HBB* −28 (A>G) mutation was also successfully corrected in HSPCs from a heterozygous β-thalassemia patient with a null β^0 *HBB* allele and the *HBB* −28 (A>G) mutation in the other allele (Zeng et al., 2020). Electroporation of RNPs containing eA3A(N57Q)-BE3 complexed with the same sgRNA used in the previous study (Gehrke et al., 2018) led to 68% of corrective C>T edits, 28% of non-corrective C>G/A edits, 3.6% of unedited alleles and 14% of bystander edits at position *HBB* −25. This low bystander editing frequency could unlikely lead to the generation of β-thalassemic phenotype. Analysis of single erythroid progenitors demonstrated that

TABLE 1 | Base editing strategies for the treatment of blood disorders.

		Model	Delivery	Target	BE	Efficiency	References
β-hemoglobinopathies	Cell line	β^S/β^S HEK293T cells	Plasmid chemical transfection	SCD mutation	ABE-NRCH	41%	Miller et al., 2020
		HEK293T cells		−198 *HBG1/2* (HPFH)	ABE7.10	30%	Gaudelli et al., 2017
		HEK293T cells		−175/−113/−116 *HBG1/2* (HPFH)	ABEmax	27–52%	Koblan et al., 2018
		HEK293T cells		−198 and −175 *HBG1/2* (HPFH)	ABE8e	24%	Richter et al., 2020
		HEK293T cells		Erythroid-specific *BCL11A* enhancer	ABE8e	54.4%	Richter et al., 2020
		HUDEP2-$\Delta^G\gamma$	Lentiviral transduction	−117 *HBG1/2* (HPFH)	hyeA3A-BE4max	50%	Zhang et al., 2020a
	Primary cells	$\beta^{-28(A>G)}/\beta^{-28(A>G)}$ patients fibroblasts and cloned embryos	Plasmid electroporation (fibroblasts) and intracytoplasmic injection of BE3 mRNA (embryos)	*HBB* −28 (A>G) mutation	BE3 YEE-BE3	23%	Liang et al., 2017
		HD HSPCs	mRNA electroporation	−198 and −199 *HBG1/2* (HPFH)	ABE8 variants	50%	Gaudelli et al., 2020
		HD and β-thalassemia patient HSPCs	RNP electroporatin	−114 and −115 *HBG1/2* (HPFH)	hA3A-BE3	20%	Wang et al., 2020
		$\beta^-/\beta^{-28(A>G)}$ erythroid precursors		*HBB* −28 (A>G) mutation	eA3A(N57G)-BE3 eA3A(N57Q)-BE3	22%	Gehrke et al., 2018
		$\beta^-/\beta^{-28(A>G)}$ HSPCs		*HBB* −28 (A>G) mutation	eA3A(N57Q)-BE3	68%	Zeng et al., 2020
		SCD and β-thalassemia patient HSPCs*		Erythroid-specific *BCL11A* enhancer	eA3A(N57Q)-BE3	86–93%	Zeng et al., 2020
		SCD patient HSPCs*		−175 *HBG1/2* (HPFH)	ABE7.10	58%	Mayuranathan et al., 2020
		SCD patient HSPCs*	mRNA/RNP electroporation	SCD mutation	ABE8e-NRCH	80/44%	Yen et al., 2020
CAR T-cell therapy	Primary cells	Human primary T-cells	mRNA/RNP electroporation	*TRAC*, *B2M*, and *PDCD1*	BE4 coBE4	35/80% 90%/ND	Webber et al., 2019
		Human primary T-cells	mRNA electroporation	*B2M*, *CD7*, *PDCD1*, *CIITA*, *TRAC*, and *CBLB*	ABE8.20-m	98%	Gaudelli et al., 2020

*tested in vitro and in xenotransplantation experiments in immunodeficient mice.
HD, healthy donor; ND, non-determined.

corrective C>T edits in position −28 restored β-globin expression. These results demonstrate that base editing can produce efficient and therapeutic edits in primary human HSPCs and, therefore, is a conceivable therapeutic approach to treat β-hemoglobinopathies.

Correcting the SCD-Causing β^S-Globin Allele With ABEs

Miller et al. used novel BE variants to edit the previously inaccessible pathogenic SCD mutation in the *HBB* gene in HEK293T cells (Miller et al., 2020). The mutated allele harbors at position 6 a GTG codon that codes for a valine instead of the wild-type GAG codon translated to a glutamic acid.

With the current base editing technology, this A>T mutation cannot be reverted. However, the GTG codon can be converted to a GCG triplet coding for an alanine. This mutation is present in the Makassar allele (HbG) and is non-pathogenic in both heterozygous and homozygous individuals (Viprakasit et al., 2002; Mohamad et al., 2018). Miller et al. tested the ABE-NRRH, ABE-NRTH, and ABE-NRCH variants (compatible with NRRH, NRTH, and NRCH PAMs, respectively), and the previously reported NG-ABEmax [compatible with an NG PAM (Huang et al., 2019)] and sgRNAs targeting protospacer sequences followed by CATG and CACC PAMs in HEK293T cells homozygous for the β^S-allele. These novel ABEs showed higher on-target base editing activity when using sgRNAs targeting protospacer sequences followed by CACC PAM with ABE-NRCH variant being the most efficient (conversion rate: 41 ± 4%).

A combination of the engineered deaminase of ABE8e and the Cas9n-NRCH led to the creation of ABE8e-NRCH enzyme. This BE efficiently generated 80 and 45% of HbG alleles after RNA or RNP electroporation of SCD HSPCs, respectively. After erythroid differentiation, the high HbG expression (76 and 52% of the total Hb types in samples treated with RNA or RNP electroporation, respectively), and the concomitant decrease of HbS expression, rescued the RBC sickling phenotype. Importantly, editing of the SCD mutation was maintained in xenotransplanted mice (Yen et al., 2020). Altogether, these results show that base editing can be used to modify the SCD-causing β^S-allele in order to generate a non-pathogenic variant.

Base Editing Strategies for Reactivating Fetal Hemoglobin to Treat β-Hemoglobinopathies

Correcting the SCD point mutation is a feasible therapeutic approach as all the SCD patients have the same mutation. However, since β-thalassemia is associated with >300 mutations, this approach seems inconceivable to treat this disease as many mutation-specific therapeutic products should be developed. Interestingly, the clinical course of β-hemoglobinopathy patients is ameliorated in the presence of genetic mutations causing a condition termed hereditary persistence of fetal hemoglobin [HPFH (Forget, 1998)]. Therefore, an approach aimed at reactivating the γ-globin genes (HBG1 and 2) and fetal hemoglobin (HbF) could represent a universal strategy for treating not only β-thalassemia but also SCD patients. HPFH mutations in the promoter of the γ-globin genes either generate de novo DNA motifs recognized by transcriptional activators (e.g., KLF1, TAL1, and GATA1) or disrupt binding sites for transcriptional repressors (e.g., BCL11A and LRF).

Base editing strategies have been developed to reactivate HbF either by generating HPFH mutations or by downregulating the HbF repressor BCL11A via disruption of its erythroid-specific enhancer. It is noticeable that, differently from CRISPR/Cas9 nuclease, base editing allows also the generation of HPFH mutations that create binding sites for transcriptional activators.

Inserting HPFH Mutations in the HBG1/2 Promoters

Gaudelli and colleagues designed a sgRNA that allows ABE7.10 to generate a C-to-T conversion at position −198 in both HBG1 and HBG2 promoters in HEK293T cells with 29 and 30% of efficiency, respectively (Gaudelli et al., 2017). This point mutation is known to cause HPFH in adults by recruiting the KLF1 transcriptional activator. Similarly, Koblan et al., used ABEmax to install the following HPFH and HPFH-like mutations in HEK293T cells: (1) −175 T>C (generating a binding site for TAL1); (2) −113 A>G (generating a binding site for GATA1); and (3) −116 A>G (HPFH-like mutation in the BCL11A binding site) with efficiencies ranging from 27 to 52% in HEK293T cells (Koblan et al., 2018).

The highly efficient ABE8e variant was also capable of installing HPFH mutations in the HBG1/2 promoters in

HEK293T cells (Richter et al., 2020). Interestingly, both ABE8e and ABEmax could successfully generate the −198 and −175 HPFH mutations, but only ABE8e was capable of simultaneously generating both conversions with a frequency of up to 24%. These results indicate that ABE8e can be used for multiplex base editing. Indeed, the generation of multiple HPFH mutations or the simultaneous targeting of genomic regions involved in HBG1/2 silencing (e.g., the HBG1/2 promoters and the BCL11A gene) could further increase HbF levels.

The −117 G>A HPFH mutation (disrupting the BCL11A binding site) was inserted in an adult erythroid progenitor cell line (HUDEP2-$\Delta^G\gamma$) via lentiviral delivery of hyeA3A-BE4max (Zhang et al., 2020a). This enzyme was generated by inserting the N57G mutation into hyA3A-BE4max, to narrow the editing window and avoid bystander editing that was detrimental on the activity of the HBG1/2 promoters (Zhang et al., 2020a). An editing frequency of up to 50% led to substantial elevation of γ-globin mRNA expression.

More importantly, HPFH mutations have been inserted using BEs in HSPCs. Wang et al. introduced the −115 C>T and −114 C>T HPFH/HPFH-like mutations (disrupting the BCL11A binding site) in healthy donor and β-thalassemia patient HSPCs via electroporation of RNP containing hA3A-BE3 and a sgRNA targeting the HBG1/2 promoters (Wang et al., 2020). Editing frequency was ∼20% with C>non-T editing events (themselves being HPFH mutations) representing one-fifth of the total edits. HbF reactivation was observed in the erythroid progeny of edited HSPCs. Interestingly, this base editing strategy avoided the deletion of the 5.2-kb region between HBG1 and HBG2 promoters. This genomic deletion is commonly observed upon Cas9 nuclease-mediated cleavage of the two identical HBG1 and HBG2 promoters and results in the loss of HBG2 gene expression (Traxler et al., 2016; Li et al., 2018a).

Gaudelli et al. used the novel ABE8s to insert the −198 HPFH mutation (generating a KLF1 binding site) in the HBG1/2 promoters (Gaudelli et al., 2020). HSPCs derived from healthy donors were electroporated with mRNA encoding either ABE8 or ABEmax and a sgRNA targeting the −198 nucleotide of the HBG1/2 promoters. ABE8 treatment led to higher editing efficiencies (∼50%) compared to ABEmax (∼30%) at position −198. Furthermore, only ABE8s were able to simultaneously edit positions −198 and −199. The Authors observed a 3.5-fold average increase in γ-globin expression in erythrocytes differentiated from HSPCs treated with ABE8 compared to mock-treated cells. A statistically significant increase of median γ-globin levels was also observed in all ABE8-treated cells compared to ABEmax-treated samples. These results suggest that simultaneous editing at position −198 and −199 by ABE8s contributed to γ-globin induction.

Recently, the −175 HPFH mutation has been efficiently introduced in up to 58% of HBG promoters upon ABE7.10-RNP electroporation of SCD HSPCs. Reactivation of HbF expression was obtained in 60% of erythroid cells differentiated from edited HSPCs (14% expression in control cells). This resulted in a 2-fold decrease in the fraction of sickled RBCs. After xenotransplantation in immunodeficient mice, despite the reduced editing frequency, HbF was detectable in 32% of erythroblasts (Mayuranathan et al., 2020).

Disrupting the Erythroid-Specific BCL11A Enhancer

CRISPR/Cas9 nuclease-mediated disruption of the binding site for the GATA1 transcription activator within the *BCL11A* erythroid-specific enhancer is associated with potent *BCL11A* downregulation and γ-globin upregulation. Therefore, this GATA1 binding site represents a potent target for inducing HbF. Ongoing clinical trials aim at evaluating the safety and efficacy of this approach in patients with transfusion dependent β-thalassemia (NCT03655678) and SCD (NCT03745287). One year after cell infusion, the two first patients showed a high editing efficiency, strong HbF de-repression and 100% of F-cells in the peripheral blood resulting in transfusion-independence and elimination of vaso-occlusive crises in the SCD patient (Frangoul et al., 2020) Long-term follow-up studies are necessary to confirm safety and efficacy of this therapeutic strategy (Frangoul et al., 2020).

An alternative approach relies on BEs to precisely edit the GATA1 BS while substantially limiting DSBs. The evolved ABE8e variant was employed in HEK293T cells to install simultaneously two A>G edits in the GATA1 binding site of the *BCL11A* enhancer. ABE8e substantially outperformed ABEmax (54% efficiency for ABE8e vs. 8% for ABEmax) (Richter et al., 2020).

Zeng et al. used RNP containing eA3A(N57Q)-BE3 to achieve high frequency of cytosine base edits at the same GATA1 binding site (86%-93%). This resulted in therapeutically relevant HbF induction in erythroid cells derived from β-thalassemia and SCD patient HSPCs (Zeng et al., 2020). In particular, the erythroid progeny of edited SCD HSPCs exhibited high level of HbF expression (up to 32%), and β-thalassemic erythroid cells showed potent HbF induction that led to improved erythropoiesis. Importantly, xenotransplantation experiments in immunodeficient mice showed efficient C>T editing in *bona fide* human HSCs, while the frequency of C>non-T edits was significantly reduced compared to *in vitro*-treated HSPCs. Finally, multiplex editing of erythroid cells from a β-thalassemia patient to simultaneously disrupt the *BCL11A* erythroid enhancer and correct the *HBB* −28 A>G promoter mutation, led to further improvement of the β-thalassemic phenotype, compared to individual editing of the two regions (*BCL11A* enhancer or *HBB* −28 only).

In conclusion, base editing approaches represent a promising new modality for treating patients with β-thalassemia and SCD by reactivating fetal globin gene expression.

Developing Safe Allogeneic CAR-T Cell-Based Therapies Using Base Editing

Chimeric antigen receptor (CAR)-T cell therapy is based on the engineering of T-cells to attack tumor cells. The current CAR-T cell-based therapies are effective against hematological malignancies, but limited by their autologous nature (Qasim, 2019; Kim and Cho, 2020). Nuclease-based strategies aimed at inactivating multiple genes involved in alloreactivity allowed the generation of allogeneic CAR-T cells. However, DSBs resulting from multiplex nuclease-based genome editing can lead to large

genomic rearrangements such as translocations (Stadtmauer et al., 2020). BEs can be employed to inactivate genes (e.g., by generating premature stop codons or by disrupting splice sites). Thus, BEs have been successfully used to develop safe allogeneic CAR-T cell-based therapies (Webber et al., 2019; Gaudelli et al., 2020), virtually eliminating the genotoxic risks associated to DSBs (**Figure 2**, **Table 1**).

Webber et al. exploited CBEs to simultaneously target three loci involved in alloreactivity: the T-cell receptor α constant (*TRAC*) locus, β-2 microglobulin (*B2M*), and programmed cell death 1 (*PDCD1*). The ultimate goal was to generate CD19-targeted CAR-T cells without inducing DSBs and potential translocations (Webber et al., 2019). Targeting each locus separately by electroporating BE4 mRNA and individual sgRNAs (targeting splice donor or acceptor sites) was efficient. However, multiple base editing frequency was modest even when using a higher mRNA dose. RNP delivery of BE4 and more significantly mRNA delivery of a codon-optimized BE4 (coBE4) led to considerably higher efficiencies with 90% of protein loss for all the targets and a proportion of triple knockout cells of up to 90%. Importantly, no translocation event was detected in base-edited T cells compared to samples treated with SpCas9 nuclease inactivating the three targets via DSB generation. Multiplex base editing did not affect cell differentiation, expansion and functionality and cytokine production (Webber et al., 2019).

Similarly, Gaudelli et al. used ABE8s to disrupt genes involved in alloreactivity (*B2M*, *CD7*, *PDCD1*, *CIITA*, *TRAC*, and *CBLB*) by targeting their splice sites. ABE8.20-m was the best performing enzyme, achieving base editing efficiencies of 98-99% for each of the 6 genes targeted individually and a median protein loss of 60% in primary T cells. ABE8.20-m mRNA electroporation of T cells resulted in efficient multiplex editing of three genes (*B2M*, *CIITA*, and *TRAC)* (with frequencies >98% for each gene) and concomitant reduced protein expression (Gaudelli et al., 2020).

These studies demonstrate the crucial role of base editing in the development of DSB-free and safe allogeneic CAR T-cell-based therapies.

CHALLENGES OF BASE EDITING APPROACHES

BE Delivery

Different methods have been reported to deliver BEs in cell lines and primary cells (**Figure 3**). Plasmid DNA transfection is an easy, cheap and fast way to produce and deliver BEs to the target cells. Many proof-of-concept studies have used this method to achieve efficient base editing and potentially develop new therapeutic strategies for blood disorders (Gaudelli et al., 2017; Liang et al., 2017; Koblan et al., 2018; Miller et al., 2020; Richter et al., 2020). However, plasmid transfection faces some limitations, such as poor efficiency and toxicity in primary cells (e.g., HSPCs and T cells) (Lattanzi et al., 2019). Moreover, compared to more transient delivery systems (i.e., mRNA and RNP delivery), transfection of BE-expressing plasmids generates more likely

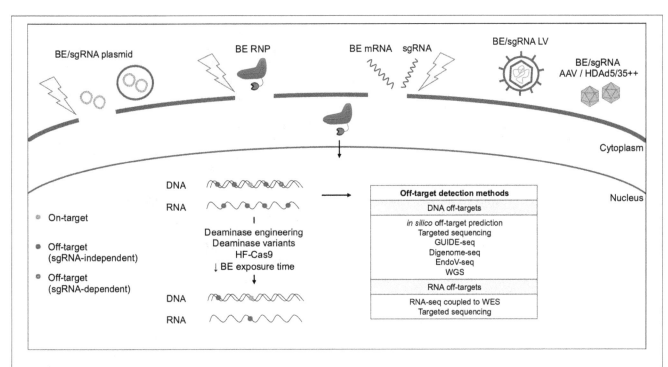

FIGURE 3 | Base editing delivery systems and potential off-target activity. BEs are delivered by plasmid chemical transfection (e.g., lipofectamine) or electroporation (yellow thunder), RNP or mRNA electroporation or LV/AAV transduction. BEs can cause RNA and DNA off-target effects in a sgRNA-independent (red dots) or -dependent (blue dots) manner. Off-target activity can be reduced by modifying the deaminase and/or the Cas9. Current methods used to predict and detect DNA and RNA off-targets are indicated in the table. WGS, Whole Genome Sequencing; WES, Whole Exome Sequencing.

off-target effects due to their prolonged expression (Rees et al., 2017).

Lentiviral-mediated BE delivery has also been explored in proof-of-principle studies (Zhang et al., 2020a,b); however, prolonged expression of BEs in hematopoietic cells must be avoided to prevent immune response and off-target editing.

Therefore, transient BE delivery via mRNA or RNP electroporation has been exploited by many research groups to avoid or reduce limitations associated with plasmid and lentiviral delivery. This type of delivery is preferred for the development of clinically-relevant therapeutic strategies (Kouranova et al., 2016).

Several studies aimed at developing treatments for blood disorders have been conducted by delivering mRNAs coding for BEs in T cells and HSPCs [BE3 (Webber et al., 2019), BE4 (Webber et al., 2019), ABEmax (Gaudelli et al., 2020), ABE8 (Gaudelli et al., 2020), and ABE8e-NRCH (Yen et al., 2020)]. Webber et al. showed that codon optimization of BE4 mRNA substantially increases base editing efficiency (Webber et al., 2019). Interestingly, chemical modification of the ABE mRNA (5′capping, uridine depletion and replacement of all remaining uridines with 5-methoxyuridine) and the sgRNA (2′-O-methyl 3′-phosphorothioate modification at first and last three nucleotides) drastically improved ABE protein expression and base editing efficiency in cell lines (Jiang et al., 2020). Therefore, these modifications can potentially increase base editing efficiency in primary cells after BE mRNA delivery.

BE protein production and electroporation in patient-derived HSPCs has been performed successfully for APOBEC3A-based

BEs [eA3A-BE3 (Gehrke et al., 2018), eA3A(N57Q)-BE3 (Gehrke et al., 2018; Zeng et al., 2020), and hA3A-BE3 (Wang et al., 2020)]. On the contrary, only Webber et al. have described the delivery of an APOBEC1-based BE as RNP (BE4) in clinically-relevant CD3$^+$ T-cells. Furthermore, this study showed that mRNA electroporation outperformed RNP electroporation in terms of base editing efficiency (Webber et al., 2019). However, successful delivery of APOBEC1-based BEs as RNPs was reported in cell lines [BE3 (Kim et al., 2017a; Park et al., 2017; Rees et al., 2017; Yeh et al., 2018), HF-BE3 (Rees et al., 2017), enAsCas12a-BE (Kleinstiver et al., 2019)] although in some cases extensive optimization of the protein production was required (Rees et al., 2017). Regarding ABEs, both ABE7.10 and ABE8e-NRCH were electroporated as RNP complexes in SCD HSPCs, but mRNA electroporation of ABE8e-NRCH led to higher editing efficiencies (Mayuranathan et al., 2020; Yen et al., 2020).

Data on cytotoxicity observed upon BE mRNA or RNP delivery in primary hematopoietic cells are limited (Zeng et al., 2020). Interestingly, two cycles of BE RNP electroporation were required to achieve high frequency of base editing in human HSPCs. This reduced cell viability from 83% (1 round of transfection) to 47% (2 rounds of transfection) and engraftment (Zeng et al., 2020). These results suggest that BE delivery requires further optimization before moving to clinical studies.

As base editing is a recently emerged technology and given the large variety of BEs, BE mRNAs and proteins are not yet commercially available, thus limiting the testing of new therapeutic strategies in primary hematopoietic cells.

Lastly, to overcome the limitations of *ex vivo* HSC-based gene therapy approaches (namely, the loss of the long-term repopulating capacity due to the prolonged culture, and the need for myeloablation and a specialized bone marrow transplantation center), *in vivo* gene therapy strategies have been proposed to deliver BEs to HSCs (Li et al., 2020). To this aim, a suitable *in vivo* delivery system, such as AAV or HDAd5/35++ adenovirus vectors should be used. So far, several studies have established a system to deliver *in vivo* ABEs or CBEs using AAV vectors (Winter et al., 2019; Chen et al., 2020; Hu et al., 2020; Levy et al., 2020). As BEs are large enzymes that cannot be packaged in a single AAV, many groups used a split-intein system based on the use of two AAV vectors harboring the two moieties of a SpCas9-based CBE fused to intein fragments that are reassembled *in vivo* via *trans*-splicing. However, this system is still inefficient, therefore the use of smaller BEs able to be packaged in a single AAV [such as SauriBE4max (Hu et al., 2020)] is preferable. Notably, AAV-mediated delivery specifically to HSCs has not yet been performed and is highly challenging. Intravenous injection of HDAd5/35++ vectors has been used to deliver the CRISPR/Cas9 nuclease system to murine HSCs mobilized in the bloodstream (Li et al., 2020). These vectors can accommodate large expression cassettes, although a selection system needs to be used to reach therapeutically relevant efficiencies of genetic correction in HSCs. Recently, this system has been exploited to deliver into HSCs BEs introducing HPFH point mutations in the *HBG1/2* promoters in a humanized mouse model (Li et al., 2020).

BE Off-Target Activity

The use of base editing system may lead to undesired DNA and RNA off-target effects. Many efforts have been done to increase the specificity of the Cas9 and the deaminase and eliminate off-targets (**Figure 3**).

DNA Off-Targets

The DNA off-target effects of BEs can be sgRNA-independent or -dependent (Rees et al., 2019).

The sgRNA-independent off-target effects occur at unpredicted sites and are due to the intrinsic DNA affinity of the deaminase domain. Different studies compared the sgRNA-independent off-target activity of CBEs and ABEs and showed a higher frequency of off-targets for CBEs than for ABEs (Zuo et al., 2019; Doman et al., 2020; Lee et al., 2020; Yu et al., 2020). Modifications in the deaminase domain or the use of alternative deaminases allowed the development of CBE variants that exhibit low DNA sgRNA-independent off-target activity and maintain high on-target efficiency (YE1-BE4, R33A-BE4, YE1-BE4-CP1028, and YE1-BE4-NG; (Doman et al., 2020); AmAPOBEC1, SsAPOBEC3B^{R54Q}, BE3^{R132E}, YE1-BE3, and FE1-BE3; (Yu et al., 2020; Zuo et al., 2020). An alternative way to achieve a high on-target/off-target ratio is to provide the BEs as RNPs. This limits the BE exposure time and reduces the extent of sgRNA-independent off-target editing (Doman et al., 2020). Similarly, BE mRNA delivery decreases off-target editing by limiting BE expression in time (Yu et al., 2020). Therefore, transient BE RNP and mRNA delivery should be preferred

compared to plasmid transfection and lentiviral transduction to avoid off-target effects.

Whole genome sequencing is used to evaluate the sgRNA-independent off-target effects, although the coverage is insufficient to detect rare events.

The sgRNA-dependent off-target effects rely on the ability of the Cas9n domain to bind via the sgRNA to genomic sites similar to the on-target site as well as on the presence of an A or a C in the suitable base editing window and in the suitable context for each BE (Gaudelli et al., 2017). Some initial studies suggested that CBEs and ABEs have a lower DNA sgRNA-dependent off-target activity compared to the Cas9 nuclease (Gaudelli et al., 2017; Kim et al., 2017) and that CBEs are in general more prone than ABEs to generate this type of off-target events (Liu et al., 2018; Doman et al., 2020). The use of high-fidelity versions of the Cas9n [e.g., HF-BE3 (Rees et al., 2017), Sniper-Cas9 BE3 (Lee et al., 2018), HF1-eA3A-BE3 and Hypa-eA3A-BE3 (Gehrke et al., 2018)], the BE delivery as RNP (Richter et al., 2020), or even the reduced RNP exposure (Zeng et al., 2020) can minimize the sgRNA-dependent off-target effects.

The *in silico* Cas-off finder software followed by targeted deep sequencing of the predicted off-targets (Gehrke et al., 2018; Wang et al., 2020; Zeng et al., 2020; Zhang et al., 2020a) and experimental methods such as GUIDE-seq (Gehrke et al., 2018; Webber et al., 2019; Gaudelli et al., 2020; Richter et al., 2020; Zeng et al., 2020), Digenome-seq (Kim et al., 2019; Zhang et al., 2020a), and EndoV-seq (Liang et al., 2019; Richter et al., 2020) have been mainly used to evaluate the potential sgRNA-dependent DNA off-target effects of BEs.

RNA Off-Targets

BEs may also cause off-target effects at RNA level in a sgRNA-independent manner. The first studies revealed that both CBEs and ABEs can modify the RNA, resulting in tens of thousands of C>U and A>I edits, respectively (Grünewald et al., 2019a; Rees et al., 2019). The RNA edits were spread throughout the transcriptome. To overcome this issue, specific mutations (R33A/K34A) that are known to reduce the RNA C>U base conversion activity of rAPOBEC1 were inserted in CBEs. The resulting BE (BE3-R33A/K34A) presents RNA off-target activity reduced to baseline levels, while maintaining an on-target DNA activity similar to the original BEs (Grünewald et al., 2019a). Furthermore, new rAPOBEC1-containing CBE variants (BE3^{R132E}, YE1-BE3, and FE1-BE3) caused a remarkable reduction in the RNA off-target effects (Zuo et al., 2020).

A variety of deaminases and deaminase variants have been used instead of the rAPOBEC1, such as hA3A, eA3A, human AID (hAID), and PmCDA1, to abolish the RNA C-to-U activity of CBEs. hA3A-BE3 showed substantial RNA editing (Grünewald et al., 2019b); however, the use of hA3A harboring amino acid substitutions in the RNA binding domain (R128A) and in the ssDBD (Y130F) abolished RNA off-target effects (Zhou et al., 2019). eA3A induced a number of RNA edits slightly increased compared to controls, while hAID and PmCDA1 had no RNA editing activity (Grünewald et al., 2019b). The use of other deaminases and their simultaneous engineering led to the generation of novel CBEs (backbone of the BE4 with either RrA3F^{F130L}, AmAPOBEC1, SsAPOBEC3B^{R54Q}, or PpAPOBEC1$^{H122A/R33A}$) with a high ratio of on-target to off-target activity (Yu et al., 2020).

In the case of ABEs, even though the RNA off-target activity was lower in comparison with CBEs, the insertion of point mutations in the TadA domain (E59A or E59Q) and in the engineered TadA* domain (V106W) led to the development of ABE variants (ABEmaxAW and ABEmaxQW) with greatly reduced RNA off-target activity and normal DNA on-target activity (Rees et al., 2019) (Gaudelli et al., 2020)(Richter et al., 2020). Other mutations, such as the F148A mutation in the TadA domain (ABE7.10^{F148A}), have also been proved to eliminate the RNA A>I activity of ABEs (Zhou et al., 2019). The removal of the wild-type TadA domain from the classical ABEmax gave rise to a smaller variant (miniABEmax). Its subsequent mutagenesis (in positively charged residues of the engineered TadA* domain that may interact with the phosphate backbone of a nucleic acid) generated miniABEmax$^{K20A/R21A}$ and miniABEmax^{V82G} showing lower off-target activity (Grünewald et al., 2019b).

Notably, some BEs can also modify their own transcripts, leading to a set of heterogeneous base editing proteins. This issue can be eclipsed by employing BE variants with less RNA off-target activity or by using RNPs as a delivery system (Grünewald et al., 2019b).

RNA-seq is commonly used to analyze RNA off-target effects. This analysis should be coupled to whole exome sequencing to exclude that RNA edits are not caused by the editing of the corresponding DNA regions. Alternatively, RNA off-target analysis can be performed by targeting sequencing of RT-PCR amplicons corresponding to commonly edited cellular mRNAs.

Promisingly, in most of the studies focused on the exploitation of BEs for the treatment of a blood disorder, the few detected DNA off-target effects had no predicted functional importance (Gehrke et al., 2018; Webber et al., 2019; Wang et al., 2020; Zeng et al., 2020; Zhang et al., 2020a). In parallel, RNA off-target effects were either undetectable (Webber et al., 2019), or very few (Zhang et al., 2020a), or possibly avoided by deaminase mutations that reduce the RNA editing (Zeng et al., 2020).

NOVEL EDITING SYSTEMS

Dual-Function BEs

The variety of base editing tools was further expanded in three different studies describing BEs that are able to perform A>G and C>T concurrent substitutions in the same target site (**Figure 4**). These enzymes [SPACE (Grünewald et al., 2020), Target-ACEmax, ACBEmax (Sakata et al., 2020), and A&C-BEmax (Zhang et al., 2020b)] show either increased or similar editing efficiency compared to the combination of separate ABE and CBE, while displaying similar or even reduced RNA-editing and sgRNA-dependent DNA off-target activity (Grünewald et al., 2020; Sakata et al., 2020; Zhang et al., 2020b). These dual-deaminase BEs expand the targeting spectrum of base editing, allowing more codon changes and TG>CA and CA>TG multi-nucleotide variant modifications, all in the context of a unique protospacer (Grünewald et al., 2020; Sakata et al., 2020; Zhang et al., 2020b).

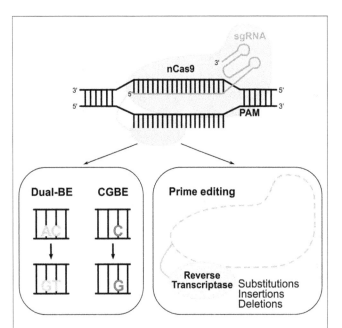

FIGURE 4 | Novel base and prime editors. Novel BEs with a modified deaminase, such as dual functioned BE and CGBE, convert AC-to-GT or CA-to-TG, and C-to-G, respectively. In the prime editing system, a reverse transcriptase uses a pegRNA to install substitutions, insertions, and deletions.

Interestingly, the A&C-BEmax allowed the installation of two different HPFH point mutations in the *HBG1/2* promoters in an adult erythroid progenitor cell lin. These mutations disrupt the BCL11A binding site and generate a DNA motif recognized by the GATA1 transcriptional activator (Zhang et al., 2020b).

C>G Base Editing

Out of the total pathogenic point mutations [ClinVar database (Rees and Liu, 2018)], 47% can be reverted by ABEs (A>G) and 14% by CBEs (C>T). The generation of a novel BE that performs C>G transversions (CGBE; **Figure 4**) increased the scope of base editing, allowing the correction of an additional 11% of the total pathogenic point mutations (Rees and Liu, 2018). The development of CGBE was based on: (1) the removal of the UGI from the BE4max architecture to enable the cytosine glycosylation and (2) the addition of an *E.coli*-derived uracil DNA glycosylase that allows C>G transversions (Kurt et al., 2020). CGBE efficiently induced C>G edits with good efficiencies and very few C>T and C>A byproducts. Furthermore, the insertion of the R33A amino acid substitution decreased the RNA off-target edits and the sgRNA-dependent DNA off-target effects. Finally, the targeting range of CGBE was further enlarged by using Cas9 variants with altered or relaxed PAM recognition specificities (Kurt et al., 2020). Overall, CGBE enables 14 different amino acid substitutions that cannot be generated by CBEs or ABEs, and allows the correction of additional disease-causing mutations in both coding and non-coding regions (Kurt et al., 2020).

Prime Editing

The diversity of base editing tools allows A>G, C>T, and C>G substitutions, with either regular, or more flexible to minimum PAM requirements. The prime editing (PE) system contains a prime editing extended guide RNA (pegRNA)-guided reverse transcriptase instead of a deaminase. The development of PE was a breakthrough as it requires no PAM sequence adjacent to the target site and it can accomplish not only all 12 types of point mutations, but also insertions (of up to 44 bp) and deletions (of up to 80 bp), or even combination of substitutions, insertions and deletions (**Figure 4**; Anzalone et al., 2019). Importantly, PE showed less DNA off-target activity compared to the CRISPR/Cas9 nuclease system. However, the modestly higher InDel frequency of prime editing compared to base editing should always be taken into consideration and further safety studies need to be performed. A proof-of-principle for the treatment of SCD by PE was provided in HEK293T cells by correcting the disease-causing A>T transversion mutation, which cannot be reverted by the current BEs (Anzalone et al., 2019).

CONCLUSIONS AND PERSPECTIVES

In conclusion, BEs exhibit plenty of advantages compared to classical approaches of genome editing based on designer nucleases. The low frequency of DSBs generated by BEs is undoubtedly one of the most significant advantages, placing base editing in the top spot amongst the different genome editing tools in terms of safety. Avoiding p53-mediated apoptosis that can result from DSBs formation allows the safe genetic manipulation of p53-sensitive cells, such as HSCs (Milyavsky et al., 2010), and therefore the safe treatment of genetic blood disorders. Moreover, the low frequency of DSB formation prevents the generation of large chromosomal rearrangements, thus maintaining DNA integrity. Importantly, the multiplex editing of two or more loci is feasible with base editing and has been proved very

promising in the case of blood disorders. Multiplex base editing led to greater therapeutic effects in β-thalassemic HSPCs edited to simultaneously correct a β-thalassemia-causing mutation and inactivate the *BCL11A* erythroid-specific enhancer. Concomitant editing of 3 loci involved in alloreactivity using BEs allowed the safe production of allogeneic CAR-T cells. In addition, while the CRISPR/Cas9 nuclease system is efficiently used for disrupting genomic regions by generating small InDels (e.g., to disrupt transcription factor binding sites), the base editing system can also be exploited to introduce precise point mutations that either revert disease-causing point mutations or generate *de novo* transcription factor binding sites. These types of modifications can be inserted into the genome through HDR-based strategies, though less efficiently and mainly in target cells that are dividing. Base editing overcomes this obstacle as it is efficacious even in quiescent cells, such as HSCs. Nevertheless, some barriers still exist for base editing, such as the DNA and RNA of-target activity. However, the DNA off-target activity of BEs can be eliminated by using high fidelity Cas enzymes. Similarly, the RNA off-target effects can be abolished by using engineered deaminase variants. Furthermore, the current pool of BEs enables A>G, C>T, and C>G conversions, thus more enzymes need to be created to generate all the different types of conversions, with PE being the current alternative solution to this issue. Last but not least, the delivery of BEs as mRNA or RNP in clinically-relevant cells needs to be further optimized to allow base editing therapeutic approaches to enter the clinical realm.

AUTHOR CONTRIBUTIONS

PA, AM, and MB wrote and edited the manuscript. All authors contributed to the article and approved the submitted version.

REFERENCES

Amaya-Uribe, L., Rojas, M., Azizi, G., Anaya, J.-M., and Gershwin, M. E. (2019). Primary immunodeficiency and autoimmunity: a comprehensive review. *J. Autoimmun.* 99, 52–72. doi: 10.1016/j.jaut.2019.01.011

Antony, J. S., Latifi, N., Haque, A. K. M. A., Lamsfus-Calle, A., Daniel-Moreno, A., Graeter, S., et al. (2018). Gene correction of HBB mutations in CD34+ hematopoietic stem cells using Cas9 mRNA and ssODN donors. *Mol. Cell. Pediatr.* 5:9. doi: 10.1186/s40348-018-0086-1

Anzalone, A. V., Randolph, P. B., Davis, J. R., Sousa, A. A., Koblan, L. W., Levy, J. M., et al. (2019). Search-and-replace genome editing without double-strand breaks or donor DNA. *Nature* 576, 149–157. doi: 10.1038/s41586-019-1711-4

Blattner, G., Cavazza, A., Thrasher, A. J., and Turchiano, G. (2020). Gene editing and genotoxicity: targeting the off-targets. *Front. Genome Ed.* 2:613252. doi: 10.3389/fgeed.2020.613252

Cappellini, M. D., Porter, J. B., Viprakasit, V., and Taher, A. T. (2018). A paradigm shift on beta-thalassaemia treatment: how will we manage this old disease with new therapies? *Blood Rev.* 32, 300–311. doi: 10.1016/j.blre.2018.02.001

Castagnoli, R., Delmonte, O. M., Calzoni, E., and Notarangelo, L. D. (2019). Hematopoietic stem cell transplantation in primary immunodeficiency diseases: current status and future perspectives. *Front. Pediatr.* 7:295. doi: 10.3389/fped.2019.00295

Cavazzana, M., Antoniani, C., and Miccio, A. (2017). Gene therapy for β-hemoglobinopathies. *Mol. Ther. J. Am. Soc. Gene Ther.* 25, 1142–1154. doi: 10.1016/j.ymthe.2017.03.024

Cavazzana, M., Bushman, F. D., Miccio, A., André-Schmutz, I., and Six, E. (2019). Gene therapy targeting haematopoietic stem cells for inherited diseases: progress and challenges. *Nat. Rev. Drug Discov.* 18, 447–462. doi: 10.1038/s41573-019-0020-9

Chatterjee, P., Jakimo, N., and Jacobson, J. M. (2018). Minimal PAM specificity of a highly similar SpCas9 ortholog. *Sci. Adv.* 4:eaau0766. doi: 10.1126/sciadv.aau0766

Chen, Y., Zhi, S., Liu, W., Wen, J., Hu, S., Cao, T., et al. (2020). Development of highly efficient dual-AAV split adenosine base editor for *in vivo* gene therapy. *Small Methods* 2020:2000309. doi: 10.1002/smtd.202000309

Cromer, M. K., Vaidyanathan, S., Ryan, D. E., Curry, B., Lucas, A. B., Camarena, J., et al. (2018). Global transcriptional response to CRISPR/Cas9-AAV6-based genome editing in CD34+ hematopoietic stem and progenitor cells. *Mol. Ther. J. Am. Soc. Gene Ther.* 26, 2431–2442. doi: 10.1016/j.ymthe.2018.06.002

Cullot, G., Boutin, J., Toutain, J., Prat, F., Pennamen, P., Rooryck, C., et al. (2019). CRISPR-Cas9 genome editing induces megabase-scale chromosomal truncations. *Nat. Commun.* 10:1136. doi: 10.1038/s41467-019-09006-2

Dever, D. P., Bak, R. O., Reinisch, A., Camarena, J., Washington, G., Nicolas, C. E., et al. (2016). CRISPR/Cas9 β-globin gene targeting in human haematopoietic stem cells. *Nature* 539, 384–389. doi: 10.1038/nature20134

Doman, J. L., Raguram, A., Newby, G. A., and Liu, D. R. (2020). Evaluation and minimization of Cas9-independent off-target DNA editing by cytosine base editors. *Nat. Biotechnol.* 38, 620–628. doi: 10.1038/s41587-020-0414-6

Forget, B. G. (1998). Molecular basis of hereditary persistence of fetal hemoglobin. *Ann. N. Y. Acad. Sci.* 850, 38–44. doi: 10.1111/j.1749-6632.1998.tb10460.x

Frangoul, H., Altshuler, D., Cappellini, M. D., Chen, Y.-S., Domm, J., Eustace, B. K., et al. (2020). CRISPR-Cas9 gene editing for sickle cell disease and β-thalassemia. *N. Engl. J. Med.* doi: 10.1056/NEJMoa2031054. [Epub ahead of print].

Gaudelli, N. M., Komor, A. C., Rees, H. A., Packer, M. S., Badran, A. H., Bryson, D. I., et al. (2017). Programmable base editing of A•T to G•C in genomic DNA without DNA cleavage. *Nature* 551, 464–471. doi: 10.1038/nature24644

Gaudelli, N. M., Lam, D. K., Rees, H. A., Solá-Esteves, N. M., Barrera, L. A., Born, D. A., et al. (2020). Directed evolution of adenine base editors with increased activity and therapeutic application. *Nat. Biotechnol.* 38, 892–900. doi: 10.1038/s41587-020-0491-6

Gehrke, J. M., Cervantes, O., Clement, M. K., Wu, Y., Zeng, J., Bauer, D. E., et al. (2018). An APOBEC3A-Cas9 base editor with minimized bystander and off-target activities. *Nat. Biotechnol.* 36, 977–982. doi: 10.1038/nbt.4199

Grünewald, J., Zhou, R., Garcia, S. P., Iyer, S., Lareau, C. A., Aryee, M. J., et al. (2019a). Transcriptome-wide off-target RNA editing induced by CRISPR-guided DNA base editors. *Nature* 569, 433–437. doi: 10.1038/s41586-019-1161-z

Grünewald, J., Zhou, R., Iyer, S., Lareau, C. A., Garcia, S. P., Aryee, M. J., et al. (2019b). CRISPR DNA base editors with reduced RNA off-target and self-editing activities. *Nat. Biotechnol.* 37, 1041–1048. doi: 10.1038/s41587-019-0236-6

Grünewald, J., Zhou, R., Lareau, C. A., Garcia, S. P., Iyer, S., Miller, B. R., et al. (2020). A dual-deaminase CRISPR base editor enables concurrent adenine and cytosine editing. *Nat. Biotechnol.* 38, 861–864. doi: 10.1038/s41587-020-0535-y

Haapaniemi, E., Botla, S., Persson, J., Schmierer, B., and Taipale, J. (2018). CRISPR-Cas9 genome editing induces a p53-mediated DNA damage response. *Nat. Med.* 24, 927–930. doi: 10.1038/s41591-018-0049-z

Hu, J. H., Miller, S. M., Geurts, M. H., Tang, W., Chen, L., Sun, N., et al. (2018). Evolved Cas9 variants with broad PAM compatibility and high DNA specificity. *Nature* 556, 57–63. doi: 10.1038/nature26155

Hu, Z., Wang, S., Zhang, C., Gao, N., Li, M., Wang, D., et al. (2020). A compact Cas9 ortholog from *Staphylococcus auricularis* (SauriCas9) expands the DNA targeting scope. *PLoS Biol.* 18:e3000686. doi: 10.1371/journal.pbio.3000686

Huang, T. P., Zhao, K. T., Miller, S. M., Gaudelli, N. M., Oakes, B. L., Fellmann, C., et al. (2019). Circularly permuted and PAM-modified Cas9 variants broaden the targeting scope of base editors. *Nat. Biotechnol.* 37, 626–631. doi: 10.1038/s41587-019-0134-y

Ihry, R. J., Worringer, K. A., Salick, M. R., Frias, E., Ho, D., Theriault, K., et al. (2018). p53 inhibits CRISPR-Cas9 engineering in human pluripotent stem cells. *Nat. Med.* 24, 939–946. doi: 10.1038/s41591-018-0050-6

Jeong, Y. K., Yu, J., and Bae, S. (2019). Construction of non-canonical PAM-targeting adenosine base editors by restriction enzyme-free DNA cloning using CRISPR-Cas9. *Sci. Rep.* 9:4939. doi: 10.1038/s41598-019-41356-1

Jiang, T., Henderson, J. M., Coote, K., Cheng, Y., Valley, H. C., Zhang, X.-O., et al. (2020). Chemical modifications of adenine base editor mRNA and guide RNA expand its application scope. *Nat. Commun.* 11:1979. doi: 10.1038/s41467-020-15892-8

Kato, G. J., Piel, F. B., Reid, C. D., Gaston, M. H., Ohene-Frempong, K., Krishnamurti, L., et al. (2018). Sickle cell disease. *Nat. Rev. Dis. Primer* 4:18010. doi: 10.1038/nrdp.2018.10

Kim, D., Lim, K., Kim, S.-T., Yoon, S.-H., Kim, K., Ryu, S.-M., et al. (2017). Genome-wide target specificities of CRISPR RNA-guided programmable deaminases. *Nat. Biotechnol.* 35, 475–480. doi: 10.1038/nbt.3852

Kim, D. W., and Cho, J.-Y. (2020). Recent advances in allogeneic CAR-T cells. *Biomolecules* 10:263. doi: 10.3390/biom10020263

Kim, H. S., Jeong, Y. K., Hur, J. K., Kim, J.-S., and Bae, S. (2019). Adenine base editors catalyze cytosine conversions in human cells. *Nat. Biotechnol.* 37, 1145–1148. doi: 10.1038/s41587-019-0254-4

Kim, K., Ryu, S.-M., Kim, S.-T., Baek, G., Kim, D., Lim, K., et al. (2017a). Highly efficient RNA-guided base editing in mouse embryos. *Nat. Biotechnol.* 35, 435–437. doi: 10.1038/nbt.3816

Kim, Y. B., Komor, A. C., Levy, J. M., Packer, M. S., Zhao, K. T., and Liu, D. R. (2017b). Increasing the genome-targeting scope and precision of base editing with engineered Cas9-cytidine deaminase fusions. *Nat. Biotechnol.* 35, 371–376. doi: 10.1038/nbt.3803

Kleinstiver, B. P., Sousa, A. A., Walton, R. T., Tak, Y. E., Hsu, J. Y., Clement, K., et al. (2019). Engineered CRISPR-Cas12a variants with increased activities and improved targeting ranges for gene, epigenetic and base editing. *Nat. Biotechnol.* 37, 276–282. doi: 10.1038/s41587-018-0011-0

Koblan, L. W., Doman, J. L., Wilson, C., Levy, J. M., Tay, T., Newby, G. A., et al. (2018). Improving cytidine and adenine base editors by expression optimization and ancestral reconstruction. *Nat. Biotechnol.* 36, 843–846. doi: 10.1038/nbt.4172

Komor, A. C., Kim, Y. B., Packer, M. S., Zuris, J. A., and Liu, D. R. (2016). Programmable editing of a target base in genomic DNA without double-stranded DNA cleavage. *Nature* 533, 420–424. doi: 10.1038/nature17946

Komor, A. C., Zhao, K. T., Packer, M. S., Gaudelli, N. M., Waterbury, A. L., Koblan, L. W., et al. (2017). Improved base excision repair inhibition and bacteriophage Mu Gam protein yields C:G-to-T:A base editors with higher efficiency and product purity. *Sci. Adv.* 3:eaao4774. doi: 10.1126/sciadv.aao4774

Kosicki, M., Tomberg, K., and Bradley, A. (2018). Repair of double-strand breaks induced by CRISPR/Cas9 leads to large deletions and complex rearrangements. *Nat. Biotechnol.* 36, 765–771. doi: 10.1038/nbt.4192

Kouranova, E., Forbes, K., Zhao, G., Warren, J., Bartels, A., Wu, Y., et al. (2016). CRISPRs for optimal targeting: delivery of CRISPR components as DNA, RNA, and protein into cultured cells and single-cell embryos. *Hum. Gene Ther.* 27, 464–475. doi: 10.1089/hum.2016.009

Kurt, I. C., Zhou, R., Iyer, S., Garcia, S. P., Miller, B. R., Langner, L. M., et al. (2020). CRISPR C-to-G base editors for inducing targeted DNA transversions in human cells. *Nat. Biotechnol.* 39, 41–46. doi: 10.1038/s41587-020-0609-x

Lapinaite, A., Knott, G. J., Palumbo, C. M., Lin-Shiao, E., Richter, M. F., Zhao, K. T., et al. (2020). DNA capture by a CRISPR-Cas9-guided adenine base editor. *Science* 369, 566–571. doi: 10.1126/science.abb1390

Lattanzi, A., Meneghini, V., Pavani, G., Amor, F., Ramadier, S., Felix, T., et al. (2019). Optimization of CRISPR/Cas9 delivery to human hematopoietic stem and progenitor Cells for therapeutic genomic rearrangements. *Mol. Ther. J. Am. Soc. Gene Ther.* 27, 137–150. doi: 10.1016/j.ymthe.2018.10.008

Lee, H. K., Smith, H. E., Liu, C., Willi, M., and Hennighausen, L. (2020). Cytosine base editor 4 but not adenine base editor generates off-target mutations in mouse embryos. *Commun. Biol.* 3:19. doi: 10.1038/s42003-019-0745-3

Lee, J. K., Jeong, E., Lee, J., Jung, M., Shin, E., Kim, Y.-H., et al. (2018). Directed evolution of CRISPR-Cas9 to increase its specificity. *Nat. Commun.* 9:3048. doi: 10.1038/s41467-018-05477-x

Leibowitz, M. L., Papathanasiou, S., Doerfler, P. A., Blaine, L. J., Yao, Y., Zhang, C.-Z., et al. (2020). Chromothripsis as an on-target consequence of CRISPR-Cas9 genome editing. *bioRxiv.* doi: 10.1101/2020.07.13.200998

Leonard, A., and Tisdale, J. F. (2018). Stem cell transplantation in sickle cell disease: therapeutic potential and challenges faced. *Expert Rev. Hematol.* 11, 547–565. doi: 10.1080/17474086.2018.1486703

Levy, J. M., Yeh, W.-H., Pendse, N., Davis, J. R., Hennessey, E., Butcher, R., et al. (2020). Cytosine and adenine base editing of the brain, liver, retina, heart and skeletal muscle of mice via adeno-associated viruses. *Nat. Biomed. Eng.* 4, 97–110. doi: 10.1038/s41551-019-0501-5

Li, C., Georgakopoulou, A., Gil, S., Lieber, A. (2020). *In Vivo* HSC gene therapy with base editors allows for efficient reactivation of fetal globin in beta-yac mice. *Blood.* 136, 22–22. doi: 10.1182/blood-2020-141492

Li, C., Psatha, N., Sova, P., Gil, S., Wang, H., Kim, J., et al. (2018a). Reactivation of γ-globin in adult β-YAC mice after *ex vivo* and *in vivo* hematopoietic stem cell genome editing. *Blood* 131, 2915–2928. doi: 10.1182/blood-2018-03-838540

Li, X., Wang, Y., Liu, Y., Yang, B., Wang, X., Wei, J., et al. (2018b). Base editing with a Cpf1-cytidine deaminase fusion. *Nat. Biotechnol.* 36, 324–327. doi: 10.1038/nbt.4102

Liang, P., Ding, C., Sun, H., Xie, X., Xu, Y., Zhang, X., et al. (2017). Correction of β-thalassemia mutant by base editor in human embryos. *Protein Cell* 8, 811–822. doi: 10.1007/s13238-017-0475-6

Liang, P., Xie, X., Zhi, S., Sun, H., Zhang, X., Chen, Y., et al. (2019). Genome-wide profiling of adenine base editor specificity by EndoV-seq. *Nat. Commun.* 10:67. doi: 10.1038/s41467-018-07988-z

Liu, Z., Chen, S., Shan, H., Jia, Y., Chen, M., Song, Y., et al. (2020). Efficient base editing with high precision in rabbits using YFE-BE4max. *Cell Death Dis.* 11:36. doi: 10.1038/s41419-020-2244-3

Liu, Z., Lu, Z., Yang, G., Huang, S., Li, G., Feng, S., et al. (2018). Efficient generation of mouse models of human diseases via ABE- and BE-mediated base editing. *Nat. Commun.* 9:2338. doi: 10.1038/s41467-018-04768-7

Liu, Z., Shan, H., Chen, S., Chen, M., Song, Y., Lai, L., et al. (2019). Efficient base editing with expanded targeting scope using an engineered Spy-mac Cas9 variant. *Cell Discov.* 5:58. doi: 10.1038/s41421-019-0128-4

Locatelli, F., Crotta, A., Ruggeri, A., Eapen, M., Wagner, J. E., Macmillan, M. L., et al. (2013). Analysis of risk factors influencing outcomes after cord blood transplantation in children with juvenile myelomonocytic leukemia: a EUROCORD, EBMT, EWOG-MDS, CIBMTR study. *Blood* 122, 2135–2141. doi: 10.1182/blood-2013-03-491589

Locatelli, F., Merli, P., and Strocchio, L. (2016). Transplantation for thalassemia major: alternative donors. *Curr. Opin. Hematol.* 23, 515–523. doi: 10.1097/MOH.0000000000000280

Magrin, E., Miccio, A., and Cavazzana, M. (2019). Lentiviral and genome-editing strategies for the treatment of β-hemoglobinopathies. *Blood* 134, 1203–1213. doi: 10.1182/blood.2019000949

Marktel, S., Scaramuzza, S., Cicalese, M. P., Giglio, F., Galimberti, S., Lidonnici, M. R., et al. (2019). Intrabone hematopoietic stem cell gene therapy for adult and pediatric patients affected by transfusion-dependent ß-thalassemia. *Nat. Med.* 25, 234–241. doi: 10.1038/s41591-018-0301-6

Mayuranathan, T., Yen, J. S., Newby, G. A., Yao, Y., Porter, S. N., Woodard, K. J., et al. (2020). *Adenosine Base Editing of Γ-Globin Promoters Induces Fetal Hemoglobin and Inhibit Erythroid Sickling.* ASH. Available online at: https://ash.confex.com/ash/2020/webprogram/Paper141498.html (accessed December 8, 2020).

Miccio, A., Cesari, R., Lotti, F., Rossi, C., Sanvito, F., Ponzoni, M., et al. (2008). *In vivo* selection of genetically modified erythroblastic progenitors leads to long-term correction of β-thalassemia. *Proc. Natl. Acad. Sci. U.S.A.* 105, 10547–10552. doi: 10.1073/pnas.0711666105

Miller, S. M., Wang, T., Randolph, P. B., Arbab, M., Shen, M. W., Huang, T. P., et al. (2020). Continuous evolution of SpCas9 variants compatible with non-G PAMs. *Nat. Biotechnol.* 38, 471–481. doi: 10.1038/s41587-020-0412-8

Milyavsky, M., Gan, O. I., Trottier, M., Komosa, M., Tabach, O., Notta, F., et al. (2010). A distinctive DNA damage response in human hematopoietic stem cells reveals an apoptosis-independent role for p53 in self-renewal. *Cell Stem Cell* 7, 186–197. doi: 10.1016/j.stem.2010.05.016

Mohamad, A. S., Hamzah, R., Selvaratnam, V., Yegapan, S., and Sathar, J. (2018). Human hemoglobin G-Makassar variant masquerading as sickle cell anemia. *Hematol. Rep.* 10:7210. doi: 10.4081/hr.2018.7210

Nishimasu, H., Shi, X., Ishiguro, S., Gao, L., Hirano, S., Okazaki, S., et al. (2018). Engineered CRISPR-Cas9 nuclease with expanded targeting space. *Science* 361, 1259–1262. doi: 10.1126/science.aas9129

Park, D.-S., Yoon, M., Kweon, J., Jang, A.-H., Kim, Y., and Choi, S.-C. (2017). Targeted base editing via RNA-guided cytidine deaminases in xenopus laevis embryos. *Mol. Cells* 40, 823–827. doi: 10.14348/molcells.2017.0262

Pattabhi, S., Lotti, S. N., Berger, M. P., Singh, S., Lux, C. T., Jacoby, K., et al. (2019). *In vivo* outcome of homology-directed repair at the HBB gene in HSC using alternative donor template delivery methods. *Mol. Ther. Nucleic Acids* 17, 277–288. doi: 10.1016/j.omtn.2019.05.025

Piel, F. B., Steinberg, M. H., and Rees, D. C. (2017). Sickle cell disease. *N. Engl. J. Med.* 376, 1561–1573. doi: 10.1056/NEJMra1510865

Qasim, W. (2019). Allogeneic CAR T cell therapies for leukemia. *Am. J. Hematol.* 94, S50–S54. doi: 10.1002/ajh.25399

Ran, F. A., Cong, L., Yan, W. X., Scott, D. A., Gootenberg, J. S., Kriz, A. J., et al. (2015). *In vivo* genome editing using *Staphylococcus aureus* Cas9. *Nature* 520, 186–191. doi: 10.1038/nature14299

Rees, H. A., Komor, A. C., Yeh, W.-H., Caetano-Lopes, J., Warman, M., Edge, A. S. B., et al. (2017). Improving the DNA specificity and applicability of base editing through protein engineering and protein delivery. *Nat. Commun.* 8:15790. doi: 10.1038/ncomms15790

Rees, H. A., and Liu, D. R. (2018). Base editing: precision chemistry on the genome and transcriptome of living cells. *Nat. Rev. Genet.* 19, 770–788. doi: 10.1038/s41576-018-0059-1

Rees, H. A., Wilson, C., Doman, J. L., and Liu, D. R. (2019). Analysis and minimization of cellular RNA editing by DNA adenine base editors. *Sci. Adv.* 5:eaax5717. doi: 10.1126/sciadv.aax5717

Richter, M. F., Zhao, K. T., Eton, E., Lapinaite, A., Newby, G. A., Thuronyi, B. W., et al. (2020). Phage-assisted evolution of an adenine base editor with improved Cas domain compatibility and activity. *Nat. Biotechnol.* 38, 883–891. doi: 10.1038/s41587-020-0453-z

Romero, Z., Lomova, A., Said, S., Miggelbrink, A., Kuo, C. Y., Campo-Fernandez, B., et al. (2019). Editing the sickle cell disease mutation in human hematopoietic stem cells: comparison of endonucleases and homologous donor templates. *Mol. Ther. J. Am. Soc. Gene Ther.* 27, 1389–1406. doi: 10.1016/j.ymthe.2019.05.014

Sakata, R. C., Ishiguro, S., Mori, H., Tanaka, M., Tatsuno, K., Ueda, H., et al. (2020). Base editors for simultaneous introduction of C-to-T and A-to-G mutations. *Nat. Biotechnol.* 38, 865–869. doi: 10.1038/s41587-020-0509-0

Schiroli, G., Conti, A., Ferrari, S., Della Volpe, L., Jacob, A., Albano, L., et al. (2019). Precise gene editing preserves hematopoietic stem cell function following transient p53-mediated DNA damage response. *Cell Stem Cell* 24, 551–565.e8. doi: 10.1016/j.stem.2019.02.019

Stadtmauer, E. A., Fraietta, J. A., Davis, M. M., Cohen, A. D., Weber, K. L., Lancaster, E., et al. (2020). CRISPR-engineered T cells in patients with refractory cancer. *Science* 367:eaba7365. doi: 10.1126/science.aba7365

Taher, A. T., Weatherall, D. J., and Cappellini, M. D. (2018). Thalassaemia. *Lancet* 391, 155–167. doi: 10.1016/S0140-6736(17)31822-6

Tan, J., Zhang, F., Karcher, D., and Bock, R. (2019). Engineering of high-precision base editors for site-specific single nucleotide replacement. *Nat. Commun.* 10:439. doi: 10.1038/s41467-018-08034-8

Thompson, A. A., Walters, M. C., Kwiatkowski, J., Rasko, J. E. J., Ribeil, J.-A., Hongeng, S., et al. (2018). Gene therapy in patients with transfusion-dependent β-thalassemia. *N. Engl. J. Med.* 378, 1479–1493. doi: 10.1056/NEJMoa1705342

Thuronyi, B. W., Koblan, L. W., Levy, J. M., Yeh, W.-H., Zheng, C., Newby, G. A., et al. (2019). Continuous evolution of base editors with expanded target compatibility and improved activity. *Nat. Biotechnol.* 37, 1070–1079. doi: 10.1038/s41587-019-0193-0

Traxler, E. A., Yao, Y., Wang, Y.-D., Woodard, K. J., Kurita, R., Nakamura, Y., et al. (2016). A genome-editing strategy to treat β-hemoglobinopathies that recapitulates a mutation associated with a benign genetic condition. *Nat. Med.* 22, 987–990. doi: 10.1038/nm.4170

Viprakasit, V., Wiriyasateinkul, A., Sattayasevana, B., Miles, K. L., and Laosombat, V. (2002). Hb G-makassar [β 6(A3)Glu→ Ala; codon 6 (G A G→ G C G)]: molecular characterization, clinical, and hematological effects. *Hemoglobin* 26, 245–253. doi: 10.1081/HEM-120015028

Walton, R. T., Christie, K. A., Whittaker, M. N., and Kleinstiver, B. P. (2020). Unconstrained genome targeting with near-PAMless engineered CRISPR-Cas9 variants. *Science* 368, 290–296. doi: 10.1126/science.aba8853

Wang, L., Li, L., Ma, Y., Hu, H., Li, Q., Yang, Y., et al. (2020). Reactivation of γ-globin expression through Cas9 or base editor to treat β-hemoglobinopathies. *Cell Res.* 30, 276–278. doi: 10.1038/s41422-019-0267-z

Wang, X., Li, J., Wang, Y., Yang, B., Wei, J., Wu, J., et al. (2018). Efficient base editing in methylated regions with a human APOBEC3A-Cas9 fusion. *Nat. Biotechnol.* 36, 946–949. doi: 10.1038/nbt.4198

Weatherall, D. J. (2001). Phenotype-genotype relationships in monogenic disease: lessons from the thalassaemias. *Nat. Rev. Genet.* 2, 245–255. doi: 10.1038/35066048

Webber, B. R., Lonetree, C.-L., Kluesner, M. G., Johnson, M. J., Pomeroy, E. J., Diers, M. D., et al. (2019). Highly efficient multiplex human T cell engineering without double-strand breaks using Cas9 base editors. *Nat. Commun.* 10:5222. doi: 10.1038/s41467-019-13007-6

Weber, L., Frati, G., Felix, T., Hardouin, G., Casini, A., Wollenschlaeger, C., et al. (2020). Editing a γ-globin repressor binding site restores fetal hemoglobin synthesis and corrects the sickle cell disease phenotype. *Sci. Adv.* 6:eaay9392. doi: 10.1126/sciadv.aay9392

Weber, L., Poletti, V., Magrin, E., Antoniani, C., Martin, S., Bayard, C., et al. (2018). An optimized lentiviral vector efficiently corrects the human sickle cell disease phenotype. *Mol. Ther. Methods Clin. Dev.* 10, 268–280. doi: 10.1016/j.omtm.2018.07.012

Winter, J., Luu, A., Gapinske, M., Manandhar, S., Shirguppe, S., Woods, W. S., et al. (2019). Targeted exon skipping with AAV-mediated split adenine base editors. *Cell Discov.* 5:41. doi: 10.1038/s41421-019-0109-7

Wu, Y., Zeng, J., Roscoe, B. P., Liu, P., Yao, Q., Lazzarotto, C. R., et al. (2019). Highly efficient therapeutic gene editing of human hematopoietic stem cells. *Nat. Med.* 25, 776–783. doi: 10.1038/s41591-019-0401-y

Xie, F., Ye, L., Chang, J. C., Beyer, A. I., Wang, J., Muench, M. O., et al. (2014). Seamless gene correction of β-thalassemia mutations in patient-specific iPSCs using CRISPR/Cas9 and piggyBac. *Genome Res.* 24, 1526–1533. doi: 10.1101/gr.173427.114

Yang, L., Zhang, X., Wang, L., Yin, S., Zhu, B., Xie, L., et al. (2018). Increasing targeting scope of adenosine base editors in mouse and rat embryos through fusion of TadA deaminase with Cas9 variants. *Protein Cell* 9, 814–819. doi: 10.1007/s13238-018-0568-x

Yeh, W.-H., Chiang, H., Rees, H. A., Edge, A. S. B., and Liu, D. R. (2018). *In vivo* base editing of post-mitotic sensory cells. *Nat. Commun.* 9, 2184. doi: 10.1038/s41467-018-04580-3

Yen, J. S., Newby, G. A., Mayuranathan, T., Porter, S. N., Yao, Y., Woodard, K. J., et al. (2020). *Base Editing Eliminates the Sickle Cell Mutation and Pathology in Hematopoietic Stem Cells Derived Erythroid Cells.* ASH. Available online at: https://ash.confex.com/ash/2020/webprogram/Paper139016.html (accessed December 8, 2020).

Yu, Y., Leete, T. C., Born, D. A., Young, L., Barrera, L. A., Lee, S.-J., et al. (2020). Cytosine base editors with minimized unguided DNA and RNA off-target events and high on-target activity. *Nat. Commun.* 11:2052. doi: 10.1038/s41467-020-15887-5

Zeng, J., Wu, Y., Ren, C., Bonanno, J., Shen, A. H., Shea, D., et al. (2020). Therapeutic base editing of human hematopoietic stem cells. *Nat. Med.* 26, 535–541. doi: 10.1038/s41591-020-0790-y

Zhang, J.-P., Li, X.-L., Li, G.-H., Chen, W., Arakaki, C., Botimer, G. D., et al. (2017). Efficient precise knockin with a double cut HDR donor after CRISPR/Cas9-mediated double-stranded DNA cleavage. *Genome Biol.* 18:35. doi: 10.1186/s13059-017-1164-8

Zhang, X., Chen, L., Zhu, B., Wang, L., Chen, C., Hong, M., et al. (2020a). Increasing the efficiency and targeting range of cytidine base editors through fusion of a single-stranded DNA-binding protein domain. *Nat. Cell Biol.* 22, 740–750. doi: 10.1038/s41556-020-0518-8

Zhang, X., Zhu, B., Chen, L., Xie, L., Yu, W., Wang, Y., et al. (2020b). Dual base editor catalyzes both cytosine and adenine base conversions in human cells. *Nat. Biotechnol.* 38, 856–860. doi: 10.1038/s41587-020-0527-y

Zhou, C., Sun, Y., Yan, R., Liu, Y., Zuo, E., Gu, C., et al. (2019). Off-target RNA mutation induced by DNA base editing and its elimination by mutagenesis. *Nature* 571, 275–278. doi: 10.1038/s41586-019-1314-0

Zuo, E., Sun, Y., Wei, W., Yuan, T., Ying, W., Sun, H., et al. (2019). Cytosine base editor generates substantial off-target single-nucleotide variants in mouse embryos. *Science* 364, 289–292. doi: 10.1126/science.aav9973

Zuo, E., Sun, Y., Yuan, T., He, B., Zhou, C., Ying, W., et al. (2020). A rationally engineered cytosine base editor retains high on-target activity while reducing both DNA and RNA off-target effects. *Nat. Methods* 17, 600–604. doi: 10.1038/s41592-020-0832-x

14

Normal Iron Homeostasis Requires the Transporter SLC48A1 for Efficient Heme-Iron Recycling in Mammals

William R. Simmons[1†], Lily Wain[1], Joseph Toker[1], Jaya Jagadeesh[1], Lisa J. Garrett[2], Rini H. Pek[3†], Iqbal Hamza[3] and David M. Bodine[1*]

[1] Hematopoiesis Section, Genetics and Molecular Biology Branch, National Human Genome Research Institute (NHGRI), Bethesda, MD, United States, [2] National Human Genome Research Institute (NHGRI) Embryonic Stem Cell and Transgenic Mouse Core Facility, Bethesda, MD, United States, [3] Department of Animal & Avian Sciences, University of Maryland, College Park, MD, United States

*Correspondence:
David M. Bodine
tedyaz@mail.nih.gov

†Present address:
William R. Simmons,
Human Genetics Program,
Department of Genetic Medicine, The
Johns Hopkins University School of
Medicine, Baltimore, MD,
United States
Rini H. Pek,
BioHealth Innovation Inc., Rockville,
MD, United States

In mammals over 65% of the total body iron is located within erythrocytes in the heme moieties of hemoglobin. Iron homeostasis requires iron absorbed from the diet by the gut as well as recycling of iron after the destruction of senescent erythrocytes. Senescent erythrocytes are engulfed by reticuloendothelial system macrophages where hemoglobin is broken down in the lysosomes, releasing heme for iron recovery in the cytoplasm. We recently showed that the SLC48A1 protein is responsible for transporting heme from the lysosome to the cytoplasm. CRISPR generated SLC48A1-deficient mice accumulate heme in their reticuloendothelial system macrophages as hemozoin crystals. Here we describe additional features of SLC48A1-deficient mice. We show that visible hemozoin first appears in the reticuloendothelial system macrophages of SLC48A1-deficient mice at 8 days of age, indicating the onset of erythrocyte recycling. Evaluation of normal and SLC48A1-deficient mice on iron-controlled diets show that SLC48A1-mediated iron recycling is equivalent to at least 10 parts per million of dietary iron. We propose that mutations in human SLC48A1 could contribute to idiopathic iron disorders.

Keywords: gene editing (CRISPR-Cas9), erythrocyte phagocytosis, erythropoiesis, mouse model, anemia

INTRODUCTION

Hemoglobin within erythrocytes of an average adult human male contain about 2.5 g of iron, representing about 65% of the total body iron. The continuous production of new erythrocytes requires iron, some of which is absorbed from the diet by the gut. Absorbed iron is then bound to transferrin, which enters the circulation from where it is imported into developing orthochromic erythroblasts (Andrews, 2008; Giger and Kalfa, 2015). As erythrocytes senesce, the majority of iron is recovered from hemoglobin by reticuloendothelial system (RES) macrophages. After engulfing senescent erythrocytes, RES macrophages digest the hemoglobin, releasing heme. In the cytoplasm, the enzyme heme oxygenase processes heme to remove the iron atom, which is exported from the cell by ferroportin and bound by transferrin for passage to the bone marrow to produce new erythrocytes (Kong et al., 2013). In erythroblasts, imported transferrin-bound iron is subsequently incorporated into heme by a series of enzymes associated with the mitochondrial membrane (Chung et al., 2012; Kong et al., 2013). From there heme rapidly associates with nascent alpha and beta globin chains which are assembled into a heterotetrameric hemoglobin molecule (2 alpha chains with their associated heme molecules and 2 beta chains with their associated heme molecules).

The levels of heme synthesis and nascent globin chain translation are carefully regulated to allow efficient production of hemoglobin while avoiding toxicity due to excess heme (Ponka et al., 1998; Chung et al., 2012; Chen, 2014). There are contrasting views about how heme synthesis and hemoglobin assembly are coordinated. The original view is that the heme synthesis pathway and hemoglobin translation are co-regulated to synthesize exactly as much heme as is needed for the amount of globin chains present (Chen, 2014; Ponka et al., 2017). Genetic support for this view comes from the fact that mutations in the genes encoding the heme synthesis pathway enzymes are well-known and are causally related to a wide variety of hematologic disorders (Fontenay et al., 2006; Peoc'h et al., 2019). Similarly, heme has been shown to regulate the translation of erythroid proteins including globin chain translation through the action of Heme-regulated eIF2α kinase (HRI) (Keerthivasan et al., 2011; Zhang et al., 2019).

An emerging view posits that developing red cells also express heme transporters to keep the levels of heme and globin chains balanced. Early erythroblasts maintain stoichiometric amounts of heme and globin by expressing heme exporters to prevent free heme from exceeding globin levels, while reticulocytes, which have extruded their mitochondria, import heme needed for hemoglobin synthesis (Keerthivasan et al., 2011). Support for this view come from the discovery of a heme exporter, FLVCR, which has been shown to be expressed at high levels at the CFU-E stage before declining during terminal erythroid maturation (Quigley et al., 2004; Keel et al., 2008). While variants in *FLVCR* have been proposed to play a role in a wide variety of disorders, no causal relationship between an *FLVCR* variant and a disease has been discovered (Quigley et al., 2005; Gnana-Prakasam et al., 2011; Nieuwenhuizen et al., 2013). However, in animal models, deficiency of FLVCR causes a lethal anemia due to heme toxicity (Keel et al., 2008). A heme importer, HRG1 (encoded by the mammalian gene *SLC48A1*), was originally discovered in *C. elegans* (Rajagopal et al., 2008; White et al., 2013). Subsequently, the heme transport function of orthologs of HRG1 has been demonstrated in yeast models and for mammalian SLC48A1, in tissue culture models. Recently we described a mouse model of *SLC48A1* deficiency. *SLC48A1*-deficient mice are unable to transport heme from RES phagolysosomes into the cytoplasm. *SLC48A1*-deficient animals avoid heme toxicity because the lysosomal heme crystalizes into hemozoin, a supposedly inert form of heme. Prior to this finding, hemozoin had only been observed in the food vacuoles or lysosomes of blood-feeding parasites such as *Plasmodium* (Pek et al., 2019).

In this report we present additional phenotypic characterization of the SLC48A1 deficient animals. These include a complete analysis of the highly efficient gene editing at the *Slc48a1* locus (15 mutations in 36 founder animals; 41%) and the range of gene-edited mutations recovered. We also demonstrate that hemozoin begins to accumulate in RES macrophages 8 days after birth, which we propose correlates with the beginning of erythrocyte recycling in the mouse. Finally, we show that SLC48A1-deficient mice require more dietary iron to maintain erythropoiesis than littermate control animals.

METHODS

Animals

All mice were housed in a 12 h light-dark cycle. Both male and female mice were used in all studies. No differences between the genders were observed. All animal protocols were approved by the NHGRI Animal Care and Use Committee and the Institutional Animal Care and Use Committee at the University of Maryland, College Park.

Generation of HRG1$^{-/-}$ Mice

Guide and Cas9 RNAs: Three guide RNAs (1 = 5′ TAGGG ACGGTGGTCTACCGACAACCGG 3′; 2 = 5′ CGGTGGTCT ACCGACAACCG 3′; 3 = 5′ AACCGGGGACTGCGGCGAT G 3′) were purchased from Sage Laboratories 2033 Westport Center Drive, St Louis, MO. Cas 9 RNA was purchased from Trilink Biotechnologies, San Diego, CA. The guide RNA and Cas9 RNA were combined at a concentration of 5 ng/μl (each) in 10 mM Tris, 0.25 mM EDTA (pH 7.5) for pronuclear injection. Pronuclear injection was performed using standard procedures (Behringer et al., 2014). Briefly, fertilized eggs were collected from superovulated C57BL/6J females ~9 h after mating to 129/SvJ male mice (resulting animals are B6129F$_1$). In a second set of experiments, fertilized eggs were collected from superovulated C57BL/6J females mated to C57BL/6N males (resulting animals are B6JB6NF$_1$). In these experiments, Guide 1 RNA and Cas9 protein were combined at a concentration of 5 ng/μl (Guide 1) and 10 ng/ μl (Cas9) in 10 mM Tris, 0.25 mM EDTA (pH 7.5) to form a ribonuclear protein complex. All pronuclei were injected with a capillary needle with a 1–2 μm opening pulled with a Sutter P-1000 micropipette puller. The RNAs or ribonuclear protein were injected using a FemtoJet 4i (Eppendorf) with continuous flow estimated to deposit ~2 pl of solution. Injected eggs were surgically transferred to pseudo-pregnant BALB/cByJ x C57BL/6ByJ (CB6F$_1$) recipient females.

DNA was obtained from founder (F$_0$) animals by tail biopsy, amplified by PCR (Forward 5′-TGCACCTGTGACTCGGCG-3′ Reverse 5′-TAGGTCCCGCCACGTTCATAA-3′ and sequenced to determine the genotype. F$_0$ animals carrying mutations were crossed to C57BL/6 animals and the resulting heterozygous F$_1$ animals were either intercrossed to generate homozygous mutant animals or back crossed to C57BL/6 mice for propagation.

Western Blot

Western Blots were performed as described previously (Pek et al., 2019). Spleen tissue was frozen in liquid nitrogen and ground using an ice cold mortar and pestle. The powdered spleen tissue was added to prep buffer (250 mM Sucrose, 1 mM EDTA, 10 mM Tris-HCl pH 7.4, 3X protease inhibitor cocktail) in a dounce homogenizer for further homogenization. Homogenates were centrifuged at 800 g for 10 min at 4°C, then at 100,000 g for 2 h at 4°C. The pellet was resuspended in lysis buffer (150 mM NaCl, 1 mM EDTA, 20 mM HEPES pH 7.4, 2% Triton-X, 3X protease inhibitor), sonicated and centrifuged at 11,000 g for 30 min at 4°C. The protein concentration of the supernatant was determined using the BCA assay (Pierce BCA Protein Assay Kit, Thermo Fisher Scientific, cat. Number 23225). Samples were mixed with SDS-loading buffer and separated on a 4–20% Criterion TGX Precast Midi Protein Gel (Bio-rad, cat. number 5671094). After transfer to a nitrocellulose membrane the proteins were cross-linked by UV treatment and stained with Ponceau S before incubation in blocking buffer (5% non-fat dry milk in 0.05% Tris-buffered saline-Tween 20) for 1 h at room temperature. Blots were then incubated overnight at 4°C in blocking buffer containing rabbit anti-SLC48A1 antibody (1:300 dilution). After three washes in 0.05% Tris-buffered saline-Tween 20, the blots were incubated 1 h with horseradish peroxidase (HRP)-conjugated goat anti-rabbit IgG secondary antibody (1:20000; Invitrogen cat. Number 31460) in blocking buffer. After the secondary antibody incubation, the membranes were washed five times with 0.05% Tris-buffered saline-Tween 20 and the signals visualized by using enhanced chemiluminescence (SuperSignal West Pico, Pierce) and detected using ChemiDoc Imaging Systems (Bio-Rad).

Diet Study

The iron-controlled diets were custom ordered from Envigo (Madison, WI) and contained 5, 10, or 20 ppm iron, as measured by ICP-MS. Three breeding units consisting of M13 heterozygous littermates provided the $Slc48a1^{+/+}$, $Slc48a1^{+/-}$ and $Slc48a1^{-/-}$ mice used in these studies. At least 31 from each breeding unit were used.

The parental cages were manitained on an iron replete diet (400 ppm) and the date of birth of the litters was recorded. At least 31 from each breeding unit were used. Tail biopsies were collected from the pups at 10 days of age (P10) for genotyping. At 15 days, when pups first begin to eat solid food, the food in the parental cages was switched to one of the three iron restricted diets (5, 10, or 20 ppm). On day 21, the pups were weaned into special cages containing the iron restricted diets and the 400 ppm diet was restored to the parental cages. Since mice derive ~25% of their nutrition from copography, the pups were placed in cages with wire bottoms to prevent feeding on feces. In addition, to prevent iron in the feces of wild type or heterozygors animals from rescuing SLC48A1 deficiency, the animals were segregated by genotype.

CBC Studies

Fifty microliters of peripheral blood was collected at weaning (P21) and every week thereafter until week 14 by retro-orbital bleeding and the complete blood counts were determined. Retro-orbitally blood was drawn into heparinized capillary tubes (Fisher Scientific). Immediately after blood collection, it was ejected into EDTA tubes (Beckton Dickenson). Complete blood counts were performed using the Element HT5 Veterinary Hematology Analyzer (Heska). Data were aggregated in Microsoft Excel and analyzed using R Studio.

Histology

Prenatal mice were harvested from timed C57BL/6 $SLC48a1^{+/-}$ intercross matings at days E12.5 to birth. Post-natal animals were euthanized at days P0–21. The fetal liver, fetal spleen, postnatal spleen, and bone marrow were harvested and fixed in formalin.

Paraffin-embedded tissue sections stained with hematoxylin and eosin by Histoserve (Rockville, MD).

RESULTS

Generation of Mutations at the *Slc48a1* Locus

Initially we evaluated three different guide RNAs, which were injected into $B6129F_1$ zygotes along with Cas9 protein. Guides 1 and 2 targeted overlapping regions of *Slc48a1* exon 1, while guide 3 targeted exon 2. At E14.5, embryos were analyzed for evidence of editing at the *Slc48a1* locus. Guide 1 generated 3/12 embryos with evidence of editing at the *Slc48a* locus, while Guide 2 generated 3/13 embryos with evidence of targeting. No animals with evidence of gene targeting were identified in the Guide 3 experiments.

The SLC48A1 protein has four predicted membrane-spanning domains. Guide 1 targets the *Slc48a1* locus in the region of the first transmembrane domain of SLC48A1 (**Figure 1**), which we hypothesized would be more likely to cause loss-of-function mutations. Therefore, we repeated the Guide 1 injections and obtained 7/15 F_0 (~47%) $B6129F_1$ animals with edits in the *Slc48a1* locus. To generate mice on a more uniform background we performed a second round of injections with Guide 1/Cas9 ribonucleoprotein into $B6BNF_1$ embryos. From a total of 21 F_0 mice, we identified eight $B6BNF_1$ F_0 animals (~37%). In all cases, F_0 animals were crossed to C57BL/6J mice for propagation. All analyses described were performed on animals backcrossed at least four generations to C57BL/6 before intercrossing.

Of the 15 mutations in the region targeted by Guide 1, we observed 13 deletions and two insertions. Five of the 15 gene edited sites were at or within 1 base of the PAM sequence. We observed two examples of different founder animals carrying identical mutations; a 7-base pair deletion (M1; B1) and an 18-base pair deletion (M3; B3).

Characterization of *Slc48a1* Deficient Mice

The 12 lines with insertions or deletions had frame shifts beginning at ~amino acid 30 depending on the location of the editing. These frame shifts led to premature termination, truncating the SLC48A1 protein between amino acids 50 and 125. Homozygous mutant animals of all of the deletion/insertion lines had similar hemozoin accumulation in their spleens, marrow and liver. As we have previously reported, mice homozygous for *Slc48a1* frame shift mutations were born in a Mendelian ratio. Western blotting of spleen and liver tissue from homozygous mutant mice of the M6, M4, B10, and B13 lines showed a complete lack of SLC48A1 protein (Pek et al., 2019) (**Supplementary Figure 1**). Similarly, Slc48a1 mRNA was absent from homozygous mutant mice of multiple lines (Pek et al., 2019). The M3, B3, and B11 lines, all of which had in-frame deletions, were cryopreserved, but not evaluated.

SLC48A1-deficient mice fed the standard laboratory rodent diet (~400 ppm iron) had peripheral blood counts that were all within the normal range, including the red cell indices shown in **Table 1**. No differences were observed between male and female animals. As described previously, we did observe an ~15%

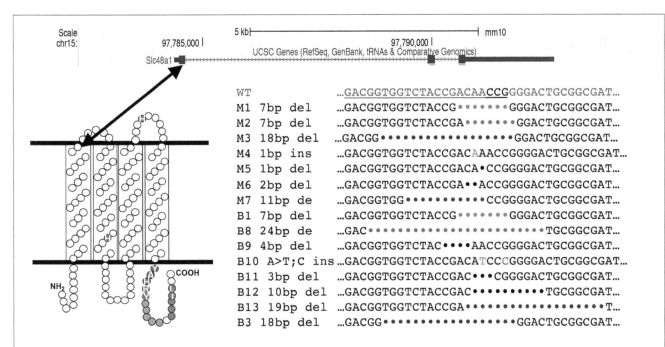

FIGURE 1 | CRISPR generated mutations in the mouse *Slc48a1* gene. The top panel shows the mouse *Slc48a1* locus. Large boxes indicate coding sequence (exons), smaller boxes transcribed, non-coding sequence. The lines between exons represent introns. The first exon encodes the first transmembrane domain (lower left). The sequence of CRISPR Guide RNA 1 is shown in blue text at the top of the bottom right panel. The sequence of the mutations in the 15 transgenic mouse founder lines are shown in black text.

TABLE 1 | Red cell indices of control and *Slc48a1* mutant mice.

Genotype	RBC (10^6)	Hemoglobin (g/dL)	HCT (%)	MCV (fL)	n F/M
+/+ C57BL/6	9.052 (0.42)	15.2 (0.50)	46.50 (1.91)	48.76 (1.45)	9
+/+ Littermate	10.186 (0.37)	15.54 (0.50)	44.22 (1.65)	43.48 (2.37)	5 3/2
+/Slc48a1 Littermate	10.763 (0.28)	16.26 (1.25)	45.91 (3.41)	44.60 (2.28)	8 4/4
Slc48a1/Slc48a1 Littermate	10.150 (0.63)	15.38 (0.98)	44.10 (2.80)	43.48 (1.84)	10 5/5

Mean and Standard Deviation (parentheses) for each value are shown. The number of animals analyzed and the sex distribution are shown in the right column. We did not observe any differences in males and females so the data are pooled.

increase in the size of the spleen in SLC48A1-deficient animals (Pek et al., 2019).

Accumulation of Hemozoin in SLC48A1-Deficient Mice

We have previously reported that the spleens, bone marrow, and livers of adult SLC48A1-deficient mice contained large amounts of black pigmented granules. Chemical extraction of this material followed by high resolution X-ray powder diffraction demonstrated that the dark pigment was identical to malarial hemozoin (Slater et al., 1991; Coronado et al., 2014; Pek et al., 2019). Immunohistochemistry, flow cytometry, and

electron microscopy showed that the hemozoin crystals were present in RES macrophages (Pek et al., 2019).

We hypothesized that heme concentrated in the lysosomes of RES macrophages would begin to crystalize as soon as the recycling of senescent red cells begins in in SLC48A1-deficient animals. To test this hypothesis, we examined the reticuloendothelial tissues of animals homozygous for the B13 mutation (19 base pair deletion; **Figure 1**) at different ages beginning prenatally and extending through birth (P0) to adulthood (>6 weeks). H and E staining of fetal liver and fetal spleen along with the spleen and bone marrow of newborn animals revealed no visible hemozoin, compared to the large amount of hemozoin visible in the spleens of adult animals (**Figure 2**). The first evidence of visible hemozoin was observed in the spleens of 8-day old animals (P8; **Figure 2** and higher magnifications in **Supplementary Figure 2**). The hemozoin crystals at P8 were infrequent, but were shown to contain iron by Perl's staining (**Supplementary Figure 2**). Beyond P8, the number of visible hemozoin crystals increased steadily (**Figure 2**). We conclude that the recycling of senescent red blood cells occurs by at least 8 days of age.

Deficiency of SLC48A1 Increases the Dietary Iron Requirement

We have previously shown that both wild type and SLC48A1-deficient mice become severely anemic when placed on a diet containing ~2 ppm iron (standard mouse diets contain ~400 ppm iron) (Pek et al., 2019). To determine more precisely the dietary iron requirements of wild type and SLC48A1 deficient mice, we analyzed the iron dependence of +/+, +/*Slc48a1⁻*, and *Slc48a1⁻*/*Slc48a1⁻* animals maintained on diets containing 20, 10, or 5 ppm iron. One of the three diets was introduced into the parental cage at P15, the time at which pups first eat solid food. At weaning (P21), the animals were segregated by genotype and were housed on wire grids to prevent recovery of iron by coprophagy. The animals' complete blood counts were monitored weekly beginning at weaning and extending over an 80-day period of observation. Animals of all three genotypes, +/+, +/*Slc48a1⁻*, and *Slc48a1⁻*/*Slc48a1⁻*, demonstrated the

typical mild anemia of the post-weaning period (http://www.informatics.jax.org/greenbook/frames/frame17.shtml). On the 20 ppm diet, the red cell indices of animals of all three genotypes increased to normal levels over the course of observation (**Figure 3** and **Supplementary Figure 3**). On the 10 ppm diet the red blood cell counts (RBC), hemoglobin (Hb; **Figure 3**) and hematocrit (**Supplementary Figure 3**) of animals of all three genotypes increased to normal levels, but the mean cell volume (MCV) of +/+ and +/*Slc48a1⁻* mice remained at the post-weaning levels and did not increase. On the 10 ppm diet the MCV of *Slc48a1⁻*/*Slc48a1⁻* mice decreased, indicating iron

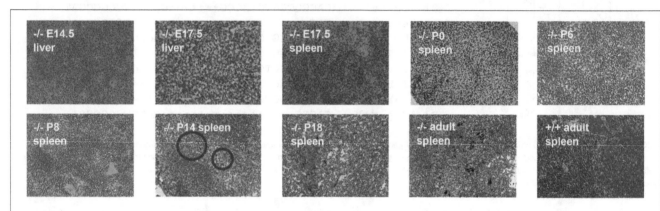

FIGURE 2 | Hemozoin accumulation in SLC48A1 deficient mice. Hematopoietic tissues were collected at the indicated times, fixed, sectioned and stained with Hematoxylin and Eosin. Hemozoin appears as a black pigment, first visible on postnatal day 8 (P8; orange arrow). No hemozoin is observed prior to P8, in prenatal tissues or in wild type adult (8 week) spleen. Magnification 20X.

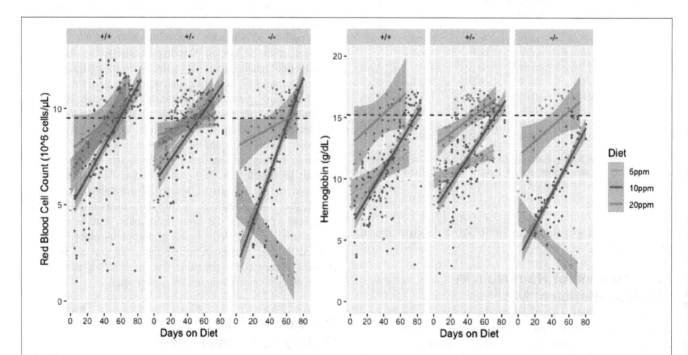

FIGURE 3 | Red Blood Cell Counts (RBC; left panel) and Hemoglobin levels (Hb; right panel) of mice on iron restricted diets. The RBC or Hb values are shown on the Y-axis and the days on the iron restricted diet is shown on the X-axis. Genotypes are shown at the top of the panels. Animals were sampled weekly and each dot represents one observation. Linear models of the y values and 95% confidence intervals are shown as lines or shaded areas, respectively. The green lines represent animals on the 20 ppm diet. Orange lines represent animals on the 10 ppm diet and blue lines represent animals on the 5 ppm diet. The dotted line is the mean value for adult C57BL/6 mice.

deficiency. We conclude that animals of all three genotypes become sensitive to dietary iron restriction at 10 ppm, and that the 10 ppm diet is not sufficient to sustain erythropoiesis in $Slc48a1^-/Slc48a1^-$ mice (**Supplementary Figure 3**). On the 5 ppm diet, the RBC of $+/+$ and $+/Slc48a1^-$ mice increased to normal levels (**Figure 3**), but $Slc48a1^-/Slc48a1^-$ mice became severely anemic. The low post-weaning Hb levels persisted throughout the course of observation in $+/+$ and $+/Slc48a1^-$ mice while the Hb levels of $Slc48a1^-/Slc48a1^-$ decreased (**Figure 3**). The MCV of $+/+$ and $+/Slc48a1^-$ mice on the 5 ppm diet decreased while the MCV of $Slc48a1^-/Slc48a1^-$ mice increased due to the severe anemia and reticulocytosis (**Supplementary Figure 3**). Finally, on a 5 ppm diet the hematocrits of $+/+$ and $+/Slc48a1^-$ mice stayed at the post-weaning levels and were severely decreased in $Slc48a1^-/Slc48a1^-$ mice. We conclude that the sequestering of heme as hemozoin in the RES macrophage phagolysomes In SLC48A1 deficient mice is responsible for the progressive anemia.

DISCUSSION

Prior to our discovery of hemozoin in SLC48A1-deficient RES macrophages, hemozoin had only been observed in the lysosomal-like organelles of blood-feeding organisms that digest hemoglobin such as malaria parasites of the genus *Plasmodium* (Francis et al., 1997; Egan, 2008; Pek et al., 2019). A search of the data available on the UCSC genome browser (https://genome.ucsc.edu/cgi-bin/hgGateway) revealed that *Plasmodium* sp. and other blood feeding parasites have no orthologs of *SLC48A1* to import heme from the lysosomes to the cytoplasm and hence would be expected to be sensitive to heme toxicity. Biochemically, the sequestering of heme in the form of non-toxic hemozoin allows the parasite to avoid heme toxicity (Schwarzer et al., 1993; Basilico et al., 2003). In cell-free systems, heme crystallization into hemozoin has been shown to be a pH and concentration-dependent reaction (Chong and Sullivan, 2003; Huy et al., 2006; Stiebler et al., 2010). In the acidic-environment of the lysosome, heme has been proposed to crystallize into hemozoin after a critical concentration has been reached (Chong and Sullivan, 2003; Stiebler et al., 2010). Our observation that hemozoin does not accumulate in the reticuloendothelial tissues of prenatal and early post-natal mice indicates the critical concentration of heme in the lysosomes of RES macrophages of SLC48A1 deficient mice is not attained until ~8 days of age (P8).

The number of erythrocytes in the post-natal mouse increases 15–20-fold in the first 28 days of life (http://www.informatics.jax.org/greenbook/frames/frame17.shtml), while the mass of the animal increases 10-fold. We propose that during the first 8 days of life, the iron needed to generate heme and hemoglobin comes mainly from maternal sources. Using the presence of hemozoin in SLC48A1-deficient mice as an indicator of erythrocyte recycling, we propose that significant erythrocyte recycling begins at approximately P8. This time-point is ~17 days after the first definitive erythrocytes enter the circulation

from the fetal liver (Craig and Russell, 1964). Since the life-span of adult mouse erythrocytes has been measured between 33 and 60 days (Horký et al., 1978; Beutler, 2005; Wang et al., 2010), 17 days is consistent with detectable erythrocyte recycling beginning at 1/3–1/2 of the life span of the earliest erythrocytes.

The inability to recycle heme caused by SLC48A1 deficiency predicts that SLC48A1-deficient neonatal and adolescent mice would become increasingly dependent on dietary iron. Our data indicate that a diet of 20 ppm iron is sufficient to maintain mouse erythropoiesis, even in the absence of iron from recycled erythrocytes in SLC48A1-deficient mice. On a 10 ppm iron diet, wildtype and $+/Slc48a1$ mice can supply the necessary iron for erythropoiesis, although they show signs of mild anemia. In SLC48A1-deficient mice on a 10 ppm iron diet we observed a progressive anemia that first becomes significant after 45 days on a low-iron diet. This would represent a full erythrocyte life span for those erythrocytes present at birth and the halfway point for erythrocytes present at 21 days when maternal dietary iron is no longer available (Horký et al., 1978; Beutler, 2005; Wang et al., 2010). We conclude that iron recovered from recycled red blood cells is equivalent to feeding ~10 ppm of dietary iron.

To date no genetic variants in the human *SLC48A1* gene have been associated with anemia or any other disease in humans. The SLC48A1-mediated transport of heme has been shown to be dependent on several highly conserved amino acids in the membrane-spanning domains (Yuan et al., 2012; Korolnek et al., 2014; Marciano et al., 2015). We predict that, particularly in areas of the world with iron-poor diets, idiopathic anemia may be caused by *SLC48A1* variants. In regions where dietary iron is not limiting, we predict that variants in the *SLC48A1* gene could lead to iron loading in RES macrophages, as has been described for Bantu siderosis or African Iron Overload (AIO) (Walker and Arvidsson, 1950, 1953; Bothwell, 1964; Gordeuk, 2002; Camaschella, 2015; Liu et al., 2016).

ETHICS STATEMENT

All animal protocols were approved by the NHGRI Animal Care and Use Committee and the Institutional Animal Care and Use Committee at the University of Maryland, College Park.

AUTHOR CONTRIBUTIONS

IH and DB designed the experiments and edited the manuscript. LG generated the mutant mice. JJ performed the initial genotyping. WS, LW, JT, and RP performed the experiments and wrote the manuscript. All authors contributed to the article and approved the submitted version.

ACKNOWLEDGMENTS

We thank Xuedi Zhang for help with the Western Blotting.

REFERENCES

Andrews, N. C. (2008). Forging a field: the golden age of iron biology. *Blood* 112, 219–230. doi: 10.1182/blood-2007-12-077388

Basilico, N., Tognazioli, C., Picot, S., Ravagnani, F., and Taramelli, D. (2003). Synergistic and antagonistic interactions between haemozoin and bacterial endotoxin on human and mouse macrophages. *Parassitologia* 45, 135–140.

Behringer, R., Gertsenstein, M., Nagy, K. V., and Nagy, A. (2014). *Manipluating the Mouse Embryo: A Laboratory Manual, Fourth Edition.* Cold Spring Harbor, NY: Cold Spring Harbor Laboratory Press.

Beutler, E. (2005). "Destruction of erythrocytes," in *Williams Hematology, 7th Edn,* eds M. A. Lichtman, E. Beutler, K. Kaushansky, T. J. Kipps, U. Seligsohn and J. T. Prchal (New York, NY: McGraw-Hill Book Co.), 405–410.

Bothwell, T. H. (1964). "Iron overload in the Bantu," in *Iron Metabolism,* ed F. Gross (Berlin; Heidelberg: Springer). doi: 10.1007/978-3-642-87152-8_20

Camaschella, C. (2015). Iron-deficiency anemia. *N. Engl. J. Med.* 372, 1832–1843. doi: 10.1056/NEJMra1401038

Chen, J.-J. (2014). Translational control by heme-regulated eIF2α kinase during erythropoiesis. *Curr. Opin. Hematol.* 21:172. doi: 10.1097/MOH.0000000000000030

Chong, C. R., and Sullivan, D. J. Jr. (2003). Inhibition of heme crystal growth by antimalarials and other compounds: implications for drug discovery. *Biochem. Pharmacol.* 66, 2201–2212. doi: 10.1016/j.bcp.2003.08.009

Chung, J., Chen, C., and Paw, B. H. (2012). Heme metabolism and erythropoiesis. *Curr. Opin. Hematol.* 19:156. doi: 10.1097/MOH.0b013e328351c48b

Coronado, L. M., Nadovich, C. T., and Spadafora, C. (2014). Malarial hemozoin: from target to tool. *Biochim. Biophys. Acta General Subj.* 1840, 2032–2041. doi: 10.1016/j.bbagen.2014.02.009

Craig, M. L., and Russell, E. S. (1964). A developmental change in hemoglobins correlated with an embryonic red cell population in the mouse. *Dev. Biol.* 10, 191–201. doi: 10.1016/0012-1606(64)90040-5

Egan, T. J. (2008). Haemozoin formation. *Mol. Biochem. Parasitol.* 157, 127–136. doi: 10.1016/j.molbiopara.2007.11.005

Fontenay, M., Cathelin, S., Amiot, M., Gyan, E., and Solary, E. (2006). Mitochondria in hematopoiesis and hematological diseases. *Oncogene* 25, 4757–4767. doi: 10.1038/sj.onc.1209606

Francis, S. E., Sullivan, D. J., and Goldberg, D. E. (1997). Hemoglobin metabolism in the malaria parasite *Plasmodium falciparum. Annu. Rev. Microbiol.* 51, 97–123. doi: 10.1146/annurev.micro.51.1.97

Giger, K. M., and Kalfa, T. A. (2015). Phylogenetic and ontogenetic view of erythroblastic islands. *BioMed. Res. Int.* 2015:873628. doi: 10.1155/2015/873628

Gnana-Prakasam, J. P., Reddy, S. K., Veeranan-Karmegam, R., Smith, S. B., Martin, P. M., and Ganapathy, V. (2011). Polarized distribution of heme transporters in retinal pigment epithelium and their regulation in the iron-overload disease hemochromatosis. *Invest. Ophthalmol. Vis. Sci.* 52, 9279–9286. doi: 10.1167/iovs.11-8264

Gordeuk, V. R. (2002). African iron overload. *Semin. Hematol.* 39, 263–269. doi: 10.1053/shem.2002.35636

Horký, J., Vácha, J., and Znojil, V. (1978). Comparison of life span of erythrocytes in some inbred strains of mouse using 14C-labelled glycine. *Physiol. Bohemoslov.* 27, 209–217.

Huy, N. T., Uyen, D. T., Sasai, M., Trang, D. T., Shiono, T., Harada, S., et al. (2006). A simple and rapid colorimetric method to measure hemozoin crystal growth *in vitro. Anal. Biochem.* 354, 305–307. doi: 10.1016/j.ab.2005.08.005

Keel, S. B., Doty, R. T., Yang, Z., Quigley, J. G., Chen, J., Knoblaugh, S., et al. (2008). A heme export protein is required for red blood cell differentiation and iron homeostasis. *Science* 319, 825–828. doi: 10.1126/science.1151133

Keerthivasan, G., Wickrema, A., and Crispino, J. D. (2011). Erythroblast enucleation. *Stem Cells Int.* 2011:139851. doi: 10.4061/2011/139851

Kong, W. N., Lei, Y. H., and Chang, Y. Z. (2013). The regulation of iron metabolism in the mononuclear phagocyte system. *Expert Rev. Hematol.* 6, 411–418. doi: 10.1586/17474086.2013.814840

Korolnek, T., Zhang, J., Beardsley, S., Scheffer, G. L., and Hamza, I. (2014). Control of metazoan heme homeostasis by a conserved multidrug resistance protein. *Cell Metab.* 19, 1008–1019. doi: 10.1016/j.cmet.2014.03.030

Liu, J., Pu, C., Lang, L., Qiao, L., Abdullahi, M. A., and Jiang, C. (2016). Molecular pathogenesis of hereditary hemochromatosis. *Histol. Histopathol.* 8, 833–840. doi: 10.14670/HH-11-762

Marciano, O., Moskovitz, Y., Hamza, I., and Ruthstein, S. (2015). Histidine residues are important for preserving the structure and heme binding to the *C. elegans* HRG-3 heme-trafficking protein. *J. Biol. Inorg. Chem.* 20, 1253–1261. doi: 10.1007/s00775-015-1304-0

Nieuwenhuizen, L., Schutgens, R. E., van Asbeck, B. S., Wenting, M. J., van Veghel, K., Roosendaal, G., et al. (2013). Identification and expression of iron regulators in human synovium: evidence for upregulation in haemophilic arthropathy compared to rheumatoid arthritis, osteoarthritis, and healthy controls. *Haemophilia* 19, e218–e227. doi: 10.1111/hae.12208

Pek, R. H., Yuan, X., Rietzschel, N., Zhang, J., Jackson, L., Nishibori, E., et al. (2019). Hemozoin produced by mammals confers heme tolerance. *elife* 8:e49503. doi: 10.7554/eLife.49503

Peoc'h, K., Nicolas, G., Schmitt, C., Mirmiran, A., Daher, R., Lefebvre, T., et al. (2019). Regulation and tissue-specific expression of δ-aminolevulinic acid synthases in non-syndromic sideroblastic anemias and porphyrias. *Mol. Genet. Metab.* 128, 190–197. doi: 10.1016/j.ymgme.2019.01.015

Ponka, P., Beaumont, C., and Richardson, D. R. (1998). Function and regulation of transferrin and ferritin. *Semin. Hematol.* 35, 35–54.

Ponka, P., Sheftel, A. D., English, A. M., Scott Bohle, D., and Garcia-Santos, D. (2017). Do mammalian cells really need to export and import heme? *Trends Biochem. Sci.* 42, 395–406. doi: 10.1016/j.tibs.2017.01.006

Quigley, J. G., Gazda, H., Yang, Z., Ball, S., Sieff, C. A., and Abkowitz, J. L. (2005). Investigation of a putative role for FLVCR, a cytoplasmic heme exporter, in Diamond-Blackfan anemia. *Blood Cells Mol. Dis.* 35, 189–192. doi: 10.1016/j.bcmd.2005.01.005

Quigley, J. G., Yang, Z., Worthington, M. T., Phillips, J. D., Sabo, K. M., Sabath, D. E., et al. (2004). Identification of a human heme exporter that is essential for erythropoiesis. *Cell* 118, 757–766. doi: 10.1016/j.cell.2004.08.014

Rajagopal, A., Rao, A. U., Amigo, J., Tian, M., Upadhyay, S. K., Hall, C., et al. (2008). Haem homeostasis is regulated by the conserved and concerted functions of HRG-1 proteins. *Nature* 453, 1127–1131. doi: 10.1038/nature06934

Schwarzer, E., Turrini, F., Giribaldi, G., Cappadoro, M., and Arese, P. (1993). Phagocytosis of P. falciparum malarial pigment hemozoin by human monocytes inactivates monocyte protein kinase C. *Biochim. Biophys. Acta* 118, 51–54. doi: 10.1016/0925-4439(93)90089-J

Slater, A. F., Swiggard, W. J., Orton, B. R., Flitter, W. D., Goldberg, D. E., Cerami, A., et al. (1991). An iron-carboxylate bond links the heme units of malaria pigment. *Proc. Natl. Acad. Sci. U.S.A.* 88, 325–329. doi: 10.1073/pnas.88.2.325

Stiebler, R., Hoang, A. N., Egan, T. J., Wright, D. W., and Oliveira, M. F. (2010). Increase on the initial soluble heme levels in acidic conditions is an important mechanism for spontaneous heme crystallization *in vitro*. *PLoS ONE* 5:e12694. doi: 10.1371/journal.pone.0012694

Walker, A. R., and Arvidsson, U. B. (1950). Iron intake and haemochromatosis in the Bantu. *Nature* 166, 438–439. doi: 10.1038/166438a0

Walker, A. R., and Arvidsson, U. B. (1953). Iron overload in the South African Bantu. *Trans. R. Soc. Trop. Med. Hyg.* 47, 536–548. doi: 10.1016/S0035-9203(53)80006-4

Wang, S., Dale, G. L., Song, P., Viollet, B., and Zou, M. H. (2010). AMPKalpha1 deletion shortens erythrocyte life span in mice: role of oxidative stress. *J. Biol. Chem.* 285, 19976–19985. doi: 10.1074/jbc.M110.102467

White, C., Yuan, X., Schmidt, P. J., Bresciani, E., Samuel, T. K., Campagna, D., et al. (2013). HRG1 is essential for heme transport from the phagolysosome of macrophages during erythrophagocytosis. *Cell Metab.* 17, 261–270. doi: 10.1016/j.cmet.2013.01.005

Yuan, X., Protchenko, O., Philpott, C. C., and Hamza, I. (2012). Topologically conserved residues direct heme transport in HRG-1-related proteins. *J. Biol. Chem.* 287, 4914–4924. doi: 10.1074/jbc.M111.326785

Zhang, S., Macias-Garcia, A., Ulirsch, J. C., Velazquez, J., Butty, V. L., Levine, S. S., et al. (2019). HRI coordinates translation necessary for protein homeostasis and mitochondrial function in erythropoiesis. *Elife* 8:e46976. doi: 10.7554/eLife.46976

15

Using Synthetically Engineered Guide RNAs to Enhance CRISPR Genome Editing Systems in Mammalian Cells

Daniel Allen[†], Michael Rosenberg[†] and Ayal Hendel[*]

Institute of Nanotechnology and Advanced Materials, The Mina and Everard Goodman Faculty of Life Sciences, Bar-Ilan University, Ramat-Gan, Israel

*Correspondence:
Ayal Hendel
ayal.hendel@biu.ac.il

[†] These authors have contributed equally to this work

CRISPR-Cas9 is quickly revolutionizing the way we approach gene therapy. CRISPR-Cas9 is a complexed, two-component system using a short guide RNA (gRNA) sequence to direct the Cas9 endonuclease to the target site. Modifying the gRNA independent of the Cas9 protein confers ease and flexibility to improve the CRISPR-Cas9 system as a genome-editing tool. gRNAs have been engineered to improve the CRISPR system's overall stability, specificity, safety, and versatility. gRNAs have been modified to increase their stability to guard against nuclease degradation, thereby enhancing their efficiency. Additionally, guide specificity has been improved by limiting off-target editing. Synthetic gRNA has been shown to ameliorate inflammatory signaling caused by the CRISPR system, thereby limiting immunogenicity and toxicity in edited mammalian cells. Furthermore, through conjugation with exogenous donor DNA, engineered gRNAs have been shown to improve homology-directed repair (HDR) efficiency by ensuring donor proximity to the edited site. Lastly, synthetic gRNAs attached to fluorescent labels have been developed to enable highly specific nuclear staining and imaging, enabling mechanistic studies of chromosomal dynamics and genomic mapping. Continued work on chemical modification and optimization of synthetic gRNAs will undoubtedly lead to clinical and therapeutic benefits and, ultimately, routinely performed CRISPR-based therapies.

Keywords: CRISPR-Cas9, engineered nuclease, gRNA, chemical modifications, genome editing, gene therapy, CRISPR therapeutics

INTRODUCTION

Up until the discovery of the Clustered Regularly Interspaced Short Palindromic Repeats (CRISPR) system, genome editing was limited in its capabilities. CRISPR is simpler and more versatile than other genome editing tools, such as zinc-finger nucleases (ZFNs) and Transcription-Activator-Like-Effector-Nucleases (Porteus and Carroll, 2005; Carroll, 2011, 2014). The CRISPR system components are modified from the prokaryotic adaptive immune system. Throughout evolution, bacteria and archaea acquired the ability to store copies of portions of invading foreign genetic material such as plasmids, phage genomes, or RNA, as segments between clustered repetitive sequences in the genome. These sequences are transcribed together into CRISPR RNAs (crRNAs), which are subsequently utilized to recognize and destroy the invading complementary DNA or RNA molecules by Cas nucleases (Horvath and Barrangou, 2010; Terns and Terns, 2011; Morange, 2015). The current nomenclature identifies two classes of the CRISPR-Cas systems, Class 1 and

2 (Makarova et al., 2020). Class 2 is distinguished by a multi-domain effector Cas nuclease and uses trans-activating CRISPR RNA (tracrRNA), in addition to crRNA, for target recognition and cleavage (Makarova et al., 2020). With three types in each class and more than a dozen subtypes, the CRISPR-Cas system represents a fruitful field for developing bioengineering tools.

Since it was first reported in 2013 that the CRISPR system could be repurposed into a reliable and straightforward genome editing technique in mammalian cells (Cong et al., 2013; Mali et al., 2013; Hsu et al., 2014), the CRISPR-Cas system has championed the field of gene editing. The most popular tool developed based on the CRISPR-Cas system is CRISPR-Cas9 (Jiang and Doudna, 2017), derived from *Streptococcus pyogenes*. Cas9 belongs to the Class 2 type II system and is a multi-domain endonuclease that requires both crRNA and tracRNA to introduce a double-strand break (DSB) at the target genomic site. After crRNA and tracrRNA anneal together to form a guide RNA (gRNA), they assemble a ribonucleoprotein (RNP) complex with a Cas9 molecule to direct site-specific DNA cleavage. The complex then scans the DNA for a complementary sequence to the 20 nucleotides on its $5'$ end, termed the guide region (spacer region), with an adjacent upstream protospacer adjacent motif (PAM) sequence ($5'$-NGG-$3'$ in *S. pyogenes*) (Jiang and Doudna, 2017). Once the PAM is recognized, the guide region of the gRNA undergoes seed nucleation to form an A-form-like helical RNA:DNA hybrid duplex. Only once the RNA and DNA complete R-loop formation, also known as the zipped conformation, and structural rearrangement of the nuclease domains commence, can the endonuclease cut the DNA creating a DSB (Jiang et al., 2015; Jiang and Doudna, 2017). One of the benefits of the two-component system is that the gRNA can be modified independently from the Cas nuclease, making the alteration of CRISPR as a genome-editing tool easy and flexible with almost unlimited target capability and high efficiency (Hsu et al., 2014; Moon et al., 2019). The guide can be adapted to the target by switching the 20 nucleotides with any sequence complementary to a desired target site in the genome (providing the genomic sequence is flanked by a PAM sequence). In addition to Cas9 (Type II), other members of the Class 2 system have also been exploited for targeted editing, including Cas12a (formally Cpf1), that belongs to Type V, and Cas13a (Type VI). In contrast to Cas9, Cas12a utilizes a single molecule gRNA with a $3'$ oriented spacer region and a $5'$ pseudoknot ($5'$ handle). Additionally, Cas12a nuclease cleavage produces cohesive double-strand breaks (DSBs) (compared to the predominantly blunt-end DSB created by Cas9) and relies on different PAM recognition sequences. Similar to Cas12a, Cas13a utilizes a single-molecule gRNA with a $3'$ oriented spacer region; however, in contrast to Cas12a, it targets complementary RNA sequences instead of DNA (Chylinski et al., 2014; Shmakov et al., 2017; Tang and Fu, 2018). Together, these CRISPR-Cas formulations confer a convenient technology for researchers to conduct sequence-specific editing of nucleic acids in a wide variety of cell types and experimental set-ups.

Due to CRISPR's wide-ranging applications, as well as its relative simplicity and highly flexible nature, it has been catapulted to the forefront of research in a remarkably vast number of organisms, from bacteria to humans (Wang et al., 2013; Guo and Li, 2015; Sid and Schusser, 2018; Xue et al., 2018; Yao et al., 2018; Ge et al., 2019; Munoz et al., 2019; Song et al., 2019; Soni, 2020). The CRISPR system can be utilized to knock-out genes by creating a DSB at the site of interest in the genome. Following the CRISPR-induced DSB, the endogenous cellular DNA repair mechanism, called non-homologous end joining (NHEJ), can repair the break, often resulting in small insertions or deletions (indels), which can lead to frameshift mutations, thereby inactivating the target gene (Yang et al., 2020). Hence, measuring the extent of indels on the site of interest, following CRISPR-mediated editing, is considered a gold standard for assessing the CRISPR activity in cultured cells and *in vivo*. Researchers also have used the CRISPR system to knock-in specific genes by taking advantage of the homology-directed repair (HDR) pathway (Yang et al., 2020), where the cell uses a template to repair the DSB. Naturally, the cell can use the sister chromatid or the homologous chromosome as a template for HDR; however, researchers have shown the ability to use an exogenous donor template to introduce genes into the CRISPR cut site (Porteus, 2016).

One of the main challenges facing researchers since the beginning of the CRISPR era is how to optimize the CRISPR system for translation to clinical therapies (Zhang, 2020). One promising direction in which CRISPR-based gene editing is currently being exploited is *ex vivo* gene therapy using cells of hematopoietic origin. In this procedure, hematopoietic stem and progenitor cells (HSPCs) or T lymphocytes are isolated from the patient's blood, undergo the desired gene correction *ex vivo*, and are then transfused back to the patient's bloodstream. Disorders that can be treated by this method include β-globin-associated diseases such as sickle-cell anemia and β-thalassemia (Dever et al., 2016; DeWitt et al., 2016; Park et al., 2019; Romero et al., 2019; Wu et al., 2019), as well as Severe Combined Immunodeficiency (SCID) (Pavel-Dinu et al., 2019), Polyendocrinopathy Enteropathy X-linked Syndrome (IPEX) (Goodwin et al., 2020), Wiskott-Aldrich Syndrome (Rai et al., 2020), X-linked chronic granulomatous disease (De Ravin et al., 2017), and Mucopolysaccharidosis Type 1 (Gomez-Ospina et al., 2019). Furthermore, T lymphocytes can be engineered using CRISPR to recognize and attack tumor cells (Gao et al., 2019; Stadtmauer et al., 2020). However, since the majority of genetic diseases and tumors occur in tissues that cannot be conveniently isolated and edited *ex vivo,* other therapeutic options must be explored. One such direction that is pursued using CRISPR-based genome editing is *in vivo* delivery of the editing complexes to the target tissues, with a focus on more accessible tissues such as the eye, liver, muscle, and cervix (Hirakawa et al., 2020). This could potentially lead to treatments for a number of diseases including cervical cancer (Zhen and Li, 2017), an inherited form of blindness Leber congenital amaurosis type 10 (LCA10) (Maeder et al., 2019), among others. Albeit, the application of the CRISPR-Cas9 system for clinical purposes still faces significant obstacles. First and foremost, safety is a critical parameter. The popular method for CRISPR-mediated gene editing in cultured cells involves transfection with plasmid DNA that expresses both gRNA and Cas9 protein under constitutive promoters (Ran et al., 2013). However, the plasmid system is problematic for use in clinical applications since plasmid DNA, as well as any foreign DNA, can trigger an innate intracellular immune response, especially in primary cells (Sun et al., 2013). Unregulated constitutive expression of integrated CRISPR-Cas9 can also destabilize the genome through persistent DSB generation. Therefore, for clinical purposes, the CRISPR-Cas9 system must possess a limited intracellular lifespan to allow for quick and efficient gene editing while minimizing off-target effects. To that end, clinically relevant CRISPR-Cas9 systems must be developed that would avoid triggering the innate immune response and increase specificity in primary cells. The current solution to these issues is to use formulations of gRNAs together with Cas9 mRNA or protein instead of plasmid DNA. Together, these drawbacks have garnered a tremendous concerted effort from researchers to modify the CRISPR-Cas9 system to improve its editing capabilities as well as its ability to be tolerated in human cells. Although equally as much work has been done to modify the Cas9 protein to improve on its characteristics, herein, we discuss the chemical modifications that have been used specifically on the gRNA to adapt this bacterial element to a more effective, accurate, and versatile genome-editing tool while concurrently attempting to improve safety in order to achieve therapeutic relevance.

PRODUCTION OF gRNAs

Like other types of RNA, gRNAs consist of ribonucleotides covalently bound together by phosphodiester bonds. To be able to complex with the Cas protein, gRNAs can come in one of two basic formulations: a two-part molecule or a single-guide molecule (sgRNA). In nature, gRNA is found as a two-part molecule consisting of crRNA (~36–42 nt), which contains the DNA-binding spacer sequence, and the tracrRNA (~67–89 nt) (Jinek et al., 2012). The crRNA sequence can be divided into a guide region and a repeat region, while the tracrRNA sequence consists of an anti-repeat region and three stem-loop (numbered 1–3) structures. The guide region forms the gRNA:DNA heteroduplex through Watson and Crick base pairing with the DNA target site, while the repeat region and the anti-repeat region form the repeat:anti-repeat duplex also through Watson and Crick base pairing (Jinek et al., 2012; Nishimasu et al., 2014) (**Figure 1A**). The second type of gRNA that can complex with Cas is a synthetic sgRNA (~100 nt) where the bridged portion between the crRNA and the tracrRNA is covalently linked by an artificial tetraloop (Jinek et al., 2012) (**Figure 1B**). The synthetic sgRNA system has been shown to achieve equivalent or higher efficiency compared to the two-part RNA system (Kelley et al., 2016; Shapiro et al., 2020).

There are a few conventional ways to produce gRNAs (Moon et al., 2019), including chemical synthesis using oligonucleotide synthesizers, *in vitro* transcription (IVT), and intracellular production via gRNA-expressing DNA vectors which hijack the host cell's transcription machinery. However, since primary cells are known to mount an innate immune response to the foreign DNA (Sun et al., 2013), as well as to the *in vitro*

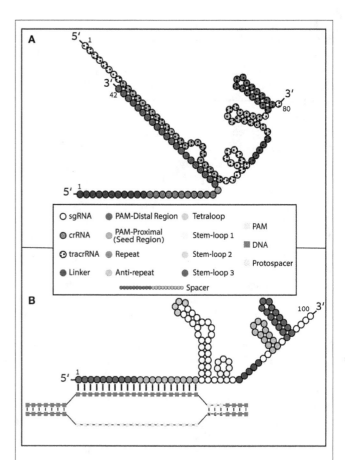

FIGURE 1 | Type II CRISPR formulations. gRNAs contain 4 loop structures: tetraloop (green), Stem-loop 1 (yellow), Stem-loop 2 (orange), and Stem-loop 3 (magenta). Stem-loop 2 and tetraloop do not interact with Cas9 as they protrude from the nuclease (Konermann et al., 2015). The spacer region of the guide undergoes Watson and Crick base pairing with the complimentary stand to the DNA protospacer. The spacer region (also known as guide region) is typically 20 nucleotides long but it has been shown that it can be shortened or lengthened (to include hairpin structures) at the 5′ end. The spacer region can be divided into two regions: the PAM-proximal (seed) region and the PAM-distal region. **(A)** Naturally occurring crRNA [~42 nt (striped nucleotides)] containing the DNA-binding spacer sequence and the trans-activating tracrRNA [80 nt (Rahdar et al., 2015) (checkered nucleotides)] annealed together through Watson and Crick base-pairing by the repeat (brown) and anti-repeat (gray) regions. **(B)** Synthetic sgRNA formulation where the crRNA and tracrRNA are covalently fused by a tetraloop. R-loop formation is depicted with Watson and Crick base pairing of the RNA:DNA heteroduplex.

transcribed gRNAs (as discussed below), chemical synthesis represents a cost-effective, expeditious alternative that produces highly purified gRNA at scalable quantities. Due to the short length of the gRNA, chemical synthesis allows for the swift and uncomplicated formational changes as well as the addition of different moieties. Recently, Taemaitree and colleagues presented a simplified method for producing sgRNAs via synthesis of the variable guide sequence (20 nt) and subsequently ligating the product to the remaining constant region (79 nt) by a triazole linkage (Taemaitree et al., 2019). Together, these advancements in the engineering of synthetically modified

TABLE 1 | gRNA modifications to improve CRISPR-Cas9 efficiency in cultured mammalian cells.

Modification(s)	Modification location	Effect on genome editing efficiency	References
M	Terminal residues	↑[#]	Hendel et al., 2015a; Rahdar et al., 2015
MS	Terminal residues	↑[#]	Hendel et al., 2015a; Basila et al., 2017; Finn et al., 2018
	Spacer (PAM-distal region)	↑[*]	Yin et al., 2017; Finn et al., 2018; Mir et al., 2018
	Spacer (tracrRNA-binding region)	↑[*]	Yin et al., 2017; Finn et al., 2018; Mir et al., 2018
	Spacer (Seed region)	↓	Yin et al., 2017; Mir et al., 2018
MSP	Terminal residues	↑[#]	Hendel et al., 2015a
cEt	Spacer (PAM-distal region)	↑	Rahdar et al., 2015
	Spacer (tracrRNA-binding region)	↑	Rahdar et al., 2015
	Spacer (Seed region)	↓	Rahdar et al., 2015
2′-F	Spacer (PAM-distal region)	↑	Rahdar et al., 2015
	Spacer (tracrRNA-gbinding region)	↑	Rahdar et al., 2015
	Spacer (Seed region)	↓	Rahdar et al., 2015; O'Reilly et al., 2019
2′-F + PS	Spacer (PAM-distal region)	↑	Yin et al., 2017; Mir et al., 2018
	Spacer (tracrRNA-binding region)	↑	Yin et al., 2017; Mir et al., 2018
	Spacer (Seed region)	↓	Yin et al., 2017; Mir et al., 2018
	Spacer (Seed region, Cas9-non-interacting residues)	↑[*]	Yin et al., 2017; Mir et al., 2018
PS	Whole crRNA	↑	Rahdar et al., 2015

[*]additionally validated in vivo.
[#]additionally validated in human primary cells.
2′-O-methyl (M or 2′-O-Me); 2′-O-methyl 3′phosphorothioate (MS); 2′-O-methyl-3′-thioPACE (MSP); S-constrained ethyl (cEt); 2′-fluoro (2′-F); and phosphorothioate (PS).

gRNA have enabled tremendous improvements in CRISPR-mediated genome editing's stability, specificity, and safety. These improvements have also expanded the applications of CRISPR-Cas9, such as techniques for enhanced HDR and improved genome imaging tools.

INCREASING CRISPR EFFICIENCY THROUGH STABILIZATION OF THE gRNA

In order to use CRISPR-Cas9 genome editing in a therapeutic setting, the first problem that needs to be addressed is gRNA stability. RNA is highly unstable compared to DNA and is extremely vulnerable to both endo- and exo-nucleases. The many years of progress in enhancing small RNA-based technologies, such as antisense RNA and RNA interference (RNAi) (Levin, 2019), includes improving RNA stability by incorporating chemical modifications onto the small RNAs (Braasch et al., 2003; Chiu and Rana, 2003; Behlke, 2008; Bennett and Swayze, 2010; Deleavey and Damha, 2012; Lennox and Behlke, 2020). Likewise, a pioneering study by Hendel et al. demonstrated that for optimal gRNA efficiency, the guide must be modified in a way

that protects it from degradation by RNA nucleases. This can be achieved by chemically modifying the gRNA ends to reduce degradation by exonucleases, thus improving the guide's stability (Hendel et al., 2015a). Modifications can be made both on the ribose ring as well as on the phosphodiester bond to reduce nuclease susceptibility. Research has also shown that the order in which the gRNA and Cas9 are delivered can change gRNA stability, as the Cas9 itself seems to confer the gRNA some level of protection from degradation when delivered as an RNP complex. However, the major contribution of Hendel et al. was proof that chemically modified gRNAs work efficiently in concert with Cas9 mRNA or protein in primary cells, which do not tolerate the introduction of plasmid DNA. The ability to chemically modify gRNAs opened the door for the development of more efficient and safer gene-editing methods that can be appropriate for clinical applications in primary cells. Nonetheless, caution should be exercised when introducing RNA modifications since further analysis found that over modification of the gRNA in the seed region, the ten nucleotides in the spacer region that recognize the target DNA closest to the PAM sequence, also known as the PAM-proximal portion, inhibits proper DNA:RNA hybridization and can significantly hinder efficiency (Rahdar et al., 2015; Basila et al., 2017; Yin et al., 2017). Another possible side effect of gRNA modification can be increased cytotoxicity, leading to cellular death, a major problem many researchers are actively seeking to solve (Basila et al., 2017). Several studies have shown that gRNA modifications in Type V CRISPRs (Cas12a), including 3′ terminal chemical modifications (Li et al., 2017; McMahon et al., 2018) and crRNA elongation (Bin Moon et al., 2018; Park et al., 2018), stabilize the complex and enhance editing efficiency. Additionally, in Cas12a, modifications in the seed region or on the 5′ handle were not well-tolerated (Safari et al., 2019). New formulations of Cas9-gRNA complexes with various RNA modifications are continually being developed to achieve the proper balance between benefits and side effects. Below we review the types of chemical modifications and their impact on various aspects of CRISPR-Cas9 applications *in vitro* and *in vivo* (**Table 1**).

Chemical Modifications on gRNA Termini

As mentioned above, a significant issue with gRNAs is their marked tendency to be degraded by exonucleases. Hendel et al. showed that sgRNAs with three different independent chemical modifications at both termini increased editing efficacy by protecting the exposed ends from degradation (Hendel et al., 2015a). Chemical modifications comprising of 2′-O-methyl (M or 2′-O-Me), 2′-O-methyl 3′phosphorothioate (MS), or 2′-O-methyl-3′-thioPACE (MSP) (**Figure 2**) were incorporated at three terminal nucleotides at both the 5′ and 3′ ends of individual sgRNAs. These modifications, specifically MS and MSP, substantially increased stability, resulting in a high level of indels at the on-target site compared to the indel frequencies obtained with the unmodified sgRNA. Moreover, with few exceptions, the increase in the on-target activity was accompanied by only a minor effect on off-target activity, thus achieving favorable on-target:off-target ratios. This was the first time it was shown that sgRNA chemical modifications enhance intracellular stability, thereby increasing genome editing efficacy when Cas9 and sgRNAs are co-delivered into human primary cells (Hendel et al., 2015a). A later study by Basila et al. systematically evaluated several combinations of MS end modifications in both the two-part system and sgRNA as well as two types of intracellular delivery mechanisms for the editing complexes: electroporation and cationic lipid transfection (Basila et al., 2017). The cationic lipid delivery technique previously suggested that liposomes protect gRNA molecules from RNase degradation in the cytosol or culture medium (Anderson et al., 2015; Liang et al., 2015). Basila et al. demonstrated that one MS modification at the 5′ and 3′ ends of the sgRNA molecule, or two MS modifications at the 5′ end of the crRNA and 3′ end of the tracrRNA were enough to improve editing efficiency when electroporated with Cas9 mRNA into K562 cells (Basila et al., 2017). However, when electroporated as an RNP complex, these modifications did not significantly increase editing efficiency. They also observed only a small increase in editing efficiency when gRNAs were delivered together with Cas9 mRNA into HeLa or U2OS cell lines, while the number and placement of modifications on gRNA termini showed a significant effect on cellular toxicity (Basila et al., 2017). Taken together, the mode of

intracellular delivery of gRNA-Cas9 complexes, whether gRNA is delivered with Cas9 mRNA or protein, and the number and positions of chemical modifications are all key factors that must be considered when planning CRISPR-Cas9 gene editing experiments. Recently, a thoroughly optimized protocol for using end-modified sgRNA in human primary HSPCs was evaluated, demonstrating high editing efficiency and specificity through the delivery of the CRISPR system as an RNP complex (Shapiro et al., 2020, 2021). This method can potentially be adapted for therapeutic purposes in other hematopoietic cells such as T and B lymphocytes, and Natural Killer (NK) cells.

Extensive and Complete Chemical Modification of gRNA Backbone

Adding modifications only on the 3′ and 5′ ends of gRNAs would protect the gRNA from exonucleolytic but not endonucleolytic activity inside the cells, which also may impair the editing efficiency by reducing gRNA stability. To address this, a study by Rahdar et al. focused on modifying the crRNA while expressing tracrRNA and Cas9 separately from plasmid DNA in HEK293T cells (Rahdar et al., 2015). They demonstrated that using a phosphorothioate (PS) (**Figure 2**) modified backbone in tandem with 2′-O-Me modifications on the terminal five nucleotides on both ends of the crRNA enhanced the editing activity, presumably by diminishing crRNA susceptibility to nucleolytic cleavage. In addition, adding modifications known to increase RNA affinity to DNA, such as 2′-fluoro (2′-F) and S-constrained ethyl (cEt) (**Figure 2**), on the crRNA inside of the PAM-distal and tracrRNA-binding regions, respectively, further increased editing activity. On the contrary, any modifications on the 2′ carbon in the ribose ring were not tolerated in the PAM-proximal (seed) region, presumably since the seed region is critical for target DNA recognition by Cas9 (Jiang et al., 2015). Lastly, they noted that it is possible to shorten the crRNA down to 29 nucleotides and still maintain its efficiency (Rahdar et al., 2015). However, in this study, the tracrRNA remained unmodified, and the potential of using these chemical modifications *in vivo* was not explored. To address this, Finn et al. examined the impact of sgRNA modifications on genome editing efficiency in mouse and rat liver *in vivo* (Finn et al., 2018). They designed lipid nanoparticles containing Cas9 mRNA and sgRNA and discovered that 2′-O-Me and PS chemical modifications on both termini of sgRNA [similar to the MS used by Hendel et al. (2015a)], as well as on the internal residues in the crRNA and tracrRNA regions, resulted in more efficient *in vivo* genome editing compared to the unmodified sgRNA or sgRNA with only terminal modifications (Finn et al., 2018). Yin et al. also performed an extensive study of gRNA modifications in *in vivo* gene editing in mouse livers using lipid nanoparticles (Yin et al., 2017); however, they used the crystal structure of the CRISPR-Cas9 RNP complex to guide the optimization of combinations of sgRNA modifications. Previous work has shown that there are ~20 positions of nucleotides in both crRNA and tracrRNA that interact with the Cas9 protein via the 2′-OH group, and thus do not tolerate any 2′-OH modifications. To show the significance of maintaining these

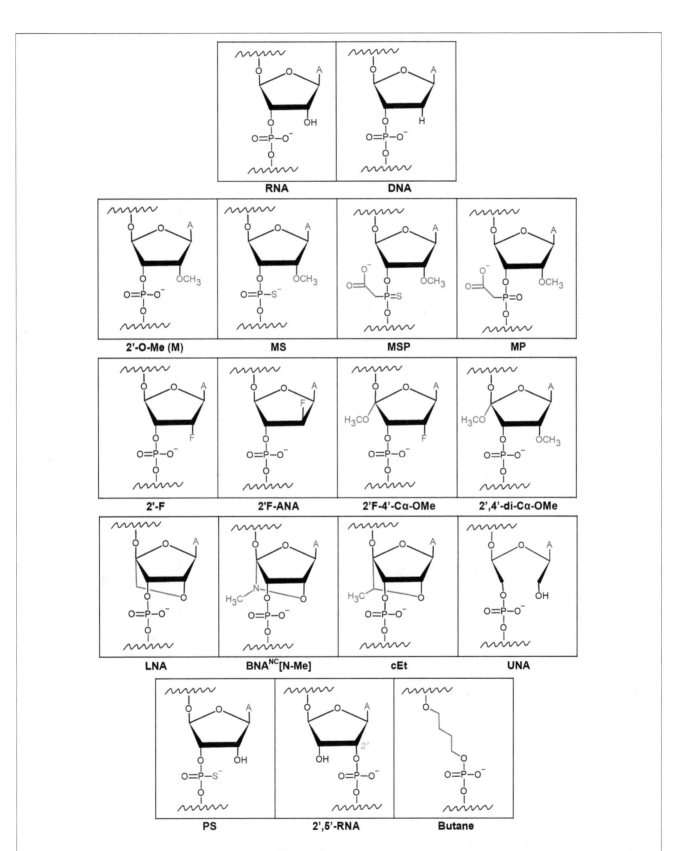

FIGURE 2 | Chemical modifications on the ribose rings and phosphate backbone of gRNAs. Ribose modifications are typically placed at the 2′OH as it is readily available for manipulation. Simple modifications at the 2′OH include 2′-O-Me, 2′-F, and 2′F-ANA. More extensive ribose modifications such as 2′F-4′-Cα-OMe and

(Continued)

FIGURE 2 | 2′,4′-di-Cα-OMe combine modification at both the 2′ and 4′ carbons. Phosphodiester modifications include sulfide-based Phosphorothioate (PS) or acetate-based phosphonoacetate alterations. Combinations of the ribose and phosphodiester modifications have given way to formulations such as 2′-O-methyl 3′phosphorothioate (MS), or 2′-O-methyl-3′-thioPACE (MSP), and 2′-O-methyl-3′-phosphonoacetate (MP) RNAs. Locked and unlocked nucleotides such as locked nucleic acid (LNA), bridged nucleic acids (BNA), S-constrained ethyl (cEt), and unlocked nucleic acid (UNA) are examples of sterically hindered nucleotide modifications. Modifications to make a phosphodiester bond between the 2′ and 5′ carbons (2′,5′-RNA) of adjacent RNAs as well as a butane 4-carbon chain link between adjacent RNAs have been described. 'A' symbolizes the nitrogen base of the RNA.

gRNA-Cas9 interactions, Yin et al. highlighted the complete abolishment of genome-editing capability when all 2′-OH sites were modified. By avoiding those 2′-OH sites, a sgRNA was designed with a pattern of PS, 2′-F, and 2′-O-Me modifications on the remaining non-Cas9-interacting nucleotides that maximized the editing efficiency both in HEK293 cells and in live animals. This underscored the importance of avoiding modifications on the endonuclease-interacting 2′-OH groups, maintaining the sgRNA-Cas9 hydrogen bonding, and modifying the other nucleotides to increase editing efficiency (Yin et al., 2017). Similar work was performed by Mir et al. where the modification pattern relied on the CRISPR-Cas9 complex crystal structure (Mir et al., 2018). Based on prior work in the field of RNA therapeutics, Mir et al. hypothesized that maximal 2′-modified ribose rings and modified backbone phosphate groups inside the crRNA and tracrRNA should generate the required gRNA formulation for clinical studies; albeit, all of the work in the study was conducted on HEK293 cells, without *in vivo* validation. They were able to obtain complete gRNA modification by combining the PS, 2′-F, and 2′-O-Me modifications which resulted in decreased Cas9 activity and as well as overall efficiency. Interestingly, they showed that the combination of heavily modified tracrRNA with completely modified crRNA exhibited satisfactory editing activity (Mir et al., 2018). An additional study by O'Reilly et al. utilized a broader variety of chemical modifications and linkers to test the compatibility and structure-activity relationships of engineered gRNAs with Cas9-mediated editing activity to try and lay out the foundation for a rational design of modified gRNAs (O'Reilly et al., 2019). The study focused solely on modifying crRNA while being mindful of the impact on the RNA's helix conformation. Modifications included: 2′F, 2′F-ANA, 2′,5′-RNA, 2′F-4′-Cα-OMe, 2′,4′-di-Cα-OMe, unlocked nucleic acids (UNA), locked nucleic acids (LNA), and butane linkers (**Figure 2**). The analysis of the relationship between these extensive modifications, the resulting structure of the RNA and RNP complex, and the subsequent intrinsic complex activity *in vitro* emphasized the necessity for maintaining an A-form-like helical structure of the crRNA in both the guide and the repeat regions. They also concluded that the guide region of crRNA, and especially the seed region, favor modifications that closely resemble the native RNA nucleotides, such as 2′-F, while more bulky modifications were less tolerable. Nevertheless, there was a clear discrepancy between the Cas9 activity in *in vitro* activity assays vs. in cultured cells after 2′-OH modification. Contrary to the *in vitro* activity assays, in cultured cells, any hydrogen-bond-disrupting modifications on the Cas9-interacting nucleotides reduced editing activity (O'Reilly et al., 2019). This highlighted the necessity for proper hydrogen bonding for Cas9-gRNA complexes in cultured cells. Therefore, when translating these discoveries to the clinic, the

relevant modifications must be validated in primary cells and animal models.

INCREASING CRISPR SPECIFICITY BY LIMITING OFF-TARGET EDITING

It is important to remember that CRISPR-Cas endonucleases did not naturally evolve to function as a highly specific gene-editing tool to edit mammalian genomes. In some cases, these bacterial nucleases have demonstrated significant off-target activity, leading to unintended DNA breaks at ectopic sites in the genome with only partial complementarity to the gRNA sequence (Li et al., 2019). While mutations or mismatches within the PAM sequence ostensibly abrogate Cas9 endonuclease activity (O'Geen et al., 2015a; Jiang and Doudna, 2017), mismatches within the guide region may be permitted (O'Geen et al., 2015b) resulting in the undesired cleavage of off-target DNA sequences. This creates a potential major pitfall for CRISPR-based therapies due to the well-understood correlation between increased DSBs to increased cellular toxicity and elevated immune response (Obe et al., 1992; Lips and Kaina, 2001; Nakad and Schumacher, 2016; Bednarski and Sleckman, 2019). Therefore, quantifying (Hendel et al., 2014, 2015b) and improving the accuracy, precision, and specificity of these nucleases (Tsai and Joung, 2016) is of major significance. Indeed, more accurate genome editing has been achieved via Cas9 nuclease modification itself (Kleinstiver et al., 2016; Slaymaker et al., 2016; Chen et al., 2017; Vakulskas et al., 2018). Additionally, Cas12a has been shown to be more specific than Cas9 at certain genomic sites (Kim et al., 2016) and may be more useful in particular settings. However, the orthogonal approach attempts to elevate CRISPR-Cas9 genome editing precision via chemical modifications on the gRNA, as discussed below (**Table 2**).

Chemical Modifications on Internal gRNA Residues

The aforementioned work by Yin et al. revealed that although PS, 2′-F, and 2′-O-Me modifications are tolerated in all of the non-Cas9 interacting nucleotides to improve gRNA stability, the extent of off-target editing between unmodified and modified sgRNA was comparable in both cultured cell lines and mice liver cells (Yin et al., 2017). Two independent studies systematically assessed the effect of modifying internal gRNA residues on Cas9 cleavage specificity. Ryan et al. sought to increase Cas9 cleavage specificity by altering the thermodynamic and kinetic properties of the gRNA-DNA heteroduplex formation, such as melting temperature (Ryan et al., 2018). They aimed to preserve sufficient duplex stability and relatively low dissociation

TABLE 2 | gRNA modifications to improve CRISPR-Cas9 specificity in cultured mammalian cells.

Modification(s)	Modification location	Effect on genome editing specificity	References
Deoxyribonucleotide substitution	crRNA 3′	↑	Kartje et al., 2018
	Spacer (PAM-distal region)	↑	Yin et al., 2018
MP	Spacer (positions 5 and 11)	↑[#]	Ryan et al., 2018
LNA	Spacer (positions 10-14)	↑	Cromwell et al., 2018
BNA^{NC}	Spacer (positions 10-14)	↑	Cromwell et al., 2018
tru-gRNA	5′ end of the spacer	↑	Fu et al., 2014
ggXX$_{20}$ gRNA	5′ end of the spacer	↑	Cho et al., 2014

[#]additionally validated in human primary cells.
2′-O-methyl-3′-phosphonoacetate (MP); locked nucleic acids (LNA); N-methyl substituted BNAs (2′,4′-BNA^{NC}[N-Me]); truncated gRNA (tru-gRNA); and two added guanine residues on the 5′ end of the spacer sequence (ggXX$_{20}$ gRNA).

rate on the fully complementary on-target genomic site while simultaneously decreasing the duplex stability and increasing the dissociation rate on the off-target sites with only partial gRNA complementarity. They first examined the on- and off-target editing by testing gRNA modifications 2′-O-Me, 2′-O-methyl-3′-phosphonoacetate (MP), MS, and MSP (**Figure 2**) in *in vitro* cleavage assays and then continued to assess the editing by NHEJ in cultured K562 cells, primary CD34^{+} HSPCs, and induced pluripotent stem cells. It was shown that MP modifications, incorporated at select sites in the ribose phosphate backbone of gRNAs (positions 5 and 11), along with modifications which protect the terminal positions (Hendel et al., 2015a), can reduce off-target cleavage activities while maintaining on-target cleavage editing (Ryan et al., 2018). Additionally, it has been shown that adding two types of bridged nucleic acids (BNAs), N-methyl substituted BNAs (2′,4′-BNA^{NC}[N-Me]) and, to a lesser extent, locked nucleic acids (LNAs) (**Figure 2**), within the central portion of the guide region (positions 10–14) of crRNAs, considerably increases mismatch discrimination in the PAM-proximal and PAM-distal regions (Cromwell et al., 2018). Cromwell et al. conducted an extensive, high-throughput analysis of Cas9 cleavage specificity both *in vitro* and in cultured cells, combined with mechanistic studies to identify the precise stage during the Cas9-cleavage reaction that was affected by the BNA^{NC} and LNA substitutions (Cromwell et al., 2018). LNAs are conformationally restricted RNA nucleotides in which the 2′ oxygen on the ribose forms a covalent bond with the 4′ carbon (You et al., 2006). LNAs display improved base stacking and thermal stability compared to unmodified RNA, resulting in highly efficient binding to complementary nucleic acids and improved mismatch discrimination (You et al., 2006). BNA^{NC}s are molecules with a six-membered bridged structure where the 2′ oxygen and the 4′ carbon are linked by a methyl-bound nitrogen. Even more effective than LNAs, BNA^{NC}s can provide additional conformational flexibility for nucleic acid binding and greater nuclease resistance. In addition, BNA^{NC} nucleotides have been shown to be less toxic than LNA nucleotides when delivered to cultured cells (Manning et al., 2017). Both BNAs mentioned above improve specificity by inducing a more dynamic RNA-DNA duplex, thereby reducing the time the nuclease spends in the zipped conformation where cleavage is activated. The shorter

interaction time in this conformation resulted in slower cleavage kinetics on the on-target sites but resulted in lowered Cas9-induced off-target DNA cleavage by several orders of magnitude (Cromwell et al., 2018), which on an overall scale was beneficial for the specificity of the genome editing.

RNA Secondary Structures and Modified Spacer Length

There are at least five stages in the gRNA-mediated Cas9 cleavage reaction, most of which involve conformational changes both within the Cas9 protein and in the RNA-DNA helix (Lim et al., 2016). R-loop formation is particularly critical for the conformational change of Cas9, turning it into an active nuclease (Josephs et al., 2015; Sternberg et al., 2015). Since, as mentioned earlier, the chemical modifications that affect zipped conformation influence Cas9-gRNA complex off-target activity (Cromwell et al., 2018), it is plausible that manipulating the secondary structure or the length of the gRNA may improve genome editing precision as well. Accordingly, Fu et al. demonstrated that manipulating the spacer length reduced off-target editing (Fu et al., 2014). Truncated gRNAs (tru-gRNAs), as short as seventeen nucleotides, have been shown to destabilize the cleavage complex formation and reduce the time spent in the zipped conformation, allowing for more specific editing (Fu et al., 2014). However, it should be emphasized that manipulating the cleavage complex stability via truncated gRNAs is obtained at the expense of on-target activity (Pavel-Dinu et al., 2019) such that the balance between efficiency and specificity of genome editing should be carefully weighed. Furthermore, adding two extra guanine residues on the 5′ end of the spacer sequence (ggXX$_{20}$ gRNA) had a variable effect on gene-editing performance in cultured cells, enhancing the guide specificity at specific genomic sites by significantly reducing off-target activity while maintaining the on-target efficiency (Cho et al., 2014). Nahar et al. demonstrated that introducing G-quadruplex (G4) structure at the 3′ end of the sgRNA resulted in increased *in vitro* serum stability and higher editing efficiency in the zebrafish embryos, compared to the unmodified sgRNA (Nahar et al., 2018). A much less pronounced effect was observed with G-rich hairpin at the 3′ end. On the other hand, G-rich hairpins or

G4 structures at the 5′ end completely abolished Cas9-mediated cleavage (Nahar et al., 2018). A later study by Kocak et al. revealed that at off-target sites where RNA:DNA mispairing exists, and binding affinity is reduced, R-loop formation is hindered, while R-loop formation can commence normally at on-target sites (Kocak et al., 2019). In fact, it has been found that modifying the RNA secondary structure by engineering a hairpin onto the 5′ end of the sgRNA spacer sequence (hp-sgRNAs) significantly increases gene editing specificity in cells when complexed with various CRISPR effector nucleases (Kocak et al., 2019). In addition, the researchers achieved higher specificity using the engineered hairpin structures than with the tru-gRNA analog when tested side by side. However, the extended sgRNAs showed a tendency to undergo intracellular digestion back to the original size. To that end, a combination of the truncated or hairpin-modified sgRNAs in tandem with the previously discussed terminal chemical modifications could prevent hairpin removal by intrinsic intracellular nuclease activity, thus maximizing the editing capabilities of engineered sgRNAs. It is important to note that the hairpin structures' design must meet stringent constraints for thermodynamic stability since below a specific free energy cut-off, the nuclease activity is severely impaired. Interestingly, the hairpin structures had a strong negative effect on the *in vitro* nuclease activity due to the slower kinetics of the cleavage reaction. On the other hand, after sufficient time in cultured cells, the reduced cleavage rate proved beneficial for the overall specificity of the modified sgRNA-mediated editing.

Partial DNA gRNA

It is well-documented that RNA residues in the crRNA and tracrRNA can be partially substituted for DNA residues without significantly impairing Cas9 activity both in *in vitro* cleavage assays and cultured cells (Rueda et al., 2017; Kartje et al., 2018; Yin et al., 2018; O'Reilly et al., 2019). The partial replacement of RNA nucleotides with DNA nucleotides in the crRNA has emerged as a potential approach to enhance CRISPR-Cas9 complex specificity by reducing off-target activity (Rueda et al., 2017; Kartje et al., 2018; Yin et al., 2018). The lower thermodynamic stability of the DNA-DNA duplex compared to the RNA-DNA duplex renders the partially DNA-substituted guide sequence of crRNA less tolerable to mismatches when interacting with genomic DNA. Kartje et al. demonstrated that *in vitro* cleavage of DNA duplexes by Cas9 could be facilitated by chimeric DNA-RNA crRNAs. Contrary to expectations, they showed that DNA substitutions inside the crRNA 3′ end, but not within the guide sequence, resulted in the Cas9-mediated cleavage being less tolerant of mismatches in the target sequence (Kartje et al., 2018). Conversely, Rueda et al. observed an increase in specificity in *in vitro* cleavage by replacing RNA residues with DNA residues inside of the guide sequence (Rueda et al., 2017). Yin et al. conducted a genome editing screen in Cas9 expressing HEK293T cells, which revealed that in living cells, the tail region, or the PAM-distal portion of the guide sequence was more amenable to DNA replacement than the seed region. They showed that replacing the ten RNA nucleotides in the PAM-distal region with DNA residues maintained on-target genome-editing activity (Yin et al., 2018). On the contrary, Cas9 endonuclease capability

was severely impaired when crRNAs underwent substitutions inside the seed region. Incorporating more than twelve DNA nucleotides at the 5′ end or four DNA nucleotides at the 3′ end of the guide region was not tolerated (Yin et al., 2018). Hence, DNA-RNA hybrid crRNAs seem to present a plausible and cost-effective formulation for efficient and more accurate *in vitro* gene editing; however, it has yet to be validated in primary cells and animal models.

INCREASING THE SAFETY OF CRISPR-MEDIATED GENE EDITING BY CURBING CELLULAR TOXICITY AND IMMUNE RESPONSES

CRISPR-Cas systems are bacterial mechanisms that researchers have worked determinedly to adapt to mammalian cells. However, as mentioned earlier, the CRISPR-Cas systems can evoke unwanted cellular and immune responses. Mammalian cells recognize the CRISPR complex as foreign and mount an immune response as a result (Cromer et al., 2018; Kim et al., 2018; Moon et al., 2019). Extensive research has been done on other nucleic acids therapies, such as siRNAs, mRNAs, and antisense oligodeoxynucleotides (ODNs) (Robbins et al., 2009; Burel et al., 2012; Kaczmarek et al., 2017; Meng and Lu, 2017) which can trigger immune responses; however, less is known about the immune recognition of gRNAs and the CRISPR system. Through a deeper understanding of the cause of the immune response, researchers have made strides to circumvent these deleterious side-effects by modifying the structure of the gRNAs.

Removal of 5′ Triphosphate and Introduction of 2′-O-Me Uridine or Guanosine Residues

In human cells, foreign RNAs are recognized in the cytosol by pathogen-associated molecular pattern (PAMP) binding receptors, Retinoic acid-inducible gene 1 (RIG-1), also known as DExD/H-Box Helicase 58 (DDX58), and melanoma differentiation-associated gene 5 (MDA5). Upon encountering a PAMP motif on an RNA molecule, these proteins trigger a signaling cascade, eventually resulting in the upregulation of type 1 interferons and interferon-stimulated genes (Kell and Gale, 2015). Recently, in order to reduce the costs of producing a large amount of gRNAs, IVT by T7/SP6 phage RNA polymerases has become a popular method. However, since 5′-triphosphate (5′-ppp), which remains on the 5′-end of IVT RNA, is recognized as a PAMP, introducing IVT gRNA species into human cells can potentially trigger an innate immune response. Indeed, multiple research groups have reported cytotoxicity due to RNA-sensing, specifically via the RIG-1 pathway, and innate immune responses in human cells triggered by the 5′-triphosphate groups present on CRISPR gRNAs (Kim et al., 2018; Schubert et al., 2018; Wienert et al., 2018). Wienert et al., Kim et al., and Schubert et al. each examined various cell lines as well as different clinically relevant primary cells such as HSPCs, human peripheral blood monocytic cells (PBMCs), and CD4$^+$ T cells. All cell types eventually exhibited a similar immune response to

5′-ppp gRNAs. Interestingly, the intracellular delivery method was deterministic in the immune response with nucleofection in HEK293 cells triggering a weaker and short-lasting type 1 interferon response, compared to lipofection (Wienert et al., 2018). Removal of the 5′-ppp groups by *in vitro* phosphatase treatment yielded 5′-hydroxyl gRNAs that could, in complex with Cas9 or Cas12a, achieve a high degree of mutagenesis in cell lines and primary human cells. This is actuated while triggering a reduced immune response similar to the synthesized gRNA species which are manufactured lacking 5′-ppp groups (Kim et al., 2018; Wienert et al., 2018). Furthermore, Schubert et al. demonstrated that the addition of 2′-O-Me and PS groups on the 2′-OH and phosphate backbone within synthesized gRNAs completely abolished any immune response (Schubert et al., 2018). This finding supported an earlier study that showed that the introduction of as few as two 2′-O-Me uridine or guanosine residues into either strand of a siRNA duplex eliminated any immune response (Judge et al., 2006). Hence, synthesized and chemically-modified gRNAs represent an optimal and clinically appropriate option for CRISPR-mediated gene editing in primary cells.

MODIFYING gRNA TO INCREASE HDR EFFICIENCY

CRISPR-mediated DSBs can be repaired via the HDR pathway to allow for precise editing of DNA sequences, to correct genetic mutations, or to introduce novel genetic fragments. HDR uses a homologous DNA template, either endogenous (sister chromatid or homologous chromosomes) or exogenously introduced (donor template) sequences for genetic manipulation, and is, therefore, significantly less error-prone (Rouet et al., 1994; Porteus, 2016; Rodgers and McVey, 2016). By taking advantage of this endogenous repair pathway, efficient gene editing and gene knock-in are possible. Plasmid donors are problematic in clinical applications due to the risk of insertional mutagenesis and of triggering an immune response to foreign DNA. Therefore, Adeno Associated Virus (AAV) vectors have become a method of choice to introduce donor templates (Gaj et al., 2017). However, AAV vectors can also elicit immune responses, especially when used in primary cells or in human subjects, posing a critical caveat for gene therapy (High and Roncarolo, 2019). Therefore, to improve HDR efficiency and eliminate virus-induced immune responses, non-viral donor DNA delivery is crucial. In addition to engineering the Cas9 protein (Aird et al., 2018; Savic et al., 2018; Ling et al., 2020) or the DNA donor (Renaud et al., 2016) to improve HDR efficiency, modifications on the gRNA itself have great potential to enhance HDR efficiency in a non-viral manner to increase the relevance of the CRISPR-Cas9 gene-editing tool for many biotechnological applications.

gRNA and Donor DNA Conjugates

In order to improve the CRISPR-Cas9 system to actuate more efficient HDR two parameters must be improved upon: increasing the transfection efficiency of the DNA donor to the edited cells (Lee et al., 2017a) and localizing the DNA donor

to the immediate vicinity of the DSB. To address these issues simultaneously, conjugated gRNA-donor DNAs, which ensures the proximity of the DNA donor to the cut site, have been engineered and have indeed showed improved HDR efficiency. These modified RNA-DNA hybrid molecules were engineered by conjugating an azide terminated DNA molecule with an alkyne modified crRNA. The engineered crRNA carrying the donor DNA was then annealed to standard tracrRNA and complexed with Cas9. The enhanced efficacy of the subsequent HDR showed that the conjugated gRNA could simultaneously act as a functional gRNA and donor DNA without the need for viral transduction (Lee et al., 2017b) (**Figure 3A**).

Using RNA Aptamers on gRNA Backbone

Another approach that has been shown to increase HDR efficiency without the need to conjugate the gRNA to the donor DNA utilizes RNA aptamers. Adding RNA aptamers on either the tetraloop or stem-loop 2, which both protrude from the Cas9 protein, leaving them free of any interactions with the nuclease itself, are well-tolerated (Konermann et al., 2015). By exploiting these RNA aptamers, CRISPR-Display was established to introduce a targeted localization method to deploy large cargo, including protein-binding cassettes, to specific DNA loci (Shechner et al., 2015). Taking advantage of the strong natural interaction between streptavidin and biotin, it was shown that the addition of a streptavidin-binding RNA aptamer on the loop domains of the gRNA along with biotinylated single-stranded oligodeoxynucleotides (ssODNs) formed a highly effective tertiary complex (streptavidin-gRNA, biotin-ssODN, and Cas9). Using this tertiary complex they highlighted an improvement in both total HDR as well as in precise HDR efficiency (Carlson-Stevermer et al., 2017) (**Figure 3B**).

MODIFYING gRNA TO UTILIZE CRISPR-Cas9 AS A ROBUST METHOD FOR NUCLEAR IMAGING

Another application that modified gRNAs seek to improve upon is the existing imaging tools of chromosomal dynamics and genomic mapping, which are essential for comprehending a plethora of basic cellular nuclear processes. Previous attempts relied on the fusion of nuclease-deficient dead Cas9 (dCas9) with fluorescent proteins (Chen et al., 2013; Ma et al., 2015), which would be directed to the target loci by expressed sgRNAs. Furthermore, in order to improve the assay sensitivity by increasing sgRNA expression, Chen et al. modified the sgRNA sequence by conducting an A-U flip to remove a potential RNA PolIII terminator sequence, as well as extending a Cas9-binding hairpin structure (Chen et al., 2013). A different approach relied on simultaneously expressing engineered gRNAs containing MS2/PCP aptamers, MS2/PCP binding proteins fused to fluorescent proteins, and dCas9. This method provided efficient and reliable live-cell multicolor labeling of multiple chromosomal loci at the same time in live cells (Shao et al., 2016; Wang et al., 2016). By utilizing only one type of Cas protein (Cas9) and one type of gRNA, the systems developed by Shao

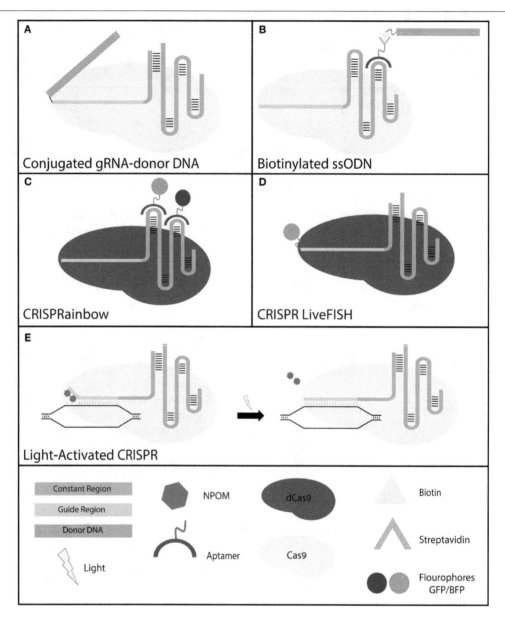

FIGURE 3 | Various applications of engineered gRNAs. **(A,B)**–gRNA modifications to improve HDR: **(A)** crRNA-donor DNA conjugate. The donor DNA is fused to the 5′ end of the guide region. **(B)** sgRNA molecule with streptavidin-binding aptamers that attach to either the tetraloop or stem-loop 2 (the two loops protruding from the Cas9 molecule). The formulation has the donor ssODN bound to a biotin molecule that binds the streptavidin tightly to ensure the proximity of the donor DNA to the break site. **(C,D)**–gRNA modifications that utilize CRISPR-dCas9 specificity for high-resolution cellular imaging: **(C)** sgRNA molecule with fluorophore-bound aptamers binding to either the tetraloop or stem-loop 2 (for the same reason as mentioned above). GFP and BFP were shown solely as examples since CRISPRainbow covers the full spectrum of combinations. **(D)** CRISPR LiveFISH method utilizes crRNAs fused to a fluorophore at the 5′ end to actuate live intracellular staining without the need for cellular fixation. **(E)** Light-activated CRISPR to allow for control over synchronous editing across a cell population. Photocaging with light-sensitive 6′-nitropiperonyloxymethyl (NPOM) thymidine modifications on the distal portion of the guide region prevents the gRNA from binding completely to its DNA target. Following exposure to light, the NPOM modifications are released and complete binding and subsequent editing commence.

et al. and Wang et al. allow greater simplicity, albeit limited to two colors unless applying additional dCas9 species fused to fluorescent proteins. The CRISPRainbow method further expanded the number of loci that can be viewed simultaneously by exploiting aptamer-carrying gRNA species (Ma et al., 2016) (**Figure 3C**). These modifications provide the CRISPR-Cas9 system the versatility to not only be used for genome editing but also for a deeper understanding of nuclear dynamics and mechanisms of action, including transcription, DNA replication, and DNA repair. In addition, the CRISPR LiveFISH method, with fluorophore-labeled gRNAs, presented a robust and novel approach using both dCas9 and dCas13 to enable real-time imaging of both DNA and RNA to track nuclear dynamics during genome editing and transcription in a wide range of live cells, including human primary cells (Wang et al., 2019) (**Figure 3D**).

MODIFYING gRNA TO PRODUCE INDUCIBLE AND CONTROLLED EDITING

Although tremendous progress in the quest to adapt the bacterial defense system to human cells has been made, much remains to be learned about the cellular response mechanisms and repair pathways in response to Cas-induced DSBs. Delivering CRISPR as an RNP complex is the most effective gene-editing method, but even then, cleavage is neither immediate nor synchronous across the treated cell population. This significantly hinders the ability to study the full spectrum of DSB formation and subsequent DNA repair dynamics. Extensive work has been done to produce inducible Cas9 systems to control nuclease activity by modifying the Cas9 protein to be activated only when induced chemically (Dow et al., 2015; Rose et al., 2017) or optically (Hemphill et al., 2015; Nihongaki et al., 2015a,b, 2017; Polstein and Gersbach, 2015; Richter et al., 2016; Zhou et al., 2018). However, a relatively simple and cost-effective method that allows optically-induced genome editing was recently demonstrated by adding photocaged light-sensitive 6'-nitropiperonyloxymethyl (NPOM) thymidine modifications on the distal portion of the gRNA (Liu et al., 2020; Moroz-Omori et al., 2020). Steric hindrance from these NPOM residues prevents binding of those residues, while the R-loop is successfully formed at the PAM-proximal residues. Due to the incomplete gRNA base pairing with the DNA site, the Cas9 remains catalytically inactive. Upon light stimulation (365 or 405 nm) that is not phototoxic to cells, as irradiation-induced damage is typically caused by wavelengths below 315 nm (Rastogi et al., 2010), photolysis of the NPOM moieties allows for complete gRNA base pairing, a conformational change in the Cas9 which in turn activates the nuclease domain, and DNA cleavage which is induced almost instantaneously. Indeed, significant DNA cleavage was generated within 30 seconds of light activation. This method of modifying the gRNA to facilitate light-induced Cas9 activation allows for synchronous DNA cleavage across a population of cells. This new CRISPR-Cas9 formulation is sure to lead to higher resolution, real-time DNA-repair analyses to better elucidate CRISPR-Cas9-induced DSB repair (Liu et al., 2020; Moroz-Omori et al., 2020) (**Figure 3E**).

CONCLUSION

The FDA, EMA, and other oversight drug approval bodies implement rigorous and demanding tests before approving a given drug or therapy. Albeit, with CRISPR-mediated genome editing being a rapidly developing field, no standardized protocol for gRNA modifications has been generated yet for clinical studies, and every gRNA should be examined on an individual basis. Hence, our goal in this review article was to elucidate the entire repertoire of gRNA chemical modifications in order to allow the researchers in the field to make educated decisions while choosing the appropriate gRNA formulation that would fit the particular study design. Although there is a wide

consensus regarding the profile of chemical modifications that improve the intracellular and intra-serum stability of guide RNAs, the proper design of the chemical gRNA modifications to improve the specificity of CRISPR-mediated genome editing is still to be determined. Notably, chemically-modified gRNAs are not restricted to the genome-editing via DSBs but can be exploited for a variety of applications involving catalytically-inactive Cas9 nucleases, Cas9 nickases, base editors and prime editors. (Anzalone et al., 2020). Though much more work remains to be done to optimize modified gRNAs for future routine human genome-editing-based therapies, there is no denying that the future of modified gRNAs and CRISPR-based therapeutics remains exceptionally bright. CRISPR-Cas systems, which can be engineered and modified with relative ease, provide a tremendous array of groundbreaking and versatile tools for programmable genome editing. The nucleic acid chemistry of gRNA enables expanding the array of nucleotide formulations from a native 4-letter RNA code to a wide range of phosphodiester, sugar ring, and nitrogen base modifications. In this review, we discussed the modifications on ribose ring and phosphodiester bonds, however, since it is well-known that RNA bases undergo a wide spectrum of modifications, such as 5-methylcytidine, or pseudouridine (Harcourt et al., 2017; Pan, 2018), which can ameliorate cellular immune responses (Hu et al., 2020), the potential to incorporate these could be a plausible future direction for engineering gRNAs. Certain modifications, such as the aforementioned MS and MSP modifications on the gRNA termini, are already being used worldwide as the quintessential standard for highly efficient genome editing. To that end, the first clinical trial, using C-C chemokine receptor type 5 (*CCR5*) knockout CD34$^+$ HSPCs edited by gRNAs with the chemical modifications described in Hendel et al. (2015a), has already been conducted in an HIV-positive patient with Acute Lymphoblastic Leukemia (Xu et al., 2019). With additional clinical trials using CRISPR-Cas9 technologies commencing [Clinicaltrials.gov, #NCT03655678, and # NCT03745287, (Frangoul et al., 2020)] we expect synthetically modified gRNA-based therapeutics to take a major leap in the years to come. Through more extensive testing and development of different gRNA modifications aimed to increase efficiency, specificity, and safety, as well as new applications such as cell imaging and payload delivery to the DSB sites, we are confident that a wide array of therapeutic and biotechnological applications of the CRISPR-Cas technology will be accelerated for the benefit of human society.

AUTHOR CONTRIBUTIONS

DA, MR, and AH contributed to the conceptualization of the review and wrote the paper. All authors approved the submitted version.

FUNDING

We gratefully acknowledge the funding support from the European Research Council (ERC) under the

Horizon 2020 Research and Innovation Program (Grant Agreement No. 755758). Additionally, we thank the Israel Science Foundation (ISF) (Grant No. 2031/19) and The Israel Cancer Research Fund (ICRF) (Grant No. 19-701-IPG) for their funding contributions. Lastly, this research was supported by the Ministry of Science, Technology & Space (Grant No. 3-14679).

ACKNOWLEDGMENTS

We thank Dr. Adi Tovin-Recht for her useful support. We thank the other members of the Hendel Lab for critically reading the manuscript and providing practical advice. Lastly, we would like to express our appreciation to Dr. Mark Behlke and Dr. Kim Lennox for reading the manuscript and providing insightful suggestions.

REFERENCES

Aird, E. J., Lovendahl, K. N., St. Martin, A., Harris, R. S., and Gordon, W. R. (2018). Increasing Cas9-mediated homology-directed repair efficiency through covalent tethering of DNA repair template. *Commun. Biol.* 1:54. doi: 10.1038/s42003-018-0054-2

Anderson, E. M., Haupt, A., Schiel, J. A., Chou, E., Machado, H. B., Strezoska, Z., et al. (2015). Systematic analysis of CRISPR-Cas9 mismatch tolerance reveals low levels of off-target activity. *J. Biotechnol.* 211, 56–65. doi: 10.1016/j.jbiotec.2015.06.427

Anzalone, A. V., Koblan, L. W., and Liu, D. R. (2020). Genome editing with CRISPR-Cas nucleases, base editors, transposases and prime editors. *Nat. Biotechnol.* 38, 824–844. doi: 10.1038/s41587-020-0561-9

Basila, M., Kelley, M. L., and Smith, A. V. B. (2017). Minimal 2′-O-methyl phosphorothioate linkage modification pattern of synthetic guide RNAs for increased stability and efficient CRISPR-Cas9 gene editing avoiding cellular toxicity. *PLoS ONE* 12:e0188593. doi: 10.1371/journal.pone.0188593

Bednarski, J. J., and Sleckman, B. P. (2019). At the intersection of DNA damage and immune responses. *Nat. Rev. Immunol.* 19, 231–242. doi: 10.1038/s41577-019-0135-6

Behlke, M. A. (2008). Chemical modification of siRNAs for *in vivo* use. *Oligonucleotides* 18, 305–319. doi: 10.1089/oli.2008.0164

Bennett, C. F., and Swayze, E. E. (2010). RNA targeting therapeutics: molecular mechanisms of antisense oligonucleotides as a therapeutic platform. *Annu. Rev. Pharmacol. Toxicol.* 50, 259–293. doi: 10.1146/annurev.pharmtox.010909.105654

Bin Moon, S., Lee, J. M., Kang, J. G., Lee, N. E., Ha, D. I., Kim, D. Y., et al. (2018). Highly efficient genome editing by CRISPR-Cpf1 using CRISPR RNA with a uridinylate-rich 3′-overhang. *Nat. Commun.* 9:3651. doi: 10.1038/s41467-018-06129-w

Braasch, D. A., Jensen, S., Liu, Y., Kaur, K., Arar, K., White, M. A., et al. (2003). RNA interference in mammalian cells by chemically-modified RNA. *Biochemistry* 42, 7967–7975. doi: 10.1021/bi0343774

Burel, S. A., Machemer, T., Ragone, F. L., Kato, H., Cauntay, P., Greenlee, S., et al. (2012). Unique O-methoxyethyl ribose-DNA chimeric oligonucleotide induces an atypical melanoma differentiation-associated gene 5-dependent induction of type I interferon response. *J. Pharmacol. Exp. Ther.* 342, 150–162. doi: 10.1124/jpet.112.193789

Carlson-Stevermer, J., Abdeen, A. A., Kohlenberg, L., Goedland, M., Molugu, K., Lou, M., et al. (2017). Assembly of CRISPR ribonucleoproteins with biotinylated oligonucleotides via an RNA aptamer for precise gene editing. *Nat. Commun.* 8:1711. doi: 10.1038/s41467-017-01875-9

Carroll, D. (2011). Genome engineering with zinc-finger nucleases. *Genetics* 188, 773–782. doi: 10.1534/genetics.111.131433

Carroll, D. (2014). Genome engineering with targetable nucleases. *Annu. Rev. Biochem.* 83, 409–439. doi: 10.1146/annurev-biochem-060713-035418

Chen, B., Gilbert, L. A., Cimini, B. A., Schnitzbauer, J., Zhang, W., Li, G. W., et al. (2013). Dynamic imaging of genomic loci in living human cells by an optimized CRISPR/Cas system. *Cell* 155, 1479–1491. doi: 10.1016/j.cell.2013.12.001

Chen, J. S., Dagdas, Y. S., Kleinstiver, B. P., Welch, M. M., Sousa, A. A., Harrington, L. B., et al. (2017). Enhanced proofreading governs CRISPR-Cas9 targeting accuracy. *Nature* 550, 407–410. doi: 10.1038/nature24268

Chiu, Y. L., and Rana, T. M. (2003). siRNA function in RNAi: a chemical modification analysis. *RNA* 9, 1034–1048. doi: 10.1261/rna.5103703

Cho, S. W., Kim, S., Kim, Y., Kweon, J., Kim, H. S., Bae, S., et al. (2014). Analysis of off-target effects of CRISPR/Cas-derived RNA-guided endonucleases and nickases. *Genome Res.* 24, 132–141. doi: 10.1101/gr.162339.113

Chylinski, K., Makarova, K. S., Charpentier, E., and Koonin, E. V. (2014). Classification and evolution of type II CRISPR-Cas systems. *Nucleic Acids Res.* 42, 6091–6105. doi: 10.1093/nar/gku241

Cong, L., Ran, F. A., Cox, D., Lin, S., Barretto, R., Habib, N., et al. (2013). Multiplex genome engineering using CRISPR/Cas systems. *Science* 339, 819–823. doi: 10.1126/science.1231143

Cromer, M. K., Vaidyanathan, S., Ryan, D. E., Curry, B., Lucas, A. B., Camarena, J., et al. (2018). Global transcriptional response to CRISPR/Cas9-AAV6-based genome editing in CD34(+) hematopoietic stem and progenitor cells. *Mol. Ther.* 26, 2431–2442. doi: 10.1016/j.ymthe.2018.06.002

Cromwell, C. R., Sung, K., Park, J., Krysler, A. R., Jovel, J., Kim, S. K., et al. (2018). Incorporation of bridged nucleic acids into CRISPR RNAs improves Cas9 endonuclease specificity. *Nat. Commun.* 9:1448. doi: 10.1038/s41467-018-03927-0

De Ravin, S. S., Li, L., Wu, X., Choi, U., Allen, C., Koontz, S., et al. (2017). CRISPR-Cas9 gene repair of hematopoietic stem cells from patients with X-linked chronic granulomatous disease. *Sci. Transl. Med.* 9:eaah3480. doi: 10.1126/scitranslmed.aah3480

Deleavey, G. F., and Damha, M. J. (2012). Designing chemically modified oligonucleotides for targeted gene silencing. *Chem. Biol.* 19, 937–954. doi: 10.1016/j.chembiol.2012.07.011

Dever, D. P., Bak, R. O., Reinisch, A., Camarena, J., Washington, G., Nicolas, C. E., et al. (2016). CRISPR/Cas9 beta-globin gene targeting in human haematopoietic stem cells. *Nature* 539, 384–389. doi: 10.1038/nature20134

DeWitt, M. A., Magis, W., Bray, N. L., Wang, T., Berman, J. R., Urbinati, F., et al. (2016). Selection-free genome editing of the sickle mutation in human adult hematopoietic stem/progenitor cells. *Sci. Transl. Med.* 8:360ra134. doi: 10.1126/scitranslmed.aaf9336

Dow, L. E., Fisher, J., O'Rourke, K. P., Muley, A., Kastenhuber, E. R., Livshits, G., et al. (2015). Inducible *in vivo* genome editing with CRISPR-Cas9. *Nat. Biotechnol.* 33, 390–394. doi: 10.1038/nbt.3155

Finn, J. D., Smith, A. R., Patel, M. C., Shaw, L., Youniss, M. R., van Heteren, J., et al. (2018). A single administration of CRISPR/Cas9 lipid nanoparticles achieves robust and persistent *in vivo* genome editing. *Cell Rep.* 22, 2227–2235. doi: 10.1016/j.celrep.2018.02.014

Frangoul, H., Altshuler, D., Cappellini, M. D., Chen, Y. S., Domm, J., Eustace, B. K., et al. (2020). CRISPR-Cas9 gene editing for sickle cell disease and beta-thalassemia. *N. Engl. J. Med.* doi: 10.1056/NEJMoa2031054. [Epub ahead of print].

Fu, Y., Sander, J. D., Reyon, D., Cascio, V. M., and Joung, J. K. (2014). Improving CRISPR-Cas nuclease specificity using truncated guide RNAs. *Nat. Biotechnol.* 32, 279–284. doi: 10.1038/nbt.2808

Gaj, T., Staahl, B. T., Rodrigues, G. M. C., Limsirichai, P., Ekman, F. K., Doudna, J. A., et al. (2017). Targeted gene knock-in by homology-directed genome editing using Cas9 ribonucleoprotein and AAV donor delivery. *Nucleic Acids Res.* 45:e98. doi: 10.1093/nar/gkx154

Gao, Q., Dong, X., Xu, Q., Zhu, L., Wang, F., Hou, Y., et al. (2019). Therapeutic potential of CRISPR/Cas9 gene editing in engineered T-cell therapy. *Cancer Med.* 8, 4254–4264. doi: 10.1002/cam4.2257

Ge, Z., Zheng, L., Zhao, Y., Jiang, J., Zhang, E. J., Liu, T., et al. (2019). Engineered xCas9 and SpCas9-NG variants broaden PAM recognition sites to generate mutations in *Arabidopsis* plants. *Plant Biotechnol. J.* 17, 1865–1867. doi: 10.1111/pbi.13148

Gomez-Ospina, N., Scharenberg, S. G., Mostrel, N., Bak, R. O., Mantri, S., Quadros, R. M., et al. (2019). Human genome-edited hematopoietic stem cells phenotypically correct Mucopolysaccharidosis type I. *Nat. Commun.* 10:4045. doi: 10.1038/s41467-019-11962-8

Goodwin, M., Lee, E., Lakshmanan, U., Shipp, S., Froessl, L., Barzaghi, F., et al. (2020). CRISPR-based gene editing enables FOXP3 gene repair in IPEX patient cells. *Sci. Adv.* 6:eaaz0571. doi: 10.1126/sciadv.aaz0571

Guo, X., and Li, X. J. (2015). Targeted genome editing in primate embryos. *Cell Res.* 25, 767–768. doi: 10.1038/cr.2015.64

Harcourt, E. M., Kietrys, A. M., and Kool, E. T. (2017). Chemical and structural effects of base modifications in messenger RNA. *Nature* 541, 339–346. doi: 10.1038/nature21351

Hemphill, J., Borchardt, E. K., Brown, K., Asokan, A., and Deiters, A. (2015). Optical control of CRISPR/Cas9 gene editing. *J. Am. Chem. Soc.* 137, 5642–5645. doi: 10.1021/ja512664v

Hendel, A., Bak, R. O., Clark, J. T., Kennedy, A. B., Ryan, D. E., Roy, S., et al. (2015a). Chemically modified guide RNAs enhance CRISPR-Cas genome editing in human primary cells. *Nat. Biotechnol.* 33, 985–989. doi: 10.1038/nbt.3290

Hendel, A., Fine, E. J., Bao, G., and Porteus, M. H. (2015b). Quantifying on- and off-target genome editing. *Trends Biotechnol.* 33, 132–140. doi: 10.1016/j.tibtech.2014.12.001

Hendel, A., Kildebeck, E. J., Fine, E. J., Clark, J., Punjya, N., Sebastiano, V., et al. (2014). Quantifying genome-editing outcomes at endogenous loci with SMRT sequencing. *Cell Rep.* 7, 293–305. doi: 10.1016/j.celrep.2014.02.040

High, K. A., and Roncarolo, M. G. (2019). Gene therapy. *N. Engl. J. Med.* 381, 455–464. doi: 10.1056/NEJMra1706910

Hirakawa, M. P., Krishnakumar, R., Timlin, J. A., Carney, J. P., and Butler, K. S. (2020). Gene editing and CRISPR in the clinic: current and future perspectives. *Biosci. Rep.* 40:BSR20200127. doi: 10.1042/BSR20200127

Horvath, P., and Barrangou, R. (2010). CRISPR/Cas, the immune system of bacteria and archaea. *Science* 327, 167–170. doi: 10.1126/science.1179555

Hsu, P. D., Lander, E. S., and Zhang, F. (2014). Development and applications of CRISPR-Cas9 for genome engineering. *Cell* 157, 1262–1278. doi: 10.1016/j.cell.2014.05.010

Hu, B., Zhong, L., Weng, Y., Peng, L., Huang, Y., Zhao, Y., et al. (2020). Therapeutic siRNA: state of the art. *Signal Transduct. Target Ther.* 5:101. doi: 10.1038/s41392-020-0207-x

Jiang, F., and Doudna, J. A. (2017). CRISPR-Cas9 structures and mechanisms. *Annu. Rev. Biophys.* 46, 505–529. doi: 10.1146/annurev-biophys-062215-010822

Jiang, F., Zhou, K., Ma, L., Gressel, S., and Doudna, J. A. (2015). STRUCTURAL BIOLOGY. a Cas9-guide RNA complex preorganized for target DNA recognition. *Science* 348, 1477–1481. doi: 10.1126/science.aab1452

Jinek, M., Chylinski, K., Fonfara, I., Hauer, M., Doudna, J. A., and Charpentier, E. (2012). A programmable dual-RNA-guided DNA endonuclease in adaptive bacterial immunity. *Science* 337, 816–821. doi: 10.1126/science.1225829

Josephs, E. A., Kocak, D. D., Fitzgibbon, C. J., McMenemy, J., Gersbach, C. A., and Marszalek, P. E. (2015). Structure and specificity of the RNA-guided endonuclease Cas9 during DNA interrogation, target binding and cleavage. *Nucleic Acids Res.* 43, 8924–8941. doi: 10.1093/nar/gkv892

Judge, A. D., Bola, G., Lee, A. C., and MacLachlan, I. (2006). Design of noninflammatory synthetic siRNA mediating potent gene silencing *in vivo*. *Mol. Ther.* 13, 494–505. doi: 10.1016/j.ymthe.2005.11.002

Kaczmarek, J. C., Kowalski, P. S., and Anderson, D. G. (2017). Advances in the delivery of RNA therapeutics: from concept to clinical reality. *Genome Med.* 9:60. doi: 10.1186/s13073-017-0450-0

Kartje, Z. J., Barkau, C. L., Rohilla, K. J., Ageely, E. A., and Gagnon, K. T. (2018). Chimeric guides probe and enhance Cas9 biochemical activity. *Biochemistry* 57, 3027–3031. doi: 10.1021/acs.biochem.8b00107

Kell, A. M., and Gale, M. Jr. (2015). RIG-I in RNA virus recognition. *Virology* 479-480, 110–121. doi: 10.1016/j.virol.2015.02.017

Kelley, M. L., Strezoska, Z., He, K., Vermeulen, A., and Smith, A. (2016). Versatility of chemically synthesized guide RNAs for CRISPR-Cas9 genome editing. *J. Biotechnol.* 233, 74–83. doi: 10.1016/j.jbiotec.2016.06.011

Kim, D., Kim, J., Hur, J. K., Been, K. W., Yoon, S. H., and Kim, J. S. (2016). Genome-wide analysis reveals specificities of Cpf1 endonucleases in human cells. *Nat. Biotechnol.* 34, 863–868. doi: 10.1038/nbt.3609

Kim, S., Koo, T., Jee, H. G., Cho, H. Y., Lee, G., Lim, D. G., et al. (2018). CRISPR RNAs trigger innate immune responses in human cells. *Genome Res.* 28, 367–373. doi: 10.1101/gr.231936.117

Kleinstiver, B. P., Pattanayak, V., Prew, M. S., Tsai, S. Q., Nguyen, N. T., Zheng, Z., et al. (2016). High-fidelity CRISPR-Cas9 nucleases with no detectable genome-wide off-target effects. *Nature* 529, 490–495. doi: 10.1038/nature16526

Kocak, D. D., Josephs, E. A., Bhandarkar, V., Adkar, S. S., Kwon, J. B., and Gersbach, C. A. (2019). Increasing the specificity of CRISPR systems with engineered RNA secondary structures. *Nat. Biotechnol.* 37, 657–666. doi: 10.1038/s41587-019-0095-1

Konermann, S., Brigham, M. D., Trevino, A. E., Joung, J., Abudayyeh, O. O., Barcena, C., et al. (2015). Genome-scale transcriptional activation by an engineered CRISPR-Cas9 complex. *Nature* 517, 583–588. doi: 10.1038/nature14136

Lee, K., Conboy, M., Park, H. M., Jiang, F., Kim, H. J., Dewitt, M. A., et al. (2017a). Nanoparticle delivery of Cas9 ribonucleoprotein and donor DNA *in vivo* induces homology-directed DNA repair. *Nat. Biomed. Eng.* 1, 889–901. doi: 10.1038/s41551-017-0137-2

Lee, K., Mackley, V. A., Rao, A., Chong, A. T., Dewitt, M. A., Corn, J. E., et al. (2017b). Synthetically modified guide RNA and donor DNA are a versatile platform for CRISPR-Cas9 engineering. *Elife* 6:e25312. doi: 10.7554/eLife.25312

Lennox, K. A., and Behlke, M. A. (2020). Chemical modifications in RNA interference and CRISPR/Cas genome editing reagents. *Methods Mol. Biol.* 2115, 23–55. doi: 10.1007/978-1-0716-0290-4_2

Levin, A. A. (2019). Treating disease at the RNA level with oligonucleotides. *N. Engl. J. Med.* 380, 57–70. doi: 10.1056/NEJMra1705346

Li, B., Zhao, W., Luo, X., Zhang, X., Li, C., Zeng, C., et al. (2017). Engineering CRISPR-Cpf1 crRNAs and mRNAs to maximize genome editing efficiency. *Nat. Biomed. Eng.* 1:0066. doi: 10.1038/s41551-017-0066

Li, D., Zhou, H., and Zeng, X. (2019). Battling CRISPR-Cas9 off-target genome editing. *Cell Biol. Toxicol.* 35, 403–406. doi: 10.1007/s10565-019-09485-5

Liang, X., Potter, J., Kumar, S., Zou, Y., Quintanilla, R., Sridharan, M., et al. (2015). Rapid and highly efficient mammalian cell engineering via Cas9 protein transfection. *J. Biotechnol.* 208, 44–53. doi: 10.1016/j.jbiotec.2015.04.024

Lim, Y., Bak, S. Y., Sung, K., Jeong, E., Lee, S. H., Kim, J. S., et al. (2016). Structural roles of guide RNAs in the nuclease activity of Cas9 endonuclease. *Nat. Commun.* 7:13350. doi: 10.1038/ncomms13350

Ling, X., Xie, B., Gao, X., Chang, L., Zheng, W., Chen, H., et al. (2020). Improving the efficiency of precise genome editing with site-specific Cas9-oligonucleotide conjugates. *Sci. Adv.* 6:eaaz0051. doi: 10.1126/sciadv.aaz0051

Lips, J., and Kaina, B. (2001). DNA double-strand breaks trigger apoptosis in p53-deficient fibroblasts. *Carcinogenesis* 22, 579–585. doi: 10.1093/carcin/22.4.579

Liu, Y., Zou, R. S., He, S., Nihongaki, Y., Li, X., Razavi, S., et al. (2020). Very fast CRISPR on demand. *Science* 368, 1265–1269. doi: 10.1126/science.aay8204

Ma, H., Naseri, A., Reyes-Gutierrez, P., Wolfe, S. A., Zhang, S., and Pederson, T. (2015). Multicolor CRISPR labeling of chromosomal loci in human cells. *Proc. Natl. Acad. Sci. U.S.A.* 112, 3002–3007. doi: 10.1073/pnas.1420024112

Ma, H., Tu, L. C., Naseri, A., Huisman, M., Zhang, S., Grunwald, D., et al. (2016). Multiplexed labeling of genomic loci with dCas9 and engineered sgRNAs using CRISPRainbow. *Nat. Biotechnol.* 34, 528–530. doi: 10.1038/nbt.3526

Maeder, M. L., Stefanidakis, M., Wilson, C. J., Baral, R., Barrera, L. A., Bounoutas, G. S., et al. (2019). Development of a gene-editing approach to restore vision loss in Leber congenital amaurosis type 10. *Nat. Med.* 25, 229–233. doi: 10.1038/s41591-018-0327-9

Makarova, K. S., Wolf, Y. I., Iranzo, J., Shmakov, S. A., Alkhnbashi, O. S., Brouns, S. J. J., et al. (2020). Evolutionary classification of CRISPR-Cas systems: a burst of class 2 and derived variants. *Nat. Rev. Microbiol.* 18, 67–83. doi: 10.1038/s41579-019-0299-x

Mali, P., Yang, L., Esvelt, K. M., Aach, J., Guell, M., DiCarlo, J. E., et al. (2013). RNA-guided human genome engineering via Cas9. *Science* 339, 823–826. doi: 10.1126/science.1232033

Manning, K. S., Rao, A. N., Castro, M., and Cooper, T. A. (2017). BNA(NC) gapmers revert splicing and reduce RNA foci with low toxicity in myotonic dystrophy cells. *ACS Chem. Biol.* 12, 2503–2509. doi: 10.1021/acschembio.7b00416

McMahon, M. A., Prakash, T. P., Cleveland, D. W., Bennett, C. F., and Rahdar, M. (2018). Chemically modified Cpf1-CRISPR RNAs mediate efficient genome editing in mammalian cells. *Mol. Ther.* 26, 1228–1240. doi: 10.1016/j.ymthe.2018.02.031

Meng, Z., and Lu, M. (2017). RNA interference-induced innate immunity, off-target effect, or immune adjuvant? *Front. Immunol.* 8:331. doi: 10.3389/fimmu.2017.00331

Mir, A., Alterman, J. F., Hassler, M. R., Debacker, A. J., Hudgens, E., Echeverria, D., et al. (2018). Heavily and fully modified RNAs guide efficient SpyCas9-mediated genome editing. *Nat. Commun.* 9:2641. doi: 10.1038/s41467-018-05073-z

Moon, S. B., Kim, D. Y., Ko, J. H., Kim, J. S., and Kim, Y. S. (2019). Improving CRISPR genome editing by engineering guide RNAs. *Trends Biotechnol.* 37, 870–881. doi: 10.1016/j.tibtech.2019.01.009

Morange, M. (2015). What history tells us XXXVII. CRISPR-Cas: the discovery of an immune system in prokaryotes. *J. Biosci.* 40, 221–223. doi: 10.1007/s12038-015-9532-6

Moroz-Omori, E. V., Satyapertiwi, D., Ramel, M. C., Hogset, H., Sunyovszki, I. K., Liu, Z., et al. (2020). Photoswitchable gRNAs for spatiotemporally controlled CRISPR-cas-based genomic regulation. *ACS Cent. Sci.* 6, 695–703. doi: 10.1021/acscentsci.9b01093

Munoz, I. V., Sarrocco, S., Malfatti, L., Baroncelli, R., and Vannacci, G. (2019). CRISPR-Cas for fungal genome editing: a new tool for the management of plant diseases. *Front. Plant Sci.* 10:135. doi: 10.3389/fpls.2019.00135

Nahar, S., Sehgal, P., Azhar, M., Rai, M., Singh, A., Sivasubbu, S., et al. (2018). A G-quadruplex motif at the 3′ end of sgRNAs improves CRISPR-Cas9 based genome editing efficiency. *Chem. Commun.* 54, 2377–2380. doi: 10.1039/C7CC08893K

Nakad, R., and Schumacher, B. (2016). DNA Damage Response and Immune Defense: Links and Mechanisms. *Front. Genet.* 7:147. doi: 10.3389/fgene.2016.00147

Nihongaki, Y., Furuhata, Y., Otabe, T., Hasegawa, S., Yoshimoto, K., and Sato, M. (2017). CRISPR-Cas9-based photoactivatable transcription systems to induce neuronal differentiation. *Nat. Methods* 14, 963–966. doi: 10.1038/nmeth.4430

Nihongaki, Y., Kawano, F., Nakajima, T., and Sato, M. (2015a). Photoactivatable CRISPR-Cas9 for optogenetic genome editing. *Nat. Biotechnol.* 33, 755–760. doi: 10.1038/nbt.3245

Nihongaki, Y., Yamamoto, S., Kawano, F., Suzuki, H., and Sato, M. (2015b). CRISPR-Cas9-based photoactivatable transcription system. *Chem. Biol.* 22, 169–174. doi: 10.1016/j.chembiol.2014.12.011

Nishimasu, H., Ran, F. A., Hsu, P. D., Konermann, S., Shehata, S. I., Dohmae, N., et al. (2014). Crystal structure of Cas9 in complex with guide RNA and target DNA. *Cell* 156, 935–949. doi: 10.1016/j.cell.2014.02.001

Obe, G., Johannes, C., and Schulte-Frohlinde, D. (1992). DNA double-strand breaks induced by sparsely ionizing radiation and endonucleases as critical lesions for cell death, chromosomal aberrations, mutations and oncogenic transformation. *Mutagenesis* 7, 3–12. doi: 10.1093/mutage/7.1.3

O'Geen, H., Henry, I. M., Bhakta, M. S., Meckler, J. F., and Segal, D. J. (2015a). A genome-wide analysis of Cas9 binding specificity using ChIP-seq and targeted sequence capture. *Nucleic Acids Res.* 43, 3389–3404. doi: 10.1093/nar/gkv137

O'Geen, H., Yu, A. S., and Segal, D. J. (2015b). How specific is CRISPR/Cas9 really? *Curr. Opin. Chem. Biol.* 29, 72–78. doi: 10.1016/j.cbpa.2015.10.001

O'Reilly, D., Kartje, Z. J., Ageely, E. A., Malek-Adamian, E., Habibian, M., Schofield, A., et al. (2019). Extensive CRISPR RNA modification reveals chemical compatibility and structure-activity relationships for Cas9 biochemical activity. *Nucleic Acids Res.* 47, 546–558. doi: 10.1093/nar/gky1214

Pan, T. (2018). Modifications and functional genomics of human transfer RNA. *Cell Res.* 28, 395–404. doi: 10.1038/s41422-018-0013-y

Park, H. M., Liu, H., Wu, J., Chong, A., Mackley, V., Fellmann, C., et al. (2018). Extension of the crRNA enhances Cpf1 gene editing *in vitro* and *in vivo*. *Nat. Commun.* 9:3313. doi: 10.1038/s41467-018-05641-3

Park, S. H., Lee, C. M., Dever, D. P., Davis, T. H., Camarena, J., Srifa, W., et al. (2019). Highly efficient editing of the beta-globin gene in patient-derived hematopoietic stem and progenitor cells to treat sickle cell disease. *Nucleic Acids Res.* 47, 7955–7972. doi: 10.1093/nar/gkz475

Pavel-Dinu, M., Wiebking, V., Dejene, B. T., Srifa, W., Mantri, S., Nicolas, C. E., et al. (2019). Gene correction for SCID-X1 in long-term hematopoietic stem cells. *Nat. Commun.* 10:1634. doi: 10.1038/s41467-019-10080-9

Polstein, L. R., and Gersbach, C. A. (2015). A light-inducible CRISPR-Cas9 system for control of endogenous gene activation. *Nat. Chem. Biol.* 11, 198–200. doi: 10.1038/nchembio.1753

Porteus, M. (2016). Genome editing: a new approach to human therapeutics. *Annu. Rev. Pharmacol. Toxicol.* 56, 163–190. doi: 10.1146/annurev-pharmtox-010814-124454

Porteus, M. H., and Carroll, D. (2005). Gene targeting using zinc finger nucleases. *Nat. Biotechnol.* 23, 967–973. doi: 10.1038/nbt1125

Rahdar, M., McMahon, M. A., Prakash, T. P., Swayze, E. E., Bennett, C. F., and Cleveland, D. W. (2015). Synthetic CRISPR RNA-Cas9-guided genome editing in human cells. *Proc. Natl. Acad. Sci. U.S.A.* 112, E7110–E7117. doi: 10.1073/pnas.1520883112

Rai, R., Romito, M., Rivers, E., Turchiano, G., Blattner, G., Vetharoy, W., et al. (2020). Targeted gene correction of human hematopoietic stem cells for the treatment of wiskott - aldrich syndrome. *Nat. Commun.* 11:4034. doi: 10.1038/s41467-020-17626-2

Ran, F. A., Hsu, P. D., Wright, J., Agarwala, V., Scott, D. A., and Zhang, F. (2013). Genome engineering using the CRISPR-Cas9 system. *Nat. Protoc.* 8, 2281–2308. doi: 10.1038/nprot.2013.143

Rastogi, R. P., Richa, K.umar, A., Tyagi, M. B., and Sinha, R. P. (2010). Molecular mechanisms of ultraviolet radiation-induced DNA damage and repair. *J. Nucleic Acids* 2010:592980. doi: 10.4061/2010/592980

Renaud, J. B., Boix, C., Charpentier, M., De Cian, A., Cochennec, J., Duvernois-Berthet, E., et al. (2016). Improved genome editing efficiency and flexibility using modified oligonucleotides with TALEN and CRISPR-Cas9 nucleases. *Cell Rep.* 14, 2263–2272. doi: 10.1016/j.celrep.2016.02.018

Richter, F., Fonfara, I., Bouazza, B., Schumacher, C. H., Bratovic, M., Charpentier, E., et al. (2016). Engineering of temperature- and light-switchable Cas9 variants. *Nucleic Acids Res.* 44, 10003–10014. doi: 10.1093/nar/gkw930

Robbins, M., Judge, A., and MacLachlan, I. (2009). siRNA and innate immunity. *Oligonucleotides* 19, 89–102. doi: 10.1089/oli.2009.0180

Rodgers, K., and McVey, M. (2016). Error-prone repair of DNA double-strand breaks. *J. Cell. Physiol.* 231, 15–24. doi: 10.1002/jcp.25053

Romero, Z., Lomova, A., Said, S., Miggelbrink, A., Kuo, C. Y., Campo-Fernandez, B., et al. (2019). Editing the sickle cell disease mutation in human hematopoietic stem cells: comparison of endonucleases and homologous donor templates. *Mol. Ther.* 27, 1389–1406. doi: 10.1016/j.ymthe.2019.05.014

Rose, J. C., Stephany, J. J., Valente, W. J., Trevillian, B. M., Dang, H. V., Bielas, J. H., et al. (2017). Rapidly inducible Cas9 and DSB-ddPCR to probe editing kinetics. *Nat. Methods* 14, 891–896. doi: 10.1038/nmeth.4368

Rouet, P., Smih, F., and Jasin, M. (1994). Expression of a site-specific endonuclease stimulates homologous recombination in mammalian cells. *Proc. Natl. Acad. Sci. U.S.A.* 91, 6064–6068. doi: 10.1073/pnas.91.13.6064

Rueda, F. O., Bista, M., Newton, M. D., Goeppert, A. U., Cuomo, M. E., Gordon, E., et al. (2017). Mapping the sugar dependency for rational generation of a DNA-RNA hybrid-guided Cas9 endonuclease. *Nat. Commun.* 8:1610. doi: 10.1038/s41467-017-01732-9

Ryan, D. E., Taussig, D., Steinfeld, I., Phadnis, S. M., Lunstad, B. D., Singh, M., et al. (2018). Improving CRISPR-Cas specificity with chemical modifications in single-guide RNAs. *Nucleic Acids Res.* 46, 792–803. doi: 10.1093/nar/gkx1199

Safari, F., Zare, K., Negahdaripour, M., Barekati-Mowahed, M., and Ghasemi, Y. (2019). CRISPR Cpf1 proteins: structure, function and implications for genome editing. *Cell Biosci.* 9:36. doi: 10.1186/s13578-019-0298-7

Savic, N., Ringnalda, F. C., Lindsay, H., Berk, C., Bargsten, K., Li, Y., et al. (2018). Covalent linkage of the DNA repair template to the CRISPR-Cas9 nuclease enhances homology-directed repair. *Elife* 7:e33761. doi: 10.7554/eLife.33761.032

Schubert, M. S., Cedrone, E., Neun, B., Behlke, M. A., and Dobrovolskaia, M. A. (2018). Chemical modification of CRISPR gRNAs eliminate type I interferon responses in human peripheral blood mononuclear cells. *J. Cytokine Biol.* 3:121. doi: 10.4172/2576-3881.1000121

Shao, S., Zhang, W., Hu, H., Xue, B., Qin, J., Sun, C., et al. (2016). Long-term dual-color tracking of genomic loci by modified sgRNAs of the CRISPR/Cas9 system. *Nucleic Acids Res.* 44:e86. doi: 10.1093/nar/gkw066

Shapiro, J., Iancu, O., Jacobi, A. M., McNeill, M. S., Turk, R., Rettig, G. R., et al. (2020). Increasing CRISPR efficiency and measuring its specificity in hspcs using a clinically relevant system. *Mol. Ther. Methods Clin. Dev.* 17, 1097–1107. doi: 10.1016/j.omtm.2020.04.027

Shapiro, J., Tovin, A., Iancu, O., Allen, D., and Hendel, A. (2021). Chemical modification of guide RNAs for improved CRISPR activity in CD34+ human hematopoietic stem and progenitor cells. *Methods Mol. Biol.* 2162, 37–48. doi: 10.1007/978-1-0716-0687-2_3

Shechner, D. M., Hacisuleyman, E., Younger, S. T., and Rinn, J. L. (2015). Multiplexable, locus-specific targeting of long RNAs with CRISPR-display. *Nat. Methods* 12, 664–670. doi: 10.1038/nmeth.3433

Shmakov, S., Smargon, A., Scott, D., Cox, D., Pyzocha, N., Yan, W., et al. (2017). Diversity and evolution of class 2 CRISPR-Cas systems. *Nat. Rev. Microbiol.* 15, 169–182. doi: 10.1038/nrmicro.2016.184

Sid, H., and Schusser, B. (2018). Applications of gene editing in chickens: a new era is on the horizon. *Front. Genet.* 9:456. doi: 10.3389/fgene.2018.00456

Slaymaker, I. M., Gao, L., Zetsche, B., Scott, D. A., Yan, W. X., and Zhang, F. (2016). Rationally engineered Cas9 nucleases with improved specificity. *Science* 351, 84–88. doi: 10.1126/science.aad5227

Song, R., Zhai, Q., Sun, L., Huang, E., Zhang, Y., Zhu, Y., et al. (2019). CRISPR/Cas9 genome editing technology in filamentous fungi: progress and perspective. *Appl. Microbiol. Biotechnol.* 103, 6919–6932. doi: 10.1007/s00253-019-10007-w

Soni, S. (2020). Cautious progress toward clinical application of human gene editing. *CRISPR J* 3, 3–4. doi: 10.1089/crispr.2020.29083.sso

Stadtmauer, E. A., Fraietta, J. A., Davis, M. M., Cohen, A. D., Weber, K. L., Lancaster, E., et al. (2020). CRISPR-engineered T cells in patients with refractory cancer. *Science* 367:eaba7365. doi: 10.1126/science.aba7365

Sternberg, S. H., LaFrance, B., Kaplan, M., and Doudna, J. A. (2015). Conformational control of DNA target cleavage by CRISPR-Cas9. *Nature* 527, 110–113. doi: 10.1038/nature15544

Sun, L., Wu, J., Du, F., Chen, X., and Chen, Z. J. (2013). Cyclic GMP-AMP synthase is a cytosolic DNA sensor that activates the type I interferon pathway. *Science* 339, 786–791. doi: 10.1126/science.1232458

Taemaitree, L., Shivalingam, A., El-Sagheer, A. H., and Brown, T. (2019). An artificial triazole backbone linkage provides a split-and-click strategy to bioactive chemically modified CRISPR sgRNA. *Nat. Commun.* 10:1610. doi: 10.1038/s41467-019-09600-4

Tang, Y., and Fu, Y. (2018). Class 2 CRISPR/Cas: an expanding biotechnology toolbox for and beyond genome editing. *Cell Biosci.* 8:59. doi: 10.1186/s13578-018-0255-x

Terns, M. P., and Terns, R. M. (2011). CRISPR-based adaptive immune systems. *Curr. Opin. Microbiol.* 14, 321–327. doi: 10.1016/j.mib.2011.03.005

Tsai, S. Q., and Joung, J. K. (2016). Defining and improving the genome-wide specificities of CRISPR-Cas9 nucleases. *Nat. Rev. Genet.* 17, 300–312. doi: 10.1038/nrg.2016.28

Vakulskas, C. A., Dever, D. P., Rettig, G. R., Turk, R., Jacobi, A. M., Collingwood, M. A., et al. (2018). A high-fidelity Cas9 mutant delivered as a ribonucleoprotein complex enables efficient gene editing in human hematopoietic stem and progenitor cells. *Nat. Med.* 24, 1216–1224. doi: 10.1038/s41591-018-0137-0

Wang, H., Nakamura, M., Abbott, T. R., Zhao, D., Luo, K., Yu, C., et al. (2019). CRISPR-mediated live imaging of genome editing and transcription. *Science* 365, 1301–1305. doi: 10.1126/science.aax7852

Wang, H., Yang, H., Shivalila, C. S., Dawlaty, M. M., Cheng, A. W., Zhang, F., et al. (2013). One-step generation of mice carrying mutations in multiple genes by CRISPR/Cas-mediated genome engineering. *Cell* 153, 910–918. doi: 10.1016/j.cell.2013.04.025

Wang, S., Su, J. H., Zhang, F., and Zhuang, X. (2016). An RNA-aptamer-based two-color CRISPR labeling system. *Sci. Rep.* 6:26857. doi: 10.1038/srep26857

Wienert, B., Shin, J., Zelin, E., Pestal, K., and Corn, J. E. (2018). *In vitro*-transcribed guide RNAs trigger an innate immune response via the RIG-I pathway. *PLoS Biol.* 16:e2005840. doi: 10.1371/journal.pbio.2005840

Wu, Y., Zeng, J., Roscoe, B. P., Liu, P., Yao, Q., Lazzarotto, C. R., et al. (2019). Highly efficient therapeutic gene editing of human hematopoietic stem cells. *Nat. Med* 25, 776–783. doi: 10.1038/s41591-019-0401-y

Xu, L., Wang, J., Liu, Y., Xie, L., Su, B., Mou, D., et al. (2019). CRISPR-edited stem cells in a patient with HIV and acute lymphocytic leukemia. *N. Engl. J. Med.* 381, 1240–1247. doi: 10.1056/NEJMoa1817426

Xue, T., Liu, K., Chen, D., Yuan, X., Fang, J., Yan, H., et al. (2018). Improved bioethanol production using CRISPR/Cas9 to disrupt the ADH2 gene in Saccharomyces cerevisiae. *World J. Microbiol. Biotechnol.* 34:154. doi: 10.1007/s11274-018-2518-4

Yang, H., Ren, S., Yu, S., Pan, H., Li, T., Ge, S., et al. (2020). Methods favoring homology-directed repair choice in response to CRISPR/Cas9 induced-double strand breaks. *Int. J. Mol. Sci.* 21:6461. doi: 10.3390/ijms21186461

Yao, R., Liu, D., Jia, X., Zheng, Y., Liu, W., and Xiao, Y. (2018). CRISPR-Cas9/Cas12a biotechnology and application in bacteria. *Synth. Syst. Biotechnol.* 3, 135–149. doi: 10.1016/j.synbio.2018.09.004

Yin, H., Song, C. Q., Suresh, S., Kwan, S. Y., Wu, Q., Walsh, S., et al. (2018). Partial DNA-guided Cas9 enables genome editing with reduced off-target activity. *Nat. Chem. Biol.* 14, 311–316. doi: 10.1038/nchembio.2559

Yin, H., Song, C. Q., Suresh, S., Wu, Q., Walsh, S., Rhym, L. H., et al. (2017). Structure-guided chemical modification of guide RNA enables potent non-viral *in vivo* genome editing. *Nat. Biotechnol.* 35, 1179–1187. doi: 10.1038/nbt.4005

You, Y., Moreira, B. G., Behlke, M. A., and Owczarzy, R. (2006). Design of LNA probes that improve mismatch discrimination. *Nucleic Acids Res.* 34: e60. doi: 10.1093/nar/gkl175

Zhang, B. (2020). CRISPR/Cas gene therapy. *J. Cell Physiol.* doi: 10.1002/jcp.30064. [Epub ahead of print].

Zhen, S., and Li, X. (2017). Oncogenic human papillomavirus: application of CRISPR/Cas9 therapeutic strategies for cervical cancer. *Cell. Physiol. Biochem.* 44, 2455–2466. doi: 10.1159/000486168

Zhou, X. X., Zou, X., Chung, H. K., Gao, Y., Liu, Y., Qi, L. S., et al. (2018). A single-Chain photoswitchable CRISPR-Cas9 architecture for light-inducible gene editing and transcription. *ACS Chem. Biol.* 13, 443–448. doi: 10.1021/acschembio.7b00603

16

The Evolving Role of Next-Generation Sequencing in Screening and Diagnosis of Hemoglobinopathies

Ahlem Achour[1,2]*, Tamara T. Koopmann[1], Frank Baas[1] and Cornelis L. Harteveld[1]

[1] Department of Clinical Genetics/LDGA, Leiden University Medical Center, Leiden, Netherlands, [2] Department of Congenital and Hereditary Diseases, Charles Nicolle Hospital, Tunis, Tunisia

*Correspondence:
Ahlem Achour
ahlemachour2@gmail.com;
A.Bach_Hamba@lumc.nl

During the last few years, next-generation sequencing (NGS) has undergone a rapid transition from a research setting to a clinical application, becoming the method of choice in many clinical genetics laboratories for the detection of disease-causing variants in a variety of genetic diseases involving multiple genes. The hemoglobinopathies are the most frequently found Mendelian inherited monogenic disease worldwide and are composed of a complex group of disorders frequently involving the inheritance of more than one abnormal gene. This review aims to present the role of NGS in both screening and pre- and post-natal diagnostics of the hemoglobinopathies, and the added value of NGS is discussed based on the results described in the literature. Overall, NGS has an added value in large-scale high throughput carrier screening and in the complex cases for which common molecular techniques have some inadequacies. It is proven that the majority of thalassemia cases and Hb variants can be diagnosed using routine analysis involving a combined approach of hematology, hemoglobin separation, and classical DNA methods; however, we conclude that NGS can be a useful addition to the existing methods in the diagnosis of these disorders.

Keywords: NGS, WES, WGS, β-thalassemia, sickle cell disease, α-thalassemia, hemoglobinopathy diagnostics

INTRODUCTION

Hemoglobinopathies are a heterogeneous group of disorders comprising the most common recessive diseases encountered worldwide and are posing a major health problem. Therefore, they comprise one of the most studied examples of Mendelian inherited monogenic diseases. Diseases resulting from Mendelian inheritance are caused by single-gene mutations and have an overall estimated frequency of 40–82 per 1,000 live births (Christianson and Howson, 2006; Weatherall and Clegg, 1996; Weatherall, 2010; Piel et al., 2013). The hemoglobinopathies are complex since frequently more than one type of hemoglobinopathy is inherited simultaneously. DNA variants of the globin genes may cause changes in the globin structure leading to the production of abnormal hemoglobin, while the variants affecting the gene expression result in reduced production of a globin chain (of normal structure) resulting in thalassemia. Approximately 7% of the world population is a healthy carrier of hemoglobinopathy (World Health Organization [WHO], 1987). Inheritance of some combinations of mutations gives rise to severe diseases, notably sickle cell disease and beta-thalassemia major, and causes major health problems. It is estimated that approximately 350,000 newborns (annually) are found to have either of these conditions. Although the prognosis for hemoglobinopathies has been markedly improved, in general, lifelong treatment is required. Because of the high prevalence, many countries have implemented national screening programs to detect carriers and to offer counseling to couples at risk to reduce the number of affected births (Giordano, 2009; Michlitsch et al., 2009; Lobitz et al., 2018). In the vast majority of cases, hemoglobinopathies are caused by point mutations or large deletions involving the globin genes. Occasionally, mutations in transacting genes and intergenic regions have been reported (Thein, 2013; Farashi and Harteveld, 2018). Understanding the different molecular mechanisms leading to hemoglobinopathies is important to provide an adequate molecular diagnosis. According to the EMQN best practice policy for molecular and hematology methods for carrier identification and prenatal diagnosis of the hemoglobinopathies (Traeger-Synodinos et al., 2015), the red cell hematology is followed by biochemical assays by using high pressure liquid chromatography (HPLC), isoelectric focusing (IEF), and/or capillary electrophoresis (CE) and confirmation at the DNA level. Based on hematology and biochemical results, molecular analysis is performed using Gap-PCR for the identification of DNA deletions or gene rearrangements, direct sequencing analysis, and/or multiplex ligation-dependent probe amplification (MLPA) (Traeger-Synodinos et al., 2015; Harteveld, 2018). The sequential workflow in which only one gene is investigated at a time by Sanger sequencing may be time-consuming and costly and may miss some rare causative variants, resulting in a delay in genetic counseling and unresolved cases. In addition, current screening methods may miss causative alpha mutations giving rise to severe hemoglobin H (HbH) disease (He et al., 2017). Currently, diagnosis of an increasing number of genetic diseases is performed by large-scale parallel sequencing of disease gene panels instead of a sequential gene by gene Sanger sequencing, and targeted panels or whole exome sequencing (WES) are used to increase the speed of diagnosis and reduce cost in many genetic diseases.

This review aims to present the different applications of next-generation sequencing (NGS) in prenatal, postnatal diagnosis, and screening of hemoglobinopathies described in the literature and to discuss the diagnostic utility of NGS in the most frequent recessive Mendelian inherited monogenic disease worldwide, the hemoglobinopathies (Williams and Weatherall, 2012).

The Role of NGS in the Molecular Screening of Thalassemia Carriers

Large-scale premarital carrier screening for alpha- and or beta-thalassemia has been described in the Chinese population using NGS. Preliminary data have shown that NGS may be more accurate as a first-tier DNA screening tool than conventional thalassemia screening. In addition to the higher sensitivity of carrier detection, it has also led to the identification of new variants.

He et al. (2017) used a targeted NGS approach covering the globin gene cluster for a large-scale population carrier screening program among 951 individuals of the Dai population in Yunnan. In a double-blind comparative study, the authors detected a thalassemia carrier rate of 49.5% using the direct NGS screening vs. 22% using the traditional approach, including red cell indexes combined with hemoglobin electrophoresis and subsequent DNA sequencing. Almost 74.8% of alpha-thalassemia carriers and 30.5% of combined alpha- and beta-thalassemia carriers were missed in screening by the traditional approach (He et al., 2017) due to normal or borderline values of MCV, MCH, and HbA_2 typically found in the genotypes ($-\alpha^{3.7}/\alpha$ α,$- \alpha^{4.2}/\alpha$ α, α^{CS} α/α α, α^{WS} α/α α). Not all of these minor variants of the alpha-globin genes play a role in the prevention of Hb Bart's hydrops fetalis, while on the other hand, it contributes to the increased risk for HbH disease in the offspring of couples with one partner being alpha 0-thalassemia carrier.

A large study by Shang et al. (2017) including 10,111 couples demonstrated that NGS-based screening analysis covering the globin gene cluster and four modifying genes (KLF1, BCL11A, HBS1L, and MYB) identified 4,840 mutant alleles in 4,180 individuals. In total, 186 couples at risk of having affected offspring were identified, 35/186 of which would have been missed by traditional diagnostic screening. In addition, 12.1% of variants identified by the described NGS assay, would have remained undetected by the conventional methods involving selective potential carriers based on hematology and fraction identification methods, such as HPLC or CE, followed by Gap-PCR, MLPA, reverse dot blot (RDB), and Sanger sequencing (Shang et al., 2017). Preliminary studies by PCR-NGS among 57,229 cases were performed in Guangxi, China, and revealed uncommon or novel mutations (458 mutations in total) that could not be detected by conventional methods (Munkongdee et al., 2020).

Another approach was the combined NGS and Gap-PCR screening aiming to detect the common deletions responsible for 80% of the molecular causes of alpha-thalassemia, which are not routinely identified with short-read sequencing platforms. In this study, amongst 15,807 samples, 1,704 thalassemia carriers (prevalence 10.8%) were detected using a combination of hematology assays, Gap PCR, and NGS analysis. The prevalence rates of alpha-thalassemia, beta-thalassemia, and combined alpha- and beta-thalassemia were 5.97% (943/15,807), 4.48% (708/15,807), and 0.34% (53/15,807), respectively. Combined NGS and Gap-PCR have detected 40 genomic variants, including 11 rare and novel ones. Among these variants, traditionally combined RDB and Gap-PCR could detect only three deletions and 20 types of mutations. In addition, four novel thalassemia mutations and one novel abnormal hemoglobin mutation were identified by the combined NGS-PCR approach (Zhang et al., 2019). Besides, Zhao et al. (2020) have compared the combined gap-PCR and NGS method, to the routine workflow (red cell indexes, hemoglobin electrophoresis, followed by Gap PCR, and/or DNA sequencing) among 944 couples pre-pregnancy. The hematology and biochemical assays showed a lower sensitivity of 61% and a higher missed diagnosis ratio of 39% for alpha-thalassemia mutations (Zhao et al., 2020). Thus, these two studies indicate that combined hematology, GAP PCR and

NGS, is a cost-effective approach to screen for thalassemia on a large scale.

The Role of NGS in Molecular Diagnosis

Sanger sequencing of the amplified globin gene fragments has always traditionally been the golden standard in routine molecular diagnosis of thalassemia and Hb variants, because of the small size of the alpha- and beta-globin genes (approx. 1,200 bp and 1,800 bp, respectively). When an indication of a possible hemoglobinopathy was found in the family history, microcytic hypochromic parameters or abnormal separation on IEF, HPLC, CE, or Sanger sequencing was applied to detect variants in the alpha- and beta-globin genes; however, six cases of rare anemia disorders were reported, which were diagnosed by NGS as the first-tier method (Bharadwaj et al., 2020; Rizzuto et al., 2021). Globin gene abnormalities were not expected since the results from the biochemical analysis were normal and there was no indication in the family history. Because of the clinical suspicion of hemolytic anemia, a targeted gene panel, including the globin genes or trio WES, was performed. This identified rare unstable hemoglobin variants causing severe hemolytic anemias which were missed by biochemical assays (Bharadwaj et al., 2020; Rizzuto et al., 2021). Five of the reported rare unstable hemoglobin variants were related to the beta-globin genes: Hb Köln (Bharadwaj et al., 2020), Hb Bristol, Alesha, Hb Debrousse, Hb Zunyi, and finally, a novel elongating Hb variant called Hb Mokum. Only one case was caused by a mutation in the alpha-globin gene leading to Hb Evans (Rizzuto et al., 2021). Three out of six DNA variants were *de novo*, which explained why the parents were normal and an inherited trait was not expected.

Whole exome sequencing has also led to the identification of a new *trans*-acting candidate in beta-thalassemia, acting as a genocopy. Several members of two unrelated Dutch families showing beta-thalassemia trait with a characteristic of elevated HbA$_2$ and microcytic hypochromic anemia were analyzed by Sanger sequencing, which revealed two completely normal copies of the HBB gene. WES uncovered two different pathogenic splice site variants in the *SUPT5H* gene (ENSG00000196235.14) that encodes the Spt5H protein, a component of the DSIF complex. A total of eight different pathogenic variants in the *SUPT5H* gene have been identified in 25 patients with a similar beta-thalassemia minor phenotype showing no abnormalities in the HBB gene (16, Dutch; 2, French; and 7, Greek) (Achour et al., 2020).

Finally, NGS has been used to establish the genotype- and phenotype-correlation of the alpha-thalassemia X-linked intellectual disability (ATR-X) and the ATR-16 syndrome. WES of two boys with white matter changes showed an association with ATR-X as reported by Lee et al. (2015). Likewise, Babbs et al. (2020) have reported three family members with ATR-16 syndrome presenting alpha-thalassemia, intellectual disability, developmental delay, speech delay, and facial dysmorphism. These severe phenotypes are generally caused by deletions > 1 Mb contrasting with the 967 kb deletion identified in the siblings. Whole genome sequencing (WGS) was performed on specimens from the three siblings and identified a shared non-sense variant in the SMD6 gene (chromosome 15), a negative regulator of the bone morphogenetic protein signaling pathway reported to underlie craniosynostosis, speech delay, global developmental delay, fine motor impairment, and aortic valve abnormalities with variable penetrance (Babbs et al., 2020).

The identification of copy number variation and characterization of deletion/duplication breakpoints in molecular diagnostics for hemoglobinopathies is routinely done using traditional methods, such as gap-PCR and MLPA. Recently, Rangan et al. (2019) have compared long-range read sequencing methods to standard methods to identify causative mutations in complex thalassemia cases involving the beta-globin gene cluster. This showed impressive superiority and comprehensiveness to Sanger sequencing, MLPA, array CGH, and short-range sequencing technology. First, single nucleotide variants (SNVs) have been identified with a sensitivity and specificity of 99.5%. Then, large structural variants (SVs), such as large deletions, duplications, insertions, crossovers, and fusions spanning many kilobases, were characterized in the heterozygous, homozygous, and compound heterozygous state to a precise genomic coordinate. Finally, phasing SNVs identified Hb S haplotypes (Rangan et al., 2019).

The Role of NGS in Non-invasive Prenatal Diagnosis (NIPD) and Preimplantation Diagnosis (PGD)

With the advent of massive parallel sequencing (MPS), the sensitivity and precision of NIPD) on free fetal DNA in maternal circulation has been greatly enhanced. Hence, many researchers have developed new approaches based on NGS to apply NIPD to monogenic diseases, and beta-thalassemia was one of the models intensively studied. The first approach was based on the relative haplotype dosage analysis (RHDO), either by shotgun genome-wide sequencing (Lo et al., 2010) or by targeted sequencing (Lam et al., 2012) of genomic regions of interest. The principle of RHDO is to deduce the fetal inheritance of maternally transmitted mutations by quantifying the relative dosage of haplotypes looking at single nucleotide polymorphisms (SNP) in and around the target gene. These two studies clearly showed both clinical feasibility and utility of NIPD in beta-thalassemia based on PCR methodologies and NGS strategies (Lo et al., 2010; Lam et al., 2012). Vermeulen et al. (2017) utilized target locus amplification (TLA) in NIPD to achieve robust haplotyping in parents of affected offspring without the need to analyze other first-degree family members. TLA involves an initial step to crosslink physically the proximal sequences in the parental DNA. The subsequent sequencing of the targeted crosslinked region (e.g., the HBB gene cluster) using just a few primers facilitates sequencing of 10–100 kb across the locus of interest and the subsequent derivation and phasing of parental haplotypes. Targeted deep sequencing of the phased variants in cfDNA from the pregnant mother and tailored statistical analysis have allowed robust prediction of the fetal genotype relative to the disorder under investigation (Vermeulen et al., 2017). Recently, Yang et al. (2019) have developed a novel approach termed cfBEST for NIPD of monogenic disorders. Based on NGS methodology, the authors aimed to directly deduce the fetal and maternal genotypes by counting single allelic molecules and calculating the mutation ratio in cfDNA of maternal circulation without prior knowledge of parental genotypes. This approach was validated with a blinded assay among 143 pregnant women at risk for beta-thalassemia, which revealed an allele detection sensitivity of 99.1% and a specificity of 99.9% (Yang et al., 2019).

Finally, Kubikova et al. (2018) described a novel preimplantation genetic testing protocol, based on NGS technology, for the virtual detection of all mutations in the *HBB* gene. In this study, a multiplex PCR protocol has been designed allowing simultaneous amplification of multiple overlapping DNA fragments encompassing the entire *HBB* gene sequence in addition to 17 well-characterized closely linked SNP. Amplicons were subsequently analyzed using an NGS method revealing both disease-causing mutations and SNP genotypes. The *HBB* mutation status and associated SNP haplotypes were successfully determined in all 21 embryos suggesting that the combination of trophectoderm biopsy and highly sensitive NGS may provide superior accuracy than typically achieved using traditional PGD approaches (Kubikova et al., 2018).

DISCUSSION

Over the past few years, the scientific literature has proven the efficiency of NGS in research, diagnosis, and screening for many Mendelian inherited diseases. Currently, target gene panels and WES approaches have become methods of choice to detect mutations in many heterogeneous genetic diseases and have been adopted in many clinical laboratories. Although many studies have focused on the role of MPS in Mendelian diseases (Jennings et al., 2017; Kalayinia et al., 2018; Pipis et al., 2019; Pecoraro et al., 2020), the diagnostic application of NGS in hemoglobinopathies is still not widely adopted. The cost of NGS and the small size of globin genes, which facilitates Sanger sequencing, might have contributed to this delay; however, due to the continuous reduction in the cost of NGS sequencing, this might change in the future.

Next-generation sequencing has been studied as a tool for large-scale carrier screening of thalassemia among different populations living in China. Although all of these studies suggested the high accuracy of NGS in detecting carriers, this is still not easily reproducible in other populations and cost remains high, especially, for endemic low-income countries. In addition, several mutations revealed in these large-scale screening studies do not have clinical implications which make the utility of its detection questionable.

Similarly, hemoglobinopathies are unique in comparison with other diseases in that detection of carriers is possible using hematological and biochemical tests. Thus, in the majority of the cases, low-cost hematological and biochemical assays are still preferred, especially, in endemic countries. At the same time, mutations found by NGS need phenotypic information to be interpreted properly. The hematological and biochemical analyses represent the phenotype and therefore cannot be skipped according to best-practice recommendations. Furthermore, Gap-PCR as a screening step will remain mandatory to detect deletions that cause over

80% of alpha-thalassemias (Harteveld and Higgs, 2010). In addition, it is important to mention the technical difficulties in sequencing the globin genes due to the high degree of homology with duplicated- and pseudo-genes. Indeed, the presence of high homology between HBA1 and HBA2, HBB and HBD, and HBG1 and HBG2, and the presence of Alu repeats in the alpha-gene cluster, and LINE repeats in the beta-gene cluster interfere with the specificity of NGS. However, the detection of deletions/duplications/inversions and translocations using shorthead sequencing is still challenging (Yamamoto et al., 2016). Primarily, at present time, no data on detecting CNV in hemoglobinopathies using NGS are available. Furthermore, NGS is still more expensive than conventional DNA techniques used for hemoglobinopathies screening and diagnosis. We expect that with the improvement of either long-read NGS technologies, the introduction of WGS in the clinical diagnostic setting, the improvement of copy number variant detection and decrease in costs, MPS would find a vast place in routine laboratory diagnostics of hemoglobinopathies.

On the other hand, NGS has proven to be an efficient tool in resolving complex cases of thalassemia, congenital severe anemia, and hemolytic anemia that otherwise would have remained undiagnosed. The unstable dominant hemoglobin variants, such as reported by Bharadwaj et al. (2020) and Rizzuto et al. (2021), demonstrated the importance to include both globin genes and red cell membrane genes in gene panels to diagnose congenital anemia disorders. In the example of *SUPT5H*, NGS has allowed the identification of a new *trans*-acting factor gene involved in regulating beta-globin gene expression, which results in beta-thalassemia trait when haploinsufficient. This finding did not only contribute to the diagnosis and genetic counseling for families showing atypical beta-thalassemia intermedia but also opened new opportunities for a better understanding of the erythroid-specific beta-gene regulation of expression and possibly to future perspectives of gene therapy. NGS has also contributed for a better establishment of genotype-phenotype correlation of the hemoglobinopathies by identifying modifier genes in ATR-16. Although these investigations may not have direct clinical utility in prognosis and patient management at present, they may contribute to a better understanding of the pathophysiology of the hemoglobinopathies.

Finally, during the development of NIPD for hemoglobinopathies, many of the methods employed have been based on NGS and a common feature of these studies is the necessity to detect specific paternally inherited alleles. All these studies have in common the necessity to detect specific paternally inherited alleles. Although most of these studies demonstrated good specificity and sensitivity, they have inherent limitations, such as complicated procedures, a lack of versatility, and the need for prior knowledge of parental genotypes or haplotypes. NGS-based methodology of cfBEST has been used to directly deduce the fetal and maternal genotypes by counting single allelic molecules and calculating the mutation ratio in cfDNA of maternal circulation without prior knowledge of the parental genotypes. This method and TLA may provide a potentially practical, robust, and affordable approach for NIPD.

In conclusion, we speculate that NGS-based technology is not likely to replace existing methods but can be a useful additional tool in the diagnostic strategy of hemoglobinopathies, especially for large-scale genetic screening and in the discovery of novel causes of thalassemia. Although the costs are still high, the vast majority of cases can be solved by traditional Sanger sequencing of the relatively small HBA1, HBA2, and HBB genes, while NGS analysis cannot be sufficient to diagnose the hemoglobinopathies without using traditional methods involving hematology and Hb-typing to establish a proper genotype-phenotype correlation. On the other hand, NGS could have a vast place in the diagnosis of unresolved complex cases involving factors outside the alpha- and beta-globin gene clusters and in prenatal screening. The validation of long-range sequencing to adequately characterize deletions and duplications involving the alpha- and beta-globin genes and the decrease in costs would open future opportunities for NGS in the diagnosis of the hemoglobinopathies.

AUTHOR CONTRIBUTIONS

All authors listed have made a substantial, direct and intellectual contribution to the work, and approved it for publication.

ACKNOWLEDGMENTS

The authors wanted to thank Barbara Wild for reading and editing the manuscript. This work was generated within the European Reference Network on Rare Hematological Diseases (ERNEuroBloodNet, FPA 739541).

REFERENCES

Achour, A., Koopmann, T., Castel, R., Santen, G. W. E., den Hollander, N., Knijnenburg, J., et al. (2020). A new gene associated with a β-thalassemia phenotype: the observation of variants in SUPT5H. *Blood* 136, 1789–1793. doi: 10.1182/blood.2020005934

Babbs, C., Brown, J., Horsley, S. W., Slater, J., Maifoshie, E., Kumar, S., et al. (2020). ATR-16 syndrome: mechanisms linking monosomy to phenotype. *J. Med. Genet.* 57, 414–421. doi: 10.1136/jmedgenet-2019-106528

Bharadwaj, R., Raman, T., Thangadorai, R., and Munirathnam, D. (2020). Targeted Next Generation Sequencing (NGS) to diagnose hereditary hemolytic anemias. *Int. J. Hematol-Oncol. Stem Cell Res.* 14, 177–180.

Christianson, A., and Howson, C. P. (2006). *Global Report on Birth Defects. March of Dimes Birth Defects Foundation White Plains*, New York.

Farashi, S., and Harteveld, C. L. (2018). Molecular basis of α-thalassemia. *Blood Cells Mol. Dis.* 70, 43–53.

Giordano, P. C. (2009). Prospective and retrospective primary prevention of hemoglobinopathies in multiethnic societies. *Clin. Biochem.* 42, 1757–1766. doi: 10.1016/j.clinbiochem.2009.06.027

Harteveld, C. L., and Higgs, D. R. (2010). Alpha-thalassaemia. *Orphanet. J. Rare Dis.* 5:13.

Harteveld, C. L. (2018). Diagnosis of haemoglobinopathies: new scientific advances. *Thalass Rep.* 8, 7–8.

He, J., Song, W., Yang, J., Lu, S., Yuan, Y., Guo, J., et al. (2017). Next-generation sequencing improves thalassemia carrier screening among premarital adults in a high prevalence population: the Dai nationality, China. *Genet. Med.* 19, 1022–1031. doi: 10.1038/gim.2016.218

Jennings, L. J., Arcila, M. E., Corless, C., Kamel-Reid, S., Lubin, I. M., Pfeifer, J., et al. (2017). Guidelines for validation of next-generation sequencing-based oncology panels: a joint consensus recommendation of the association for molecular pathology and college of american pathologists. *J. Mol. Diagn. JMD.* 19, 341–365. doi: 10.1016/j.jmoldx.2017.01.011

Kalayinia, S., Goodarzynejad, H., Maleki, M., and Mahdieh, N. (2018). Next generation sequencing applications for cardiovascular disease. *Ann. Med.* 50, 91–109.

Kubikova, N., Babariya, D., Sarasa, J., Spath, K., Alfarawati, S., and Wells, D. (2018). Clinical application of a protocol based on universal next-generation sequencing for the diagnosis of beta-thalassaemia and sickle cell anaemia in preimplantation embryos. *Reprod. Biomed. Online* 37, 136–144. doi: 10.1016/j.rbmo.2018.05.005

Lam, K.-W. G., Jiang, P., Liao, G. J. W., Chan, K. C. A., Leung, T. Y., Chiu, R. W. K., et al. (2012). Noninvasive prenatal diagnosis of monogenic diseases by targeted massively parallel sequencing of maternal plasma: application to β-thalassemia. *Clin. Chem.* 58, 1467–1475. doi: 10.1373/clinchem.2012.189589

Lee, J. S., Lee, S., Lim, B. C., Kim, K. J., Hwang, Y. S., Choi, M., et al. (2015). Alpha-thalassemia X-linked intellectual disability syndrome identified by whole exome sequencing in two boys with white matter changes and developmental retardation. *Gene* 569, 318–322. doi: 10.1016/j.gene.2015.04.075

Lo, Y. M. D., Chan, K. C. A., Sun, H., Chen, E. Z., Jiang, P., Lun, F. M. F., et al. (2010). Maternal plasma DNA sequencing reveals the genome-wide genetic and mutational profile of the fetus. *Sci. Transl. Med.* 2:61ra91. doi: 10.1126/scitranslmed.3001720

Lobitz, S., Telfer, P., Cela, E., Allaf, B., Angastiniotis, M., Backman Johansson, C., et al. (2018). Newborn screening for sickle cell disease in Europe: recommendations from a Pan-European consensus conference. *Br. J. Haematol.* 183, 648–660.

Michlitsch, J., Azimi, M., Hoppe, C., Walters, M. C., Lubin, B., Lorey, F., et al. (2009). Newborn screening for hemoglobinopathies in California. *Pediatr. Blood Cancer* 52, 486–490. doi: 10.1002/pbc.21883

Munkongdee, T., Chen, P., Winichagoon, P., Fucharoen, S., and Paiboonsukwong, K. (2020). Update in laboratory diagnosis of thalassemia. *Front. Mol. Biosci.* 7:74. doi: 10.3389/fmolb.2020.00074

Pecoraro, V., Mandrioli, J., Carone, C., Chiò, A., Traynor, B. J., and Trenti, T. (2020). The NGS technology for the identification of genes associated with the ALS. a systematic review. *Eur. J. Clin. Invest.* 50:e13228.

Piel, F. B., Patil, A. P., Howes, R. E., Nyangiri, O. A., Gething, P. W., Dewi, M., et al. (2013). Global epidemiology of sickle haemoglobin in neonates: a contemporary geostatistical model-based map and population estimates. *Lancet Lond. Engl.* 381, 142–151. doi: 10.1016/s0140-6736(12)61229-x

Pipis, M., Rossor, A. M., Laura, M., and Reilly, M. M. (2019). Next-generation sequencing in Charcot-Marie-Tooth disease: opportunities and challenges. *Nat. Rev. Neurol.* 15, 644–656. doi: 10.1038/s41582-019-0254-5

Rangan, A., Hein, M. S., Koganti, T., Jenkinson, W. G., Hilker, C. A., Blommel, J. H., et al. (2019). Long range sequencing shows improved resolution in the detection of beta globin cluster variants. *Blood* 134(Suppl._1), 3548–3548. doi: 10.1182/blood-2019-130652

Rizzuto, V., Koopmann, T. T., Blanco-Álvarez, A., Tazón-Vega, B., Idrizovic, A., Díaz, et al. (2021). Usefulness of NGS for diagnosis of dominant beta-thalassemia and unstable hemoglobinopathies in five clinical cases. *Front. Physiol.* 12:628236. doi: 10.3389/fphys.2021.628236

Shang, X., Peng, Z., Ye, Y., Asan, Zhang, X., Chen, Y., et al. (2017). Rapid targeted next-generation sequencing platform for molecular screening and clinical genotyping in subjects with hemoglobinopathies. *EBioMedicine* 23, 150–159.

Thein, S. L. (2013). The molecular basis of β-thalassemia. *Cold Spring Harb. Perspect. Med.* 3:a011700.

Traeger-Synodinos, J., Harteveld, C. L., Old, J. M., Petrou, M., Galanello, R., Giordano, P., et al. (2015). EMQN Best Practice Guidelines for molecular and haematology methods for carrier identification and prenatal diagnosis of the haemoglobinopathies. *Eur. J. Hum. Genet. EJHG* 23, 426–437. doi: 10.1038/ejhg.2014.131

Vermeulen, C., Geeven, G., de Wit, E., Verstegen, M. J. A. M., Jansen, R. P. M., van Kranenburg, M., et al. (2017). Sensitive monogenic noninvasive prenatal diagnosis by targeted haplotyping. *Am. J. Hum. Genet.* 7, 326–339.

Weatherall, D. J. (2010). Thalassemia as a global health problem: recent progress toward its control in the developing countries. *Ann. N. Y. Acad. Sci.* 1202, 17–23. doi: 10.1111/j.1749-6632.2010.05546.x

Weatherall, D. J., and Clegg, J. B. (1996). Thalassemia — a global public health problem. *Nat. Med.* 2, 847–849. doi: 10.1038/nm0896-847

Williams, T. N., and Weatherall, D. J. (2012). World distribution, population genetics, and health burden of the hemoglobinopathies. *Cold Spring Harb. Perspect. Med.* 2:a011692. doi: 10.1101/cshperspect.a011692

World Health Organization [WHO] (1987). "WHO working group on the feasibility study on hereditary disease community control programmes," in *Proceedings of the Meeting (5th: 1987: Herakleion G, Programme WHOHD. Report of the Vth Annual Meeting of the WHO Working Group on the Feasibility Study on Hereditary Disease Community Control Programmes (Hereditary anaemias: alpha thalassaemia, Herakleion, Crete, 21-24 October 1987*, (Geneva: WHO).

Yamamoto, T., Shimojima, K., Ondo, Y., Imai, K., Chong, P. F., Kira, R., et al. (2016). Challenges in detecting genomic copy number aberrations using next-generation sequencing data and the eXome Hidden Markov Model: a clinical exome-first diagnostic approach. *Hum. Genome Var.* 3:16025.

Yang, X., Zhou, Q., Zhou, W., Zhong, M., Guo, X., Wang, X., et al. (2019). A cell-free DNA barcode-enabled single-molecule test for noninvasive prenatal diagnosis of monogenic disorders: application to β-Thalassemia. *Adv. Sci. Weinh Baden-Wurtt Ger.* 6:1802332. doi: 10.1002/advs.201802332

Zhang, H., Li, C., Li, J., Hou, S., Chen, D., Yan, H., et al. (2019). Next-generation sequencing improves molecular epidemiological characterization of thalassemia in Chenzhou region. P.R. China. *J. Clin. Lab. Anal.* 33:e22845. doi: 10.1002/jcla.22845

Zhao, J., Li, J., Lai, Q., and Yu, Y. (2020). Combined use of gap-PCR and next-generation sequencing improves thalassaemia carrier screening among premarital adults in China. *J. Clin. Pathol.* 73, 488–492. doi: 10.1136/jclinpath-2019-206339

17

Comparative Analysis of Iron Homeostasis in Sub-Saharan African Children with Sickle Cell Disease and their Unaffected Siblings

Selma Gomez[1,2†], Aïssatou Diawara[3†], Elias Gbeha[4], Philip Awadalla[4], Ambaliou Sanni[1], Youssef Idaghdour[3]* and M. Cherif Rahimy[2]*

[1] Laboratoire de Biochimie et de Biologie Moléculaire, Faculté des Sciences et Techniques, University of Abomey-Calavi, Cotonou, Benin, [2] Centre de Prise en charge Médicale Intégrée du Nourrisson et de la Femme Enceinte atteints de Drépanocytose, Faculté des Sciences de la Santé, University of Abomey-Calavi, Cotonou, Benin, [3] Biology Program, Division of Science and Mathematics, New York University Abu Dhabi, Abu Dhabi, United Arab Emirates, [4] Sainte-Justine Research Centre, Centre Hospitalier et Universitaire Sainte Justine, Montréal, QC, Canada

*Correspondence:
Youssef Idaghdour
youssef.idaghdour@nyu.edu;
M. Cherif Rahimy
mrahimy@bj.refer.org,
mrahimy2@yahoo.fr

†Selma Gomez and Aïssatou Diawara contributed equally to this work.

Iron is an essential trace element subject to tight regulation to ensure adequate running of biological processes. In sub-Saharan Africa where hemoglobinopathies are common, iron homeostasis is likely to be impaired by these conditions. Here, we assessed and compared key serum proteins associated with iron metabolism between sub-Saharan African children with sickle cell disease (SCD) and their unaffected siblings. Complete blood counts and serum concentrations of four key proteins involved in iron regulation (ferritin, transferrin, sTfR, and hepcidin) were measured for 73 children with SCD and 68 healthy siblings in Benin, West Africa. We found significant differences in concentration of transferrin, sTfR, and ferritin between the two groups. Hepcidin concentrations were found at unusually high concentrations but did not differ among the two groups. We found a significant negative correlation between hepcidin levels and both MCH and MCV in the SCD group and report that sTfR concentrations show a correlation with MCV and MHC in opposite directions in the two groups. These results highlight the unusually high levels of hepcidin in the Beninese population and the patterns of differential iron homeostasis taking place under SCD status. These results lay the foundation for a systematic evaluation of the underlying mechanisms deregulating iron homeostasis in populations with SCD or high prevalence of iron deficiency.

Keywords: iron homeostasis, sickle cell disease, anemia, iron deficiency, hepcidin, serum iron proteins, red blood cell indices

INTRODUCTION

Sickle cell disease (SCD), an inherited disorder of hemoglobin (Hb) structure, is one of the most common severe disorders in the world (1). In 2010, sub-Saharan Africa accounted for two-third of SCD births worldwide, making it the most burdened region (2). In Benin, the under-five mortality rate of SCD was estimated at 15.5/1,000 in a cohort of patients benefiting from a tailored comprehensive clinical care program (CCCP) (3). SCD can also lead to severe complications in affected individuals, including significant homeostasis imbalance. Furthermore, imbalance in iron metabolism could be more accentuated in area where iron deficiency is a large health problem, such as in Benin (4, 5). Thus, it is of interest to study the patterns of iron homeostasis in a context in which both iron deficiency and SCD are common.

Regulation of iron supply is essential to ensure adequate running of biological processes, such as erythroid function, binding and transport of oxygen as well as cellular respiration, and DNA synthesis and reparation (6, 7). Iron deficiency in early childhood is associated with numerous adverse health effects, including immune, neurological, and cognitive development impairments that may be irreversible even after iron repletion (8, 9). Similarly, excess of iron is deleterious for health and has become a major cause of morbidity and premature mortality (10, 11). The total iron store in the human body is approximately 3–4 g and is mainly distributed in the Hb of mature red blood cells and developing erythroid cells. In normal conditions 1–2 mg of iron is absorbed daily and an equivalent amount is lost. There is no physiological system for iron elimination; however, iron metabolism, storage, and transport are tightly regulated by a key set of proteins (12, 13). The regulation of iron homeostasis depends on a complex feedback mechanism between body iron requirements and intestinal absorption. Thus, iron stores are subject to tight control from intake in the intestine to storage, turnover, redistribution, and mobilization in the body (13, 14).

In the last decades, there have been tremendous advances in deciphering the mechanisms of iron homeostasis in the body and the understanding of the interplay between serum proteins implicated in this process. Of these proteins, hepcidin, a small 25-amino-acid peptide, produced mainly by hepatocytes and secreted into the blood has been recognized as a key regulator in homeostasis. (15–17). Other key iron metabolism proteins in the serum include ferritin, transferrin, and soluble transferrin protein (sTfR). Polymorphisms in these proteins could affect iron metabolism (18, 19). However, such genetic variants have not been documented in Benin.

In this study, we compared key parameters of iron homeostasis between children with SCD (cases) and their unaffected siblings (control group) in the Republic of Benin, West Africa. We assessed and compared relevant hematological indicators and the serum proteins directly linked to iron metabolism between the two groups and evaluated the relationship between these hematological indicators and the serum iron proteins.

MATERIALS AND METHODS

Subjects

A total of 141 children were enrolled in our study in 2010, including 73 children with SCD. These children were part of a large cohort of early diagnosis for SCD and CCCP (20) at the "Centre de Prise en charge Médicale Intégrée du Nourrisson et de la Femme Enceinte atteints de Drépanocytose" (CPMI-NFED) (National Institute dedicated to caring of Infants and Pregnant Women affected by SCD) in Cotonou, The Republic of Benin. The CCCP includes an intensive socio-medical intervention program that aims to diagnose SCD early and to attenuate the effects of the disease on children as they grow up. As part of the

clinical follow-up program children orally received powdered generic containing 5 mg/kg/day of elemental iron with orange or lemon juice 30 min before meals. This iron supplementation was provided every 9 months for a period of 2 months. All children with SCD were sampled at least 1 month after they finished their iron supplementation regime and none of the unaffected children were taking iron during the course of the study. Of the 73 children with SCD, 15 were diagnosed with acute anemia and were transfused during the 4 months preceding sampling of which 8 were transfused once, two twice, one three time, and one six time. The control group consisted of 68 age-matched siblings of the recruited children with SCD. Approval for the study was obtained from the Ethical Committee of the Faculty of Health Sciences.

Procedures

Children with SCD were enrolled in the study after informed consent was obtained. All children were sampled under steady state during regular follow-up visits in the morning between 8:00 and 11:00 a.m. Based on clinical assessment, age-matched unaffected siblings, without any history of acute illness at least 3 months prior to sampling, were brought by parents for sampling after informed consent was obtained. Complete blood counts (CBC) were immediately performed using an automatic blood cell analyzer (KX-21, Sysmex Corporation, Japan) (Table S1 in Supplementary Material). Sera were frozen and stored at −30°C for subsequent measurement of ferritin, transferrin, sTfR, and hepcidin.

Serum ferritin, transferrin, sTfR, and hepcidin concentrations were measured using their respective ELISA kits following the manufacturers' recommended protocols: IBL International GMBH, Hamburg, Germany, for ferritin and Hepcidin and Prohormone, Modrice, Czech Republic, for transferrin and sTfR (Table S1 in Supplementary Material). The sTfR index was calculated as the ratio of log (sTfR) (nanogram/milliliter) to the log (serum ferritin) (nanogram/milliliter) as previously described (21). The reference ranges for iron homeostasis serum proteins indicating normal iron status were defined as follow: 25–283 ng/L for ferritin, 2–5 g/L for transferrin, 0.9–3.4 μg/mL for sTfR, 58.9–158.1 ng/mL for hepcidin, and 1.5 for the log (sTfR)/log (ferritin) ratio (22). For Hb, we used the pediatric cut off value defined by the World Health Organization (WHO) (23). The cut off values for the red blood cell indices were as follow: MCH < 25 pg and MCV < 75 fL.

Data Statistical Analysis

Quantitative data were analyzed using Kruskal–Wallis, Wilcoxon and median non-parametric tests. A linear regression model was used to test for differential association in SCD patients and the control group between key hematological parameters and the assayed iron regulation proteins. Sex and age were included in regression analyses as covariates. These analyses test the hypothesis that proteins directly involved in iron homeostasis are (a) differentially regulated between SCD patients and their unaffected siblings and (b) influence iron homeostasis through regulation of MCH and MCV, two of the indices most correlated with iron regulation in the body. Hypothesis (a) was tested by comparing the mean and variance of the concentration of the assayed proteins between SCD patients and the controls. Hypothesis *(b)* was tested by comparing the relationship between both MCH and MCV, as dependent variables, and the assayed proteins in the SCD and control groups.

RESULTS

Subject Characteristics

A total of 141 children, 73 SCD patients with Hb genotypes SS (53) or SC (20) and 68 unaffected siblings with Hb genotypes AA (21), AS (45), or AC (2) were recruited. The demographic, gender, and Hb characteristics of both groups are listed in **Table 1**. Age and sex distributions were not significantly different between the two groups ($p = 0.1518$ and $p = 0.1595$, respectively).

Hematological Profiles

Hematological details of patients in the steady state and controls are summarized in **Table 2**. As expected, the mean Hb concentration was significantly lower ($p < 0.0001$) in children with SCD (87.8 g/L) compared to the control group (110.0 g/L) with 87.7% of children having Hb values below the normal distribution. We note that in the control group 20.4% of children had a mean Hb concentration below the WHO's threshold defining anemia in the corresponding age group (23). We also note that mean concentration for both red blood cell indices MCV and MCH were significantly reduced in the control group ($p < 0.001$) as 54 and 85% of children in the control group had MCV and MCH values below the cut off value of 75 fL and 25 pg, compared to 30 and 52% in the SCD group, respectively.

Serum Iron Protein Profiles in the Control and SCD Groups

Mean concentrations of transferrin, sTfR, ferritin, and the log (sTfR)/log (ferritin) index were statistically different ($p < 0.001$)

between the SCD and control groups but hepcidin ($p = 0.6487$, **Table 3**). Testing for equal variances between SCD and control groups for the four proteins revealed that variance was significantly different except for hepcidin (**Figure 1**). In particular, we note the extreme case of ferritin that shows striking difference in variance between the two groups (**Figure 1**).

The mean values of transferrin and the log (sTfR)/log (ferritin) index were within the normal range (2–5 g/L and ≥1.5, respectively) in children with SCD (4.1 g/L and 5.9, respectively) whereas both were above the upper limit of normal values in the control group (6.9 g/L and 1.8, respectively). In addition, 67 and 79% of individuals in the control group have transferrin and sTfR index concentrations above the cut off. By contrast, in children with SCD, ferritin and sTfR levels were almost twofold above the upper limit of normal ferritin and sTfR (558.9 ng/L for ferritin and 5.9 µg/mL for sTfR), while in the control group both concentrations were within the normal ranges (59.0 ng/L for ferritin and 2 µg/mL for sTfR). We also compared ferritin concentration levels between SCD children with past history of blood transfusions and those who have never been transfused. The mean ferritin concentrations were not significantly different ($p = 0.1072$) between transfused and non-transfused children, suggesting that blood transfusion does not explain the observed high level of ferritin in children with SCD (Figure 1 in Supplementary Material). Finally, intriguingly in both SCD and control groups, mean hepcidin concentration were unexpectedly high (231.6 and 225.6 ng/mL, respectively) and above the upper limit of normal hepcidin values of 58.9–158.1 ng/mL. We should also note that within the control group, mean transferrin concentrations were found to be significantly different between AA and AS/C genotypes ($p = 0.006$) (Figure 2 in Supplementary Material).

Correlation between the Four Iron Homeostasis Serum Proteins and MCV and MCH

We performed multiple regression analyses to examine the relationship between the four serum iron proteins and MVC and MCH levels in SCD and control groups. First, we constructed a multivariate statistical model that includes all four serum proteins assayed against MCV or MCH. The predicted against actual Y plots (**Figures 2** and **3**) show that the models fit best in the SCD group ($p = 0.0004$ and $p = 0.0107$, respectively) relative to the control group where the fit is not statistically significant ($p = 0.2439$ and $p = 0.4725$, respectively). Univariate analyses showed that hepcidin concentrations were negatively correlated with MCV and MCH levels in the SCD group (Pearson correlation $r^2 = 0.1502$, $p = 0.0007$ and $r^2 = 0.0167$, $p = 0.0005$, respectively, **Figures 2** and **3**). Also, sTfR concentrations show opposite trends in the two groups being negatively correlated with MCV and MCH in the control group ($r^2 = 0.0946$, $p = 0.0127$ and $r^2 = 0.0915$, $p = 0.0143$, respectively) and positively correlated with MCV and MCH in the SCD group ($r^2 = 0.1593$, $p = 0.0005$ and $r^2 = 0.0283$, $p = 0.1548$, respectively) (**Figures 2** and **3**). We note that transferrin and ferritin show the same trend as sTfR in both groups but it is not statistically significant (Figure 3 in Supplementary Material). These findings show that the association between key

TABLE 1 | Characteristics of the study subjects.

	SCD patients	Controls
Patients, n (%)	73 (100%)	68 (100%)
Male gender	43 (58.9%)	32 (47.1%)
Female gender	30 (41.1%)	36 (52.9%)
Median age, month (range)	36 (12–72)	33.5 (6–72)
Hemoglobin (Hb) type, n (%)		
HbSS	53 (72.6%)	0
HbSC	20 (27.4%)	0
HbAA	0	30 (30.9%)
HbAS	0	45 (66.2%)
HbAC	0	2 (2.9%)

TABLE 2 | Hematological values in steady-state SCD patients and the controls.

Indicators	SCD patients, mean ± SD	Controls, mean ± SD	p-value
Hemoglobin concentration (g/L)	87.8 ± 15.8	110.0 ± 9.0	<0.0001
MCV (fL)	79.2 ± 8.2	73.6 ± 6.1	<0.0001
MCH (pg)	25.0 ± 2.8	23.2 ± 2.4	<0.0001

TABLE 3 | Iron homeostasis serum proteins profiles in SCD patients in the steady state and in controls.

Proteins	SCD patients			Controls			p-value[c]
	Mean ± SD	Subjects with values above the cut-off[a], n (%)	Median/ interquartile range[b]	Mean ± SD	Median/ interquartile range[b]	Subjects with values above the cut-off[a], n (%)	
Transferrin (g/L)	4.1 ± 1.5	16 (21.9)	–	6.9 ± 3.1	–	46 (67.6)	<0.0001
sTfR (µg/mL)	5.9 ± 2.2	56 (76.7)	–	1.8 ± 0.7	–	5 (6.8)	<0.0001
Ferritin (ng/L)	558.9 ± 434.7	48 (65.8)	445.6/(174.8–933.3)	44.0 ± 28.9	37.6/(24.3–54.5)	0	<0.0001
sTfR index	1.5 ± 0.3	25 (34.2)	–	2.1 ± 0.9	–	58 (79.4)	<0.0001
Hepcidin (ng/mL)	231.6 ± 128.2	47 (64.4)	215.2/(127.3–287.4)	225.6 ± 135.1	192.9/(130.3–296.9)	41 (56.2)	0.6487

[a]Cut-off values defined in Section "Materials and Methods."
[b]Median and interquartile range for non-normally distributed proteins ferritin and hepcidin.
[c]Wilcoxon test, means comparisons.

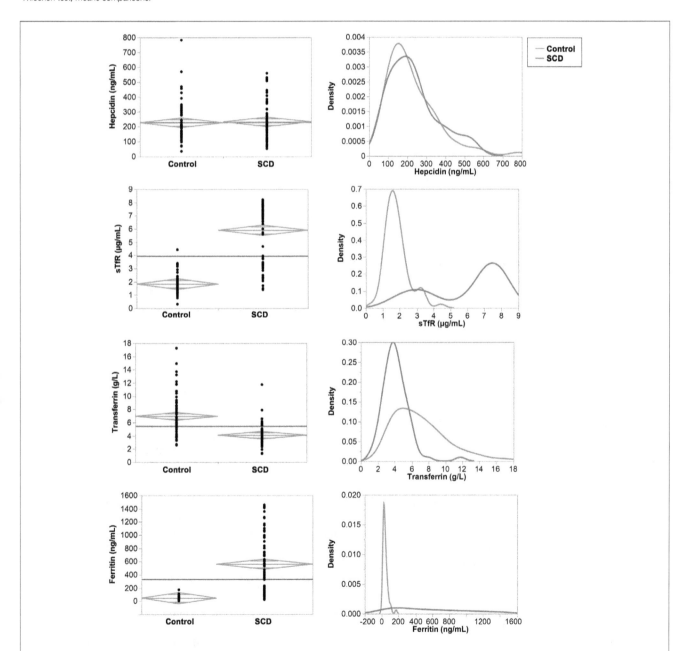

FIGURE 1 | Comparisons of means and variances of the four iron serum proteins in the control and SCD groups. Right panel: the diamonds show the 95% confidence intervals and the horizontal black line shows the mean value across the entire set of individuals. **Left panel**: the densities show the distribution of each protein in the control and SCD groups.

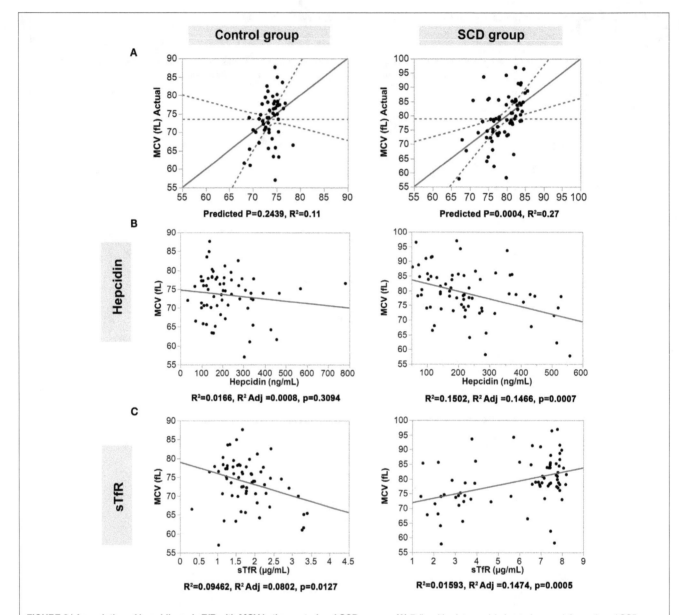

FIGURE 2 | Association of hepcidin and sTfR with MCV in the control and SCD groups. **(A)** Full multivariate models (control group, left panel, and SCD group, right panel). **(B,C)** Univariate models testing the association of each protein (control group, left panels, and SCD group, right panel). The red solid line shows the line of fit, the red dashed line represents the 95% confidence curves and the blue dashed line shows the horizontal mean reference that represents the null hypothesis.

hematological indicators (i.e., MCH and MCV) and hepcidin and sTfR is altered under the SCD condition.

To test for the effect of blood transfusion of the observed differences, we removed from the analysis the study participants who received blood transfusion and observed no significant differences in the results. To test for differences between genotypic classes within the control group, we performed the association tests by genotype (AA and AS/C groups). Of the four proteins investigated and although not statistically significant, hepcidin and ferritin concentrations showed two opposite trends in the two groups, being positively correlated with MCV and MCH in the AA group and negatively correlated in the AS/C group (Figure 4 in Supplementary Material). These findings

demonstrate that the observed differences in hepcidin and ferritin between the SCD and control groups detailed above are more pronounced when SCD patients are compared to the AA genotype group.

DISCUSSION

Sickle cell disease is common throughout much of sub-Saharan Africa. In Benin, SCD is associated with high rate of childhood mortality and morbidity (3). Although many aspects of SCD are studied, reports on proteins involved in iron homeostasis in children with SCD are scarce. Given the above, we conducted this study to document the patterns of iron metabolism in young

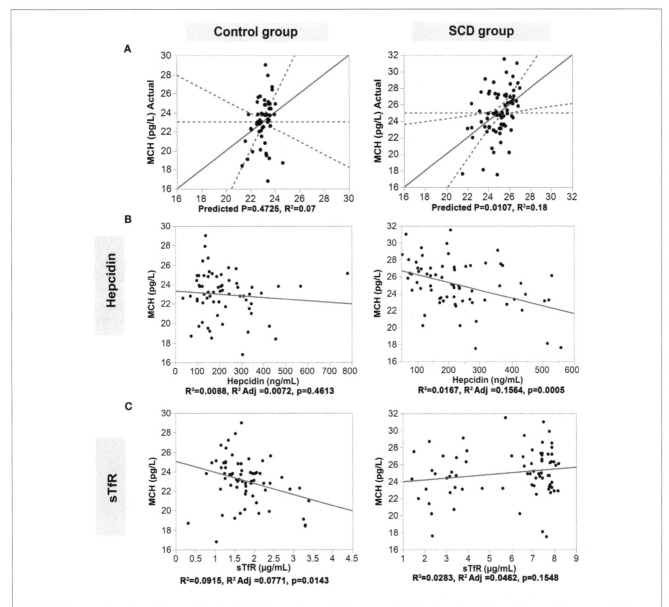

FIGURE 3 | Association of hepcidin and sTfR with MCH in the control and SCD groups. (A) Full multivariate models (control group, left panel, and SCD group, right panel). (B,C) Univariate models testing the association of each protein (control group, left panels, and SCD group, right panel). The red solid line shows the line of fit, the red dashed line represents the 95% confidence curves and the blue dashed line shows the horizontal mean reference that represents the null hypothesis.

children with and without SCD by examining hematological indices and four key serum iron metabolism-associated proteins.

The hematological indices assessed closely in our study are Hb, MCV, and MCH. Subjects with SCD had significantly lower levels of Hb compared to the controls. This observation was expected considering the physiopathology of the disease. We also note that 20.4% control children had Hb levels below the normal range but this was not associated with the sickle cell trait phenotype. In contrast to other reports (24, 25), SCD subjects in our study had higher levels of RBC indices compared to the control group. This observation could be due to the effect of the follow-up clinical program, part of which children take iron supplements (13).

These low values could be explained partly by iron deficiency, one of the main causes of anemia (26, 27). Rahimy et al. (5) previously showed that iron deficiency was a predominant condition in healthy young children in Benin. Our results are consistent with this finding, suggesting that the hematological levels in our control group are in line with the hematological profiles reported in the general pediatric population in Benin.

To assess the effect of SCD status on indicators and parameters associated with iron homeostasis (22, 28, 29), we compared the concentration of four serum iron proteins (transferrin, ferritin, sTfR, and hepcidin) and the log (sTfR)/log (ferritin) index between SCD subjects and controls. Iron balance is regulated by modulating the rate of erythropoiesis and by the amount of iron stores (30). When iron is deficient, the concentration of transferrin and sTfR increases, while that of ferritin synthesis and hepcidin declines (31, 32). In contrast to the control group, the SCD group had elevated concentrations of ferritin and sTfR and lower levels of transferrin and log (sTfR)/log (ferritin) index. Such elevated concentrations of ferritin and sTfR are usually associated with iron overload and have been reported in the case of blood transfusion (33, 34). However, this scenario is unlikely in our study as we do not observe a significant association between blood transfusion history and ferritin concentration in our cohort, suggesting the presence of an excess of intravascular hemolysis causing an increase of iron absorption as previously reported (35). Elevated levels of ferritin contrasted with normal levels of transferrin and sTfR and a normal log (sTfR)/log (ferritin) index. This observation is intriguing and warrants further investigation to unravel the underlying mechanisms.

Intriguingly, we observed high levels of hepcidin in both SCD group and controls with approximately 65 and 56% of individuals in SCD and control group, respectively, showing hepcidin levels above the upper limit of the normal range. This observation suggests that the high level of hepcidin is a common trait in Beninese children. We also observed a significant negative correlation between hepcidin levels and both MCH and MCV only in the SCD group and an opposite trend for sTfR and both MCH and MCV in the control group (negative correlation) and in the SCD group (positive correlation). We also assessed the potential effect of sickle cell trait genotype on iron homeostasis proteins by stratifying the control group by genotype (AA versus AS/C) in our association analysis. Several studies have highlighted the link between SCD trait genotypes and conditions, such as systemic inflammation (36) and oxidative stress (37). Our results show differences between AA and AS/C genotypes and demonstrate that the opposite trends observed for hepcidin and ferritin between SCD patients and the controls are driven by the AA individuals. Normal to low levels of hepcidin in SCD have been previously reported (38, 39). However, our results do not support the generalization of these findings. This observation hints to the possibility that the effect of other variables modulating the production of hepcidin might be in play in our cohort or in West African populations in general as indicated by the unusually high levels of hepcidin even in the unaffected group. High levels of hepcidin under severe iron deficiency have only been reported

in pathological conditions, such as rare hepatic adenomas and familial iron-refractory iron deficiency anemia (40, 41). In our study population, it is unlikely that the observed patterns results from pathological conditions, given our knowledge of medical history of the study subjects and given that the trend is observed in both disease and control groups. The observed relationship between hepcidin and MCH and MCV in populations such as Benin where iron deficiency is prevalent can also be modulated by diet and/or selective pressure to maintain low levels of iron in the body against infectious agents that require high levels of iron (42–45). We hypothesize that these factors contribute to the negative correlation we observe between hepcidin and both MCH and MCV, an effect exacerbated under SCD status. However, further investigations are required to confirm these hypotheses. Our study also highlights the unusually high levels of hepcidin in the Beninese population and the differential patterns of iron homeostasis through the association between hepcidin levels and key hematological parameters. Furthermore, SCD patients are more likely to suffer from nutritional deficiencies caused by increased metabolic requirements (46, 47). Polymorphisms in genes coding for iron regulation proteins can also modulate the mechanisms of iron metabolisms (48). Future studies should account for these variables that can alter the expression and/or function of the key iron metabolism proteins.

These results lay the foundation for a systematic evaluation of the underlying mechanisms deregulating iron homeostasis in populations with SCD or high prevalence of iron deficiency.

AUTHOR CONTRIBUTIONS

MCR and AS designed the study, MCR and YI supervised the study, EG and PA provided reagents, SG performed the experiments, AD analyzed the data, and MCR, YI, and AD wrote the manuscript.

ACKNOWLEDGMENTS

We would like to thank the children who participated in the study and their families.

REFERENCES

Serjeant GR. Sickle-cell disease. *Lancet* (1997) **350**:725–30. doi:10.1016/ S0140-6736(97)07330-3

Piel FB, Hay SI, Gupta S, Weatherall DJ, Williams TN. Global burden of sickle cell anaemia in children under five, 2010-2050: modelling based on demographics, excess mortality, and interventions. *PLoS Med* (2013) **10**:e1001484. doi:10.1371/journal.pmed.1001484

Rahimy MC, Gangbo A, Ahouignan G, Alihonou E. Newborn screening

for sickle cell disease in the Republic of Benin. *J Clin Pathol* (2009) **62**:46–8. doi:10.1136/jcp.2008.059113

Hercberg S, Chauliac M, Galan P, Devanlay M, Zohoun I, Agboton Y, et al. Prevalence of iron deficiency and iron-deficiency anaemia in Benin. *Public Health* (1988) **102**:73–83. doi:10.1016/S0033-3506(88)80013-1

Rahimy MC, Fanou L, Somasse YE, Gangbo A, Ahouignan G, Alihonou E. When to start supplementary iron to prevent iron deficiency in early childhood in sub-Saharan Africa setting. *Pediatr Blood Cancer* (2007) **48**:544–9. doi:10.1002/pbc.21103

Joshi RS, Moran E, Sanchez M. *Cellular Iron Metabolism. The IRP/IRE Regulatory Network. Iron Metabolism.* Barcelona: InTech (2012).

Abbaspour N, Hurrell R, Kelishadi R. Review on iron and its importance for human health. *J Res Med Sci* (2014) **19**:164–74.

Onabanjo OO, Jerling JC, Covic N, Van Graan A, Taljaard C, Mamabolo RL. Association between iron status and white blood cell counts in African schoolchildren of the North-West Province, South Africa. *J Epidemiol Glob Health* (2012) **2**:103–10. doi:10.1016/j.jegh.2012.07.003

Subramaniam G, Girish M. Iron deficiency anemia in children. *Indian J Pediatr* (2015) **82**(6):558–64. doi:10.1007/s12098-014-1643-9

Fleming RE, Ponka P. Iron overload in human disease. *N Engl J Med* (2012) **366**:348–59. doi:10.1056/NEJMra1004967

Siddique A, Kowdley KV. Review article: the iron overload syndromes. *Aliment Pharmacol Ther* (2012) **35**:876–93. doi:10.1111/j.1365-2036.2012.05051.x

Arora S, Kapoor RK. Iron metobolism in humans: an overview. In: Arora S, editor. *Iron Metabolism.* Basaidarapur: InTech (2012). 186 p.

Ganz T, Nemeth E. Iron metabolism: interactions with normal and disordered erythropoiesis. *Cold Spring Harb Perspect Med* (2012) **2**:a011668. doi:10.1101/cshperspect.a011668

Wang J, Pantopoulos K. Regulation of cellular iron metabolism. *Biochem J* (2011) **434**:365–81. doi:10.1042/BJ20101825

Nicolas G, Vaulont S. [Deciphering the action mechanism of hepcidin]. *Med Sci (Paris)* (2005) **21**:7–9. doi:10.1051/medsci/20052117

Ganz T, Nemeth E. Hepcidin and iron homeostasis. *Biochim Biophys Acta* (2012) **1823**:1434–43. doi:10.1016/j.bbamcr.2012.01.014

Ganz T. Systemic iron homeostasis. *Physiol Rev* (2013) **93**:1721–41. doi:10.1152/physrev.00008.2013

Lee PL, Halloran C, Trevino R, Felitti V, Beutler E. Human transferrin G277S mutation: a risk factor for iron deficiency anaemia. *Br J Haematol* (2001) **115**:329–33. doi:10.1046/j.1365-2141.2001.03096.x

Kasvosve I, Delanghe JR, Gomo ZA, Gangaidzo IT, Khumalo H, Wuyts B, et al. Transferrin polymorphism influences iron status in blacks. *Clin Chem* (2000) **46**:1535–9.

Rahimy MC, Gangbo A, Ahouignan G, Adjou R, Deguenon C, Goussanou S, et al. Effect of a comprehensive clinical care program on disease course in severely ill children with sickle cell anemia in a sub-Saharan African setting. *Blood* (2003) **102**:834–8. doi:10.1182/blood-2002-05-1453

Oustamanolakis P, Koutroubakis IE, Messaritakis I, Niniraki M, Kouroumalis EA. Soluble transferrin receptor-ferritin index in the evaluation of anemia in inflammatory bowel disease: a case-control study. *Ann Gastroenterol* (2011) **24**:108–14.

Infusino I, Braga F, Dolci A, Pantheghini M. Soluble transferrin receptor (sTfR) and sTfR/log ferritin index for the diagnosis of iron-deficiency anemia. A meta-analysis. *Am J Clin Pathol* (2012) **138**:642–9. doi:10.1309/AJCP16NTXZLZFAIB

WHO. *Haemoglobin Concentrations for the Diagnosis of Anaemia and Assessment of Severity.* Geneva: World Health Organization (2011). 6 p.

Valavi E, Ansari MJ, Zandian K. How to reach rapid diagnosis in sickle cell disease? *Iran J Pediatr* (2010) **20**:69–74.

Akodu SO, Kehinde OA, Diaku-Akinwumi IN, Njokanma OF. Iron deficiency anaemia among pre-school children with sickle cell anaemia: still a rare diagnosis? *Mediterr J Hematol Infect Dis* (2013) **5**:e2013069. doi:10.4084/MJHID.2013.069

Bhukhanvala DS, Sorathiya SM, Shah AP, Patel AG, Gupte SC. Prevalence and hematological profile of beta-thalassemia and sickle cell anemia in four communities of Surat city. *Indian J Hum Genet* (2012) **18**:167–71. doi:10.4103/0971-6866.100752

Payandeh M, Rahimi Z, Zare ME, Kansestani AN, Gohardehi F, Hashemian AH. The prevalence of anemia and hemoglobinopathies in the hematologic clinics of the kermanshah province, Western iran. *Int J Hematol Oncol Stem Cell Res* (2014) **8**:33–7.

Coyne D. Iron indices: what do they really mean? *Kidney Int Suppl* (2006):S4–8. doi:10.1038/sj.ki.5000404

Berlin T, Meyer A, Rotman-Pikielny P, Natur A, Levy Y. Soluble transferrin receptor as a diagnostic laboratory test for detection of iron deficiency anemia in acute illness of hospitalized patients. *Isr Med Assoc J* (2011) **13**:96–8.

Finch C. Regulators of iron balance in humans. *Blood* (1994) **84**:1697–702. Theil EC. Regulation of ferritin and transferrin receptor mRNAs. *J Biol Chem* (1990) **265**:4771–4.

Eisenstein RS, Blemings KP. Iron regulatory proteins, iron responsive elements and iron homeostasis. *J Nutr* (1998) **128**:2295–8.

Walter PB, Harmatz P, Vichinsky E. Iron metabolism and iron chelation in sickle cell disease. *Acta Haematol* (2009) **122**:174–83. doi:10.1159/000243802

Porter J, Garbowski M. Consequences and management of iron overload in sickle cell disease. *Hematology Am Soc Hematol Educ Program* (2013) **2013**:447–56. doi:10.1182/asheducation-2013.1.447

Ray D, Mondal R, Chakravarty UK, Burman DR. Assessment of iron status in patient of sickle cell disease and trait and its relationship with the frequency of blood transfusion in paediatric patients attending at B.S. Medical College & Hospital, Bankura, West Bengal, India. *Int J Sci* (2014) **2**:37–9.

Tripete J, Connes P, Hedreville M, Etienne-Julan M, Marlin L, Hue O, et al. Patterns of exercise-related inflammatory response in sickle cell trait carriers. *Br J Sports Med* (2010) **44**:232–7. doi:10.1136/bjsm.2008.047530

Faes C, Balayssac-Siransy E, Connes P, Hivert L, Danho C, Bogui P, et al. Moderate endurance exercise in patients with sickle cell anaemia: effects on oxidative stress and endothelial activation. *Br J Haematol* (2014) **164**:124–30. doi:10.1111/bjh.12594

Kearney SL, Nemeth E, Neufeld EJ, Thapa D, Ganz T, Weinstein DA, et al. Urinary hepcidin in congenital chronic anemias. *Pediatr Blood Cancer* (2007) **48**:57–63. doi:10.1002/pbc.20616

Kroot JJ, Laarakkers CM, Kemna EH, Biemond BJ, Swinkels DW. Regulation of serum hepcidin levels in sickle cell disease. *Haematologica* (2009) **94**:885–7. doi:10.3324/haematol.2008.003152

Weinstein DA, Roy CN, Fleming MD, Loda MF, Wolfsdorf JI, Andrews NC. Inappropriate expression of hepcidin is associated with iron refractory anemia: implications for the anemia of chronic disease. *Blood* (2002) **100**:3776–81. doi:10.1182/blood-2002-04-1260

Finberg KE, Heeney MM, Campagna DR, Aydinok Y, Pearson HA, Hartman KR, et al. Mutations in TMPRSS6 cause iron-refractory iron deficiency anemia (IRIDA). *Nat Genet* (2008) **40**:569–71. doi:10.1038/ng.130

Boelaert JR, Vandecasteele SJ, Appelberg R, Gordeuk VR. The effect of the host's iron status on tuberculosis. *J Infect Dis* (2007) **195**:1745–53. doi:10.1086/518040

Schaible UE, Kaufmann SH. Iron and microbial infection. *Nat Rev Microbiol* (2004) **2**:946–53. doi:10.1038/nrmicro1046

Sazawal S, Black RE, Ramsan M, Chwaya HM, Stoltzfus RJ, Dutta A, et al. Effects of routine prophylactic supplementation with iron and folic acid on admission to hospital and mortality in preschool children in a high malaria transmission setting: community-based, randomised, placebo-controlled trial. *Lancet* (2006) **367**:133–43. doi:10.1016/S0140-6736(06)67962-2

Drakesmith H, Prentice A. Viral infection and iron metabolism. *Nat Rev Microbiol* (2008) **6**:541–52. doi:10.1038/nrmicro1930

Hyacinth HI, Gee BE, Hibbert JM. The role of nutrition in sickle cell disease. *Nutr Metab Insights* (2010) **3**:57–67. doi:10.4137/NMI.S5048

Hibbert JM, Creary MS, Gee BE, Buchanan ID, Quarshie A, Hsu LL. Erythropoiesis and myocardial energy requirements contribute to the hypermetabolism of childhood sickle cell anemia. *J Pediatr Gastroenterol Nutr* (2006) **43**:680–7. doi:10.1097/01.mpg.0000228120.44606.d6

Pelusi S, Girelli D, Rametta R, Campostrini N, Alfieri C, Traglia M, et al. The A736V TMPRSS6 polymorphism influences hepcidin and iron metabolism in chronic hemodialysis patients: TMPRSS6 and hepcidin in hemodialysis. *BMC Nephrol* (2013) **14**:48. doi:10.1186/1471-2369-14-48

Usefulness of NGS for Diagnosis of Dominant Beta-Thalassemia and Unstable Hemoglobinopathies in Five Clinical Cases

Valeria Rizzuto[1,2,3], Tamara T. Koopmann[4], Adoración Blanco-Álvarez[5], Barbara Tazón-Vega[5], Amira Idrizovic[1], Cristina Díaz de Heredia[6], Rafael Del Orbe[7], Miriam Vara Pampliega[7], Pablo Velasco[6], David Beneitez[8], Gijs W. E. Santen[4], Quinten Waisfisz[9], Mariet Elting[9], Frans J. W. Smiers[10], Anne J. de Pagter[10], Jean-Louis H. Kerkhoffs[11], Cornelis L. Harteveld[4] and Maria del Mar Mañú-Pereira[1]*

[1] Translational Research in Child and Adolescent Cancer – Rare Anemia Disorders Research Laboratory, Vall d'Hebron Research Institute, ERN-EuroBloodNet Member, Barcelona, Spain, [2] Josep Carreras Leukaemia Research Institute, Badalona, Spain, [3] Department of Medicine, Universitat de Barcelona, Barcelona, Spain, [4] Department of Clinical Genetics, Leiden University Medical Center, ERN-EuroBloodNet Member, Leiden, Netherlands, [5] Hematologic Molecular Genetics Unit, Hematology Department, Hospital Universitari Vall d'Hebron, ERN-EuroBloodNet Member, Barcelona, Spain, [6] Oncohematologic Pediatrics Department, Hospital Universitari Vall d'Hebron, ERN-EuroBloodNet Member, Barcelona, Spain, [7] Hematology Department, Hospital Universitario Cruces, Barakaldo, Spain, [8] Red Blood Cell Disorders Unit, Hematology Department, Hospital Universitari Vall d'Hebron, ERN-EuroBloodNet Member, Barcelona, Spain, [9] Department of Clinical Genetics, VU Medical Center, Amsterdam, Netherlands, [10] Department of Pediatric Hematology, Leiden University Medical Center, Leiden, Netherlands, [11] Department of Hematology, HAGA City Hospital, The Hague, Netherlands

*Correspondence:
Maria del Mar Mañú-Pereira
mar.manu@vhir.org

Unstable hemoglobinopathies (UHs) are rare anemia disorders (RADs) characterized by abnormal hemoglobin (Hb) variants with decreased stability. UHs are therefore easily precipitating, causing hemolysis and, in some cases, leading to dominant beta-thalassemia (dBTHAL). The clinical picture of UHs is highly heterogeneous, inheritance pattern is dominant, instead of recessive as in more prevalent major Hb syndromes, and may occur *de novo*. Most cases of UHs are not detected by conventional testing, therefore diagnosis requires a high index of suspicion of the treating physician. Here, we highlight the importance of next generation sequencing (NGS) methodologies for the diagnosis of patients with dBTHAL and other less severe UH variants. We present five unrelated clinical cases referred with chronic hemolytic anemia, three of them with severe blood transfusion dependent anemia. Targeted NGS analysis was performed in three cases while whole exome sequencing (WES) analysis was performed in two cases. Five different UH variants were identified correlating with patients' clinical manifestations. Four variants were related to the beta-globin gene (Hb Bristol—Alesha, Hb Debrousse, Hb Zunyi, and the novel Hb Mokum) meanwhile one case was caused by a mutation in the alpha-globin gene leading to Hb Evans. Inclusion of alpha and beta-globin genes in routine NGS approaches for RADs has to be considered to improve diagnosis' efficiency of RAD due to UHs. Reducing misdiagnoses and underdiagnoses of UH variants, especially of the severe forms leading to dBTHAL would also facilitate the early start of intensive or curative treatments for these patients.

Keywords: unstable hemoglobinopathies, dominant beta-thalassemia, next generation sequencing, whole exome sequencing, rare anemia disorders

INTRODUCTION

Beta-thalassemia major (BTHAL) is a well-known life-threatening condition characterized by severe transfusion-dependent anemia. BTHAL is an autosomal recessive disorder presenting with high frequencies in populations from the Mediterranean area. Currently, up to 257 genetic variants in the beta-globin gene (*HBB*) have been identified as BTHAL disease-causing, leading to a total or partial reduction of beta-globin chain synthesis. The clinical severity of BTHAL is related to the extent of imbalance between the alpha and non-alpha-globin chains, while clinical management consists of regular life-long red blood cell (RBC) transfusions and iron chelation therapy. At present, the only definitive cure is bone marrow transplant (Efremov, 2007; Galanello and Origa, 2010). Both BTHAL patients and carriers are usually easily diagnosed through routine laboratory tests. However, there is an ultra-rare condition overlapping BTHAL clinical manifestations known as dominant beta-thalassemia (dBTHAL), which is caused by the presence of certain unstable (UH) or hyper unstable (HUH) hemoglobinopathies.

UHs are a group of congenital disorders caused by mutations in globin genes leading to destabilization of hemoglobin (Hb) molecules as a consequence of (a) amino acid substitutions within the heme pocket, (b) disruption of secondary structure, (c) substitution in the hydrophobic interior of the subunit, (d) amino acid deletions, and (e) elongation of the subunit. Thus, altering any of the steps in globin processing, including subunit folding, heme interaction, dimerization, or tetramerization (Bunn and Forget, 1986). These abnormal Hb variants undergo rapid denaturation followed by precipitation, leading to the formation of Heinz bodies, which cause hemolysis of RBCs. Clinical manifestations may vary from asymptomatic to severely affected forms. Treatment is mainly symptomatic and based on transfusion requirements as for BTHAL (Steinberg et al., 2009; Thom et al., 2013).

UHs are dominantly inherited with a significant rate of *de novo* mutations. They generally do not separate from normal Hb using standard methods. Thus, diagnosis of dBTHAL can be challenging since it requires a high index of suspicion and the diagnosis may be delayed for years hampering the access to timely treatment interventions.

The study we present herein confirms the relevance of including globin genes in next generation sequencing (NGS) approaches for the diagnosis of rare anemia disorders (RADs), especially for cases with no family history in which the anemia is not easily explained.

PATIENTS AND METHODS

Clinical Reports

Here we present five clinical cases diagnosed with UH after NGS analysis. Clinical data and laboratory findings are shown in **Table 1**.

The first case is a male pediatric patient referred with severe chronic blood dependent anemia since he was 4-month-old,

asthenia, jaundice, and short stature. No family history of hemolytic anemia. Examination of blood smear revealed polychromasia, anisopoikilocytosis, basophil stippling, Cabot rings, schistocytes, and spherocytes. Separation and quantification of Hb fractions did not reveal any extraordinary peak and showed normal values for HbA_2 and HbF. At 5-year-old he underwent splenectomy. After the surgery, Heinz bodies were present (**Figures 1, 2**) and isopropanol stability test, performed according to standard methodology, appeared positive (**Figure 3**). Family studies in both parents were strictly normal, including evaluation of Hb fractions. Enzyme activity assays, EMA-binding test, and osmotic gradient ectacytometry (LoRRca MaxSis) were performed to rule out hemolytic anemia due to RBC defects other than hemoglobinopathy. Results, although not strictly normal, did not reveal any RBC defect. However, they should be taken with caution since the patient was intensively transfused. Genetic analysis was performed on *PKLR* and *G6PD* genes failing to reveal any disease-causing mutation.

The second case is a female adult patient with mild chronic compensated hemolysis referred for diagnosis when she was 20 years old. The father also presented with mild compensated hemolysis. No further examinations were performed before referral. Although the presence of extravascular hemolysis, the examination of blood smear was not informative. Separation and quantification of Hb fractions did not reveal any extra peaks and Heinz body and stability tests were normal. Further laboratory tests were performed to rule out hemolytic anemia due to RBC enzyme and membrane defects, including enzyme activity assays, EMA-binding test, and osmotic gradient ectacytometry (LoRRca MaxSis). All of them showed normal values.

The third case is a male adult patient. He presented with several episodes of hemolytic crises during childhood requiring blood transfusion on two occasions. He underwent splenectomy at the age of 25-year-old. The patient was diagnosed with hereditary spherocytosis (HS) following a previous HS diagnosis of his mother and the absence of abnormal Hb peaks by conventional electrophoresis.

Patients who underwent splenectomy neither clinically improved nor presented complications as pulmonary hypertension, thrombosis or increased hemolysis during 10-year follow-up.

The last two cases are two unrelated children who presented with macrocephaly and severe congenital anemia. The parents of both patients had no family history for abnormal Hb or thalassemia and had normal hematological features. Therefore, conventional testing for abnormal Hb was not performed. All siblings were unaffected.

The first of these two unrelated children is a male patient presenting with large head circumference and hepatosplenomegaly. Congenital dyserythropoietic anemia was suspected. However, no genetic analysis was performed for confirmation. He underwent successfully bone marrow transplant at the age of 4.

The second child is a female patient presenting with frontal bossing, macrocephaly, and severe anemia at the age of 2. Congenital dyserythropoietic anemia was suspected. Therefore, genetic analysis of *CDAN1* and *SEC23B* genes was

TABLE 1 | Overview on clinical and genetic data of the five reported clinical cases.

Parameters	Case 1	Case 2	Case 3	Case 4	Case 5
Gender/Age	**Male/Pediatric**	**Female/Adult**	**Male/Adult**	**Male/Pediatric**	**Female/Pediatric**
Hb (120–170 g/L)	70–80	119	141	82	79
MCV (80–100 fL)	110–115	97.8	102.3	83	Not done
MCHC (27–33.5 g/dL)	28	32.1	30.8	Not done	Not done
Reticulocyte count (50–100 · 10⁹/L)	900	293	331	810	Not done
Reticulocyte count (%)	34	7.71	7.39	Not done	Not done
Lactate dehydrogenase-LDH (U/L)	4,500–5,000	243	145	186	259
Hb Fractions	Normal	Normal	Normal	Not done	Not done
Heinz bodies	Positive	Negative	Positive	Not done	Not done
Stability test	Positive	Negative	Positive	Not done	Not done
Age of onset (months)	4	Unknown	Unknown	Unknown	2
Family history	No family history	Father presents mild compensated hemolysis	Mother diagnosed with hereditary spherocytosis	No family history	No family history
Transfusion need	8 U/Year	No	2 times	Multiple	Multiple
Splenectomy	Yes (5 y)	No	Yes (25 y)	No	No
Stem cell transplant (age years)	No	No	No	Yes (4 y)	Yes (3 y)
Genotype	HBBc.202G > A (p.Val67Met)	HBA1c.187G > A (p.Val62Met)	HBBc.290T > C (p.Leu96Pro)	HBBc.442T > C (p.Ter147Glnext*21)	HBBc.442T > A (p.Ter147Lysext*21)
Hb variant name	Hb Bristol-Alesha	Hb Evans	Hb Debrousse	Hb Zunyi	Hb Mokum

*Performed after the diagnosis of UH.

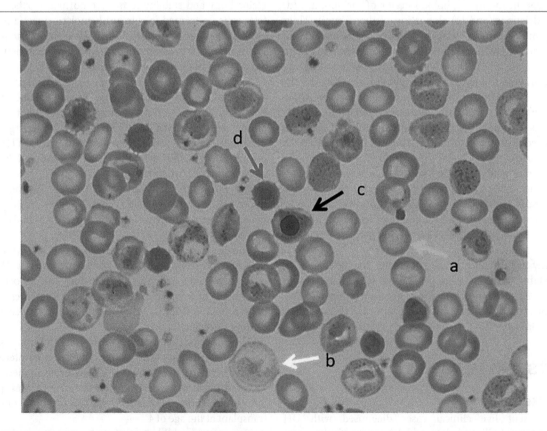

FIGURE 1 | Peripheral Blood Smear, May Grunwald Giemsa Stain. **(a)** Transfused red blood cells, **(b)** non-transfused red blood cells with hemoglobinization abnormalities, **(c)** orthochromatic erythroblast, **(d)** erythrocitary inclusions that correspond to Heinz bodies.

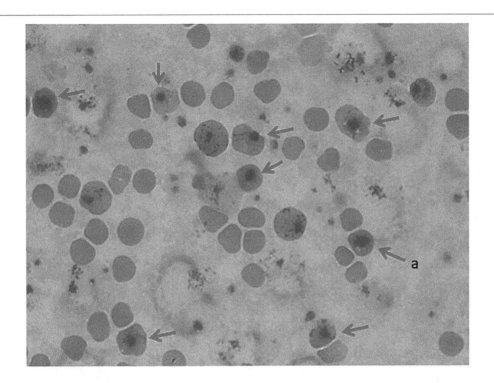

FIGURE 2 | Peripheral Blood Smear, Brilliant Cresyl Blue Stain. **(a)** Heinz bodies.

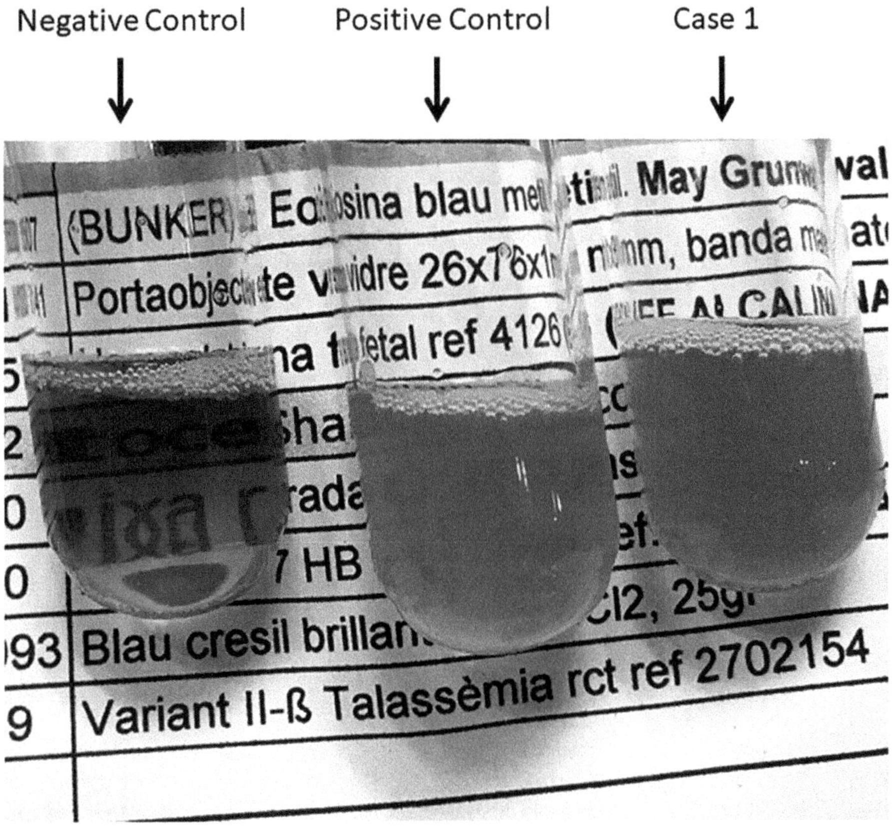

FIGURE 3 | Isopropanol Test_01. Negative control (Hb AS), Positive control (Hb F), and Case 1.

TABLE 2 | List of genes included in the t-NGS approach.

Symbol	Phenotype MIM number	Gene/Locus MIM number	Category	Description
ADA	102700	608958	Enzymopathy	Adenosine deaminase
AK1	103000	103000	Enzymopathy	Adenylate kinase 1
ALDOA	611881	103850	Enzymopathy	Aldolase, fructose-bisphosphate a
ANK1	616089	612641	Membranopathy	Ankyrin 1
ATRX	301040	300032	Alpha-thalassemia myelodysplasia syndrome, somatic; Alpha-thalassemia/mental retardation syndrome; Mental retardation-hypotonic facies syndrome, X-linked	Helicase 2, x-linked
BPGM	222800	613896	Erythrocytosis and methemoglobinemia due to enzyme alteration	Bisphosphoglycerate mutase
C15orf41	615631	615626	Congenital dyserythropoietic anemia	Chromosome 15 open reading frame 41
CDAN1	224120	224120	Congenital dyserythropoietic anemia	Codanin 1
CYB5R3	250800	613213	Methemoglobinemia, type I; Methemoglobinemia, type II	Cytochrome b5 reductase 3
EPB41	611804	130500	Membranopathy	Erythrocyte membrane protein band 4.1
EPB42	612690	177070	Membranopathy	Erythrocyte membrane protein band 4.2
EPO	617907	133170	Erythropoiesis modulator	Erythropoietin
EPOR	133100	133171	Erythropoiesis modulator	Erythropoietin receptor
G6PD	300908	305900	Enzymopathy	Glucose-6-phosphate dehydrogenase
GAPDH	*	138400	Enzymopathy	Glyceraldehyde-3-phosphate dehydrogenase
GATA1	300835	305371	Congenital dyserythropoietic anemia	Gata binding protein 1 (globin transcription factor 1)
GCLC	230450	606857	Enzymopathy	Glutamate-cysteine ligase, catalytic subunit
GPI	613470	172400	Enzymopathy	Glucose-6-phosphate isomerase
GSR	618660	138300	Enzymopathy	Glutathione reductase
GSS	266130	601002	Enzymopathy	Glutathione synthetase
GYPC	616089	110750	Membranopathy	Glycophorin c (gerbich blood group)
HBA1	617981	141800	Hemoglobinopathy	Hemoglobin–alpha locus 1
HBA2	617981	141850	Hemoglobinopathy	Hemoglobin–alpha locus 2
HBB	617980	141900	Hemoglobinopathy	Hemoglobin subunit beta
HBD	*	142000	Thalassemia due to Hb Lepore; Thalassemia, delta-	Hemoglobin–delta locus
HBG1	141900	141749	Fetal hemoglobin quantitative trait locus 1	Hemoglobin, gamma a
HBG2	613977	142250	Cyanosis, transient neonatal; Fetal hemoglobin quantitative trait locus 1	Hemoglobin, gamma g
HK1	235700	142600	Enzymopathy	Hexokinase 1
KCNN4	616689	602754	Membranopathy	Potassium channel, calcium activated intermediate/small conductance subfamily n alpha, member 4
KIF23	*	605064	Congenital dyserythropoietic anemia	Kinesin family member 23
KLF1	613673	600599	Congenital dyserythropoietic anemia	Kruppel-like factor 1 (erythroid)
NT5C3A	266120	606224	Enzymopathy	5′-nucleotidase, cytosolic iiia
PFKL	*	171860	Hemolytic anemia due to phosphofructokinase deficiency	Phosphofructokinase, liver type
PFKM	232800	610681	Enzymopathy	Phosphofructokinase, muscle
PGD	*	172200	Enzymopathy	6-phosphogluconate dehydrogenase, erythrocyte
PGK1	300653	311800	Enzymopathy	Phosphoglycerate kinase 1
PIEZO1	616089	611184	Membranopathy	Piezo-type mechanosensitive ion channel component 1
PKLR	266200	609712	Enzymopathy	Pyruvate kinase, liver and rbc
RHAG	185000	180297	Membranopathy	rh-associated glycoprotein
SEC23B	224100	610512	Congenital dyserythropoietic anemia	Sec23 homolog b, copii coat complex component

(Continued)

TABLE 2 | Continued

Symbol	Phenotype MIM number	Gene/Locus MIM number	Category	Description
SLC2A1	606777	138140	Membranopathy	Solute carrier family 2 (facilitated glucose transporter), member 1
SLC4A1	612653	109270	Membranopathy	Solute carrier family 4 (anion exchanger), member 1 (diego blood group)
SPTA1	130600	182860	Membranopathy	Spectrin alpha, erythrocytic 1
SPTB	616649	182870	Membranopathy	Spectrin beta, erythrocytic
TPI1	615512	190450	Enzymopathy	Triosephosphate isomerase 1
UGT1A1	237900	191740	Gilbert syndrome	udp glucuronosyltransferase 1 family, polypeptide a1

*Not available.

performed not revealing any disease-causing mutation. She underwent successfully bone marrow transplant when she was almost 3-year-old.

In all cases, RAD due to Hb variant was not suspected mainly due to the fact that parents did not present family history of RADs, except for case 3, RBC parameters were found to be normal and abnormal Hb fractions were absent when analyzed. Therefore, genetic testing was performed for genes associated with RADs other than globin genes, failing to show a conclusive diagnosis.

Genetics Analysis

Written informed consent was obtained from cases or legal guardian. Targeted NGS (t-NGS) analysis was performed in cases 1, 2, and 3 while whole exome sequencing (WES) analysis was performed in cases 4 and 5. For all the patients, genomic DNA was extracted from peripheral blood. For patients who underwent bone marrow transplant, DNA samples were previously stored.

The designed t-NGS panel covered 46 genes described as disease causing for RADs, including genes responsible for membrane disorders, enzyme defects, congenital dyserytrhopoietic anemia and the HBA1/HBA2 and HBB genes responsible for alpha and beta-globin chains, respectively. The full list of genes included is shown in **Table 2**. Exon and exon/intron boundaries were capture using a NimbleGen SeqCap EZ HyperCap (Roche) solution-based capture system followed by next generation sequencing on the MySeq (Illumina) with 150 bp paired-end reads. For the bioinformatics analysis, alignment to the hg38 genome was performed with BWA-MEM (Li H. 203 arXIV:1303.3997v2) and detection of changes with GATK[1]. Obtained variants were filtered and annotated based on variant effect, coverage ($>$30) and MAF ($>$0.05). Resulting variants were assessed for technique pitfalls through IGV. The nomenclature used was the recommended by HGVS[2]. Finally, disease-causing variants were prioritized based on inheritance pattern and VarSome[3] for previous evidence as disease causing mutations or predictions score information. Variants were reported according to American College of Medical Genetics (ACMG) guidelines.

For case 4, WES was performed in a trio approach (patient and both parents). Libraries were prepared using the Kapa HTP kit (Illumina, San Diego, CA, United States) and capture was performed using the SeqCap EZ Human Exome Library v3.0 (Roche NimbleGen Madison, WI, United States). Sequencing was done on an Illumina HiSeq2500 HTv4 (Illumina, San Diego, CA, United States) with paired-end 125-bp reads. Read alignment to hg19 and variant calling were done with a pipeline based on BWA-MEM0.7 and GATK 3.3.0. The median coverage of the captured target region was at least 98$\times$. Variant annotation and prioritizing were done using Cartagenia Bench Lab NGS (Agilent Technologies). Variants located outside the exons and intron/exon boundaries and variants with a minor allele frequency (MAF) of $>$1% in control databases, including dbSNP137[4], 1000 Genomes Project (phase 3)[5], and Exome Variant Server (EVS), NHLBI Exome Sequencing Project National Heart, Lung, and Blood Institute GO Exome Sequencing Project (ESP6500 release)[6] and in-house exome controls were excluded. Variants that fitted with a de novo or recessive mode of inheritance were further prioritized based on literature, predicted (deleterious) effects on protein function by e.g., truncating the protein, affecting splicing, amino acid change, and evolutionary conservation.

For case 5, WES was performed in a trio approach (patient and both parents). Exomes were captured using the Agilent SureSelectXT Human All Exon v5 (Agilent, Santa Clara, CA, United States) accompanied by Illumina paired-end sequencing on the HiSeq2000 (Illumina, San Diego, CA, United States). The in-house sequence analysis pipeline Modular GATK-Based Variant Calling Pipeline (MAGPIE) (LUMC Sequencing Analysis Support Core, LUMC) was used to call the SNVs/indels. LOVDplus (Leiden Genome Technology Center, LUMC, Leiden) was used for interpretation of variants.

RESULTS

Genetic variants in globin genes responsible for UH or HUH were found in all five cases as shown in **Table 1**. All variants were confirmed by Sanger sequencing.

In case 1, variant HBB:c.202G $>$ A (p.Val67Met) was found in exon 2 in the heterozygous state. This HBB variant is known as Hb Bristol-Alesha, a UH associated with moderate-severe hemolytic anemia. The variant was not found in the parents, suggesting a de novo variant in the patient.

---

[1]https://software.broadinstitute.org/gatk/

[2]http://www.hgvs.org

[3]https://varsome.com

[4]http://www.ncbi.nlm.nih.gov/projects/SNP

[5]http://www.internationalgenome.org/

[6]http://evs.gs.washington.edu/EVS/

In case 2, variant *HBA1*:c.187G > A (p.Val62Met) was found in exon 2 in the heterozygous state. This *HBA1* variant is known as Hb Evans and is associated wild with mild hemolytic anemia and classified as UH. Parents were not sequenced.

In Case 3, variant *HBB*:c.290T > C (p.Leu96Pro) was found in in exon 2 in the heterozygous state. This *HBB* variant is known as Hb Debrousse and is described as a moderate UH. Parents were not sequenced. Nevertheless, antecedents of hemolytic anemia are present in the mother, suggesting a dominant inheritance pattern.

In cases 4 and 5, two missense stop-loss mutations at position 422 of the *HBB* gene were found. The first variant *HBB*:c.442T > C (p.Ter147Glnext*21), found in case 4, is known as Hb Zunyi, while the second variant *HBB*:c.442T > A (p.Ter147Lysnext*21), found in case 5, constitutes a novel variant which was called Hb Mokum. Both variants cause the loss of a stop codon and elongation of the translated beta-globin chain of 21 amino acids due to a new stop codon in the 3′ untranslated region (3′UTR) of the *HBB* gene. The variants were not found in the parents suggesting *de novo* variants in the patients.

According to the ACMG guidelines, all the variants were classified as pathogenic (Richards et al., 2015).

DISCUSSION

We highlight the importance of including globin genes in the NGS analysis of RAD for enabling the diagnosis of UH. We present five clinical cases affected with RAD due to UH variants, four are related to the beta-globin gene (Hb Bristol—Alesha, Hb Debrousse, Hb Zunyi, and the novel Hb Mokum), meanwhile, one is related to the alpha-globin gene (Hb Evans). The use of NGS has been crucial for the final conclusive diagnosis.

The severity of RADs due to UHs depends on the mutation's impact on protein stability and consequently on the degree of hemolysis and inefficient erythropoiesis. Patients' RBCs typically display abnormal but unspecific morphology with microcytosis, hypochromia, moderate to severe anisopoikilocytosis, basophilic stippling, and inclusions that may become particularly prominent following splenectomy (Steinberg et al., 2009; Kent et al., 2014). UHs are commonly inherited in a dominant way or presented as *de novo*, although there are some examples of recessive inheritance leading to mild phenotypes. According to results obtained through the HbVar Query page (dated 14th January 2020), 1,534 Hb variants have been described so far due to mutations on either *HBA1/HBA2* or the *HBB* genes. Up to 251 variants (16.4%) are classified as UH or HUH based on heat or isopropanol stability tests and/or low Hb abundancy (Giardine et al., 2007, 2014). It is worthy to highlight that all the HUH variants involving the *HBB* gene reported positive stability tests, meanwhile in most of the HUH involving the alpha-globin genes, hyper instability has been only deduced from low abundance. This must be cautiously taken since mutations in alpha-globin genes are lower expressed (<25%) than in beta-globin gene due to the existence of duplicated alpha-globin genes, *HBA1* and *HBA2*, especially in mutations involving the *HBA2* gene, as it encodes

a 2-3–fold higher level of mRNA than *HBA1* (Liebhaberts et al., 1986). Thus, the beta-globin gene is the first option to investigate for disease-causing mutations leading to RADs due to UHs/HUHs especially in cases with moderate to severe phenotypes.

Interestingly, Hb Bristol-Alesha is classified as a UH variant, not as a HUH as we expected based on the severity of the patient's clinical picture. The change to methionine at position 67 of the beta-globin chain alters the hydrophobic heme pocket causing the instability of the protein (Kano et al., 2004). As described in previous clinical reports, at physical examination, splenomegaly and jaundice may be found. Iron overload and gallstones may develop due to the rapid turnover of RBCs.

Hb Debrousse, reported twice in literature, is a UH characterized by well-compensated chronic hemolytic anemia due to its high oxygen affinity. Hb Debrousse is caused by leucine to proline substitution at position 96 involving the hydrophobic environment of the proximal side of the heme. In the previously reported cases, Hb Debrousse discovery was possible after a Parvovirus B19 infection that caused a hemolytic crisis (Lacan et al., 1996). Indeed, since affected patients show a chronic well-compensated hemolytic anemia, the diagnosis of such a variant is unlikely until the globin genes are investigated. Such a study is usually performed only when some complications occur.

Hb Zunyi was recently reported for the first time as a *de novo* mutation in a Chinese child with severe anemia requiring blood transfusion, malnutrition, growth delay, splenomegaly and hepatomegaly (Su et al., 2019). In the study herein, we identified both Hb Zunyi and Hb Mokum as *de novo* mutations in the heterozygous state. Hb Zunyi and the novel Hb Mokum are stop-loss mutations at position 442 in *HBB*, resulting in an elongated beta-globin chain leading to HUHs. The extra amino acids in the elongated beta-globin chain (169 a.a.) are probably affecting its helical sequence, interfering with its tertiary structure and causing an unstable tetramer. Frameshift mutations in the *HBB* gene, resulting in the elongated beta-globin chain, have been described before but resulted in shorter beta-chains (max. 157 aa.) and milder phenotypes than the mutations described here (Su et al., 2019).

Finally, Hb Evans is classified as UH. It is consequence of a valine to methionine substitution at position 62 of the alpha2-globin chain encoding gene *HBA2*. Hb Evans has been reported in patients presenting with mild hemolytic anemia that was getting worse particularly in case of stress (Wilson et al., 1989).

The standard tests to detect abnormal anemias are High Precision Liquid Chromatography (HPLC) or conventional or capillary electrophoresis (CE). However, UHs/HUHs do not normally appear in the peak-patterns or appear as small peaks that may be mistaken for degradation products. In three of the five UH cases reported here, extra peaks were not detected. More confined methods are Heinz Bodies test or stability tests as isopropanol precipitation or heat stability tests, which are affordable screening techniques for UHs/HUHs variants. In the patient with Hb Bristol-Alesha, Heinz bodies were detected and heat stability test was positive only after splenectomy (**Figures 1**, **2**), while in the other patients, Heinz bodies and heat stability test were not performed. Genetic analysis of globin genes should be performed for diagnosis confirmation. Inclusion of *HBA1/HBA2* and *HBB* in NGS approaches will facilitate timely conclusive diagnosis. as a screening tool for hemolytic anemias will assist in reaching a definitive diagnosis sooner.

Furthermore, the occurrence of *de novo* mutations causing UHs/HUHs should also be considered in the analysis of genetic variants.

The usefulness of NGS in improving the diagnosis of RADs has already been demonstrated in several studies as well as its relevance in new gene discovery (Shang et al., 2017; Duez et al., 2018). In the case of overlapping phenotypes, which frustrate proper diagnosis, the use of NGS may be beneficial for ultra-rare RADs. In a recent publication, 36% of patients initially diagnosed with congenital dyserytrhopoietic anemia, received a final diagnosis of pyruvate kinase deficiency after NGS analysis (Russo et al., 2018). Nevertheless, in the majority of the t-NGS panels reported, globin genes are not included, since globin genes are quite short and molecular diagnosis of most common Hb disorders, such as sickle cell disease (SCD) and thalassemia syndromes, is well-established through Sanger sequencing and GAP-PCR/MLPA. Therefore, dBTHAL disorders due to UH/HUH may also benefit from NGS approaches for RADs by including globin genes, as presented herein.

Current literature on dBTHAL and UH/HUH variants is mainly composed of retrospective case reports, which makes evidenced-based management of this RAD unlikely. In addition, to benefit from the most adequate management it is necessary to achieve a diagnosis as early as possible. In conclusion, this study confirms the importance of NGS as a fundamental tool to early identify and treat UH/HUH in patients with RAD without an established diagnosis after standard methodologies.

Future challenges include a better understanding of disease characteristics and management, and consideration of bone marrow transplant as a curative option. Therefore, we encourage that these patients are referred to expert Units in referral centers for enabling basic and clinical research taking advantage of the already established European Reference Networks for rare hematological disorders, ERN-EuroBloodNet.

ETHICS STATEMENT

Written informed consent was obtained from the cases/legal guardian for the publication of any potentially identifiable images or data included in this article.

AUTHOR CONTRIBUTIONS

VR, MM-P, CLH, TK, and DB wrote the manuscript. All authors critically revised the manuscript.

ACKNOWLEDGMENTS

This work was generated within the European Reference Network on Rare Hematological Diseases (ERN-EuroBloodNet, FPA 739541).

REFERENCES

Bunn, H. F., and Forget, B. G. (1986). *Hemoglobin: Molecular, Genetic and Clinical Aspects*. Philadelphia, PA: W. B. Saunders Company, doi: 10.1016/0092-8674(87)90069-9

Duez, J., Carucci, M., Garcia-Barbazan, I., Corral, M., Perez, O., Luis Presa, J., et al. (2018). High-throughput microsphiltration to assess red blood cell deformability and screen for malaria transmission-blocking drugs. *Nat. Protoc.* 13, 1362–1376. doi: 10.1038/nprot.2018.035

Efremov, G. D. (2007). Dominantly inherited β-Thalassemia. *Hemoglobin* 31, 193–207. doi: 10.1080/03630260701290092

Galanello, R., and Origa, R. (2010). Beta-Thalassemia. *Orphanet J. Rare Dis.* 5:11. doi: 10.1186/1750-1172-5-11

Giardine, B., Borg, J., Viennas, E., Pavlidis, C., Moradkhani, K., Joly, P., et al. (2014). Updates of the hbvar database of human hemoglobin variants and Thalassemia Mutations. *Nucleic Acids Res.* 42, 1063–1069. doi: 10.1093/nar/gkt911

Giardine, B., van Baal, S., Kaimakis, P., Riemer, C., Miller, W., Samara, M., et al. (2007). HbVar database of human hemoglobin variants and thalassemia mutations: 2007 update. *Hum. Mutat.* 28:206. doi: 10.1002/humu.9479

Kano, G., Morimoto, A., Hibi, S., Tokuda, C., Todo, S., and Sugimoto, T. (2004). Hb Bristol-Alesha presenting Thalassemia-Type hyperunstable hemoglobinopathy. *Int. J. Hematol.* 80, 410–415. doi: 10.1532/IJH97.04048

Kent, M. W., Oliveira, J. L., Hoyer, J. D., Swanson, K. C., Kluge, M. L., Dawson, D. B., et al. (2014). Hb grand junction (HBB: C.348-349delinsG; P.His117IlefsX42): a new hyperunstable hemoglobin variant. *Hemoglobin* 38, 8–12. doi: 10.3109/03630269.2013.853672

Lacan, P., Kister, J., Francina, A., Souillet, G., Galactéros, F., Delaunay, J., et al. (1996). Hemoglobin debrousse (B96[FG3]Leu → Pro): a new unstable hemoglobin with twofold increased oxygen affinity. *Am. J. Hematol.* 51, 276–281. doi: 10.1002/(SICI)1096-8652(199604)51:4<276::AID-AJH5<3.0.CO;2-T

Liebhaberts, S. A., Cash, F. E., Ballad, S. K., and Human Gene Expression (1986). Human A-Globin gene expression. The dominant role of the Alpha 2-Locus in MRNA and protein synthesis. *J. Biol. Chem.* 261, 15327–15333.

Richards, S., Aziz, S., Bale, S., Bick, D., Das, S., Acmg Laboratory Quality Assurance Committee, et al. (2015). Standards and guidelines standards and guidelines for the interpretation of sequence variants: a joint consensus recommendation of the American College of Medical Genetics and Genomics and the Association for Molecular Pathology. *Genet. Med.* 17, 405–424. doi: 10.1038/gim.2015.30

Russo, R., Manna, F., Gambale, A., Marra, R., Rosato, B. E., Caforio, P., et al. (2018). Multi-Gene panel testing improves diagnosis and management of patients with Hereditary Anemias. *Am. J. Hematol.* 93, 672–682. doi: 10.1002/ajh.25058

Shang, X., Peng, Z., Ye, Y., Asan, Zhang, X., Chen, Y., et al. (2017). Rapid targeted next-generation sequencing platform for molecular screening and clinical genotyping in subjects with hemoglobinopathies. *EBioMedicine* 23, 150–159. doi: 10.1016/j.ebiom.2017.08.015

Steinberg, M. H., Forget, B. G., Higgs, D. R., and Weatherall, D. J. (2009). *Disorders of Hemoglobin: Genetics, Pathophysiology, and Clinical Management, Second Edition*, Vol. 94. Cambridge: Cambridge University Press, i–iv. doi: 10.1017/CBO9780511596582

Su, Q., Chen, S., Wu, L., Tian, R., Yang, X., Huang, X., et al. (2019). Severe thalassemia caused by Hb Zunyi [B147(HC3)Stop→Gln; HBB: C.442T>C)] on the β-Globin gene. *Hemoglobin* 43, 7–11. doi: 10.1080/03630269.2019.1582430

Thom, C. S., Dickson, C. F., Gell, D. A., and Weiss, M. J. (2013). Hemoglobin variants: biochemical properties and clinical correlates. *Cold Spring Harb. Perspect. Med.* 3, 1–22. doi: 10.1101/cshperspect.a011858

Wilson, J. B., Webber, B. B., Kutlar, A., Reese, A. L., Mckie, V. C., Lutcher, C. L., et al. (1989). Hb evans or A262(E11)Val→metβ2; an unstable hemoglobin causing a mild hemolytic anemia. *Hemoglobin* 13, 557–566. doi: 10.3109/03630268908993106

Molecular Characterization Analysis of Thalassemia and Hemoglobinopathy in Quanzhou, Southeast China

Jianlong Zhuang[1], Na Zhang[1], Yuanbai Wang[1], Hegan Zhang[2], Yu Zheng[3], Yuying Jiang[1], Yingjun Xie[4,5]* and Dongmei Chen[6]*

[1] Prenatal Diagnosis Center, Quanzhou Women's and Children's Hospital, Quanzhou, China, [2] Department of Gynecology, Quanzhou Women's and Children's Hospital, Quanzhou, China, [3] Research and Development Department, Yaneng BIOscience (Shenzhen) Co. Ltd., Shenzhen, China, [4] Key Laboratory for Major Obstetric Diseases of Guangdong Province, Department of Obstetrics and Gynecology, The Third Affiliated Hospital of Guangzhou Medical University, Guangzhou, China, [5] Key Laboratory of Reproduction and Genetics of Guangdong Higher Education Institutes, The Third Affiliated Hospital of Guangzhou Medical University, Guangzhou, China, [6] Department of Neonatal Intensive Care Unit, Quanzhou Women's and Children's Hospital, Quanzhou, China

*Correspondence:
Yingjun Xie
xieyjun@mail2.sysu.edu.cn
Dongmei Chen
chendm9090@163.com

Background: There are limited reports available on investigations into the molecular spectrum of thalassemia and hemoglobinopathy in Fujian province, Southeast China. Here, we aim to reveal the spectrum of the thalassemia mutation and hemoglobinopathy in Quanzhou prefecture, Fujian province.

Methods: We collected data from a total of 17,407 subjects with the thalassemia trait in Quanzhou prefecture. Gap-PCR, DNA reverse dot blot hybridization, and DNA sequencing were utilized for common and rare thalassemia gene testing.

Results: In our study, we identified 7,085 subjects who were carrying thalassemia mutations, representing a detection rate of 40.70% (7,085/17,407). Among them, 13 different α-thalassemia gene mutations were detected, with the most common mutation being $-^{SEA}$ (69.01%), followed by $-\alpha^{3.7}$ (21.34%) and $-\alpha^{4.2}$ (3.96%). We also discovered 26 β-thalassemia gene mutations, with the mutations of IVS-II-654 (C > T) (36.28%) and CD41/42(–TCTT) (29.16%) being the most prevalent. Besides, a variety of rare thalassemia variants were identified. Among them, the $-^{FIL}$, β^{Malay}, $\beta^{IVS-I-130}$, and $\beta^{IVS-II-672}$ mutations were identified in Fujian province for the first time. Additionally, we detected 78 cases of hemoglobinopathies, of which Hb Owari was the first reported case in Fujian province and Hb Miyashiro was the first case identified in the Chinese population.

Conclusion: Our study indicates that there is a diverse range of thalassemia mutations, and it also reveals the mutation spectrum of rare thalassemia and hemoglobinopathies in Quanzhou, Fujian province. It provides valuable data for the prevention and control of thalassemia in Southeast China.

Keywords: thalassemia, hemoglobinopathy, molecular spectrum, DNA sequencing, Southeast China

INTRODUCTION

Thalassemia is a hereditary blood disorder caused by human globin gene synthesis disorders, of which α- and β-thalassemia are the most common genotypes (Weatherall, 2001). It most commonly occurs in Mediterranean countries, the Middle East, the Indian subcontinent, Southeast Asia, and China (Modell and Darlison, 2008; Weatherall, 2008). Thalassemia is mainly distributed in the southern regions of China, especially Guangdong, Guangxi, and Hainan provinces (Zhang et al., 2010; Li et al., 2014; Yao et al., 2014; Yin et al., 2014; He et al., 2018; Lu et al., 2021).

Fujian province, which is located in Southeast China, also displays a high prevalence of thalassemia (Xu et al., 2013; Huang et al., 2019; Zhuang et al., 2020a). Quanzhou prefecture has the largest population in Fujian and possesses high population mobility, which may have led to greater diversity and complexity of thalassemia gene mutations. Recently, more rare or novel thalassemia mutations have been identified in the Quanzhou region (Zhuang et al., 2019, 2020b). To date, no effective medical treatment for thalassemia intermedia or major has been developed. Fetuses with α-thalassemia major usually die *in utero* or shortly after birth, and this condition also often leads to the mortality of the pregnant mother (Vichinsky, 2013). Fetuses with β-thalassemia major usually develop severe progressive anemia after 3–6 months and rarely survive past 5 years of age if not treated with a regular transfusion program and chelation therapy (Liaska et al., 2016). Therefore, thalassemia genetic detection before marriage or pregnancy, as well as prenatal diagnosis, is the only effective intervention to prevent the births of babies with thalassemia major or intermedia. However, there is very little knowledge on the genotypes of thalassemia, and there is a lack of information on the hemoglobinopathy mutation spectrum in the Quanzhou region.

This retrospective study was performed to analyze the spectrum of the thalassemia gene mutation and characterize the genotypes of rare thalassemia and hemoglobinopathy in Quanzhou prefecture. It aims to provide valuable reference data for the prevention and control of thalassemia in Southeast China.

MATERIALS AND METHODS

Study Subjects

A total of 17,407 subjects who were suspected of being thalassemia carriers were recruited at Quanzhou Women's and Children's Hospital between January 2013 and March 2021. The age of these subjects ranged from 1 to 67 years old. We performed thalassemia gene detection on all of the subjects who met the following inclusion criteria: (1) routine hematology examination showed abnormal mean corpuscular volume (MCV) <82 fl/or mean corpuscular hemoglobin (MCH) <27 pg; (2) abnormal hemoglobin electrophoresis; (3) parents or siblings carried the thalassemia gene mutation; (4) at least one of the couple was identified as a thalassemia carrier.

Hematological Analysis and Serum Ferritin Test

Approximately 4 ml of peripheral blood was collected from each subject and anticoagulated with EDTA-K_2 for routine blood analysis and hemoglobin electrophoresis analysis. We performed routine blood detection on all of the subjects using an automated cell counter (Sysmex XS-1000i; Sysmex Co., Ltd., Kobe, Japan) and analyzed the hemoglobin components by hemoglobin electrophoresis (Sebia, Evry Cedex, France). Positive hematological screening was defined as an MCV of less than 82 fl and/or an MCH concentration of less than 27 pg and/or hemoglobin A2 (HbA2) levels greater than 3.4% or less than 2.6% or an Hb F value of more than 2.0%. All patients with positive hematological analysis results underwent thalassemia gene testing.

For the serum ferritin test, approximately 3 ml of peripheral blood was collected from the patients. Then, it was centrifuged at 3,500 rpm for 10 min to separate the serum. The serum ferritin test was performed with Siemens Healthcare

TABLE 1 | Distribution of α-thalassemia genotypes in Quanzhou Prefecture.

Genotypes	Cases	Frequency	Class
$_{-}^{SEA}/\alpha\alpha$	3,427	70.17%	Common
$-\alpha^{3.7}/\alpha\alpha$	897	18.37%	Common
$-\alpha^{4.2}/\alpha\alpha$	163	3.34%	Common
$\alpha\alpha^{QS}/\alpha\alpha$	100	2.05%	Common
$-\alpha^{3.7}/_{-}^{SEA}$	71	1.45%	Common
$\alpha\alpha^{CS}/\alpha\alpha$	64	1.31%	Common
$\alpha\alpha^{WS}/\alpha\alpha$	46	0.94%	Common
$-\alpha^{3.7}/-\alpha^{3.7}$	30	0.61%	Common
$-\alpha^{4.2}/_{-}^{SEA}$	16	0.33%	Common
$\alpha\alpha^{WS}/-\alpha^{3.7}$	11	0.23%	Common
$-\alpha^{3.7}/-\alpha^{4.2}$	8	0.16%	Common
$\alpha\alpha^{CS}/_{-}^{SEA}$	7	0.14%	Common
$Hk\alpha\alpha/_{-}^{SEA}$	5	0.10%	Rare
$_{-}^{THAI}/\alpha\alpha$	5	0.10%	Rare
$\alpha\alpha^{IVS-II-55(T>G)}/\alpha\alpha$	5	0.10%	Rare
$\alpha\alpha^{WS}/_{-}^{SEA}$	4	0.08%	Common
$\alpha\alpha^{QS}/_{-}^{SEA}$	4	0.08%	Common
$\alpha\alpha^{QS}/-\alpha^{3.7}$	3	0.06%	Common
$\alpha\alpha^{QS}/-\alpha^{4.2}$	2	0.04%	Common
$\alpha\alpha^{CS}/-\alpha^{3.7}$	2	0.04%	Common
$-\alpha^{4.2}/-\alpha^{4.2}$	2	0.04%	Common
$\alpha\alpha^{WS}/-\alpha^{4.2}$	2	0.04%	Common
$Hk\alpha\alpha/\alpha\alpha$	2	0.04%	Rare
$\alpha\alpha^{WS}/\alpha\alpha^{WS}$	1	0.02%	Common
$\alpha\alpha^{CS}/\alpha\alpha^{WS}$	1	0.02%	Common
$\alpha\alpha^{CS}/-\alpha^{4.2}$	1	0.02%	Common
$-\alpha^{3.7}/_{-}^{THAI}$	1	0.02%	Rare
$\alpha\alpha/\alpha\alpha\alpha^{anti4.2}$	1	0.02%	Rare
$_{-}^{FIL}/\alpha\alpha$	1	0.02%	Rare
$-\alpha^{27.6}/_{-}^{SEA}$	1	0.02%	Rare
$-\alpha^{6.9}/_{-}^{SEA}$	1	0.02%	Novel
Total	4,884	100%	

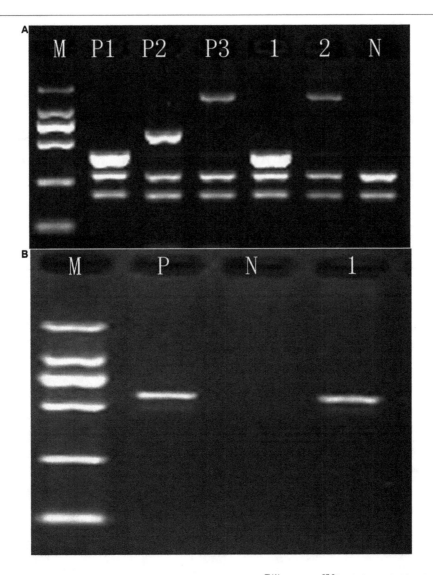

FIGURE 1 | Identification of rare α-thalassemia using gap-PCR. **(A)** Electrophoresis result of $-^{THAI}/\alpha\alpha$ and $-\alpha^{27.6}/\alpha\alpha$ thalassemia; M, maker; P1, positive control of $-^{THAI}/\alpha\alpha$; P2, positive control of $-\alpha^{21.9}/\alpha\alpha$; P3, positive control of $-\alpha^{27.6}/\alpha\alpha$; N, negative control; 1, $-^{THAI}$ thalassemia carrier; 2, $-\alpha^{27.6}$ thalassemia carrier.
(B) Electrophoresis result of $-^{FIL}/\alpha\alpha$ thalassemia; M, maker; P, positive control of $-^{FIL}/\alpha\alpha$; N, negative control; 1, $-^{FIL}/\alpha\alpha$ thalassemia carrier.

Diagnostics equipment and kit (Siemens, United States) and using the ADVIA Centaur XP Immunoassay System (Siemens, United States).

Molecular Diagnosis of Thalassemia

For each subject with positive hematological analysis results for the molecular analysis of common α- and β-thalassemia, we collected a further 2 ml of peripheral blood. An automatic nucleic acid extractor (Ruibao Biological Co., Ltd., Taiwan) was used to extract the genomic DNA of the subjects. We also used Gap-PCR to detect the three common deletional α-thalassemia mutations [Yaneng BIOscience (Shenzhen) Co. Ltd., Shenzhen]. The PCR reverse dot hybridization technique (PCR-RDB) was utilized to detect the three common non-deletional α-thalassemia mutations and 17 common β-thalassemia mutations [Yaneng

BIOscience (Shenzhen) Co. Ltd., Shenzhen]. The β-thalassemia mutations we detected were as follows: CD41-42(-TCTT), IVS-II-654(C > T), −28 (A > G), CD71/72(+ A), CD17(AAG > TAG), CD26(GAG > AAG), CD43(GAG > TAG), −29(A > G), CD31(-C), −32(C > A), IVS-I-1(G > T), CD27/28(+ C), −30(T > C), CD14-15(+ G), Cap + 40-43(−AAAC), initiation codon(ATG > AGG), and IVS-I-5(G > C). The experimental operations were performed strictly according to the protocols of the manufacturers.

Rare Thalassemia Analysis and DNA Sequencing

Rare α-thalassemia genotype screening kits ($-^{THAI}$, $-\alpha^{27.6}$, $-\alpha^{21.9}$) and rare β-thalassemia genotype screening kits [Taiwanese, $^G\gamma^+(^A\gamma\delta\beta)^0$, SEA-HPFH] were utilized for suspected

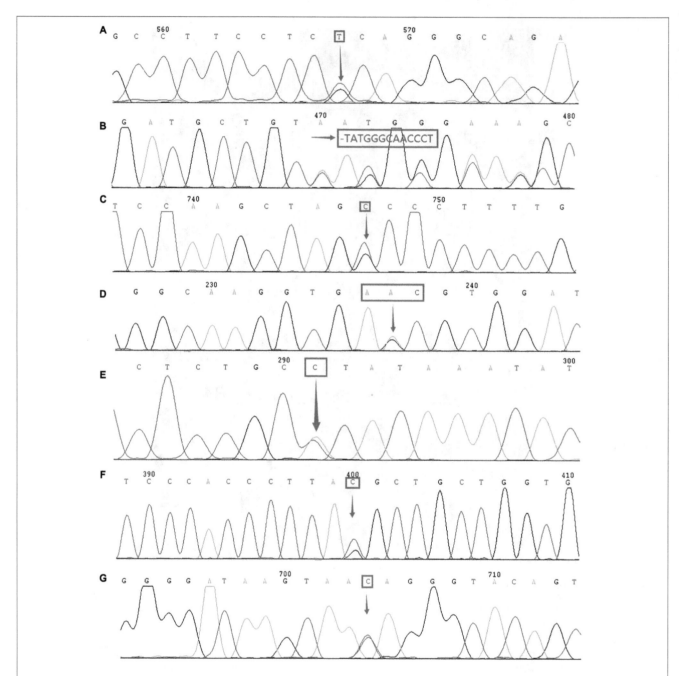

FIGURE 2 | Identification of rare α- and β-thalassemia mutations using DNA sequencing. Arrows indicate the location of the mutations. **(A)** IVS-II-55(T > G) mutation in the *HBA2* gene. **(B)** CD54-58(-TATGGGCAACCCT) mutation in the *HBB* gene. **(C)** IVS-II-806(G > C) mutation in the *HBB* gene. **(D)** Hb Malay(AAC > AGC) mutation in the *HBB* gene. **(E)** IVS-II-672(A > C) mutation in the *HBB* gene. **(F)** IVS-I-130(G > C) mutation in the *HBB* gene. **(G)** IVS-II-81(C > T) mutation in the *HBB* gene.

carriers of rare α- or β-thalassemia deletion. Indicators included low levels of Hb A2 without common α-thalassemia variants, as well as high or low levels of Hb A2 without common β-thalassemia variants.

Gap-PCR was performed to identify the deletion of $-^{FIL}$. We designed specific primers according to the known DNA sequences around the breakpoints. These primer sequences were P1: TCTAAAAATTCATCCTTAAGAGAATAA and

P2: GATCTAATGTAGTAGAGATAATAACCTTTA. All primers were synthesized at Sangon Biotech (Shanghai). The amplification conditions were 96°C for 5 min, then 35 cycles of 98°C for 30 s, 60°C for 1 min, 72°C for 2 min, and finally 72°C for 10 min. Subsequently, we performed an electrophoresis analysis.

We employed a multiplex ligation-dependent probe amplification (MLPA) assay using the SALSA MLPA Probemix

TABLE 2 | Comparison of hematological parameters among α-thalassemia silent carriers.

Groups	Cases		RBC (× 10^{12}/L)		Hb (g/L)		MCV (fl)	MCH (pg)
	M	F	M	F	M	F		
$\alpha\alpha^{QS}/\alpha\alpha$	23	27	5.51 ± 0.48	4.65 ± 0.39	138.5 ± 10.0	108.5 ± 5.8	75.20 ± 3.44	23.96 ± 1.43
$\alpha\alpha^{CS}/\alpha\alpha$	9	21	5.62 ± 0.08	4.44 ± 0.37	147.2 ± 5.6	117.7 ± 7.4	80.77 ± 4.08	26.34 ± 1.02
$\alpha\alpha^{WS}/\alpha\alpha$	6	8	5.67 ± 0.16	4.32 ± 0.28	151.3 ± 3.1	126.6 ± 5.2	82.21 ± 4.13	27.57 ± 1.80
$\alpha\alpha^{IVS-II-55(T>G)}/\alpha\alpha$	2	2	5.23 ± 0.40	4.25 ± 0.12	150.5 ± 6.4	126.0 ± 7.1	84.00 ± 2.71	29.28 ± 0.93
$-\alpha^{4.2}/\alpha\alpha$	17	51	5.65 ± 0.28	4.53 ± 0.35	148.9 ± 6.4	119.3 ± 7.8	80.79 ± 3.81	26.56 ± 1.02
$-\alpha^{3.7}/\alpha\alpha$	42	160	5.63 ± 0.35	4.56 ± 0.36	152.6 ± 7.6	119.9 ± 7.7	80.45 ± 3.06	26.53 ± 1.11
F			0.899	1.722	10.130	13.185	24.014	50.875
P			0.485	0.130	<0.001	<0.001	<0.001	<0.001

M, male; F, female; Hb, hemoglobin; MCH, mean corpuscular hemoglobin; MCV, mean corpuscular volume; RBC, red blood cell.

P140-C1HBA (MRC-Holland, Amsterdam, Netherlands) to detect the known or unknown globin gene deletions. DNA sequencing was performed when we observed suspected carriers of rare thalassemia mutations.

Statistical Analysis

The statistical analysis was conducted using SPSS19.0 software. The measurement data were expressed as $\overline{X} \pm s$, and we utilized the independent sample t-test to compare the means of the two groups. We also applied the chi-square test to compare the detection rates between the groups. A value of $p < 0.05$ was considered statistically significant.

RESULTS

Of the 17,407 suspected cases, 4,884 subjects were diagnosed with α-thalassemia, including 31 genotypes. Of these, the $-^{SEA}/\alpha\alpha$ (70.17%) mutation was the most common deletional mutation, followed by $-\alpha^{3.7}/\alpha\alpha$ (18.37%) and $-\alpha^{4.2}/\alpha\alpha$ (3.34%). The three most common non-deletional mutations were $\alpha\alpha^{QS}/\alpha\alpha$, $\alpha\alpha^{CS}/\alpha\alpha$, and $\alpha\alpha^{WS}/\alpha\alpha$, with frequencies of 2.05%, 1.31%, and 0.94%, respectively. Besides, nine genotypes of rare α-thalassemia were detected, of which $-^{THAI}/\alpha\alpha$, Hkαα/$-^{SEA}$, and $\alpha\alpha^{IVS-II-55(T>G)}/\alpha\alpha$ were the most common. Of these nine genotypes, our study was the first to detect a $-^{FIL}/\alpha\alpha$ case in Fujian province, while $-\alpha^{27.6}/-^{SEA}$ and $\alpha\alpha^{IVS-II-55(T>G)}/\alpha\alpha$ had never before been identified in Quanzhou prefecture (**Table 1** and **Figures 1, 2**).

To further analyze the hematological phenotype $\alpha\alpha^{IVS-II-55(T>G)}/\alpha\alpha$, we performed a comparison of the hematological parameters among the different genotypes of silent α-thalassemia. As **Table 2** illustrates, there are significant differences among the silent α-thalassemia groups in the hematological parameters of Hb, MCV, and MCH. Among them, $\alpha\alpha^{QS}/\alpha\alpha$-positive cases exhibited lower levels of Hb, MCV, and MCH than those of other groups, and the hematological phenotype was similar to that of α-thalassemia minor. Conversely, the rare genotype $\alpha\alpha^{IVS-II-55(T>G)}/\alpha\alpha$ displayed a milder hematological phenotype similar to $\alpha\alpha^{WS}/\alpha\alpha$.

Additionally, 2,056 cases were diagnosed with β-thalassemia. Of these, there were 2,035 cases with β-thalassemia minor

and 21 cases with β-thalassemia intermedia or major. The most common β-thalassemia variants were $\beta^{IVS-II-654}/\beta^N$ (36.19%) and $\beta^{CD41-42}/\beta^N$ (29.82%), followed by β^{CD17}/β^N (16.78%), β^{CD26}/β^N (5.35%), and β^{-28}/β^N (4.57%). These five common mutations accounted for 92.71% of β-thalassemia gene mutations. In this study, 17 cases of rare β-thalassemia variants were identified, of which $\beta^{CD54-58}/\beta^N$ and $\beta^{IVS-II-806}/\beta^N$ mutations were the first to be reported in Quanzhou, while β^{Malay}/β^N and $\beta^{IVS-II-672}/\beta^N$ had not previously been identified in Fujian province. Moreover, one subject carried two rare β-thalassemia mutations ($\beta^{IVS-I-130}/\beta^{IVS-II-81}$), which has never been encountered before (**Table 3** and **Figure 2**).

Among the suspected cases, 145 were diagnosed with compound α and β-thalassemia, while 34 of these subjects possessed the two most prevalent genotype mutations, $-^{SEA}/\alpha\alpha/\beta^{IVS-II-654}/\beta^N$ and $-\alpha^{3.7}/\alpha\alpha/\beta^{CD41-42}/\beta^N$ (**Table 4**).

Moreover, 11 subjects with low levels of Hb A2 or β-thalassemia carrier with normal levels of Hb A2 were suspected of having the δ-globin gene mutation. We confirmed that none of these subjects were suffering from iron deficiency anemia. Subsequently, we performed DNA sequencing to detect the HBD gene and discovered two δ-globin gene mutations. Two cases of known mutations [$-77(T > C)$] and one case of the novel δ-globin gene mutation [CD44(TCC > TGC) (HBD:c.134C > G)] were identified (**Figure 3**).

In this study, 39 types of mutations were identified in the allele frequencies of α(β) thalassemia mutation chromosomes, including 13 α-thalassemia gene mutations and 26 β-thalassemia mutations. Of the α-thalassemia mutant chromosomes, 5,205 chromosomes carried α-thalassemia gene mutations, of which the most frequent mutation was $-^{SEA}$ (69.01%), followed by $-\alpha^{3.7}$ (21.34), $-\alpha^{4.2}$ (3.96%), $\alpha\alpha^{QS}$ (2.19%), $\alpha\alpha^{CS}$ (1.59%), and $\alpha\alpha^{WS}$ (1.48%) (**Table 5**). Regarding the β-thalassemia mutant chromosomes, 2,223 chromosomes carrying β-thalassemia gene mutations were detected, of which the five most common mutations were IVS-II-654(C > T), CD41-42(-TCTT), CD17(A > T), CD26(G > A), and −28(A > G). The allele frequencies were 36.08%, 29.55%, 17.23%, 5.80%, and 4.77%, respectively (**Table 6**).

To further investigate the hemoglobin variants, we performed a DNA sequencing analysis. Altogether, we detected 24 cases

TABLE 3 | Distribution of β-thalassemia genotypes in Quanzhou Prefecture.

Types	Genotypes	Cases	Frequency	Class
β^0/β^N or β^+/β^N	$\beta^{IVS-II-654}/\beta^N$	744	36.19%	Common
	$\beta^{CD41-42}/\beta^N$	613	29.82%	Common
	β^{CD17}/β^N	345	16.78%	Common
	β^{CD26}/β^N	110	5.35%	Common
	β^{-28}/β^N	94	4.57%	Common
	$\beta^{CD27/28}/\beta^N$	47	2.29%	Common
	$\beta^{CD71-72}/\beta^N$	22	1.07%	Common
	β^{CD43}/β^N	18	0.88%	Common
	β^{-29}/β^N	8	0.39%	Common
	$\beta^{CAP+40-43}\beta^N$	7	0.34%	Common
	β^{Int}/β^N	4	0.19%	Common
	$\beta^{SEA-HPFH}/\beta^N$	3	0.15%	Rare
	$\beta^{IVS-I-1}/\beta^N$	3	0.15%	Common
	$\beta^{TermCD+32}/\beta^N$	3	0.15%	Rare
	β^{CD53}/β^N	2	0.10%	Rare
	β^{CD37}/β^N	2	0.10%	Rare
	$\beta^{IVS-I-5}/\beta^N$	2	0.10%	Common
	$\beta^{CD14-15}/\beta^N$	2	0.10%	Common
	β^{-90}/β^N	1	0.05%	Rare
	$\beta^{CD54-58}/\beta^N$	1	0.05%	Rare
	β^{Malay}/β^N	1	0.05%	Rare
	β^{CD3}/β^N	1	0.05%	Rare
	$\beta^{IVS-II-806}/\beta^N$	1	0.05%	Rare
	$\beta^{IVS-II-672}/\beta^N$	1	0.05%	Rare
β^+/β^+ or β^0/β^+ or β^0/β^0	$\beta^{IVS-II-654}/\beta^{IVS-II-654}$	4	0.19%	Common
	$\beta^{IVS-II-654}/\beta^{CD17}$	4	0.19%	Common
	$\beta^{CD41-42}/\beta^{CD41-42}$	2	0.10%	Common
	$\beta^{CD26}/\beta^{CD26}$	2	0.10%	Common
	$\beta^{CD17}/\beta^{CD17}$	1	0.05%	Common
	$\beta^{IVS-II-654M}/\beta^{-28}$	1	0.05%	Common
	$\beta^{IVS-II-654}/\beta^{CD27/28}$	1	0.05%	Common
	$\beta^{IVS-II-654}/\beta^{CD41-42}$	1	0.05%	Common
	$\beta^{CD41-42}/\beta^{CD17}$	1	0.05%	Common
	$\beta^{CD41-42}/\beta^{CD26}$	1	0.05%	Common
	$\beta^{IVS-II-654M}/\beta^{CD26}$	1	0.05%	Common
	$\beta^{CD41-42}/\beta^{CD43}$	1	0.05%	Common
	$\beta^{IVS-I-130}/\beta^{IVS-II-81}$	1	0.05%	Rare
	Total	2056	100%	

TABLE 4 | Distribution of compound α and β-thalassemia in Quanzhou Prefecture.

Genotypes	$-^{SEA}/$	$-\alpha^{3.7}/$	$-\alpha^{4.2}/$	$\alpha\alpha^{WS}/$	$\alpha\alpha^{CS}/$	$\alpha\alpha^{QS}/$	$-\alpha^{3.7}/-^{SEA}$	$-\alpha^{3.7}/-\alpha^{3.7}$
	$\alpha\alpha$	$\alpha\alpha$	$\alpha\alpha$	$\alpha\alpha$	$\alpha\alpha$	$\alpha\,\alpha$		
$\beta^{IVS-II-654}/\beta^N$	21	10	3	3	2	2	0	1
$\beta^{CD41-42}/\beta^N$	13	14	4	4	0	1	0	0
β^{CD17}/β^N	10	13	1	2	3	2	0	0
β^{CD26}/β^N	3	5	0	2	0	0	1	0
β^{-28}/β^N	3	6	1	0	1	0	0	0
$\beta^{CD27/28}/\beta^N$	0	2	0	0	0	0	0	0
$\beta^{CD71-72}/\beta^N$	0	3	0	0	1	0	0	0
$\beta^{CAP+40-43}\beta^N$	4	0	1	0	0	0	1	0
β^{Int}/β^N	0	1	0	0	0	0	0	0
$\beta^{CD26}/\beta^{CD26}$	0	0	0	0	1	0	0	0

the most common non-deletional α-thalassemia variant in Fujian and Jiangxi province, Guangdong and Hunan province mainly exhibited the $\alpha\alpha^{CS}$ mutation, and $\alpha\alpha^{WS}$ was the most widespread non-deletional α-thalassemia variant in Guangxi province. The IVS-II-654(C > T) and CD41-42(-TCTT) mutations were the most common β-thalassemia mutations in Fujian and its neighboring provinces, except in Guangxi province, which mainly carried CD41-42(-TCTT) and CD17(A > T) mutations.

DISCUSSION

In China, there is a high prevalence of thalassemia in the regions south of the Yangtze River, particularly in Guangdong and Guangxi. In 2019, a study showed that the prevalence of thalassemia in Fujian was 6.8% (Huang et al., 2019). Few studies are available on the genotypes of thalassemia in Quanzhou prefecture, and there have been few investigations into rare thalassemia and hemoglobinopathy. In this study, we present the spectrum mutation of rare thalassemia and hemoglobinopathy in Quanzhou, Southeast China.

We discovered 7,085 subjects who harbored thalassemia mutations; therefore, the detection rate was 40.70%. As **Table 5** displays, we identified 5,205 chromosomes carrying α-thalassemia gene mutations. The three most common deletional variants were $-^{SEA}$, $-\alpha^{3.7}$, and $-\alpha^{4.2}$, which is consistent with previous studies in Fujian province and neighboring provinces (Xu et al., 2004; Zheng et al., 2011; Lin et al., 2014, 2019; Dai et al., 2017; Cao et al., 2019; Liu et al., 2019; Chen M. F. et al., 2020). However, the non-deletional variants of α-thalassemia showed a great disparity with other regions (Xu et al., 2004; Zheng et al., 2011; Lin et al., 2014; Liu et al., 2019). Among these variants, 22 cases of rare α-thalassemia were detected, with $-^{THAI}/\alpha\alpha$ and $Hk\alpha\alpha/-^{SEA}$ being the most common. This is consistent with another study conducted in Fujian province (Huang et al., 2019). Before this study, $-^{FIL}/\alpha\alpha$ had only ever been detected in Taiwan; thus, this was the first-ever reported case in Fujian province (Chen et al., 2002). The $-^{FIL}$ deletion covers both the α1 and α2 gene, which leads to α-thalassemia major if compounded with $-^{SEA}$ deletion. We identified five cases of the $\alpha\alpha^{IVS-II-55(T>G)}/\alpha\alpha$

of Hb Q-Thailand [CD74(GAC > CAC)], two cases of Hb G-Honolulu [CD30(GAG > CAG)], and one case of Hb Owari [CD121(GTG > ATG)], all of which were induced by the α-globin gene mutation. Similarly, we identified 37 cases of Hb New York [CD113(GTG > GAG)], 12 cases of Hb J-Bangkok [CD56(GGC > GAC)], one case of Hb Miyashiro [CD23(GTT > GGT)], and one case of Hb G-Coushatta [CD22(GAA > GCA)]. These cases were caused by the β-globin gene mutation (**Figure 4**).

By analyzing the spectrum of thalassemia genotypes in Fujian and the neighboring provinces, we discovered that the highest frequency genotypes of deletional α-thalassemia were similar. However, the mutations in α-thalassemia and β-thalassemia showed distinct regional differences. As **Table 7** reveals, $\alpha\alpha^{QS}$ was

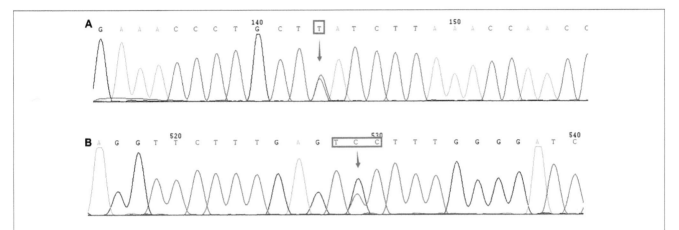

FIGURE 3 | Identification of δ-globin gene mutation using DNA sequencing. Arrows indicate the location of the mutations. **(A)** −77(T > C) (HBD:c.-127T > C) mutation in the *HBD* gene. **(B)** Novel mutation of CD44(TCC > TGC) (HBD:c.134C > G) in the *HBD* gene.

TABLE 5 | Allele frequency of α-thalassemia mutations in Quanzhou Prefecture.

Mutation type	HGVS name	Allele	Frequency
_SEA	NC_000016.9:g.215400_234700del	3592	69.01%
−α³·⁷	NC_000016.9:g.223300_227103del	1111	21.34%
−α⁴·²	NC_000016.9:g.219817_(223755_224074)del	206	3.96%
αα^QS	HBA2: c.377T > C	114	2.19%
αα^CS	HBA2: c.427T > C	83	1.59%
αα^WS	HBA2: c.369C > G	77	1.48%
Hkαα	/	7	0.13%
_THAI	NC_000016.9:g.199800_233300del	6	0.12%
αα^{IVS−II−55(T>G)}	HBA2: c.300 + 55T > G	5	0.10%
ααα^{anti 4.2}	/	1	0.02%
_FIL	NC_000016.9:g.200820_232670del	1	0.02%
−α²⁷·⁶	NC_000016.9:g.198215_225854del	1	0.02%
−α⁶·⁹	NG_000006.1:g.29785_36746del	1	0.02%
Total		5205	100%

HGVS, human genome variation society.

TABLE 6 | Allele frequency of β-thalassemia mutations in Quanzhou Prefecture.

Mutation type	HGVS name	Allele	Frequency
IVS-II-654(C > T)	HBB: c.316−197C > T	802	36.08%
CD41-42(-TCTT)	HBB: c.126_129delCTTT	657	29.55%
CD17(A > T)	HBB: c.52A > T	383	17.23%
CD26(G > A)	HBB: c.79G > A	129	5.80%
−28(A > G)	HBB: c.-78A > G	106	4.77%
CD27/28(+ C)	HBB: c.84_85insC	50	2.25%
CD71-72 (+ A)	HBB: c.216_217insA	26	1.17%
CD43 (G > T)	HBB: c.130G > T	19	0.85%
CAP + 40-43(-AAAC)	HBB: c.-11_-8delAAAC	13	0.58%
−29(A > G)	HBB: c.-79A > G	8	0.36%
Initiation codon(T > G)	HBB: c.2T > G	5	0.22%
SEA-HPFH	NC_000011.10:g.5222877_5250288del	3	0.13%
Term CD + 32(A > C)	HBB: c. + 32A > C	3	0.13%
CD53(-T)	HBB: c.162delT	3	0.13%
CD37(G > A)	HBB: c.113G > A	2	0.09%
IVS-I-1(G > T)	HBB: c.92 + 1G > T	2	0.09%
CD14-15(+ G)	HBB: c.45_46insG	2	0.09%
IVS-I-5(G > C)	HBB: c.92 + 5G > C	2	0.09%
−90(C > T)	HBB: c.-140C > T	1	0.04%
CD3(C > T)	HBB: c.10C > T	1	0.04%
CD54-58(-TATGGG CAACCCT)	HBB: c.165_177 delT ATGGGCAACCCT	1	0.04%
IVS-II-806(G > C)	HBB: c.316−45G > C	1	0.04%
IVS-I-130(G > C)	HBB: c.93-1G > C	1	0.04%
IVS-II-81(C > T)	HBB: c.315 + 81C > T	1	0.04%
Hb Malay(A > G)	HBB: c.59A > G	1	0.04%
IVS-II-672 (A > C)	HBB: c.316−179 A > C	1	0.04%
Total		2,223	100%

HGVS, human genome variation society.

mutation in this study, a mutation that was first identified in Fuzhou city and subsequently reported in the Nanping region of Fujian province (Cao et al., 2019; Chen M. F. et al., 2020). This indicates that $\alpha\alpha^{IVS-II-55(T>G)}$ may be an increasingly common mutation that will possibly become more prevalent in Fujian province. Further analysis of the hematological phenotype of $\alpha\alpha^{IVS-II-55(T>G)}/\alpha\alpha$ provided similar results as tests for $\alpha\alpha^{WS}/\alpha\alpha$.

In this study, we detected 2,223 chromosomes carrying β-thalassemia gene mutations. The most frequent mutation was IVS-II-654(C > T), which was consistent with several regions in South China (Lin et al., 2014; Dai et al., 2017; Cao et al., 2019; Liu et al., 2019; Chen M. F. et al., 2020). However, the most prevalent β-thalassemia mutation in the nearby provinces of Guangdong and Guangxi is CD41-42(-TCTT) (Xu et al., 2004; Zheng et al., 2011). Our study indicates a higher frequency of the CD26(G > A) mutation in comparison with other regions in Fujian province. A previous study demonstrated that CD26(G > A) is the most common β-thalassemia mutation

in Yunnan province, which is located in Southwestern China (Zhang et al., 2012). In this research, we detected a diverse range of rare or novel β-thalassemia variants. Among them, this was only the second time the $\beta^{IVS-II-806}/\beta^{N}$ mutation,

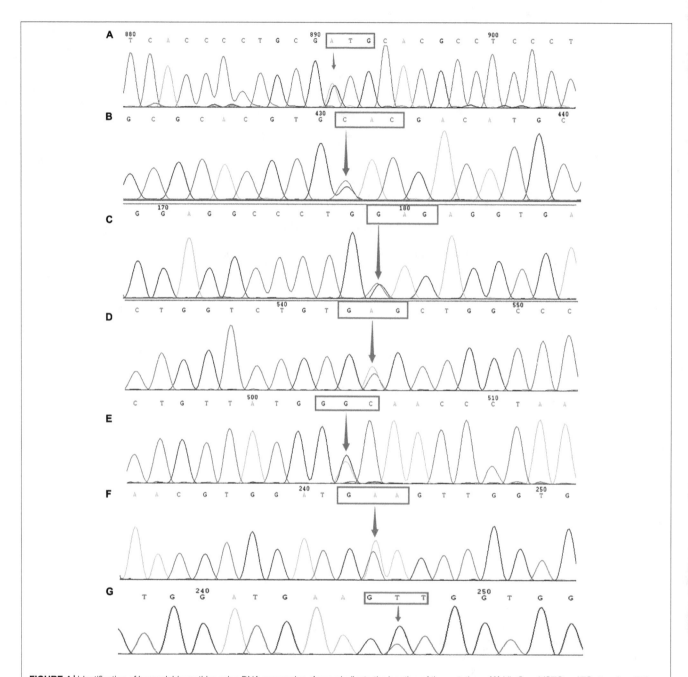

FIGURE 4 | Identification of hemoglobinopathies using DNA sequencing. Arrows indicate the location of the mutations. **(A)** Hb Owari (GTG > ATG at codon 121) mutation in the *HBA1* gene. **(B)** Hb Q-Thailand (GAC > CAC at codon 74) mutation in the *HBA1* gene. **(C)** Hb G-Honolulu (GAG > CAG at codon 30) mutation in the *HBA2* gene. **(D)** Hb New York (GTG > GAG at codon 113) mutation in the *HBB* gene. **(E)** Hb J-Bangkok (GGC > GAC at codon 56) mutation in the *HBB* gene. **(F)** Hb G-Coushatta (GAA > GCA at codon 22) in the *HBB* gene. **(G)** Hb Miyashiro (GTT > GGT at codon 23) mutation in the *HBB* gene.

which was first identified in the Nanping region north of Fujian, had been identified in humans (Chen M. F. et al., 2020). Additionally, we made the earliest discovery of the rare mutations of Hb Malay(AAC > AGC), IVS-II-672(A > C), and IVS-I-130(G > C) in Fujian province. In the Chinese population, Hb Malay is an extremely rare "Hb Knossos-like" β^+-thalassemia abnormality, with only one known recorded case (Ma et al., 2000). This mutation is thought to create an alternate splicing site between codons 17 and 18, reducing the efficiency of the

normal donor splice site at IVS-I to about 60% (Yang et al., 1989). The IVS-II-672(A > C) mutation had only been previously reported in Guangxi province, which suggests that it is a silent mutation, as the red blood cell indices are normal and there are normal or borderline Hb A2 levels (Zhao et al., 2016). However, in the case of our study, low levels of hemoglobin (106 × 10^{12} g/L) and higher levels of Hb A2 (4.5%) were observed. Thus, more research should be conducted to reveal whether the IVS-II-672(A > C) mutation causes β^+-thalassemia.

TABLE 7 | Comparison of allele frequency of thalassemia mutations in Fujian and neighboring provinces.

Genotypes	Fujian Province				Guangdong Province (Xu et al., 2004)	Guangxi Province (Zheng et al., 2011)	Jiangxi Province (Lin et al., 2014)	Hunan Province (Liu et al., 2019)
	Quanzhou (this study)	Fuzhou (Cao et al., 2019)	Longyan (Dai et al., 2017)	Nanping (Chen M. F. et al., 2020)				
α-thalassemia								
_$_SEA$	69.01%	77.58%	81.76%	72.68%	48.54%	68.50%	66.51%	52.88%
$-\alpha^{3.7}$	21.34%	14.50%	13.27%	15.30%	36.40%	16.36%	22.86%	31.73%
$-\alpha^{4.2}$	3.96%	3.29%	4.97%	4.10%	11.09%	8.40%	8.08%	9.11%
$\alpha\alpha^{QS}$	2.19%	2.69%	–	2.46%	0.42%	0.62%	1.62%	1.15%
$\alpha\alpha^{CS}$	1.59%	0.45%	–	0.82%	2.09%	3.03%	0.92%	3.25%
$\alpha\alpha^{WS}$	1.48%	1.05%	–	0.55%	–	3.09%	–	1.88%
β-thalassemia								
IVS-II-654(C > T)	36.08%	41.81%	44.95%	35.27%	24.75%	5.26%	40.70%	38.89%
CD41-42(-TCTT)	29.55%	36.10%	28.11%	25.12%	36.36%	48.37%	30.81%	27.49%
CD17(A > T)	17.23%	9.74%	9.08%	10.14%	4.04%	27.40%	5.23%	13.82%
CD26(G > A)	5.80%	1.90%	1.46%	4.35%	5.05%	4.51%	0.58%	3.13%
−28(A > G)	4.77%	4.28%	8.20%	9.18%	16.67%	5.35%	15.70%	4.70%
CD27/28(+ C)	2.25%	4.04%	5.71%	3.38%	2.02%	0.08%	5.23%	2.14%

Additionally, we identified a rare compound mutation, which is a combination of the IVS-I-130(G > C) (β^0-thalassemia) and IVS-II-81(C > T) mutations. This causes minor thalassemia, which suggests that the IVS-II-81(C > T) mutation may be a silent mutation.

Besides, we identified two δ-globin gene mutations, including -77(T > C) and CD44 (TCC > TGC) (HBD:c.134C > G). Previous studies have shown that the -77(T > C) mutation is the most common δ-globin gene mutation in China (Liu et al., 2013; Chen M. et al., 2020) and may cause δ^0- or δ^+-thalassemia. In our case, the -77(T > C) mutation was combined with the CD17(A > T) mutation, resulting in normal levels of Hb A2 (2.7%). This indicates that the diagnosis of β-thalassemia could be hindered when it is combined with δ-thalassemia. Moreover, we made the first discovery in the Chinese population of the novel δ-globin gene mutation CD44(TCC > TGC) (HBD:c.134C > G). The mutation at codon 44, which results in Ser→Cys acid substitution, is believed to cause δ^+-thalassemia.

We conducted an extensive analysis of the hemoglobinopathy spectrum for the subjects in our study and identified three types of hemoglobinopathies that were induced by an α-globin gene mutation. Among them, Hb Q-Thailand (α74: Asp→His) has previously been reported in Chinese and other Southeast Asian populations. It is invariably linked to a leftward single α-globin gene deletion ($-\alpha^{4.2}$) and causes Hb Q-H disease when associated with α-thalassemia (mainly $-^{SEA}$) (Hu et al., 2011; Zeng et al., 1992). Moreover, our study presented the first cases of Hb Owari (α121:Val→Met) in Fujian province, which was first identified in the Japanese population and exhibits normal functional properties (Harano et al., 1986). Additionally, we detected 37 cases of Hb New York, 12 cases of Hb J-Bangkok, and one case each of Hb Miyashiro and Hb G-Coushatta, all of which are induced by the β-globin gene mutation. We

detected the first cases in the Quanzhou region of Hb New York, Hb J-Bangkok, and Hb G-Coushatta in this study. Previous studies indicated that co-inheritance of Hb New York with three α-globin gene deletions could lead to a severe Hb H disease (Chan et al., 1987). In this study, we identified a male compound of Hb J-Bangkok and CD41-42(-TCTT). He exhibited normal hemoglobin values (137 × 10^{12} g/L), low levels of MCV (56 fl) and MCH (18.3 pg), and increased Hb A2 (6.0%). Our results were consistent with those of a previous study, which suggested that the coexistence of Hb J-Bangkok and β-thalassemia may not aggravate the phenotype (Zhao et al., 2013). Moreover, our study first identified the rare Hb Miyashiro mutation in the Chinese population. There is a GTT > GGT mutation at codon 23 in the β-globin gene, which can be detected by polyacrylamide gel isoelectric focusing (IEF) or reversed-phase high-performance liquid chromatography (HPLC) (Nakatsuji et al., 1981; Ohba et al., 1984). Therefore, we believe that it is essential to identify the hemoglobin variants in a population with a high prevalence of thalassemia in a routine setting.

A diverse range of rare thalassemia mutations was identified in this study, which is consistent with the location and the increasing population in Quanzhou prefecture. Notably, with thalassemia detection kits, we identified some rare thalassemia mutations that were more pervasive than the so-called common thalassemia mutations, such as CD31(-C), −32(C > A), and −30(T > C), which have never been detected in this region before. Nowadays, next-generation sequencing is being increasingly used to improve thalassemia detection (He et al., 2017; Zhao et al., 2020). Thus, DNA sequencing technology combined with gap-PCR can detect all known and unknown mutations in the α- and β-globin gene in a cost-effective way, which will greatly reduce missed diagnoses.

CONCLUSION

In this study, we conducted a comprehensive large-scale study on the thalassemia mutation in Quanzhou prefecture, which provides valuable data for the prevention and control of thalassemia. Our study is the first to reveal the spectrum of rare thalassemia mutations and hemoglobinopathies in the Quanzhou region. From this study, a diversity of rare thalassemia mutations and hemoglobinopathies was identified. This research, combined with the use of DNA sequencing and gap-PCR technology, shows great value in the investigation of rare and novel thalassemia gene mutations.

ETHICS STATEMENT

The studies involving human participants were reviewed and approved by the Ethics Committee of The Women's and Children's Hospital of Quanzhou (2020No.8). The patients/participants provided their written informed consent to participate in this study.

AUTHOR CONTRIBUTIONS

JZ designed the study and wrote the article. NZ and JZ performed conventional thalassemia analysis. YZ performed specific gap-PCR amplification and DNA sequencing. NZ and HZ analyzed the data. YX, YJ, DC, and YW revised and polished the manuscript. All authors have approved the final article.

ACKNOWLEDGMENTS

We wish to thank the subjects for agreeing to participate in this study. We would also like to express our appreciation to Quanzhou City Science and Technology Bureau for funding this work.

REFERENCES

Cao, P. J., Chen, L. Y., Jiang, L. L., Yang, Y., Chen, S. T., Huang, C. L., et al. (2019). [Analysis of Gene Mutation Types of Thalassemia in Fuzhou Area of China]. *Zhongguo Shi Yan Xue Ye Xue Za Zhi.* 27, 893–898.

Chan, V., Chan, T. K., Tso, S. C., and Todd, D. (1987). Combination of three alpha-globin gene loci deletions and hemoglobin New York results in a severe hemoglobin H syndrome. *Am. J. Hematol.* 24, 301–306. doi: 10.1002/ajh. 2830240310

Chen, M., Huang, H., Chen, L., Lin, N., Zhang, M., Lin, Y., et al. (2020). First report of the spectrum of δ-globin gene mutations among women of reproductive age in Fujian area-Discrimination of δ-thalassemia, α-thalassemia, and Iron Deficiency Anemia. *J. Clin. Lab. Anal.* 34:e23479.

Chen, M. F., Huang, M. Z., Lin, Q., Huang, J., Chen, F., Zhang, J. Y., et al. (2020). [Analysis of the Types of Thalassemia Gene Mutations in Nanping Area of Fujian, China]. *Zhongguo Shi Yan Xue Ye Xue Za Zhi.* 28, 918–926.

Chen, T. P., Liu, T. C., Chang, C. S., Chang, J. G., Tsai, H. J., and Lin, S. F. (2002). PCR-based analysis of alpha-thalassemia in Southern Taiwan. *Int. J. Hematol.* 75, 277–280. doi: 10.1007/bf02982041

Dai, Q. F., Li, X. L., Wang, Y. X., and Cao, C. F. (2017). [Analysis of Gene Mutation Types of Thalassemia in Longyan Area of Fujian Province in China]. *Zhongguo Shi Yan Xue Ye Xue Za Zhi.* 25, 498–502.

Harano, T., Harano, K., and Ueda, S. (1986). Hb Owari [alpha 121 (H 4) Val—-Met]: a new hemoglobin variant with a neutral-to-neutral amino acid substitution detected by isoelectric focusing. *Hemoglobin* 10, 127–134. doi: 10.3109/03630268609046439

He, J., Song, W., Yang, J., Lu, S., Yuan, Y., Guo, J., et al. (2017). Next-generation sequencing improves thalassemia carrier screening among premarital adults in a high prevalence population: the Dai nationality, China. *Genet. Med.* 19, 1022–1031. doi: 10.1038/gim.2016.218

He, S., Li, J., Li, D. M., Yi, S., Lu, X., Luo, Y., et al. (2018). Molecular characterization of α- and β-thalassemia in the Yulin region of Southern China. *Gene* 655, 61–64. doi: 10.1016/j.gene.2018.02.058

Hu, C., Zhang, L., Pan, J., Zeng, Z., Zhen, S., Fang, J., et al. (2011). Three cases of Hb Q-H disease found in a Cantonese family. *Mol. Med. Rep.* 4, 279–281.

Huang, H., Xu, L., Chen, M., Lin, N., Xue, H., Chen, L., et al. (2019). Molecular characterization of thalassemia and hemoglobinopathy in Southeastern China. *Sci. Rep.* 9:3493.

Li, B., Zhang, X. Z., Yin, A. H., Zhao, Q. G., Wu, L., Ma, Y. Z., et al. (2014). High prevalence of thalassemia in migrant populations in Guangdong Province, China. *BMC Public Health* 14:905. doi: 10.1186/1471-2458-14-905

Liaska, A., Petrou, P., Georgakopoulos, C. D., Diamanti, R., Papaconstantinou, D., Kanakis, M. G., et al. (2016). β-Thalassemia and ocular implications: a systematic review. *BMC Ophthalmol.* 16:102. doi: 10.1186/s12886-016-0285-2

Lin, M., Zhong, T. Y., Chen, Y. G., Wang, J. Z., Wu, J. R., Lin, F., et al. (2014). Molecular epidemiological characterization and health burden of thalassemia in Jiangxi Province, P. R. China. *PLoS One* 9:e101505. doi: 10.1371/journal.pone. 0101505

Lin, Y. H., Lin, W., and Wang, X. X. (2019). [Genotyping of Patients with α and β Thalassemia in Fujian Province Area in China]. *Zhongguo Shi Yan Xue Ye Xue Za Zhi.* 27, 899–903.

Liu, N., Xie, X. M., Zhou, J. Y., Li, R., Liao, C., and Li, D. Z. (2013). Analysis of δ-globin gene mutations in the Chinese population. *Hemoglobin* 37, 85–93. doi: 10.3109/03630269.2012.747965

Liu, Q., Jia, Z. J., Xi, H., Liu, J., Peng, Y., and Wang, H. (2019). [Analysis on the Genotype of 5018 Cases of Thalassemia in Hunan Area]. *Zhongguo Shi Yan Xue Ye Xue Za Zhi.* 27, 1938–1942.

Lu, H., Qin, Q., Li, J. H., Chen, T., Liang, S. J., and Lu, X. S. (2021). [Genetic Diagnosis of Thalassemia in Baise, Guangxi Zhuang Autonomous Region]. *Zhongguo Shi Yan Xue Ye Xue Za Zhi.* 29, 865–868.

Ma, S. K., Chow, E. Y., Chan, A. Y., Kung, N. N., Waye, J. S., Chan, L. C., et al. (2000). beta-thalassemia intermedia caused by compound heterozygosity for Hb Malay (beta codon 19 AAC-> AGC; asn-> Ser) and codons 41/42 (-CTTT) beta(0)-thalassemia mutation. *Am. J. Hematol.* 64, 206–209. doi: 10.1002/1096-8652(200007)64:3<206::aid-ajh12>3.0.co;2-#

Modell, B., and Darlison, M. (2008). Global epidemiology of haemoglobin disorders and derived service indicators. *Bull. World Health Organ.* 86, 480–487. doi: 10.2471/blt.06.036673

Nakatsuji, T., Miwa, S., Ohba, Y., Hattori, Y., Miyaji, T., Miyata, H., et al. (1981). Hemoglobin Miyashiro (beta 23[B5] val substituting for gly) an electrophoretically silent variant discovered by the isopropanol test. *Hemoglobin* 5, 653–666. doi: 10.3109/03630268108991833

Ohba, Y., Hattori, Y., Miyaji, T., Takasaki, M., Shirahama, M., Fujisawa, K., et al. (1984). Purification and properties of hemoglobin Miyashiro. *Hemoglobin* 8, 515–518. doi: 10.3109/03630268408991736

Vichinsky, E. P. (2013). Clinical manifestations of α-thalassemia. *Cold Spring Harb. Perspect. Med.* 3:a011742. doi: 10.1101/cshperspect.a011742

Weatherall, D. J. (2001). Phenotype-genotype relationships in monogenic disease: lessons from the thalassaemias. *Nat. Rev. Genet.* 2, 245–255. doi: 10.1038/35066048

Weatherall, D. J. (2008). Hemoglobinopathies worldwide: present and future. *Curr. Mol. Med.* 8, 592–599. doi: 10.2174/156652408786241375

Xu, L. P., Huang, H. L., Wang, Y., Zheng, L., Wang, L. S., Xu, J. B., et al. (2013). [Molecular epidemiological analysis of α- and β-thalassemia in Fujian province]. *Zhonghua Yi Xue Yi Chuan Xue Za Zhi.* 30, 403–406.

Xu, X. M., Zhou, Y. Q., Luo, G. X., Liao, C., Zhou, M., Chen, P. Y., et al. (2004). The prevalence and spectrum of alpha and beta thalassaemia in Guangdong Province: implications for the future health burden and population screening. *J. Clin. Pathol.* 57, 517–522. doi: 10.1136/jcp.2003.014456

Yang, K. G., Kutlar, F., George, E., Wilson, J. B., Kutlar, A., Stoming, T. A., et al. (1989). Molecular characterization of beta-globin gene mutations in Malay patients with Hb E-beta-thalassaemia and thalassaemia major. *Br. J. Haematol.* 72, 73–80. doi: 10.1111/j.1365-2141.1989.tb07655.x

Yao, H., Chen, X., Lin, L., Wu, C., Fu, X., Wang, H., et al. (2014). The spectrum of α- and β-thalassemia mutations of the Li people in Hainan Province of China. *Blood Cells Mol. Dis.* 53, 16–20. doi: 10.1016/j.bcmd.2014.01.003

Yin, A., Li, B., Luo, M., Xu, L., Wu, L., Zhang, L., et al. (2014). The prevalence and molecular spectrum of α- and β-globin gene mutations in 14,332 families of Guangdong Province, China. *PLoS One* 9:e89855. doi: 10.1371/journal.pone.0089855

Zeng, F. Y., Fucharoen, S., Huang, S. Z., and Rodgers, G. P. (1992). Hb Q-Thailand [alpha 74(EF3)Asp->His]: gene organization, molecular structure, and DNA diagnosis. *Hemoglobin* 16, 481–491. doi: 10.3109/03630269208993116

Zhang, C. M., Wang, Y., Gao, L. S., Gao, J. H., He, X. L., Feng, H. J., et al. (2010). Molecular epidemiology investigation of beta-thalassemia in Zhongshan City, Guangdong Province, People's Republic of China. *Hemoglobin* 34, 55–60. doi: 10.3109/03630260903547724

Zhang, J., Zhu, B. S., He, J., Zeng, X. H., Su, J., Xu, X. H., et al. (2012). The spectrum of α- and β-thalassemia mutations in Yunnan Province of Southwestern China. *Hemoglobin* 36, 464–473. doi: 10.3109/03630269.2012.717327

Zhao, J., Li, J., Lai, Q., and Yu, Y. (2020). Combined use of gap-PCR and next-generation sequencing improves thalassaemia carrier screening among premarital adults in China. *J. Clin. Pathol.* 73, 488–492. doi: 10.1136/jclinpath-2019-206339

Zhao, L., Qing, J., Liang, Y., and Chen, Z. (2016). A novel compound heterozygosity in Southern China: IVS-II-5 (G>C) and IVS-II-672 (A>C). *Hemoglobin* 40, 428–430. doi: 10.1080/03630269.2016.1252387

Zhao, Y., Shang, X., Xiong, F., Liu, Y. H., Lou, J. W., and Xu, X. M. (2013). [Analysis of clinical phenotypes of compound heterozygotes of Hb J-Bangkok and β-thalassemia]. *Zhonghua Yi Xue Yi Chuan Xue Za Zhi.* 30, 148–151.

Zheng, C. G., Liu, M., Du, J., Chen, K., Yang, Y., and Yang, Z. (2011). Molecular spectrum of α- and β-globin gene mutations detected in the population of Guangxi Zhuang Autonomous Region, People's Republic of China. *Hemoglobin* 35, 28–39. doi: 10.3109/03630269.2010.547429

Zhuang, J., Jiang, Y., Wang, Y., Zheng, Y., Zhuang, Q., Wang, J., et al. (2020a). Molecular analysis of α-thalassemia and β-thalassemia in Quanzhou region Southeast China. *J. Clin. Pathol.* 73, 278–282. doi: 10.1136/jclinpath-2019-206179

Zhuang, J., Tian, J., Wei, J., Zheng, Y., Zhuang, Q., Wang, Y., et al. (2019). Molecular analysis of a large novel deletion causing α+-thalassemia. *BMC Med. Genet.* 20:74. doi: 10.1186/s12881-019-0797-8

Zhuang, J., Zheng, Y., Wang, Y., Zhuang, Q., Jiang, Y., Xie, Q., et al. (2020b). Identification of a new β-thalassaemia variant Term CD+32(HBB: c.32A>C) in two Chinese families. *J. Clin. Pathol.* 73, 593–596. doi: 10.1136/jclinpath-2020-206426

Permissions

The contributors of this book come from diverse backgrounds, making this book a truly international effort. This book will bring forth new frontiers with its revolutionizing research information and detailed analysis of the nascent developments around the world.

We would like to thank all the contributing authors for lending their expertise to make the book truly unique. They have played a crucial role in the development of this book. Without their invaluable contributions this book wouldn't have been possible. They have made vital efforts to compile up to date information on the varied aspects of this subject to make this book a valuable addition to the collection of many professionals and students.

This book was conceptualized with the vision of imparting up-to-date information and advanced data in this field. To ensure the same, a matchless editorial board was set up. Every individual on the board went through rigorous rounds of assessment to prove their worth. After which they invested a large part of their time researching and compiling the most relevant data for our readers.

The editorial board has been involved in producing this book since its inception. They have spent rigorous hours researching and exploring the diverse topics which have resulted in the successful publishing of this book. They have passed on their knowledge of decades through this book. To expedite this challenging task, the publisher supported the team at every step. A small team of assistant editors was also appointed to further simplify the editing procedure and attain best results for the readers.

Apart from the editorial board, the designing team has also invested a significant amount of their time in understanding the subject and creating the most relevant covers. They scrutinized every image to scout for the most suitable representation of the subject and create an appropriate cover for the book.

The publishing team has been an ardent support to the editorial, designing and production team. Their endless efforts to recruit the best for this project, has resulted in the accomplishment of this book. They are a veteran in the field of academics and their pool of knowledge is as vast as their experience in printing. Their expertise and guidance has proved useful at every step. Their uncompromising quality standards have made this book an exceptional effort. Their encouragement from time to time has been an inspiration for everyone.

The publisher and the editorial board hope that this book will prove to be a valuable piece of knowledge for researchers, students, practitioners and scholars across the globe.

List of Contributors

Gloria Barbarani, Agata Łabedz and Antonella Ellena Ronchi
Dipartimento di Biotecnologie e Bioscienze, Università di Milano-Bicocca, Milan, Italy

Bella Banjanin
Department of Hematology, Erasmus Medical Center Cancer Institute, Rotterdam, Netherlands
Oncode Institute, Erasmus Medical Center Cancer Institute, Rotterdam, Netherlands

Rebekka K. Schneider
Department of Hematology, Erasmus Medical Center Cancer Institute, Rotterdam, Netherlands
Oncode Institute, Erasmus Medical Center Cancer Institute, Rotterdam, Netherlands
Department of Cell Biology, Faculty of Medicine, Institute for Biomedical Engineering, Rheinisch-Westfälische Technische Hochschule (RWTH) Aachen University, Aachen, German

Georges Blattner, Alessia Cavazza, Adrian J. Thrasher and Giandomenico Turchiano
Infection, Immunity and Inflammation Research and Teaching Department, Zayed Centre for Research into Rare Disease in Children, Great Ormond Street Institute of Child Health, University College London, London, United Kingdom

Alejandra Gutierrez-Guerrero, Philippe E. Mangeot, Caroline Costa, Ornellie Bernadin, Séverine Périan, Floriane Fusil, Gisèle Froment and François-Loïc Cosset
CIRI–International Center for Infectiology Research, Inserm, U1111, Université Claude Bernard Lyon 1, CNRS, UMR5308, Ecole Normale Supérieure de Lyon, Université Lyon, Lyon, France

Maria Jimena Abrey Recalde
CIRI–International Center for Infectiology Research, Inserm, U1111, Université Claude Bernard Lyon 1, CNRS, UMR5308, Ecole Normale Supérieure de Lyon, Université Lyon, Lyon, France
Laboratory of Lentiviral Vectors and Gene Therapy, University Institute of Italian Hospital, National Scientific and Technical Research Council (CONICET), Buenos Aires, Argentina

Adriana Martinez-Turtos and Adrien Krug
Université Côte d'Azur, INSERM, Nice, France

Francisco Martin and Karim Benabdellah
Centre for Genomics and Oncological Research (GENYO), Genomic Medicine Department, Pfizer/University of Granada/Andalusian Regional Government, Granada, Spain

Emiliano P. Ricci
CIRI–International Center for Infectiology Research, Inserm, U1111, Université Claude Bernard Lyon 1, CNRS, UMR5308, Ecole Normale Supérieure de Lyon, Université Lyon, Lyon, France
Laboratory of Biology and Modeling of the Cell (LBMC), Université de Lyon, Ecole Normale Supérieure de Lyon (ENS de Lyon), Université Claude Bernard, Inserm, U1210, CNRS, UMR5239, Lyon, France

Els Verhoeyen
CIRI–International Center for Infectiology Research, Inserm, U1111, Université Claude Bernard Lyon 1, CNRS, UMR5308, Ecole Normale Supérieure de Lyon, Université Lyon, Lyon, France
Université Côte d'Azur, INSERM, Nice, France

Rik Gijsbers
Laboratory for Viral Vector Technology & Gene Therapy, Department of Pharmaceutical and Pharmacological Sciences, Faculty of Medicine, Katholieke Universiteit Leuven, Leuven, Belgium

Simone Giovannozzi
Laboratory for Viral Vector Technology & Gene Therapy, Department of Pharmaceutical and Pharmacological Sciences, Faculty of Medicine, Katholieke Universiteit Leuven, Leuven, Belgium
KU Leuven, Department of Microbiology, Immunology and Transplantation, Allergy and Clinical Immunology Research Group, Leuven, Belgium

Eduard Ayuso
INSERM UMR1089, University of Nantes, Centre Hospitalier Universitaire, Nantes, France

Alex J. Félix, Anna Solé, Véronique Noé and Carlos J. Ciudad
Department of Biochemistry and Physiology, School of Pharmacy and Food Sciences, and Institute for Nanoscience and Nanotechnology (IN2UB), University of Barcelona, Barcelona, Spain

Stefanie Klaver-Flores, Kirsten Canté-Barrett, Karin Pike-Overzet and Frank J. T. Staal
Department of Immunology, Leiden University Medical Center, Leiden, Netherlands

Hidde A. Zittersteijn, Rob C. Hoeben and Manuel A. F. V. Gonçalves
Department of Cell and Chemical Biology, Leiden University Medical Center, Leiden, Netherlands

Arjan Lankester
Department of Pediatrics, Willem-Alexander Children's Hospital, Leiden University Medical Center, Leiden, Netherlands

Cornelis L. Harteveld
Department of Human and Clinical Genetics, The Hemoglobinopathies Laboratory, Leiden University Medical Center, Leiden, Netherlands
Department of Clinical Genetics, Leiden University Medical Center, ERN-EuroBloodNet Member, Leiden, Netherlands

Arjan C. Lankester
Department of Pediatrics, Stem Cell Transplantation Program, Willem-Alexander Children's Hospital, Leiden University Medical Center, Leiden, Netherlands

Samuele Ferrari and Valentina Vavassori
San Raffaele Telethon Institute for Gene Therapy (SR-Tiget), Istituto di Ricovero e Cura a Carattere Scientifico San Raffaele Scientific Institute, Milan, Italy
PhD course in Molecular Medicine, Vita-Salute San Raffele University, Milan, Italy

Daniele Canarutto
San Raffaele Telethon Institute for Gene Therapy (SR-Tiget), Istituto di Ricovero e Cura a Carattere Scientifico San Raffaele Scientific Institute, Milan, Italy
PhD course in Molecular Medicine, Vita-Salute San Raffele University, Milan, Italy
Pediatric Immunohematology and Bone Marrow Transplantation Unit, Istituto di Ricovero e Cura a Carattere Scientifico Ospedale San Raffaele, Milan, Italy

Aurelien Jacob
San Raffaele Telethon Institute for Gene Therapy (SR-Tiget), Istituto di Ricovero e Cura a Carattere Scientifico San Raffaele Scientific Institute, Milan, Italy
PhD Program in Translational and Molecular Medicine (DIMET), Milano-Bicocca University, Monza, Italy

Maria Carmina Castiello
San Raffaele Telethon Institute for Gene Therapy (SR-Tiget), Istituto di Ricovero e Cura a Carattere Scientifico San Raffaele Scientific Institute, Milan, Italy
Institute of Genetic and Biomedical Research Milan Unit, National Research Council, Milan, Italy

Attya Omer Javed
San Raffaele Telethon Institute for Gene Therapy (SR-Tiget), Istituto di Ricovero e Cura a Carattere Scientifico San Raffaele Scientific Institute, Milan, Italy

Pietro Genovese
Division of Hematology/Oncology, Boston Children's Hospital, Boston, MA, United States
Department of Pediatric Oncology, Dana-Farber Cancer Institute, Boston, MA, United States
Harvard Stem Cell Institute, Cambridge, MA, United States
Department of Pediatrics, Harvard Medical School, Boston, MA, United States

Elizabeth K. Benitez, Anastasia Lomova Kaufman, Lilibeth Cervantes, Danielle N. Clark, Paul G. Ayoub, Shantha Senadheera, Kyle Osborne, Julie M. Sanchez, Ralph Valentine Crisostomo, Roger P. Hollis, Zulema Romero and Donald B. Kohn
Department of Microbiology, Immunology & Molecular Genetics, David Geffen School of Medicine, University of California, Los Angeles, Los Angeles, CA, United States

Xiaoyan Wang
Department of General Internal Medicine and Health Services Research, University of California, Los Angeles, Los Angeles, CA, United States

Nina Reuven and Yosef Shaul
Department of Molecular Genetics, Weizmann Institute of Science, Rehovot, Israel

Cansu Koyunlar and Emma de Pater
Department of Hematology, Erasmus MC, Rotterdam, Netherlands

Giulia Pavani and Mario Amendola
INTEGRARE, UMR_S951, Genethon, Inserm, Univ Evry, Univ Paris-Saclay, Evry, France

Eleni Papanikolaou
Department of Molecular Technologies and Stem Cell Therapy, Miltenyi Biotec, Bergisch Gladbach, Germany
Laboratory of Biology, School of Medicine, National and Kapodistrian University of Athens, Athens, Greece

Andreas Bosio
Department of Molecular Technologies and Stem Cell Therapy, Miltenyi Biotec, Bergisch Gladbach, Germany

Panagiotis Antoniou, Annarita Miccio and Mégane Brusson
Université de Paris, Imagine Institute, Laboratory of Chromatin and Gene Regulation During Development, INSERM UMR 1163, Paris, France

William R. Simmons, Lily Wain, Joseph Toker, Jaya Jagadeesh and David M. Bodine
Hematopoiesis Section, Genetics and Molecular Biology Branch, National Human Genome Research Institute (NHGRI), Bethesda, MD, United States

Lisa J. Garrett
National Human Genome Research Institute (NHGRI) Embryonic Stem Cell and Transgenic Mouse Core Facility, Bethesda, MD, United States

Rini H. Pek and Iqbal Hamza
Department of Animal & Avian Sciences, University of Maryland, College Park, MD, United States

Daniel Allen, Michael Rosenberg and Ayal Hendel
Institute of Nanotechnology and Advanced Materials, The Mina and Everard Goodman Faculty of Life Sciences, Bar-Ilan University, Ramat-Gan, Israel

Ahlem Achour
Department of Clinical Genetics/LDGA, Leiden University Medical Center, Leiden, Netherlands
Department of Congenital and Hereditary Diseases, Charles Nicolle Hospital, Tunis, Tunisia

Tamara T. Koopmann and Gijs W. E. Santen
Department of Clinical Genetics, Leiden University Medical Center, ERN-EuroBloodNet Member, Leiden, Netherlands

Frank Baas
Department of Clinical Genetics/LDGA, Leiden University Medical Center, Leiden, Netherlands

Selma Gomez
Laboratoire de Biochimie et de Biologie Moléculaire, Faculté des Sciences et Techniques, University of Abomey-Calavi, Cotonou, Benin
Centre de Prise en charge Médicale Intégrée du Nourrisson et de la Femme Enceinte atteints de Drépanocytose, Faculté des Sciences de la Santé, University of Abomey-Calavi, Cotonou, Benin

Aïssatou Diawara and Youssef Idaghdour
Biology Program, Division of Science and Mathematics, New York University Abu Dhabi, Abu Dhabi, United Arab Emirates

Elias Gbeha and Philip Awadalla
Sainte-Justine Research Centre, Centre Hospitalier et Universitaire Sainte Justine, Montréal, QC, Canada

Ambaliou Sanni
Laboratoire de Biochimie et de Biologie Moléculaire, Faculté des Sciences et Techniques, University of Abomey-Calavi, Cotonou, Benin

M. Cherif Rahimy
Centre de Prise en charge Médicale Intégrée du Nourrisson et de la Femme Enceinte atteints de Drépanocytose, Faculté des Sciences de la Santé, University of Abomey-Calavi, Cotonou, Benin

Valeria Rizzuto
Translational Research in Child and Adolescent Cancer – Rare Anemia Disorders Research Laboratory, Vall d'Hebron Research Institute, ERN-EuroBloodNet Member, Barcelona, Spain
Josep Carreras Leukaemia Research Institute, Badalona, Spain
Department of Medicine, Universitat de Barcelona, Barcelona, Spain

Adoración Blanco-Álvarez and Barbara Tazón-Vega
Hematologic Molecular Genetics Unit, Hematology Department, Hospital Universitari Vall d'Hebron, ERN-EuroBloodNet Member, Barcelona, Spain

Amira Idrizovic and Maria del Mar Mañú-Pereira
Translational Research in Child and Adolescent Cancer – Rare Anemia Disorders Research Laboratory, Vall d'Hebron Research Institute, ERN-EuroBloodNet Member, Barcelona, Spain

Cristina Díaz de Heredia and Pablo Velasco
Oncohematologic Pediatrics Department, Hospital Universitari Vall d'Hebron, ERN-EuroBloodNet Member, Barcelona, Spain

Rafael Del Orbe and Miriam Vara Pampliega
Hematology Department, Hospital Universitario Cruces, Barakaldo Spain

David Beneitez
Red Blood Cell Disorders Unit, Hematology Department, Hospital Universitari Vall d'Hebron, ERN-EuroBloodNet Member, Barcelona, Spain

Quinten Waisfisz and Mariet Elting
Department of Clinical Genetics, VU Medical Center, Amsterdam, Netherlands

Frans J. W. Smiers and Anne J. de Pagter
Department of Pediatric Hematology, Leiden University Medical Center, Leiden, Netherlands

Jean-Louis H. Kerkhoffs
Department of Hematology, HAGA City Hospital, The Hague, Netherlands

Jianlong Zhuang, Na Zhang, Yuanbai Wang and Yuying Jiang
Prenatal Diagnosis Center, Quanzhou Women's and Children's Hospital, Quanzhou, China

Hegan Zhang
Department of Gynecology, Quanzhou Women's and Children's Hospital, Quanzhou, China

Yu Zheng
Research and Development Department, Yaneng BIOscience (Shenzhen) Co. Ltd., Shenzhen, China

Yingjun Xie
Key Laboratory for Major Obstetric Diseases of Guangdong Province, Department of Obstetrics and Gynecology, The Third Affiliated Hospital of Guangzhou Medical University, Guangzhou, China

Key Laboratory of Reproduction and Genetics of Guangdong Higher Education Institutes, The Third Affiliated Hospital of Guangzhou Medical University, Guangzhou, China

Dongmei Chen
Department of Neonatal Intensive Care Unit, Quanzhou Women's and Children's Hospital, Quanzhou, China

Index

Printed in the USA
CPSIA information can be obtained
at www.ICGtesting.com
JSHW051551051023
49754JS00005B/42